THE PRINCIPLES OF HORSESHOEING II

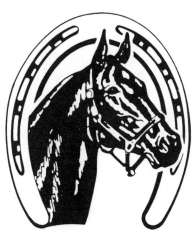

An Illustrated Textbook of
FARRIER SCIENCE
and
CRAFTSMANSHIP

by

Doug Butler, PhD, CJF, FWCF

REVISED AND ENLARGED EDITION

THE PRINCIPLES OF HORSESHOEING

Original Edition Copyright © 1974
Revised and Enlarged Edition Copyright © 1985
Second Printing 1991
Third Printing 1993
Fourth Printing 1995

KARL DOUGLAS BUTLER, JR.
All Rights Reserved

Graphics Consultant
Bert Summers

Printed by
Walsworth Co., Inc.

Published by
Butler Publishing
P.O. Box 1390
LaPorte, CO 80535

Library of Congress Catalog Card Number 73-88039
ISBN 0-916992-02-1

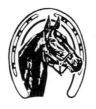

THE PRINCIPLES OF HORSESHOEING
A Textbook of Farrier Science and Craftsmanship
Revised and Enlarged Edition

TABLE OF CONTENTS

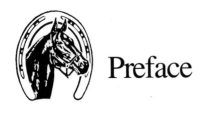

Preface

Horseshoeing has come of age. In today's leisure-oriented society, horseshoers occupy a key and prominent place. Historically, horseshoers have always held a prominent position among the tradesmen and in society because of their indispensability: *everything* moved with horse and oxen power. The animals had to be shod to work.

Today, horseshoers are important by the choice of a leisure-oriented public. Horse-oriented activities are the leading sports in America today. More people are actively involved as participants or spectators in horse sports than in any other modern sport.

Large horse numbers demand many horseshoers. The demand for competent and dependable horseshoers has never been greater than it is now. People expect and will pay for professional service.

The increase in interest and horse numbers and the pressing demand for horseshoers, coupled with availability of ready-made shoes and materials, has encouraged many unskilled persons to begin practicing the trade. Those desiring to practice farrier skills must become educated to prevent injury to our nation's horse population.

Designed to be a comprehensive textbook, *The Principles of Horseshoeing* is adaptable to courses offered by vocational schools or colleges in Horseshoeing, Blacksmithing, Farrier or Veterinary Science. It is intended that the text be a supplement to the close association of an inspiring teacher. However, the book will be of interest to horse owners who desire to gain a better appreciation of the work of the horseshoer. Veterinarians will also find this text both interesting and useful.

The principles of horseshoeing are set forth in this book. Every detail is not included—nor could it be. Horseshoeing is as much an art as it is a science and therefore must be learned and applied individually. The reader is invited to add to the principles specific instances that have been learned by his experience and study.

The principles contained in this book have been developed by years of experience and sweat at the forge and under a horse by numerous ancient and modern horseshoers. The Author does not claim to have invented all these principles. If he can be found worthy of any credit, it must be in the organization and teaching of these principles.

Experience in teaching as well as practicing horseshoeing has contributed to the design and contents of the book. Students, horseshoers, teachers, and veterinarians have all contributed to the building of this work. The first edition was nearly 10 years in the making. This revised edition has been 10 more years in preparation. Those who are quick to discover faults with the book should consider the difficulties in undertaking such a task. The Author invites constructive criticism and comment from the reader to assist him in the preparation of future editions.

The Author gratefully acknowledges the assistance of the many people that contributed their time and talents to make this book possible. Photos and drawings made by persons other than the author are acknowledged in the illustration captions. A special thanks is due Mrs. Ruth Tillett of Maryville, MO, for typing and editing the many revisions of the manuscript.

It is the sincere hope of the Author that this book will provide incentive for improvement to each individual engaged in the complicated and evolving horseshoeing profession. Others may gain a basic understanding of the work of the horseshoer. The only way to truly understand horseshoeing is to work at the anvil, get under the horse, and do it. The apprentice system may not be popular as a method of training anymore, but it still takes mental and physical effort, combined with long hours of practice and critical supervision, to master the principles of horseshoeing.

August, 1984
Doug Butler

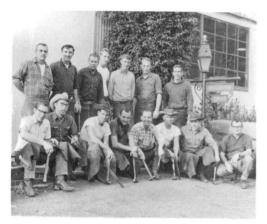

Fig. A-1. *The Author as a student with instructor Ralph Hoover (right) at the Cal Poly Horseshoeing School, San Luis Obispo, California, in 1963. Photo by California Polytechnic State University.*

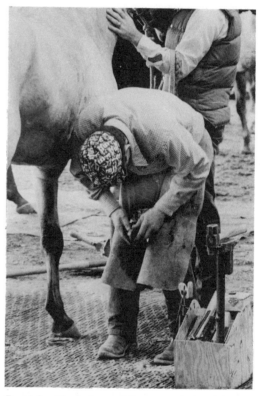

Fig. A-2. *The Author on his way to winning the North American Challenge Cup Futurity of the American Farriers' Association Convention, Jackson, Mississippi, in 1980. Photo by H. Heymering.*

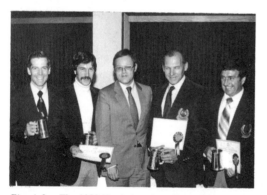

Fig. A-3. *The 1980 North American Horseshoeing Team in Dublin, Ireland. Left to right: Doug Butler, Texas; Randy Luikart, Ohio; Peter Kries, representing Mustad Nail Company; Bruce Daniels, New Jersey; and Bob Marshall, British Columbia, Canada. Photo by Lensmen, Ltd., Dublin.*

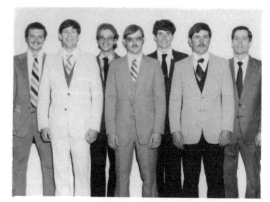

Fig. A-4. *The Author as a professor (right) with a graduating class at Northwest Missouri State University, Maryville, Missouri, in 1983. Photo by NWMSU.*

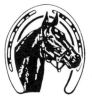

About the Author

Doug Butler was reared on a livestock farm in Upstate New York. As a young lad, he learned to ride, compete, and handle a rope. While very young, he seemed to like and have a special way with horses and tools as did many of his progenitors including his great-great-grandfather, who was a pioneer blacksmith in the great trek West during the mid-19th Century. At an early age, Doug started trimming and shoeing horses on the farm after careful observation and study of local horseshoers.

Upon graduation from high school, he went West. There he labored as a working cowboy on several ranches, and was taught by experts the elements of horse training and horseshoeing.

Later, as a student in Animal Science at Utah State University, he helped pay his way by shoeing, horse training, and working in cattle roundups. He was also active in the rodeo club.

The Author continued his studies and activities at California Polytechnic State University, San Luis Obispo, where he became an understudy of the late Ralph Hoover, outstanding authority and nationally-known horseshoeing instructor.

Even before graduation from Cal Poly, the Author, under the direction and recommendation of Mr. Hoover, assisted in blacksmithing and horseshoeing classes there, and taught several horseshoeing courses at Montana State University, The Pennsylvania State University, and elsewhere. Soon he was in demand to give demonstrations and short courses both in the U.S. and Canada. Also while an undergraduate, Mr. Butler wrote and published an illustrated booklet, *Horseshoeing Iron and Forge Work,* which was adopted by several horseshoeing schools as a textbook and was reprinted twice because of demand.

The Author earned his M.S. at The Pennsylvania State University. His thesis concerned special studies which he did on the shoeing and treatment of sandcracks in the hoofs of horses.

For several years, Mr. Butler was an Assistant Professor of Animal Science at California State Polytechnic University, Pomona, where he taught classes in horseshoeing, equitation, and horse science, and was the rodeo team coach.

The Author earned his Ph.D. at Cornell University in the Equine Research Program of the New York State Veterinary College. His thesis research was related to the effect of nutrition on hoof growth and quality. Also while a graduate student, the Author published *The Principles of Horseshoeing.* It became the most widely used textbook on the subject in the world.

As an Associate Professor of Range Animal Science, Dr. Butler directed the horse science program at Sul Ross State University, Alpine, Texas. He conducted a unique graduate program and taught basic and advanced courses in farrier training, horsemanship, and horse production.

February 29, 1980, Doug Butler won the North American Challenge Cup Futurity Horseshoeing Contest. This contest was sponsored by the American Farrier's Association in conjunction with its annual convention held in Jackson, MS. He also was priviledged to participate as a member of the North American Horseshoeing Team at the International Horseshoeing Competitions in Great Britain in 1980 and 1986.

From 1981 to 1990, Dr. Butler taught at Northwest Missouri State University where he developed both a horse science and a farrier science curriculum.

Dr. Butler has been invited to speak at professional meetings and clinics throughout the United States and Canada. In addition, he has served as a consultant to a number of race tracks, show stables, and horse farms. He was a contributing editor of the *American Farrier's Journal* for ten years. He is a Certified Journeyman Farrier in the American Farrier's Association.

To continue his own studies, Dr. Butler challenged himself to complete all three levels of the rigorous English examination system. He is the first person outside Great Britain to become a Fellow by examination of the Worshipful Company of Farriers.

Currently, Dr. Butler is Associate Professor of Animal Science at Colorado State University where he is teaching professional farrier training and horse science courses. Many of his former students are operating successful horse related businesses in various parts of the world.

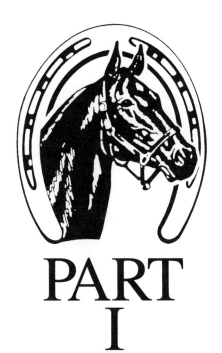

PART
I

BASIC SKILLS AND
PLEASURE HORSE SHOEING

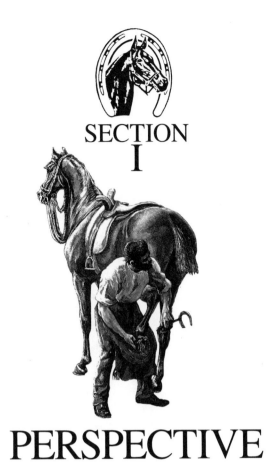

SECTION
I

PERSPECTIVE

Chapter 1

Need For Horseshoers

Unlimited Opportunity

There were two young shoe salesmen who went to the frontiers of Africa to merchandise their goods. After a week, one wired, "Am returning home. No market for shoes. Everyone goes barefoot." The other wired back, "Send two shiploads of shoes immediately. Market unlimited. Everyone goes barefoot!"

Horses have four feet instead of two! Perhaps one of the most optimistic and attractive features about the horseshoeing business is the fact that horses' feet grow and change at such a rate that they must be cared for every 2 months or less.

Opportunities in horseshoeing are unlimited. The horse industry is the fastest growing segment of the livestock business. Spectator attendance at horse-oriented sports is greater than any other. The rapid growth of pleasure and show horse numbers, horse clubs and sports, businesses related to the horse industry, and equine research make the future look very good.

Horse Numbers Increasing

Some people, particularly old-timers, say that horseshoeing is a dying trade, a lost art, a van-

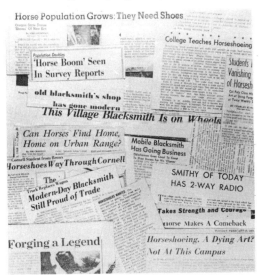

Fig. 1-1. A growing horse industry has created a demand for horseshoers. Photo by L. Sadler.

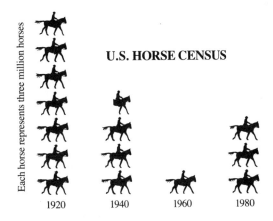

U.S. HORSE CENSUS

Each horse represents three million horses

1920   1940   1960   1980

Fig. 1-2. Horse numbers have tripled in the last two decades. U.S. horse census. United States Department of Agriculture (USDA) figures.

ishing occupation. One of the reasons for this popular belief is the tremendous change that the horse population has undergone in the past 60 years, perhaps in their lifetime.

U.S. horse numbers were at an all-time high in 1915 of 21.5 million and at an all-time low in 1960 of about 3 million. During this time of change, the nature as well as the number of horses changed. Both draft and pleasure horse numbers dropped until about 1945; then, pleasure horses began to make tremendous increases until, in 1960, they were growing at a faster rate than work horses were decreasing. Two-thirds of the horse population were grade animals in 1960. By 1981, more than one-half the horses in the U.S. were of registered quality.

In 1982, the horse population of the U.S. was estimated at nine million head. Numbers tripled in two decades! Each of these horses has four feet!

Growth has now leveled off, but at the same time there has been more emphasis placed upon quality. Horsemen with quality horses are buying more services. The horse business has been conservatively estimated as a $15 billion a year business. A recent survey (1977) estimated that 40 million people owned or rode horses and another 40 million people would like to be equestrian horsepersons.

Equine Population Growth by State

RANK	STATE	1983	1971
1	California	850,000	406,000
2	Texas	780,000	625,000
3	Oklahoma	300,000	230,000
4	Illinois	273,000	300,000
5	Montana	250,000	250,000
6	Ohio	248,000	205,000
7	Missouri	242,000	188,000
8	Michigan	222,000	169,000
9	Kentucky	220,000	170,000
10	Colorado	219,000	125,000
11	Tennessee	219,000	180,000
12	Minnesota	211,000	157,000
13	New York	205,000	250,000
14	Pennsylvania	197,000	98,000
15	Kansas	192,000	150,000
16	Iowa	188,000	120,000
17	Florida	187,000	145,000
18	Idaho	179,000	125,000
19	Louisiana	176,000	150,000
20	Arkansas	175,000	128,000
21	Washington	169,000	125,000
22	Mississippi	167,000	149,000
23	Oregon	166,000	125,000
24	Arizona	164,000	100,000
25	New Mexico	164,000	90,000
26	Indiana	159,000	75,000
27	Wisconsin	156,000	110,000
28	Virginia	156,000	118,000
29	Georgia	147,000	107,000
30	Nebraska	146,000	78,000
31	Alabama	145,000	129,000
32	North Carolina	144,000	140,000
33	South Dakota	134,000	85,000
34	Utah	125,000	95,000
35	Wyoming	104,000	48,000
36	North Dakota	84,000	35,000
37	Nevada	76,000	50,000
38	Maryland	72,000	61,000
39	South Carolina	72,000	70,000
40	New Jersey	69,000	31,000
41	West Virginia	54,000	40,000
42	Connecticut	46,000	30,000
43	Massachusetts	42,000	21,000
44	Maine	29,000	25,000
45	Vermont	25,000	12,000
46	New Hampshire	24,000	20,000
47	Washington DC & Terr.*	19,000	27,000
48	Hawaii	16,000	10,000
49	Delaware	12,000	8,000
50	Alaska	10,000	3,000
51	Rhode Island	5,000	9,000
	TOTAL	8,434,000	6,197,000

*Includes Puerto Rico, Virgin Islands, Guam, and American Samoa

Fig. 1-3. Horse numbers have increased most rapidly on the west coast. U.S. equine population growth by state. American Horse Council (AHC) figures.

There are over 75 American colleges and universities that offer horse courses as a part of their curriculum. Over a dozen offer a major in horse science. Most states employ at least one full-time horse extension specialist. Nearly 30 states have horse councils. There are over 150 equine periodicals, and over 60 breed registries, many with educational services.

The leading horse states are California and Texas. Each of these states is estimated to have over 600,000 horses. The next closest states each have about half as many as the leading states. Twelve states are estimated to have over 200,000 horses each and an additional 20 states each have over 100,000 horses. The remaining 16 states are each estimated to have an average of 25,000 horses.

Horse racing continues to be the leading spectator sport in the U.S. About 80 million people attended horse races in 1975. This nearly equaled the combined attendance of professional football and baseball.

Rodeos continue to increase in popularity. About 14 million people attended over 600 pro rodeos sponsored by the Professional Rodeo Cowboys Association (PRCA) in 1980. More than 500,000 horses are estimated to be used for stock work in the U.S.

Over 1,700 horse shows are sanctioned annually by the American Horse Shows Association (AHSA). Over 2,000 shows were sanctioned by the American Quarter Horse Association (AQHA) in 1980. The American Horse Council (AHC) estimates that over 20,000 horse shows are held annually.

While race, rodeo and show horses are a prime source of income to many of our finest farriers, the majority of the nation's horses are owned and used for recreational (pleasure) riding. Many of these horses are owned by young people whose families make an average income. Studies have repeatedly shown that the horseshoer gets more of the pleasure horseman's dollar than the veterinarian.

The state of Kentucky, one of the leading horse states with over 200,000 horses, recently did a comprehensive survey and found the following percentages by use: pleasure, 46; breeding, 18; work, 12; showing, 10; racing, 10; and other, 4 percent. Most of the other states have

Light Horse Annual Registrations

Rank	Breed	1983	1980	1975	1968	1960
1	Quarter Horse	168,346	137,090	97,723	57,000	37,000
2	Thoroughbred	47,500	36,453	28,786	22,700	12,901
3	Arabian	27,500	19,725	15,000	6,980	1,610
4	Appaloosa	22,184	25,384	20,175	12,389	4,052
5	Standardbred	20,298	15,219	12,830	10,682	6,413
6	Paint	11,128	9,654	5,287	2,390	-0-
7	Saddlebred	9,025	8,973	9,836	8,411	2,329
8	Anglo & Half-Arab	8,334	14,257	11,351	9,800	2,200
9	Tennessee Walker	5,400	6,673	6,591	8,492	2,623
10	Morgan	5,317	4,537	3,400	2,134	1,069
11	Pinto	3,404	1,502	2,229	2,258	230
12	Palomino	1,952	1,548	1,539	1,262	657
13	Hackney	631	595	1,015	656	459
		331,019	281,610	215,762	145,154	71,543

Fig. 1-4. Registered horses are becoming more popular. Light horse annual registrations in the U.S. from 1960 to 1980. American Horse Council (AHC) figures.

an even higher percentage of pleasure horses since breeding and racing are not as significant as they are in Kentucky.

Horses now provide leisure-time pleasure for one-third of the nation's population. The horse industry has continued to grow in spite of bad national economic news. The horse continues its tradition of faithful service even in the midst of our highly complex and inanimate society. And, each of these horses has four feet!

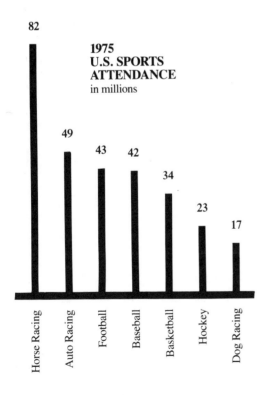

Fig. 1-5. Horse racing has been the leading spectator sport in America for over 30 years. 1975 U.S. sports attendance. Triangle Publications of Highstown, NJ figures.

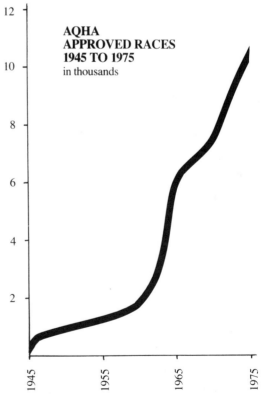

Fig. 1-6. Growth in American Quarter Horse Association (AQHA) approved races. AQHA figures.

A Comparison of Percentage of Horse Uses, Breeds, Classes and Operations in Two States

PRIMARY USE	KENTUCKY	NEW YORK
Pleasure Riding	46.1	59.2
Breeding	18.6	9.0
Racing	9.6	13.1
Showing	9.8	13.5
Working	11.8	3.2
Youth Projects	0.6	1.9
Other	3.5	0.1
LIGHT HORSE BREED		
Thoroughbred	31.4	17.1
Crossbred	17.7	26.9
Quarter Horse	13.5	19.0
Saddlebred	12.5	3.4
Standardbred	7.1	16.0
Appaloosa	4.4	7.2
Arabian	1.1	4.3
Morgan	0.8	4.4
Tennessee Walker	9.2	—
Other	2.3	1.7
CLASSES OF EQUINE		
Light Horses	71.6	77.5
Ponies	20.3	18.3
Draft Horses	2.7	3.0
Mules & Donkeys	5.4	1.2
TYPE OF HORSE OPERATION		
Farm-Horse, Live-stock or Crop	71.5	53.0
Non-Farm Residence	26.2	42.4
Public Boarding & Training Stable	1.7	2.8
Other	0.6	1.8

Fig. 1-7. A comparison of horse uses, breeds, classes and operations in two states. Kentucky Equine Survey (1977) and New York State Equine Survey (1978) figures.

Demand for Competence

Professional Horseshoers, highly-skilled and competent to meet any situation, are always in demand. In some areas, poor mechanics can get by and have much of the public satisfied with their work. It once was stated that about 30 percent of today's horse owners shoe their own horses. However, once horse owners are exposed to expertise which they can recognize, they will rarely go back to a less-skilled shoer or continue to do their own horseshoeing. A man with his knowledge in his hands as well as in his head is always in demand. The day is coming when a horseshoer will be in business because he is the best, and not because he is the only one available.

The business of horseshoeing, like many others, is becoming highly competitive and highly specialized. It used to be that the local blacksmith would do horseshoeing along with the other work in his shop. Now, the horseshoer comes to the horse in his complete mobile horseshoeing shop. Frequently, modern horseshoers in metropolitan areas further specialize in caring for one breed or type of horse, such as race horses or gaited horses.

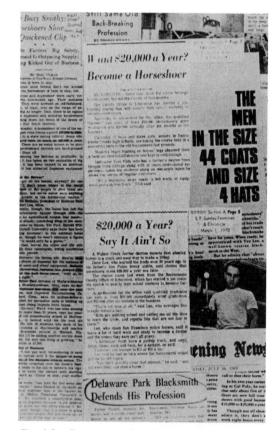

Fig. 1-8. Exaggeration by a few has encouraged incompetence. Photo by L. Sadler.

Horseshoeing as a Profession

Horseshoeing is an art or skill, but it is also a science. Horseshoers must often work closely with veterinarians in treating conditions in the legs or feet of horses. A background in the sciences, especially anatomy and physiology, becomes a necessity when diagnosing, treating and discussing such ailments with a professional like a veterinarian. For this reason, and because a horseshoer is often considered by the public as an expert on horses, many are finding it advantageous to get some formal training at a college or university.

In 1983 there were over 60 public and private schools that offered some type of training in horseshoeing. These schools vary tremendously. In Europe, horseshoeing schools are sponsored by the national government. Most countries tie the schooling to an apprenticeship system. Examination and licensing by guilds are traditional.

Horseshoeing is an art, a skill, a business, a science and a service. One of the great reasons for optimism in the future of horseshoeing is the opportunity to offer superior service. Slipshod service at sky-high prices has become the byword of our modern life. When people are offered dependable service and quality craftsmanship, they will become steady customers.

Horseshoeing has many of the characteristics of a profession.

The characteristics of a profession are:
1. It is sufficiently complex to require many years of study in a prescribed curriculum before practice is commenced.
2. An internship (apprenticeship) and years of practice are necessary to achieve competency.
3. A board examination and certification are required to practice and to advance standing.
4. A patient or client risks serious injury to self or property due to malpractice.
5. It has unique traditions and vocabulary including a code of conduct and dress.
6. A large investment is required in state of the art technology (equipment) and ancillary (support) personnel.
7. The potential exists for making an above average income per hour while making a positive contribution to society.

Farrier science and craftsmanship (commonly called horseshoeing) includes the following highly skilled specialties:
1. Restoring and maintaining the ideal form and normal function (balancing) of the horse's foot by trimming.
2. Protecting the horse's foot from wear and trauma by shoeing.
3. Altering the horse's foot and limb position (stance) to minimize stress by corrective shoeing.
4. Relieving pain from the horse's foot or limb to restore soundness by therapeutic shoeing.
5. Increasing traction and providing safety for the horse (and rider) when performing on various surfaces by performance, race, road and draft horse shoeing.

6. Enhancing the natural and acquired movements (gaits) of the horse to maximize performance by gaited show horse shoeing.

Professional farriers (horseshoers) practice their profession by:
1. Analyzing the horse's stance and movement and relating it to the performance required. This may be compared to making a diagnosis.
2. Selecting an appropriate treatment for the diagnosed condition. This may be compared to writing a prescription.
3. Performing trimming operations on the living hoof. This may be compared to practicing orthopedic surgery or dentistry.
4. Designing, constructing, and applying horseshoes. This may be compared to designing and fitting orthopedic prostheses or capping teeth.
5. Educating the horse owner concerning the horse's limitations and the necessity of regular hoof care. This may be compared to monitoring postoperative care and wound or tooth hygiene.
6. Conferring with specialists in related fields. This may be compared to a multidisciplinary medical consultation team.

Exaggeration and Incompetence

Horseshoeing is a profession, and there is good reason to be excited about its future. But—a word of caution: horseshoeing is not what it is frequently made out to be by the press. In the last few years, some false ideas and information have been published over and over again which make horseshoeing out to be "easy money". Prices quoted have been incorrect and yearly income figures have been grossly exaggerated. Such publicity has encouraged many people to enter the field with little or no training. This development is unfortunate, and it will take some time for the profession to get over it.

This situation is not new. J.G. Holmstrom (1904) discussed the problem at the turn of the century:

When a young man has worked a few months in a shop, he will succeed in welding a toe calk on a horseshoe that sometimes will stay, and at once he begins to think he knows it all. There will always be some fool ready to flatter him, and the young man believes that he is now competent to start on his own hook. The result is, he hangs out his shingle, begins to practice horseshoeing and general blacksmithing, and he knows nothing about either. Let me state here that horseshoeing is a trade by itself, and so is blacksmithing. In the large cities there are black-smiths who know nothing about horseshoeing, as well as horseshoers who know nothing about blacksmithing, except welding on toe calks, and in many instances even that is very poorly done. In small places it is different. There the black-smith is both blacksmith and horseshoer. Some-times you will find a blacksmith that is a good horseshoer, but you will never find a horseshoer that is a good blacksmith. This is not generally understood. To many blacksmithing seems to mean only horseshoeing, and our trade journals are not much better posted. Whenever a black-smith is alluded to, or pictured you will always find a horseshoe in connection with it. Yet there are thousands of blacksmiths that never made a horseshoe in all their lives. Horseshoeing has developed to be quite a trade, and if a man can learn it in a few years he will do well. I would not advise any young man to start out for himself with less than three or four years' experience. Every horseshoer should make an effort to learn blacksmithing. He will be expected to know it, people don't know the difference; besides this, it will, in smaller cities, be hard to succeed with horseshoeing alone. On the other hand, every blacksmith should learn horseshoeing, for the same reasons. Therefore, seven or even ten years is a short time to learn it in. But, who has patience and good sense enough to persevere for such a course, in our times, when everybody wants to get to the front at once? Let every young man remember that the reputation you get in the start will stick to you. Therefore be careful not to start before you know your business, and the years spent in learning it will not be lost, but a foundation for your success. Remember, that if a thing is not worth being well done it is not worth being done at all. It is better to be a first-class bootblack or chimney sweep, than be a third-class of anything else.

Don't be satisfied by simply being able to do the work so as to pass, let it be first-class. Thou-sands of mechanics are turning out work just as others are doing it, but you should not be sat-isfied to do the work as others are doing it, but do it right.

The public should be able to feel as confident about having a horseshoer work on their horses as they do a veterinarian. It takes time and study and diligent practice to become a skilled horseshoer.

Some states, in an effort to overcome the problem of incompetency, have initiated licen-sing legislation for horseshoers. This could hap-pen in all states, if the profession doesn't take care of the problem itself by encouraging com-petency and dependability among its members.

The American Farriers' Association[1] has taken the lead in promoting certification of its mem-bers at various levels. Candidates must pass both practical and written tests. Certification is now available at the basic and journeyman level.

It takes time and training, close supervision and a lot of practice to obtain skill in horse-shoeing. These must be coupled with a great desire to learn and the other traits listed in the next Chapter. Then, depending on the area, it takes a great deal of time, patience and work to build up a business. Capital is required to as-semble a set of tools and equipment and an inventory of shoes and supplies.

Great Future

Walt Taylor, president and founder of the American Farrier's Association, was recently asked to comment on the future of the farrier profession:

The farrier's status as a full-fledged profes-sional—an expert in the anatomy, physiology and care of the lower leg and foot—will emerge. Our link with veterinarians will be much closer, each dependent on the other and both working in harmony with horse owners.

To maintain that high level of professional-ism, the farrier will be part of a dynamic edu-cational process. Farrier schools will be fewer in number, longer in course conduct and re-sponsible for their product. The curriculum will be more standardized in the basics, with varia-tions only for specialties pursued by that school.

The student will develop special skills in shoeing draft horses, gaited horses, racehorses, etc., by choosing a school strong in that area. Farrier schools will be accredited by the profes-sional association, with those schools failing to produce competent farriers losing their accre-ditation. The farrier of tomorrow will be certi-fied and licensed by the American Farrier's Association. Those shoers not willing to submit to this demand for excellence or unable to meet its standards will ultimately be eliminated from practice.

Competent farriers are in demand today everywhere there are horses; this shouldn't change. With the expected increase in perfor-mance horses and the weeding out of incom-petence, even more farriers will be needed in 2001 than today.

Horseshoeing has a great future for those who like the work and are willing to become skilled

[1]*P.O. Box 695, Albuquerque, NM 87103*

at it. There will always be room for a horseshoer who is competent and dependable.

If you choose to enter the profession, decide to be that kind of horseshoer!

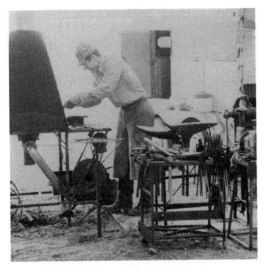

Fig. 1-9. Horseshoeing has a great future for those who are willing to become highly skilled. Photo by T. Reichert.

References

Bradley, M. 1981. Horses: A Practical and Scientific Approach. McGraw-Hill, Inc., New York.

Cunha, T.J. 1980. Horse Feeding and Nutrition. Academic Press, New York.

Educator's Division of American Farriers Association. 1981. Directory of Farrier Schools. Amer. Farriers' J. 7(1):37.

Estimated U.S. Equine Population by State. 1976. Tack and Togs Special Report. Miller Publishing Co., Minneapolis.

Evans, J.W. 1981. Horses. Freeman, San Francisco.

Governing Board of the Educator's Division of the American Farriers' Assn. 1983. Directory of farrier schools. American Farriers' J. 9(1):49.

Holmstrom, J.G. 1904. Modern Blacksmithing. Frederick J. Drake & Co., Chicago.

Perry, P.M. 1974. The horseman's pocketbook—vets 'n farriers. Amer. Horseman. (Aug):34.

Perry. P.M. 1974. Horseman's pocketbook—annual upkeep. Amer. Horseman. (Sept):35.

Taylor, W. 1981. Farriery forges ahead—the horse in the year 2001. Equus. 44:48.

Taylor, W. 1983. The importance of proper shoeing for show horses. Amer. Farriers' J. 9(2):106.

Ulman, N. Jan. 5, 1967. The busy smithy: horseshoers shoe at a quickened clip. Wall Street Journal. 169:1.

NOTES:

PERSPECTIVE

Chapter 2

Prequisites For Horseshoers

Desire to Learn

Once the master teacher, Socrates, was confronted by a young man who said he wanted to learn all Socrates knew. "Socrates," he said, "you are the wisest man in the world. I want to be learned and wise. So I have come to you to be taught wisdom and learning."

Socrates took the young man down to the sea and led him out into the water until it was up to their waists. Immediately, Socrates grabbed him about the neck and shoulders and submerged him in the sea. He struggled, and kicked violently at first but shortly became quite peaceable, as anyone will do who is held under water very long!

Socrates dragged him out of the water and laid him down on the seashore to dry out. The wise old teacher then returned to town and the business he was about before the young man had confronted him.

Sometime later, the puzzled young man reached Socrates and questioned him again. "What's the

idea, Socrates? I came to you to be taught wisdom and learning, and you tried to drown me!"

Socrates turned and looked him straight in the eye and said, "What did you want most when you were under water?"

"...Why...air," he said, somewhat bewildered.

"How badly did you want air?" asked Socrates.

"I wanted air like I've never wanted anything in my life," said the student.

Then Socrates made this classic statement: "When you want wisdom and learning like you wanted air, you won't need me to teach it to you."

The desire to learn and to be is the greatest prerequisite a person can have for anything, including horseshoeing. When a person has the desire to learn as strongly as the young man in the story had the desire for air, he will not need a master teacher in order to learn. And until this desire is cultivated, the process of transferring knowledge from the head to the hands will be slow, if not impossible, no matter who is the teacher.

There are few "naturals" in this business. A good craftsman is always one who has his knowledge in his hands. It is seldom that a person can't do something. It's usually that he doesn't *want* to do something.

As one's curiosity and desire to learn grow, one must remember that all information is not of equal value, and it must be used wisely to be of value.

There is some information that you need to know, some that you should know, and a lot that is interesting to know. Prime time should be given to the first two areas, and then the third will fall into its rightful place.

Wisdom must be applied to knowledge. Someone has said, "Knowledge, when wisdom is too weak to guide her, is like a headstrong horse that throws the rider." Another has said, "Learning without wisdom is a load of books on an ass's back." Experience is a vital part of wisdom.

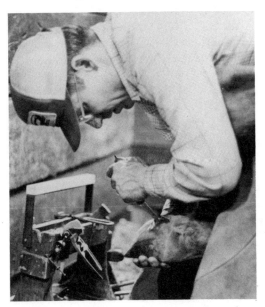

Fig. 2-1. Horseshoeing requires concentration and precision as well as being physically hard work. Photo by J. Graves.

Someone has said that to be a horseshoer, one must have the strength of Samson, the patience of Job, and the wisdom of Solomon. Others say that all that is necessary is a strong back and a weak mind so that a Size 4 hat and a Size 44 coat fit rather well and that he can look through a keyhole with both eyes at once. Actually, it requires a little more than that!

The practice of horseshoeing spans many trades and fields. A horseshoer needs to be a horseman, blacksmith, businessman and outdoorsman. A horseshoer should be a horse trainer, horse foot veterinarian, welder and a public relations man. And a horseshoer can be a specialist in corrective, therapeutic or breed type shoeing and a student of all phases of horse care and management. Obviously the "smith" is not just a "mighty man", as Longfellow said, but he must also be mighty smart!

This business of being an eternal student and having a thirst for learning and applying it cannot be over-emphasized. The more a person knows, the more he can do. The more you learn, the more you earn.

Perhaps the comment made most frequently by horseshoeing students is: "Why didn't I listen closer and try harder when I was in school?" Things come much easier there than in the school of hard kicks and knocks. Such statements of remorse make the old Arabian proverb ring loud and clear; "Four things come not back; the spoken word, the sped arrow, the past life, and the neglected opportunity."

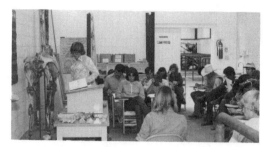

Fig. 2-2. Cultivate the desire to learn and learn all you can.

Make the most of every opportunity to learn. Read, watch others, try new things and then evaluate and apply them to your situation.

Desire and Ability to Work Hard

Another major trait that must be present or developed is the desire and ability to work and work hard. There is no way to get around it; horseshoeing is hard work! As a matter of fact, there are few jobs that require more concentration and at the same time require so much physically hard work.

In addition to the work involved in the job itself, there is also the consideration that it is piecework. When you don't work you don't get paid. So it is all work. This is the thing which washes out a lot of prospective horseshoers. They haven't developed a desire and ability to work. Actually, it's very simple, if you believe what someone once said, "Nothing is ever work unless you'd rather be doing something else."

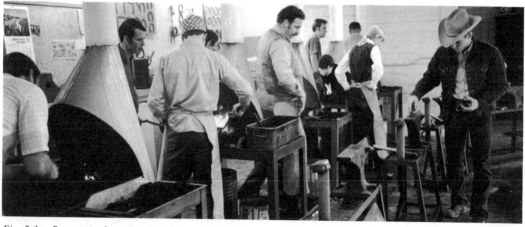

Fig. 2-3. Persons (male or female) who can handle the demands of horseshoeing should not be discouraged. Photo by R. Rankin.

In recent years, a number of women have aspired to be horseshoers. Often, the most conscientious and motivated students are women. They usually exhibit more concern for a horse's welfare than men. Women students are naturally just as smart (or smarter) than men students. The Author has had several outstanding women students.

However, it is a rare woman who is physically strong enough to consistently, day after day, stand the physical labor of horseshoeing. A woman's craftsmanship may even be superior to a man's, but her earning ability as a professional is usually hampered by the physical work involved. (Of course, this is also true for men who are not physically capable of prolonged hard work.)

Those persons (male or female) who can handle the physical and mental demands of horseshoeing should not be discouraged. Those who cannot should recognize their limitations.

Effective Teacher(s)

Evaluate carefully those who teach you. Good teachers are effective. Do they cultivate in you the desire to learn and improve yourself? Do they understand all they profess to know? Do they believe what they teach? Are they constantly learning, trying new things and improving themselves? Are they open to new ideas and innovations? These questions and others are important because any teacher, no matter who he is, teaches what he is.

Joseph Gamgee, in a textbook for horseshoers published in 1871, made this statement concerning the subject of teaching:

> Horseshoers are not, as their maligners aver, less teachable than men composing other sections of the community. The difference has consisted in the teaching which they have received, for that teaching has been conducted by those who, never having learned the art, as every art should be learned, by practice, have forgotten that to teach, one must possess knowledge, of that accurate and positive kind, which is only attainable by personal observation and study; and that in teaching any art, "example is better than precept."

Bracy Clark, one of the great horseshoeing experts and teachers of his time (the early 1800's), said:

Public institutions (teachers and books) in themselves cannot, it is obvious, create knowledge; they can only afford convenient opportunities for study to those who are disposed to employ them; and it must still be from individual exertion that improvement (learning) will spring.

Anton Lungwitz, writing at the turn of the century, said: "Horseshoeing is an industry which requires, in equal degree, knowledge and skill."

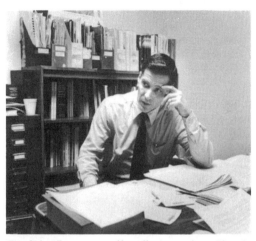

Fig. 2-4. *Expose yourself to effective teachers. Photo by R. Rogers.*

Another great teacher defined skill as accuracy plus speed.

In 1775 James Clark, "The King of Farriers," and often referred to as the Father of Modern Farriery said, "Reading alone is not sufficient to qualify a man either for the profession of physician or farrier."

Professor Henry Asmus of Cornell University instructed classes for horseshoeing and veterinary students for more than 25 years until his death in 1939. He maintained, "The science of horseshoeing must be studied the same as any other science if you wish to become a successful farrier."

William Russell, one of the most prominent men in the field at its zenith around the turn of the century, stated:

> Horseshoeing is not only an art; it is also a science. It has for its objects the surgical treatment, if you please, of the foot, as well as the mechanical work of shoeing. Three-fourths of the successful work of the farrier depends upon his knowledge of the anatomy of the foot and practical acquaintanceship with its diseases, their causes and cures.

Balance is the key. The instructor must achieve balance in his teaching; the student must achieve balance in his training. The effective teacher must be a balanced person.

Dr. George Fleming, a veterinary researcher and dedicated student of horseshoeing, summarized the challenge over 100 years ago:

> It is impossible in any art—and shoeing is no exception to this rule—to acquire a veritable (true, genuine) superiority, if its theory as well as its practice be not combined and exercised together. Practice without theory is simply routine without improvement, and theory alone is often impotent to confer advantages without the crucial test of experience.

Select an effective teacher. Work hard to please him. A teacher's best "pay" is what he sees his students become.

Quality Horseshoeing School(s)

Ideally, a several year apprenticeship to an expert teacher and craftsman would be desirable. However, in our modern American society this has become nearly impossible for the following reasons: first, very few expert teachers and craftsmen who are willing to work with students exist in the same person; second, very few students are conditioned to spend the time necessary to learn a skill from ground up at an early age; and third, complementary knowledge and skills from other areas are needed to succeed in today's society.

The apprenticeship system is still the rule in Europe, but in America it has nearly been completely replaced by schools of various types.

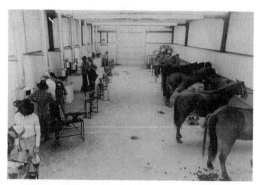

Fig. 2-5. There are tremendous differences in horseshoeing schools. Photo by C. Dillard.

In 1983, there were over 60 American public and private schools which offered some type of training in horseshoeing. There are tremendous differences in these schools. The quality of a program can be evaluated by a prospective student on the basis of five important factors:

1. The Instructor
   a. Can he teach? Does he care and want to teach? Does he have time to teach?
   b. Has he the proper credentials including above average training and experience in the field? Is his area of specialty the same as your interest?
   c. Is his craftsmanship judged superior by his peers? Is he respected by the profession?
   d. Is he continually improving and upgrading his knowledge and skills?
2. The Curriculum
   a. Does it provide the time necessary to develop skills to a competent and marketable level?
   b. Is it detailed and does it provide essential and useful information?
   c. Is it well organized and does it follow a systematic progression?
   d. Does it provide for learning of skills in related areas, such as welding, business management, horsemanship, blacksmithing, equipment construction and lameness diagnosis?
3. The Facilities
   a. Is the student/teacher ratio low?
   b. Is the instructional equipment adequate and in good repair?
   c. Are adequate supplies and animals available to practice on?
   d. Are adequate and reasonable room and board arrangements available?
4. The Community
   a. Does the local community tolerate students working on their animals?
   b. Is there a wide variety of specialized horse types for students to shoe?
   c. Are special problem type horses shod by the instructor with student assistance?
   d. Does the community respect and support the school?
5. The Cost
   a. Compare schools on the basis of equal value. Are all costs listed?
   b. Consider value for investment. Does less cost mean less value or a bargain?
   c. Consider the economic penalty you have to pay to attend school. Are savings, loans, grants or part-time work available?
   d. Consider the distance to travel to school. Do regional or cultural differences affect you?

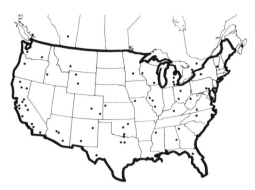

Fig. 2-6. Location of farrier schools in the U.S. in 1983. Map by the American Farrier's Journal.

Presently, the best sources of information on the quality of a school are the recommendations of former students and successful professional horseshoers. A comparison chart of all schools on the basis of the above five considerations would be ideal. Accreditation of schools by a committee of professional farrier educators may come in the future.

Other Important Considerations

The character traits preferred by horse owners are quite different from those listed as essential by horseshoers. Horseowners want a person that is dependable (keeps appointments), honest and sober.

In short, they want someone who is 1) service-oriented, 2) takes pride in himself and his craftsmanship, and 3) cares about them and their horse(s).

Other desirable traits are:

1. Age not over 35 or so to start due to the long time it takes to learn the skills involved.
2. Able-bodied and fairly strong (male or female), agile, not too tall and no major physical handicaps (especially back problems).
3. Like horses and be concerned for their welfare.
4. Unafraid of horses.
5. Like people and feel comfortable talking and dealing with them.
6. Desire to be a self-employed, independent, unique individual who takes pride in his work.
7. Desire to work with your hands and some inherent dexterity.
8. Like outdoor work.
9. "Horse sense," including good judgment and intelligence.
10. Desire to improve and excel.

Belief in Yourself

In summary, let us consider a formula for learning horseshoeing and, for that matter, for learning any trade:

1. Cultivate the desire to learn.
2. Expose yourself to a learning situation (teachers, schools, books, clinics, conventions and contests).
3. Evaluate the things learned from the situation.
4. Apply these things by practicing them until they are part of you, i.e., until the knowledge is transferred from your head to your hands. Remember: "Most things are easy to learn, but hard to master." Work at mastering the trade!
5. Realize it takes time and effort for this "transfer" of knowledge to take place. Be patient!

William Laporte, a blacksmith and horseshoer for more than 70 years and in whose shop over 100 horses were shod in a day in bygone years, left us this reminder:

> Why today the young folks think they can learn a trade overnight and if they aren't earning as much as their boss (teacher) in a couple of years they think they are failures. Old as I am, I know I never learned all there is about this profession.

6. Dedicate yourself to the service of horses and horsemen.

Effective teachers and quality horseshoeing schools are important but should be only the beginning of your learning in the trade. Allow them to help you educate yourself, but then *continue* this process of self-education *every day*.

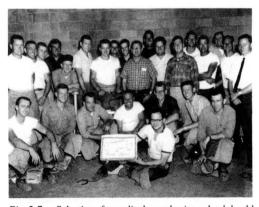

Fig. 2-7. Selection of a quality horseshoeing school should be only the beginning of your learning adventure. A 1965 class of horseshoers at The Pennsylvania State University. Photo by PSU.

The following poem may be helpful if you doubt your ability to succeed. Read it frequently and "get ahold of yourself and say I *can*!"

EQUIPMENT
Edgar A. Guest

Figure it out for yourself my lad,
You have all the greatest have had,
Two arms, two legs, two hands, two eyes,
And a brain to use if you'd be wise.
With this equipment they all began,
So start for the top and say, "I can."

Look them over, the wise and great,
They take their food from a common plate,
And similar knives and forks they use,
With similar laces they tie their shoes,
The world considers them brave and smart,
But you have all they had when they made
    their start.

You can triumph and come to skill
You can be great if you only will.
You're well equipped for the fight you choose,
You have arms and legs and a brain to use,
And men who have risen great deeds to do
Began their life with no more than you.

You are the handicap you must face,
You are the one who must choose your place,
You must say where you want to go,
How much you'll study the truth to know.
God has equipped you for life, but He
Lets you decide what you want to be.

The courage must come from the soul within,
The man must furnish the will to win.
So figure it out for yourself, my lad.
You were born with all the great have had,
With your equipment they all began
So get hold of yourself, and say: "I can."

Either you think you can or you think you can't—either way you are right!

Horseshoers! Love your trade, keep learning and improving, and pass on your best to those entering the profession! Let us follow the example of the most venerable blacksmith of all time:

THE VILLAGE BLACKSMITH
Henry Wadsworth Longfellow

Under a spreading Chestnut-tree
    The village smithy stands;
The smith, a mighty man is he,
    With large and sinewy hands;
And muscles of his brawny arms
    Are strong as iron bands.

His hair is crisp, and black, and long,
    His face is like the tan;
His brow is wet with honest sweat,
    He earns what 'er he can,
And looks the whole world in the face,
    For he owes not any man.

Week in, week out, from morn till night,
    You can hear his bellows blow;
You can hear him swing his heavy sledge,
    With measured beat and slow,
Like a sexton ringing the village bell,
    When the evening sun is low.

And children coming home from school
    Look in at the open door;
They love to see the flaming forge,
    And hear the bellows roar,
And catch the burning sparks that fly
    Like chaff from a threshing floor.

He goes on Sunday to the church,
    And sits among his boys;
He hears the parson pray and preach,
    He hears his daughter's voice,
Singing in the village choir,
    And it makes his heart rejoice.

It sounds to him like her mother's voice,
    Singing in Paradise!
He needs must think of her once more,
    How in the grave she lies;
And with his hard, rough hand he wipes
    A tear out of his eyes.

Toiling, rejoicing, sorrowing,
    Onward through life he goes;
Each morning sees some task begun,
    Each evening sees it close;
Something attempted, something done,
    Has earned a night's repose.

Thanks, thanks to thee, my worthy friend,
    For the lesson thou has taught!
Thus at the flaming forge of life
    Our fortunes must be wrought;
Thus on its sounding anvil shaped
    Each burning deed and thought.

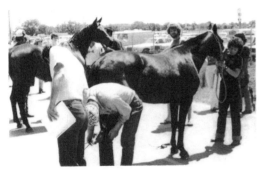 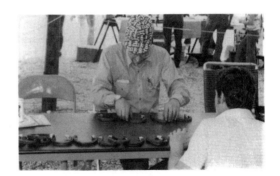

Fig. 2-8. Attendance at conventions and participation in contests will help you continue the process of self education. Judging shoeing (left) and shoes (right) at the 1979 Florida State Fair. Photos by H. Heymering.

References

Asmus, H. 1916. Anatomy of the horse's foot and the science of horseshoeing. The American Blacksmith. 15:185.

Butler, D. 1982. Checklist for farrier schools. Amer. Farriers' J. 8(6):355.

Crouthamel, D. 1983. Apprenticeship. Amer. Farriers' J. 9(2):121.

Fleming, G. 1870. Observations on the anatomy and physiology of the horse's foot. The Veterinarian. 43:13.

Gamgee, J. 1871. A Treatise on Horseshoeing and Lameness. Longmans, Green and Co., London.

Russell, W. 1892. Scientific Horseshoeing. Robert Clarke and Co., Cincinnati. p. xxv.

Smith, H.R.B. 1966. Blacksmiths' and Farriers' Tools at Shelburne Museum. The Shelburne Museum, Inc., Shelburne, VT.

Smithcors, J.F. 1957. Evolution of the Veterinary Art. Veterinary Medicine Publ. Co., Kansas City, MO.

NOTES:

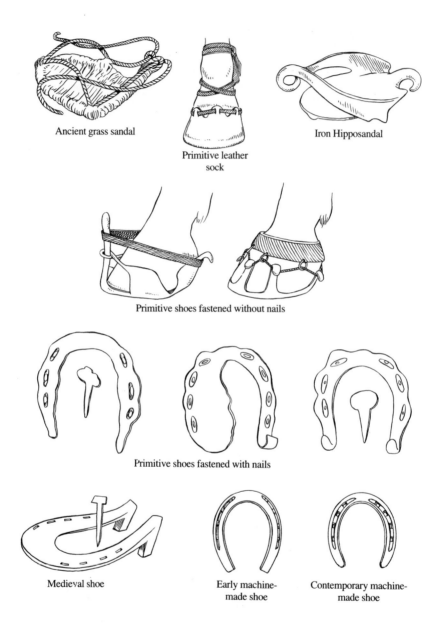

Ancient grass sandal

Primitive leather
sock

Iron Hipposandal

Primitive shoes fastened without nails

Primitive shoes fastened with nails

Medieval shoe

Early machine-
made shoe

Contemporary machine-
made shoe

*Fig. 3-1. The development of the horseshoe. Drawings by
L. Sadler.*

Chapter 3

Horseshoeing's Heritage

Horseshoeing has had a long and exciting history. Its history is interwoven with the history of man and of the earth. The horseshoeing trade is dependent upon other trades for its existence and so its history necessarily involves the history of the horse, iron and steel, weapons, horseshoe, nail and tool manufacture, and veterinary medicine.

Earliest Known Horseshoes

The first Egyptians and Persians are credited with the invention of the earliest known horseshoes. They probably were invented out of necessity soon after the horse was domesticated and used for prolonged work or war.

Scholars have theorized that the horse has been domesticated since about 3000 B.C. and used extensively for riding and draft since about 1580 B.C.

The first simple horseshoes were made from woven grass and reeds, and tied on the hoof. This type of shoeing was used in the Orient up until the 19th Century and may still be used in some parts of the world.

The Egyptians are also believed to have used the skins of animals to protect the hoof much the same as moccasins were used for humans. Genghis Khan, the fierce military genius of the 12th Century, refined this technique in his horse cavalry by using a unique rawhide cup. It fit over the hoof and when dry was extremely tough and wear resistant. This, in part, accounted for the great mobility of his Mongolian striking force.

The early Romans and Greeks made use of sandals, boots, and socks of leather and woven fiber or coarse cloth to protect their horse's hoofs. The Romans are credited with inventing the "hipposandal" which was a kind of leather sandal with an iron sole. It was fastened around the fetlock by means of leather thongs and could be easily removed. Xenophon the Greek, writing *circa* 400 B.C., discussed the importance of frog pressure and hard hoofs. Apparently, shoeing was unknown in his time.

First Horseshoeing with Nails

Horseshoeing with iron shoes and nails was invented, in all probability, by different nations at about the same time. One nation influenced another until all practiced it in one form or another.

The first blacksmith we have any evidence of was named Tubal-cain as recorded in Genesis, Chapter 4, verse 22. However, no mention of the practice of horseshoeing was made at this early date.

Recently, China has been suggested as the country of origin for the iron shoe. Horseshoes with nails have been used there for more than 2000 years. The Mongolians had a good knowledge of the treatment of various metals and may have produced the first horseshoes.

There is some inconclusive evidence to indicate that the practice of horseshoeing as we know it, with iron shoes and nails, was practiced in the 5th or 6th Century B.C. Some scholars insist that shoes and nails, which are thought to be of Greek and Roman origin, can be dated to that period.

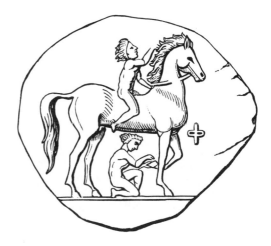

Fig. 3-2. A drawing of a silver coin found at Tarentum and dated to circa *300 B.C. The coin is now in the British Museum. It is about the size of a quarter.* From Horse Shoes and Horse-Shoeing *by G. Fleming.*

19

A silver coin discovered on the location of the ancient island town of Tarentum, now Taranto, in Southern Italy, and dated to 300 B.C., appears to depict a horse's foot being examined, but by no means conclusively demonstrates the act of horseshoeing. However, the ancestors of the founders of this ancient Greek colony were noted for their love of horses and excellent horsemanship.

The earliest known evidence in the form of a written record of horses being shod are lists of cavalry equipment from the 8th and 9th Century which list lunar or crescent-shaped iron horseshoes and their nails. Tradition has it that they were available at an earlier time, but they don't seem to have been applied as a regular practice and served mainly as a remedy for sore feet on war horses.

Archeological evidence indicates that the Celts or Gauls had horseshoes sometime before the Romans. They are reported to have had cavalries which were far superior to those of the early Roman armies.

Although horseshoeing may have had an early beginning, the practice of using iron shoes and nails appears not to have been widely known until sometime after 400 A.D., and not in regular use until around 1000 A.D. Before 1000 A.D., horseshoes were used mainly for decoration and adornment and occasionally on war horses. The Roman ruler, Nero (37-68 A.D.), is reported to have had his horses shod with silver and those of his wife, Poppaea, with gold. Even as late as the 9th Century in France, horses are said to have been shod with iron only on special occasions.

Some scholars maintain that the Romans had horseshoes and nails with them when they invaded England in 55 B.C. However, William the Conqueror, the Norman who came in 1066 A.D., is also credited with introducing the practice into England in his day.

In fact, a possible origin of the word farrier is directly related to him. Shortly after the England invasion, William the Conqueror commissioned Wakelin von Ferrariis his "Master of the Horse". This man was later promoted to be Count of Ferrers and Derby. As chief farrier, he was entrusted with the inspection and regulation of the Kingdom's farriers. The heraldic shield of the Ferrer's family displays six black shoes on a silver background. "Farrier" was a title in England after this time.

Farriers and Veterinarians

The word farrier has several possible origins. One that is frequently quoted is taken from the Low Latin word *ferraius*, meaning a worker in iron, and from the Old French *ferrer*, to shoe a horse. Pliny, the Roman scholar, used the word,

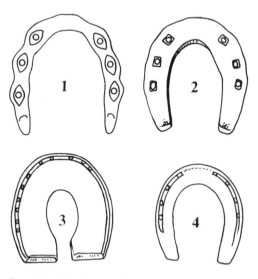

Fig. 3-4. Classification of early nail-on horseshoes. (1) Celtic or Romano-British with large bulging countersunk nail holes, B.C. to 1066 A.D.; (2) Medieval with tapered branches, calks and square nail holes, 1066 to 1550; (3) Renaissance and Keyhole with fullering and no clip, 1550 to 1800; (4) Modern with clips and machine-made, 1800 to present. From On Dating Old Horse-Shoes by G. Ward.

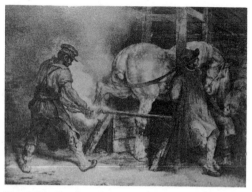

Fig. 3-3. Hot horseshoe being fit to a draft horse in a stock. The Flemish Farrier by Theodore Gericault (1791-1824). From the National Gallery of Art in Washington, DC.

ferrer, Falayan used *ferrour* in the late 15th Century and Cotgrave called a farrier *mareschal ferrant*. The Latin *ferratus* means iron-shod, while *ferramenta* refers to tools made of iron.

The word veterinarian is said to have been derived from the name of Vegitus, an early Roman practitioner of and writer on the subject of veterinary medicine.

As early as the Greek and Roman eras, the care of animals was relegated to veterinarians. They were said to be of "less figure and character" than those who practiced human medicine. Public prejudice existed against them. These veterinarians became a prosperous and indulgent class. They eventually disappeared as a separate class or profession and left a void in a society dependent upon healthy and sound horses.

By 1000 A.D., the blacksmith (worker with iron) and the horseshoer, who were often the same person in rural communities, began to practice animal medicine (such as it was) by popular demand or out of necessity.

"Farriers," as those specializing in the treatment of horse diseases (including shoeing) were called, were looked down upon with great abhorrence by those practicing the other professions. Even horsemen breathed contempt and cynicism for this class of quacks. Incredible ignorance and butchery were the order of the day. The following paraphrased summary of a treatment for founder was quite typical:

> Take out the sole of the foot. Cause the sole to fester so it will come out easier. Knife the hoof to the quick, raise the sole at the toe, and take hold of it with a pair of pinchers and pull it out, then apply hare's wool to stop the blood. Wash the sole of the foot with urine, and set on the ·shoe, and put in pitch, turpentine, and hog's grease.

A "sure-fire" treatment for ringbone was no less nefarious:

> ...cut down to the exostosis, apply a red hot iron, pour turpentine in the wound and set it afire.

One author summed up the situation by presenting the following description of farriers in his day (1838):

> Being ignorant of anatomy and physiology, they never improve beyond a certain point. Most of them have a few books, of which the bad mislead them and the good puzzle them...Give them a telescope to view the moon and they instantly become astronomers. To such people

the world is indebted for all kinds of quackery and a good deal of knavery...Among an ignorant people they may carry the imposition pretty well, and for a good while; but the day seems to be coming when quackery must expire.

In Germany, the farrier title wasn't popular. Part of the reason was a conscious effort to avoid the stereotyping that made farriery synonymous with quackery. The title of *hufbeschlag-schmiede*, meaning horseshoe smith or horseshoer, has been applied to specialists. Some have used the shorter term, *hufschmied*, literally— "hoof smith". Traditionally, the German craftsmen enjoyed as much prestige as specialized veterinarians. Later, their training schools were associated with the veterinary schools and were the finest in the world.

A few dedicated students began to make the break from the ignorant butchery that belonged to farriers not more than 200 years ago. At first they retained the name farrier, but later scrapped the term in favor of the title "veterinary surgeon".

This enlightened vanguard was instrumental in forming the first veterinary schools. Short term and inadequate as they were, these schools were the beginning of the eventual break between the two trades of veterinarian and horseshoer from that of the ancient farrier. Of course, many highly commercialized (what we would call "fly by night") schools also appeared at this time—their main interest being to capitalize on an idea whose time had come.

The more progressive schools were careful to instruct their students in more hours of horseshoeing theory and practice than the average apprenticed farrier of the day received. In fact, when veterinary colleges were founded, first in France and then in England, the main object was the improvement of horseshoeing. Medical treatment was secondary and incidental. One of the first professors of an English veterinary college declared:

> A proper method of shoeing horses is of more importance than the treatment of any, or perhaps all, diseases incidental to the horse.

Soon after 1900, the dream of these early pioneers was realized when the director of one of the first 3 year (later 4 yr.) state veterinary colleges stated that,

> Veterinary education has been lifted from the school of the tradesman to the college of a truly professional character.

Previously, a few-months to a year-long course was deemed sufficient preparation for a veterinarian. Through the efforts of a few dedicated people with high ideals, veterinary medicine gained professional status. It took a number of years to do this. One of the biggest problems to overcome was getting the veterinarians to consider themselves as and to act like professionals.

The word practitioner replaced the veterinary surgeon title in America. It had special significance for both medical doctors and veterinarians previous to the establishment of professional standards. A "doctor" would go to school for a few months and go into "practice." After killing a few folks or horses while "practicing," he would get run out of town and go to the next town to "practice" some more. After getting run out of four or five towns, he at last could convince the public he was competent enough to settle down and "practice" medicine.

Horseshoers, as a rule, were unwilling to improve themselves by college training and remained in ignorance. This created an initial split of farriers into veterinarians and horseshoers. The horseshoers carried the ignorant stigma of the farrier with them while veterinary medicine progressed to professional status. The horseshoers' (farriers') own arrogance and unwillingness to learn caused the separation. One evidence of the attitude prevalent at this time is stated in this comment made by a man in charge of the British Army farriers in India (*circa* 1870):

> My experience of farriers in the service is that it is impossible to teach them the rudiments of professional knowledge; their education has been slight, and we get them at an age when they are no longer teachable.

There were efforts made to establish professional training for horseshoers but none lasted but a short while. Some said it was because horseshoers were unteachable. Others maintained it was because of the teaching they received:

> Horseshoers are not as their maligners aver, less teachable than men composing other sections of the community. The difference has consisted in the teaching which they have received...

By the late 1800's, virtually all professional training in horseshoeing was conducted as a part of the curriculum in veterinary colleges. Horseshoers were left to learn their skills through apprenticeships from blacksmiths and aged farriers. Finally, due to the introduction of mechanized agriculture and transportation, horseshoeing became a lost art only occasionally passed on, and then only through one-to-one apprenticeships.

Horseshoeing Guilds Highly Respected

Iron horseshoes were sold made-up, hand-turned and punched, as early as the 13th and 14th Centuries to blacksmiths and farriers in England and Europe. Nails were usually made in the individual shops before the 19th Century but could also be bought "ready-made" previous to that time.

The horseshoeing and blacksmithing trades became highly respected as the chief craft guilds during this period because they required a great deal of time and skill to master, and without them nothing else functioned.

Alfred the Great, who was king of the West Saxons during the last quarter of the 9th Century, is said to have called together several of his principal craftsmen. He announced that he would appoint as Chief the one of them who could longest do without the assistance of the others. The blacksmith was soon chosen since no one could work without the tools he made or the sound horses he shod. And, the other craftsmen found it impossible to do the blacksmith's work without extensive training and experience.

There is an old legend that probably originated about this time—that the world was made at the blacksmith's forge, shaped upon an anvil from some eternal star.

Today, it is generally understood that a farrier is a horseshoer, and that a blacksmith is an iron worker. It has always been well understood in London, and some other cities in Europe, where shoeing forges were separate from smith's forges. Often, blacksmiths were farriers as well, but few farriers were skilled blacksmiths. In 1912, one master shoer and smith in the U.S. advised young apprentices to thoroughly learn both trades if they desired real proficiency, a task that he believed would take at least 10 years.

The Worshipful Company of Farriers of London is one of the oldest active guilds in the world. It has been in existence since 1356 A.D. The Farriers (Registration) Act of 1975 prohibits the shoeing of horses by unqualified persons and provides for the training and examining of farriers by the Worshipful Company of Farriers. The Company examines and certifies members at three levels. These are: Diploma of the Worshipful Company of Farriers (dip. W.F.C.), Associate of the Farriers Company of London (A.F.C.L.), and Fellowship of the Worshipful Company of Farriers (F.W.C.F.). The National Master Farriers', Blacksmiths' and Agricultural Engineers' Association is also organized in Great Britain.

The International Union of Journeymen Horseshoers of the United States and Canada (JHU) was organized in Philadelphia in 1874. The Master Horseshoers' Association (National) preceded the JHU but was gradually overshadowed by it. Today, the JHU primarily involves race track horseshoers. A comprehensive forging and horseshoeing test is required for entrance.

The American Farrier's Association (AFA) was organized in 1971. Certification tests have been adopted since 1979. Present levels are: Certified Farrier and Certified Journeyman Farrier.

Superstitions and Horseshoeing

During the Dark Ages and Medieval times, superstition reigned supreme in the horseshoeing trade as well as in other facets of life. The horseshoe was crescent-shaped and resembled a snake which was thought to be divine and keep witches away. Roman horseshoe nails were said to keep away the plague, and horses were supposed to keep nightmares away. Superstitious medieval blacksmiths believed in tapping the anvil once every few blows "to keep the devil away," and in giving it three blows at the end of the day to keep the devil chained up.

The tradition of putting a horseshoe over the door to bring good luck and keep the devil away was popular at this time. The story behind this tradition has many variations. This is one of them:

> Once upon a time, a wise old blacksmith was hard at work making horseshoes. The sound of the anvil attracted the attention of the devil. He saw that the smith was making horseshoes, and he thought it would be a good idea to get his own hoofs shod. So the devil made a deal with the smith and stood to be shod.
>
> The wise blacksmith saw with whom he was dealing, and so he nailed on a red-hot shoe, driving the nails right square into the center of the devil's hoof. The devil then paid him and left, but the honest blacksmith threw the money into the forge fire, knowing it would bring him bad luck.

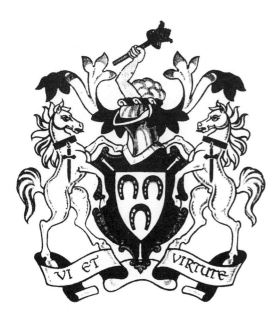

Fig. 3-5. Symbol of the Worshipful Company of Farriers of London. From The Farrier and His Craft *by L. B. Prince.*

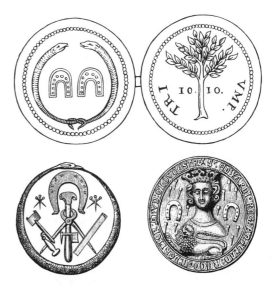

Fig. 3-6. Emblems that demonstrate the superstition surrounding horseshoes among early peoples. From Horseshoes and Horse-Shoeing *by G. Fleming.*

Meanwhile, the devil walked some distance and began to suffer the greatest torture from the new shoes. The more he danced and pranced and kicked and swore, the more they hurt him. Finally, after he had gone through the most fearful agony, he tore them off and threw them away.

From that time to this, whenever the devil sees a horseshoe he turns and runs—anxious to keep out of the way of those torturous devices.

First Books Spread Truth and Error

Very few advances were made in horseshoeing from the time of the introduction of the use of iron shoes and nails until the invention of the printing press in the 15th Century. Many authors then began to publish on the subject, and there was an opportunity for a widespread exchange of ideas from which improvements could come.

However, errors were also perpetuated by the widespread circulation of books and ideas. Some of the errors expressed then have, in varying degrees, carried down to today. They have become universally accepted and will not easily be eliminated. In 1764, E.G. LaFosse, Jr., the Farrier to the King of France, said:

> The errors of farriery are as ancient as farriers. These errors are the prime children of ignorance; through ignorance they are perpetuated.

The early writers of the horseshoeing trade coined many of the phrases we commonly use today. Blundeville, an Englishman writing in 1566, is credited with the saying: "Fit the shoe to the foot, not the foot to the shoe." A Frenchman, Solleysel, writing in 1664, was the first to describe "pointing" as an aid to diagnosing lameness. He also described the use of clips and advocated the use of light shoes and nails—something unheard of before that time. Jeremiah Bridges published the first known description of the elastic mechanism of the horse's foot in 1751 and is said to have originated the saying: "No foot, no horse."

Horseshoeing in Early America

The blacksmith was the head of the tradesmen in early America, and he "charged accordingly." Not much horse or oxen shoeing was done before 1750 in America because iron was very expensive and hard to get. The price of shoeing was very high due to the dependence upon imported iron and European guild horseshoers.

In 1779, price ceilings were placed on horseshoers and continued throughout the Revolution. The maximum price allowable was 6 pounds for shoeing a horse all around and 48 shillings for

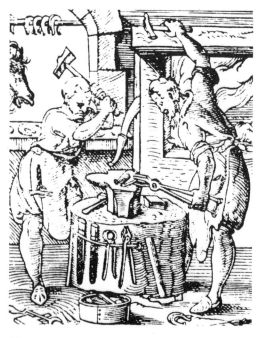

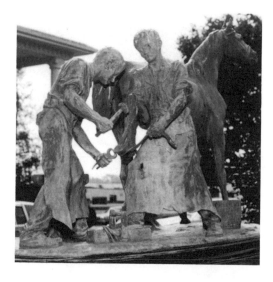

Fig. 3-7. Horseshoeing on the continent of Europe evolved as a two-man job. (Left) old woodcut, (right) statue at the Lexington Horse Center, Lexington, KY.

"shifting a set of shoes" (reset). The price of refined iron was set at 37 pounds per hundred weight. Comparatively, a felt hat sold for four pounds and the best beaver hat for 35 pounds.

In 1842, the price of shoeing a horse was five dollars and it took a load of corn to pay for it. Thus came the statement, "...a man who knows how to hammer iron can make more money than a member of Congress." Congressmen were receiving about eight dollars per day; a very high wage for the time.

There is an old saying among blacksmiths: "There are only two things a blacksmith will go to hell for, one is hammering cold iron, the other is not charging enough!"

The great Westward Movement of mid-19th Century America trekked along on horse and oxen shoes. Almost every company had its blacksmith for shoeing animals and repairing wagons.

Inventions Revolutionize Horseshoeing Techniques

Several inventions brought about some major changes in the nature of the work of horseshoeing in the mid-1800's. Henry Burden of Troy, New York, invented a machine to forge horseshoes and patented it in 1834. By 1857, he had improved the machine to the extent that it could make a shoe from a piece of hot iron in a single operation. His factory was then able to turn out 60 shoes a minute. The victory of the Union armies in the Civil War has been partially attributed to Mr. Burden's invention. The Confederate armies were limited to handmade shoes applied by a few farriers.

Daniel Dodge, also of New York, patented a machine to make horseshoe nails in 1848 and perfected it in 1862. Silas Putnam also invented a nail-making machine about this time. George Capewell invented his sometime later, and since 1881 the company he started has consistently manufactured horseshoe nails. Shoes, nails and tools for horseshoeing could all be bought ready-made by the late 1800's.

1936. Burden, H. Aug. 19.

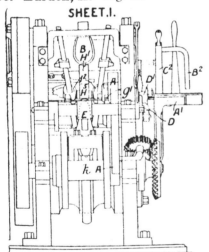

Making. In the manufacture of horse-shoes, bars are taken directly from the rolling-mill, and, without being re-heated, are passed through a machine, in which lengths are cut off, bent to a **U**-shape, swaged by revolving dies, creased, punched, and flattened, the finished shoes being discharged on to a travelling chain or belt, which carries them to the store-room. The bar is guided to the machine through a trough A¹ (Sheet 1), and passes between feed-rollers D, D¹ mounted on inclined shafts.

Fig. 3-8. Abridgment of patent specifications of Henry Burden's improved horseshoe making machine patented August 19, 1856. From the Great Britain Patent Office, London.

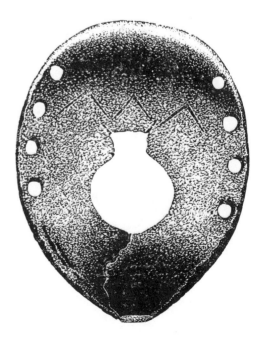

Fig. 3-9. Shoe from an Arabian stallion presented to former President U.S. Grant in 1879 by the Sultan of Turkey. This style of shoe has been used in the middle east for centuries. From Artistic Horseshoeing *by G. Rich.*

Shoes, Tools and Nails Are Mass Produced

The Phoenix Horseshoe Company, formerly of Poughkeepsie, New York, and Joliet, Illinois, was the largest manufacturer of horseshoes in the world at the turn of the Century. They went out of business in the late 1960's. Diamond Tool and Horseshoe Co., of Duluth, Minnesota, which first made horseshoes in 1908, is now the world's largest manufacturer of horseshoes.

Today, there are many foreign as well as domestic specialty shoe and tool companies marketing shoes and tools in the United States.

Capewell Manufacturing Company, of Hartford, Connecticut, is America's largest manufacturer of horseshoe nails. During the first half of this century, Capewell was a world-wide supplier of horse nails. Each nation required a particular style of head and blade of nail. At one time, Capewell manufactured over 400 different styles and varieties of horse nails. Capewell horse nails reached their peak production in 1913. They declined steadily until 1957. Since then, there

has been a slow but steady increase. By 1968, they reached a production level of about 10 per cent of the 1913 peak volume.

Mustad Horse Nail Company of Sweden is now the largest horseshoe nail manufacturer in the world. Mustad began in Norway in 1832 by pioneering the mechanization of wire-transforming processes. Mustad factories were soon established all over Europe. High custom duties and the desire of governments to be independent, especially regarding items of strategic value including military (cavalry) and agricultural (draft horses and oxen) animals, led to the establishment of factories inside the main markets. By 1930 plants were established throughout Europe. Over 800 head styles were manufactured. After World War II, roughly two-thirds of the Mustad factories including 8,000 employees were lost. At the same time, the declining numbers of horses drastically reduced the demand for horseshoe nails. For example, the production of Mustad France in the late 1930's would be sufficient for the whole world today. The last 30 years have been devoted to rebuilding plants and streamlin-

A RECORD BREAKING ACHIEVEMENT
BY
THE PHOENIX HORSESHOE COMP'Y,
AN ILLUSTRATED DESCRIPTION OF WHICH SPEAKS FOR ITSELF.

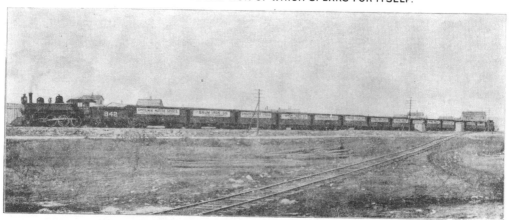

LARGE SHIPMENT OF HORSE SHOES.

The Phoenix Horseshoe Company, Joliet, Ill., made an extraordinary shipment of horseshoes December 30th, 1897, to the Baum Iron Company, of Omaha and Denver. It consisted of over 3,500 kegs, and required fourteen large-sized freight cars. The company reports that this is their largest single shipment of shoes made during the year. The train was photographed after the cars were prepared for shipment, as the company desired a momento of the occasion. The shipment covered a general assortment of the company's line of horseshoes. This heavy purchase is a striking illustration of the enterprise displayed by the Baum Iron Company, which is evidently determined to occupy a prominent place in the western heavy hardware trade. It may be well imagined that with such a shipment going out the Phoenix Horseshoe Company report their trade good. The fair treatment by the Phoenix company of their patrons, along with the superior quality of the goods, enables them to lead all other competitors and make them the peer of their respective line.

That this firm is enterprising is proven by the manner in which they try to excel in all their undertakings. This is likewise true in the material and make-up of their famous Phoenix shoes, and that the horseshoers throughout the country appreciate this fact is evinced by their liberal patronage of this make, which keep the two factories (at Poughkeepsie, N. Y., and Joliet, Ill.) constantly busy supplying the demand.

Fig. 3-10. An 1897 rail shipment of 3500 kegs of horseshoes by the 15 year old Phoenix Horseshoe Company. From an old ad by The Phoenix Horseshoe Company.

ing production methods. Recently, plants have been built in Singapore, Brazil and Turkey. Today, two out of every three horseshoe nails used throughout the world are made by Mustad.

Horseshoeing Peaks

Horseshoeing reached its peak in America in the early 1900's when horse numbers reached an all-time high. There were many qualified authorities in the field. The apprentice system was fast dying out and horseshoeing schools were initiated.

Perhaps the most famous school of instruction was set up by the U.S. Cavalry at Fort Riley, Kansas. For many years it was the largest training school for horseshoers in the United States. Its design and methods were copied by many private and public schools.

In addition, the Army trained what they called "farriers." These were veterinary aides or technicians, not horseshoers. They administered emergency veterinary treatment to cavalry horses under the supervision of a veterinarian.

The first horseshoeing schools, essentially extension programs of universities sponsoring a veterinary college, trained army horseshoers prior to and during World War I to supplement the Army School at Fort Riley, Kansas.

Horse numbers gradually dropped due to farm and transportation mechanization until they reached an all-time low in 1960. Since then, they have been steadily increasing. All indications are that pleasure horses will continue to increase as more and more leisure time becomes available.

Horseshoeing Revived

A great restoration in interest in horseshoeing has accompanied the recent increase in horse numbers.

For many years there were only two places in America where horseshoeing training could be obtained other than at the Army School or by individual apprenticeship. Both of them were connected with veterinary colleges. A "short course" (6 mo. in length) in horseshoeing was initiated at Michigan State University and during the 40's and 50's educated many horseshoers. Another college hired a former Michigan State student to start a school on the west coast in the early 50's. By 1960, there were still only a few places where training could be obtained.

During the last two decades, a virtual explosion in so called "horseshoeing schools" has paralleled a phenomenal increase in horse population. Many colleges and private schools now offer horseshoeing courses.

There were only three horseshoeing schools in the United States in 1960. There were approximately 25 in 1970. By 1973, over 50 institutions offered some form of instruction in horseshoeing. In 1975, nearly 100 courses were available in the U.S. and Canada. The number of courses stabilized around 65 by 1983. These courses are tremendously varied in content. Three veterinary schools (Auburn, Cornell and the University of Pennsylvania) have horseshoeing instruction as part of their curriculum.

Well-balanced professional training programs which combine both art and science are available for those desiring to be competent horseshoers.

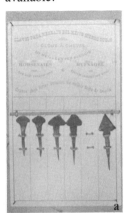 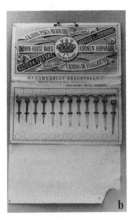 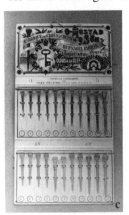 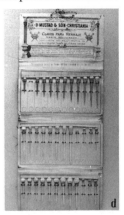

Fig. 3-11. Old Mustad nails. (a) old handmade Mustad nails, (b) Mustad-Crown brand for export to India, (c) Mustad-keg brand for export to Argentina, and (d) Mustad-Crown brand for export to Spain. Photos by H. Nilsson.

However, in all cases, further study and practice are necessary to become a qualified horseshoer. Education of the eyes and hands takes years of study and practice.

Modern Techniques

Many new developments have been introduced into the horseshoeing field in recent years. The method of making, heating and fitting shoes had changed very little for centuries until recently, even though the quality and understanding of the trimming and shoeing process had improved. Today, tools of improved design made from high-quality steel, gas forges and finished ready-made shoes have made the horseshoer's work much easier.

New products and methods of surgery for treating lamenesses and hoof diseases have been developed. Self-polymerizing acrylic plastics are used for treating quarter cracks and founder. The electron microscope, radiation biology and ther-

mography have been used to study founder. New drugs have been used to treat founder and joint diseases. Surgery and corrective shoes have been used with some success to correct severely deformed legs and feet. New plastics have been used for cushion pads and shoes. Plastic horseshoes and pads have been introduced. Slip-on and glue-on shoes are available. New products are being introduced each year.

Exciting Future

The future of horseshoeing looks very bright. Interest in horses continues to grow. Horseshoeing is an honorable and rewarding profession. Advances have been made which remove some of the handwork from the process. However, the practice of horseshoeing is still physically hard work done by hand much the same as it was centuries ago. Interest in reviving pride in craftsmanship is both alive and well.

References

Asmus, H. 1916. Anatomy of the horse's foot and the science of horseshoeing. The American Blacksmith. 15:185.

Butler, D. 1975. Horseshoeing Course Survey. Unpublished, Ithaca, N.Y.

Dollar, J. A. W. 1898. A Handbook of Horse-shoeing. William R. Jenkins, New York.

Elvinge, F. 1975. On the origin of the horseshoe. Nord. Vet. Med. 27:389.

Fleming, G. 1869. Horse Shoes and Horse-Shoeing. Chapman and Hall, London.

Fleming, G. 1870. Observations on the anatomy and physiology of the horse's foot. The Vet. 43:13.

Gamgee, J. 1871. A Treatise of Horse-shoeing and Lameness. Longmans, Green, and Co., London.

Governing Board of the Educator's Division of the American Farriers' Assn. 1983. Directory of farrier schools. Amer. Farriers' J. 9(1):49.

Grossbauer, J. and F. Habacher. 1928. Der Huf-und Klauenbeschlag. Urban and Schwarzenberg, Berlin.

Hewitt, B.1972. Horseshoeing history. The Western Horseman. October:44.

Hickman, J. 1977. Farriery. J. A. Allen, London.

Hippogriff. 1870. Army farriers and shoeing smiths. The Vet. 43:829.

Kreis, P. 1984. Personal Communication. Mustad Nail Co., I.I. Fastener AG, Zug, SWITZERLAND.

Lewis, C. T. 1918. An Elementary Latin Dictionary. American Book Co., New York.

Miller, R. M. 1976. Mind over Miller. Vet. Med. 71:16.

Moore, V. A. 1908. Special Report to the President of Cornell University by the Director of the New York State

Veterinary College. Cornell, Ithaca, NY.

Moore, V. A. 1918. Annual Report of the New York State Veterinary College. Cornell University, Ithaca, NY.

Norton, I. H. 1968. Personal Communication. Capewell Nail Co., Hartford, CT.

Pride, W. F. 1926. The History of Fort Riley. Fort Riley. Fort Riley, KS.

Prince, L. B. 1980. The Farrier and His Craft. J. A. Allen, London.

Rich, G. E. 1890. Artistic Horseshoeing. M. T. Richardson, New York.

Russell, W. 1892.Scientific Horseshoeing. Robert Clarke and Co., Cincinnati.

Skeat, W. W. 1882. An Etymological Dictionary of the English Language. Clarendon Press, Oxford.

Smith, F. 1919. The Early History of Veterinary Literature (Vol. I.), London.

Smithcors, J. F. 1957. Evolution of the Veterinary Art. Veterinary Medicine Publishing Co., Kansas City, MO.

Smithcors, J. F. 1963. The American Veterinary Profession. Iowa State University Press, Ames.

Sparks, I. G. 1976. Old Horseshoes. Shire Album No. 19. Shire Publications Ltd., Aylesbury, ENGLAND.

United States War Department. 1914. Manual for Farriers, Horseshoers, Saddlers and Wagoners or Teamsters. USWD Doc. No. 486. U.S. Government Printing Office, Washington, D.C.

Ward. G. 1939. On Dating Old Horse-Shoes. Hull Museum Publ. No. 205. Hull, ENGLAND.

White, D. S. 1917. Problems of the profession. Practitioners Short Course in Veterinary Medicine. 2:278.

Chapter 4

Public Relations For Horseshoers

People become very attached to their animals. Once, the horse was a work animal. Horses served man by expending muscular energy in behalf of their owners. Now, horses provide recreation and are treated like companion animals or pets.

Pet or "family" horses present several public relations problems. First, the animals are not as well trained or even as gentle as most animals that are worked daily. Many modern owners do not know how to care for and train their horses and/or they don't have a constant concern for their welfare because they don't depend upon them. Second, the owners have not worked with horses enough or done the hard work of shoeing to know what to expect from the horse and the horseshoer. In addition, horseshoers tend to become a scapegoat for problems that develop due to natural causes, breeding, poor management, or veterinary malpractice.

Problems relating to performance horses, as distinguished from pet horses, are usually quite different. The owners and trainers are more knowledgeable and the horses are better behaved. Horseshoers must make the trainer, owner or veterinarian subtly aware that they can do what needs to be done.

Misunderstandings and problems may occur.

Accidents will happen. A good reputation is earned by many positive impressions and may be lost by one negative one. Be honest in your dealings with others and expect them to be honest with you. Following are some principles to consider as you develop your business.

Every person you work with or associate with has a feeling or attitude about you. One has said, "There is very little difference in people, but that little difference makes a big difference. The little difference is attitude. The big difference is whether it is positive or negative."

Reilly (1952) has called these attitude differences mental levels. Each person we associate with has placed us on one of these four levels. It is desirable to determine where we stand so we can be most effective in our relations with each person.

The four levels are described as a closed mind, an open mind, confidence and belief. A closed mind must be opened by a favorable impression. A person who is open-minded needs plenty of evidence. The confidence level is the best. One who believes in you doesn't need any proof at all. In fact, it is often a mistake to go into long explanations with such a person.

Most people are offended by an ignorant or a know-it-all attitude. Try, in your dealings with

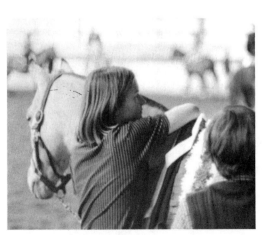

Fig. 4-1. Today, most horses are treated as pets.

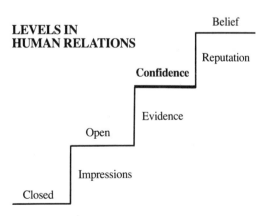

LEVELS IN HUMAN RELATIONS

Fig. 4-2. The four attitude levels of horseshoeing customers tell how people feel about you. From Successful Human Relations *by W. Reilly.*

others, to develop wisdom. It will serve you well. The person who confesses his or her ignorance is on the road to wisdom. Solomon has said, "Wisdom is the principle thing...therefore get wisdom." William Cowper said, "Knowledge is proud that he has learned so much; wisdom is humble that he knows no more." Never stop learning and improving.

Success in business has been said to be only 15 percent dependent upon technical knowledge and 85 percent dependent upon one's ability to get along with people. What you know is not as important as what you do. Your horseshoeing skill cannot be appreciated unless you can communicate it to the horse owner. There are skills that must be developed if you are to get along with people. These talents must be studied and practiced just like the mechanical skills of blacksmithing and shoeing. Those who don't recognize this fact early may have all their shoeing at one time—the first time and the last time.

Dale Carnegie's book, *How to Win Friends and Influence People,* and other self-improvement books are important reading. Treat people in a considerate, businesslike manner. As you work on yourself, your business will improve. You may spend many years perfecting the technical skills of shoeing and horse handling skills. Wisdom would suggest equal time to be devoted to developing people handling skills. Effective phone appointment making is especially important.

The following techniques have proven useful in dealing with horse owners:

1. Present a professional image. This includes grooming, dress, language and outfit.
2. Be concerned about the horse—ask about his habits, history, needs, proposed use.
3. Display prices with extras for special features, irregular conditions, training, etc. Treat everyone the same.
4. Request a clean, safe, well-lighted area to work or, if they cannot provide such, suggest they bring the horses to your shop to help you better serve them.
5. Give a conservative guarantee on your work with conditions and a time limit.
6. Set conditions on authoritative statements and avoid expressing opinions that can't be verified.
7. Never intentionally hurt a horse—rather control yourself, advise of the need for training, veterinary service or a more specialized

horseshoer. Get by a bad horse as fast as you can.
8. Praise your customers, their horses and your competition. Most people don't think they are wrong and don't want to be told they are.
9. Express appreciation to customers for their business. Give helpful literature or helps (e.g., hoof pick) to them. Inexpensive literature can be obtained from a USDA extension office.
10. Use a checklist at the phone for new customers.

Use of the Telephone

The telephone can help or hurt your business. Be courteous but be firm. Learn not to waste time on the phone. For those horseshoers that work alone, an answering service or phone attachment is a necessity. Since many people don't like to talk to a tape, a special time each night should be scheduled for receiving and making calls. Recording appointments in one book is especially important. You may want to make the next appointment at the time of the shoeing job. Or you may schedule several in advance for some customers.

A checklist by the phone is handy, especially when dealing with new customers. Some horseshoers do this by filling out a card on the person and horse(s) as they talk. Others may enter information into a computer. Have several maps of your area near the phone and with your appointment book.

A check list of things that should be covered in the conversation follows:

1. Name (person responsible for payment)
2. Address (for billing or appointment reminder)
3. Service needed (how many to trim or shoe, extras)
4. Location of horse (directions)
5. Appointment (day and approximate time, "Will someone be there?")
6. Phone number (in case have to notify of time change, follow up)
7. Identification of horse(s) (Age, color, sex and markings)
8. Past behavioral, disease or gait problems the horse may have had
9. How referred—"Whom may I thank for this business?" (Send card or call to thank them)
10. Payment discussion (approximate cost, how plan to pay, "Will you be there?" or how billed)

Once appointments are made, a follow-up call the night before or a few days before is good business. If it has been sometime since the appointment was made, you may want to say, "Did we say 8:00 or 8:30 tomorrow to do those horses of yours?" If you say, "Is tomorrow still okay?" they may use the follow-up call as an opportunity to cancel an appointment. Such wording should be avoided. Learn to ask questions that get you the answers and commitments you want.

Service Charges

The price for shoeing service in your area is mostly a matter of tradition. Normally, you should not charge less than anyone else in your area. Perhaps your knowledge and service should allow you to charge more. Other shoers may then follow your example. Price cutting makes the other shoers angry and causes the horse owner to lose respect for you and your work.

A displayed price list saves a lot of problems. Extra charges for things that take time and annoy you can be included. For example, excessive distance, emergency call, training session(s), catching, special materials, holder, consulting and missed appointment fees can all be included. You can always waive the fee if the number of horses or the size of the account warrants it. But, you must learn to control time wasters. Time is money.

A rule of thumb for setting the price in your area is the Barber Shop Formula. At the turn of the century a shave and haircut was $.25. New horse shoes all around were $2.00. If hair cuts in your town are $4.00, then that number multiplied by eight should be a fair price for horseshoeing. In this example, horseshoeing should be $32.00. Trimming is usually about one third the price of shoeing.

Another method of establishing price is to charge each part of the job by an hourly rate. Determine how much it should cost to do each type of job and make a schedule much like mechanics have for working on cars.

Discounts may be given for a large number of horses and should be given to encourage people to bring horses to your shop. Most people take their horse(s) to the veterinarian. They will bring them to your shop if you request it, especially if you give them a discount for doing so.

Ideally, work should be paid for when it is completed. However, this is not always possible. Professional billing procedures are a necessity. For example, no new work should be done until the old bill is paid. It is best to have stable management collect money when working at public barns. The trainer has the horse if the bill isn't paid. You don't have the same lien leverage. Most people will work with you if you inform them of your policy upon your first meeting.

PRO HORSESHOEING BY APPOINTMENT PRICE LIST

Shoeing (Reset)	_____		
Shoes @ _____ to			
_____ each	_____	to	_____
Shoeing with New Shoes	_____	to	_____
Trim (Weanling to Draft)	_____	to	_____
Light Pads or Bar Wedges (leather or plastic)/pair	_____	to	_____
Borium @ _____ to			
_____/shoe	_____	to	_____
Studs @ _____ to			
_____/shoe	_____	to	_____
Draft Horse Shoeing (Reset)/pair	_____		
Draft Horse Shoes @_____to_____ each	_____	to	_____
Draft Horse Shoeing with New Shoes	_____	to	_____
Gaited Horse Shoeing (Reset)/pair	_____		
Double Nail Job extra/ pair (incl. pads)	_____		
Heavy Leather pads/pair	_____		
Heavy Plastic pads, full wedges/pair	_____		
Weighted Shoes/pair	_____	to	_____
Bands/pair	_____		
Reset Bands/pair	_____		
Rework weighted shoes	_____	to	_____
Welded clips, spoons or grabs/pair shoes	_____		
Lead attached to or set in pads/pair	_____		
Lead/pair	_____		
Hoof Repair with 10X or Justi kit	_____	to	_____
Hospital Shoes or Braces/shoe	_____	to	_____
Corrective Shoeing/foot or/pair	_____	to	_____
Race Horse Plating	_____		
Racing Plates @ _____	_____		

Fig. 4-3. Itemize and display your prices.

Horseshoer—Horse Owner Responsibilities

The horseshoer's responsibility:

1. Schedule and keep appointments. Try to group appointments geographically to cut down travel time.
2. Be professional; use professional language and tact. Avoid profanity and temper tantrums.
3. Be prepared to present a bill for services rendered. Explain fees and credit terms.
4. Constantly look for ways to improve and become more efficient.
5. Study farriery in depth and keep posted on the trade. Educate the owner at appropriate moments.
6. Be well stocked and equipped for all types of shoeing.
7. Be pleasant and noncritical of other's work, horses, facilities and personalities.
8. Know your capabilities, be honest with the owner, be unafraid to refer the horse to a more specialized shoer or a veterinarian. Admit your mistakes (everyone makes them). Promptly do what must be done to make them right. Obtain liability insurance to protect yourself, especially if you shoe in a shop.
9. Make a good efficient job a foremost concern, rather than profit. This done, speed will come naturally and profit will increase.
10. Pace yourself. Take on only that which you can handle. Since shoeing is hard work and you want to continue to work each day, you should not try to do more than you are physically capable of doing.

The horse owner's responsibility:

1. Make appointments one or two weeks in advance and keep them.
2. Have the horse caught and held in a dry, accessible area.
3. Provide a good place to work—level and dry, plenty of light, shade if hot, safe and no "spooks" (small children, pets, machinery, etc.) or wire traps.
4. Be available to hold the horse. If this is not possible, provide someone who is familiar with the horse. A horse will generally stand better for someone it is familiar with, and the horseshoer may need to consult with someone who knows the horse's special needs.
5. Handle the horse's feet regularly. Keep them free of disease. Tie the horse for long periods to teach it to stand quietly for shoeing.
6. Inform the horseshoer of any behavioral or foot problems the horse may have.
7. Have the horse's feet clean and soft before the shoer comes. Overflow the water tank—

it may take several days in dry weather. Hoof dressing is usually not necessary. When it is used, apply it to a clean, washed hoof. Stabled horses generally require no preparation; however, don't apply hoof dressing for at least 24 hours before the shoer is to come. (It makes for a greasy mess!)

8. Take care of the horse. Schedule a reshoeing before the hoofs become overgrown and the shoes lost. Realize shoeing is a regular event.
9. Pay the horseshoer when he does the work.
10. Be loyal to your horseshoer! Remember the best horseshoer available is the cheapest in the long run.

Timeless Public Relations Advice

J. G. Holmstrom (1904) has given us some timeless advice on the art of public relations:

ADVICE TO HORSE OWNERS

It is cruelty to animals to raise a colt and not train him for shoeing, and the horse-shoer must suffer for this neglect also. Many a valuable horse has been crippled or maltreated, and thousands of horse-shoers suffer hardships, and many are crippled, and a few killed every year for the horse owner's carelessness in this matter. A law should be enacted making the owner of an ill-bred horse responsible for the damage done to the horse-shoer by such an animal. Every horse-raiser should begin while the colt is only a few days old to drill him for the shoeing. The feet should be taken, one after the other, and held in the same position as a horse-shoer does, a light hammer or even the fist will do, to tap on the foot with, and the feet should be handled and manipulated in the same manner the horseshoer does when shoeing. This practice should be kept up and repeated at least once a week and the colt when brought to the shop for shoeing will suffer no inconvenience. The horse-shoer's temper, as well as muscles, will be spared and a good feeling all around prevails.

Horse-raisers, remember this.

ADVICE TO YOUNG MEN

In every profession and trade it is a common thing to hear beginners say; I know, I know. No matter what you tell them, they will always answer, I know. Such an answer is never given by an old, learned or experienced man, because, as we grow older and wiser we know that there is no such thing as knowing it all. Besides this we know that there might be a better way than the way we have learned of doing the work. It is only in few cases that we can say that this is the best way, therefore we should never say, I know: first, because no young man ever had an experience wide enough to cover the whole thing; second, it is neither sensible nor polite. Better not say anything, but simply do what you have been told to do.

Every young man thinks, of course, that he has learned from the best men. This is selfish and foolish. You may have learned from the biggest botch in the country. Besides this, no matter how clever your master was, there will be things that somebody else has a better way of doing. I have heard an old good blacksmith say, that he had never had a helper but what he learned some good points from him.

Don't think it is a shame, or anything against you, to learn. We will all learn as long as we live, unless we are fools, because fools learn very little. Better to assume less than you know than to assume more.

Thousands of journeymen go idle because many a master would rather hire a greenhorn than hire a "knowing-it-all" fellow. Don't make yourself obnoxious by always telling how your boss used to do this or that. You may have learned it in the best way possible, but you may also have learned it in the most awkward way. First find out what your master wants, then do it, remembering there are sometimes many ways to accomplish the same thing. Don't be stubborn. Many mechanics are so stubborn that they will never change their ways of doing things, nor improve on either tools or ideas.

Don't be a one-idea man; and remember the maxim, "A wise man changes his mind, a fool never."

Be always punctual, have the same interest in doing good work and in drawing customers as you would were the business yours. Be always polite to the customers, no matter what happens. Never lose your temper or use profane language. Don't tell your master's competitors his way of doing business, or what is going on in his dealings with people. You are taking his money for your service, serve as you would be served.

HINTS TO BLACKSMITHS AND HORSE-SHOERS

Don't burn the shoe on.
Don't rasp under the clinchers.
Don't rasp on the outer side of the wall more than is absolutely necessary.
Don't rasp or file the clinch heads.
Don't make the shoes too short. Don't make high calks. Don't pare the frog.
Don't cut down the bars. Don't load the horse down with iron.
Don't lose your temper. Don't hit the horse with the hammer.
Don't run down your competitor. Don't continually tell how smart you are.

Don't smoke while shoeing. Don't imbibe in the shop. Don't run outdoors while sweaty. Don't know it all. Always be punctual in attendance to your business. Allow your customers to know something. No man is such a great fool but that something can be learned of him.

Be always polite. Keep posted on everything belonging to your trade. Read much. Drink little. Take a bath once a week. Dress well. This done, the craft will be elevated, and the man respected.

Good Accounts Have To Be Earned

Make people feel important and good about themselves. You must like people as well as horses to be successful. One horseshoer has said, "How can I help but like people—they give me their money!"

Try the positive, "I care" approach. Take time to explain or teach new horse owners about their responsibilities to the horse. This includes things that shoes can or cannot do for the horse. For example, when something that has been tried doesn't work, you might say, "That's what I would have done first, now let's try this." If the horse is good with you but has been bad, "The last shoer must have taught him a lesson." Or if he acts up, "This could be a nice horse if he was taught some manners."

Clean grooming and workmanlike clothes do much for your image. You only have one chance to make a first impression. Most horses are family horses. Good manners and clean language are often more important than your manual skills in getting and keeping accounts.

Be punctual. When you are not on time, you are saying your time is more valuable than the client's. They don't think so.

Do your best each time. If you don't feel good about your performance, it's not good enough. If you haven't time to do it right, you haven't time to do it over. If you make a distinction as to whether a customer can tell the difference between good and bad work, very soon you won't be able to tell the difference. C.M. Holmes (1928) said of horseshoeing: "...it is only by giving one's best that the best results are attained, and no man, as yet, has done his work too well."

Profanity is a crutch people use who don't have a vivid imagination. It is associated with a lack of education, especially a lack of reading.

In fact, studies have shown that 80 percent of people who don't read are extremely profane. One who does not read has no advantage over one who cannot read. Profanity has been called the effort of a feeble mind to express itself forcibly.

The best place for alcohol is in a bottle with the cork on. Alcohol has ruined many good horseshoers. It seems to be an occupational hazard. Studies have shown that the chances of a person becoming an alcoholic if he or she takes one drink are about one in fourteen. Those aren't very good odds for something as destructive and deadly as alcohol.

Rest or diversion is important to a horseshoer. One day a week to rest from this hard physical work is wisdom. If you can't make it in six days, you can't make it in seven. Learn to say no. Study time management techniques. Schedule your time. Take time for yourself and your family.

Personal development must be scheduled. Conventions, contests, courses, meetings, subscriptions, books all have an important role in helping you become all you can be.

In summary, Gil Reaume has said, "All good accounts have to be earned by 1) quality of work, 2) quality of personality, and 3) quality of good business habits." Horse, owner, shoer, profession and business all prosper when good ethics are practiced.

Your best advertisement is a good recommendation from a satisfied customer.

To a horse owner, the most important attribute you possess is your compassion for his horse. Professional records, statements, cards, phone book ads are helpful. Feature articles in your local newspaper are very effective. Talks at local 4H or saddle clubs, donations to horse shows or activities present an image of concern and involvement with the horse industry.

Aspire to be the best. Average is the worst of the best and the best of the worst. You can be more than that! Be all you can be! Be a winner!

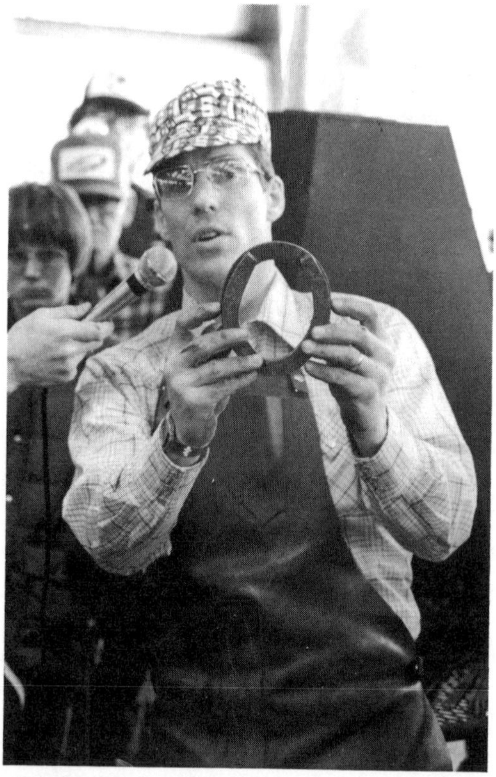

BUSINESS FORECAST
Wheelwright Lithographing Company

BUSINESS will continue to go where invited and remain where appreciated.

REPUTATIONS will continue to be made by many acts and be lost by one.

PEOPLE will go right on preferring to do business with friends.

GO-GIVERS will become the best go-getters.

THE "EXTRA-MILE" will have no traffic jams.

PERFORMANCE will continue to outsell promises.

ENTHUSIASM will be as contagious as ever.

KNOW-HOW will surpass guess-how.

TRUST, not tricks, will keep customers loyal.

QUALITY will be prized as a precious possession.

Fig. 4-4. Conventions, clinics, contests, courses and periodicals all have an important role in helping you become all you can be. Photo by H. Heymering.

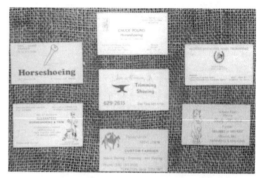

Fig. 4-5. Professional cards and feature articles will help advertise your business.

HOW TO TELL A WINNER FROM A LOSER
Vernon B. Carr

1. A winner says, "Let's find out;" a loser says, "Nobody knows."
2. When a winner makes a mistake, he says, "I was wrong;" when a loser makes a mistake, he says, "It wasn't my fault."
3. A winner goes THROUGH a problem; a loser goes AROUND it, and never gets past it.
4. A winner makes commitments; a loser makes promises.
5. A winner says, "I'm good, but not as good as I ought to be;" a loser says, "I'm not as bad as a lot of other people."
6. A winner tries to learn from those who are superior to him; a loser tries to tear down those who are superior to him.
7. A winner says, "There ought to be a better way to do it;" a loser says, "That's the way it's always been done here."

QUALITY IS LIKE BUYING OATS

IF YOU WANT NICE CLEAN OATS, YOU MUST PAY A FAIR PRICE; HOWEVER IF YOU CAN BE SATISFIED WITH OATS THAT HAVE ALREADY BEEN THROUGH THE HORSE . . . THAT COMES A LITTLE CHEAPER.

Fig. 4-6. Strive for quality in your work. Prosperity will follow.

References

Carnegie, D. 1936. How to Win Friends and Influence People. Simon & Schuster, New York.

Clevenger, B. 1979. How to give your farrier a migraine. Horseman. (Apr.):82.

Darling, R. and W. Willis. 1978. Farrier facts for new owners. Horseman. (May):64.

Dowell, M.D. 1970. Today's Horseman—Who Is He and What Is He Like? Merck Market Research Dept., Pennsylvania State University, University Park.

Duggins, G.H.1980. Fred Farrier's finances. Amer. Farriers' J. 6(1):18.

Garff, R.L. 1956. You Can Learn to Speak. Wheelwright Lithographing Co., Salt Lake City.

Garvan, F. 1983. What does your business card say about you? Amer. Farriers' J. 9(2):125.

Green, E.H. 1975. The Law and Your Horse. Wilshire Book Co., No. Hollywood, CA.

Green, L. 1979. Why not shoe horses inside? Amer. Farriers' J. 5(4):113.

Hannah, H.W. and D.F. Storm. Law for the Veterinarian and Livestock Owner. Interstate, Danville, IL.

Holmes, C.M. 1949. The Principles and Practice of Horse-Shoeing. The Farrier's Journal Publishing Co., Leeds, ENGLAND.

Holmstrom, J.G. 1904. Modern Blacksmithing. Frederick J. Drake & Co., Chicago.

Lawrence, T.H. 1975. This Thing Called Leadership. Lawrence Leiter and Co., Kansas City, MO.

Levoy, R.P. 1966. The $100,000 Practice and How to Build It. Prentice-Hall, Inc., Englewood Cliffs, NJ.

Levoy, R.P. 1976. How to handle complaints. Vet. Med./S.A.C. (Jan.):102.

Maltz, M. 1960. Psycho-Cybernetics. Wilshire Book Co., N. Hollywood, CA.

Miller, B. 1980. Paper work. Amer. Farriers' J. 6(1):12.

Miller, R.M. 1976. Mind over Miller. Vet. Med./S.A.C. (Jan.):16.

Moates, E. 1980. Law of contracts for farriers. Amer. Farriers' J. 6(3):94.

Moates, E. 1983. The farrier and the law: civil liability. Amer. Farriers' J. 9(4):312.

O'Flattery, D. 1982. Let's take the mystery out of shoeing prices. Amer. Farriers' J. 8(6):358.

Reaume, G. 1976. Ethics. Michigan Horseshoers Assn. Newsletter, Oscada, MI.

Reilly, W.J. 1952. Successful Human Relations. Harper and Row, New York.

Schwartz, D.J. 1965. The Magic of Thinking Big. Prentice-Hall, Inc., New York.

Schwartz, D.J. 1983. The Magic of Getting What You Want. William Morrow and Co., Inc., New York.

Solomon. Proverbs. The Holy Bible. Cambridge Press, ENGLAND.

Sproles, J. 1982. The cost of professionalism. Amer. Farriers' J. 8(6):356.

Staff Report. 1975. What counts with the DVM choosing public? Mod. Vet. Pract. 56:819.

Staff Report. 1975. Inflation and fees: how can you keep up? Mod. Vet. Pract. 56:825.

Staff Report. 1975. A dozen and one reasons clients complain. Norden News. (Feb.):20.

Ziglar, Z. 1982. See You at the Top. Pelican Press. Gretna, LA.

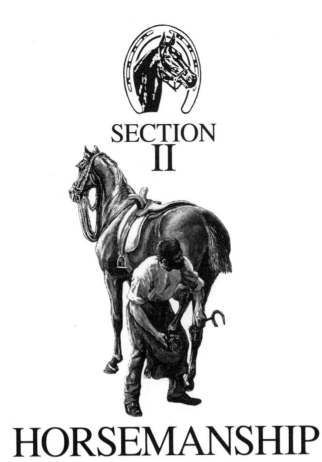

SECTION
II

HORSEMANSHIP

HORSE REGIONS

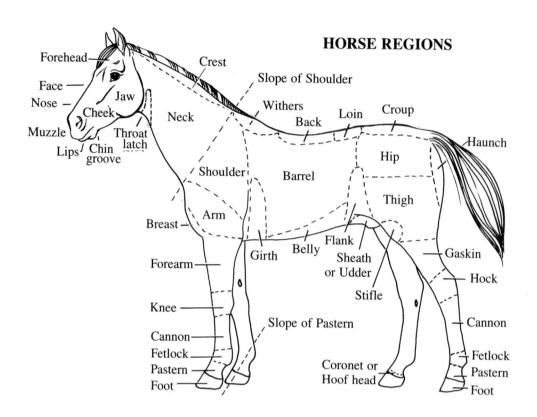

Forehead
Crest
Slope of Shoulder
Face
Jaw
Nose
Cheek
Withers
Loin
Croup
Neck
Back
Muzzle
Throat latch
Lips
Chin groove
Haunch
Shoulder
Barrel
Hip
Arm
Thigh
Breast
Flank
Girth
Belly
Sheath or Udder
Gaskin
Forearm
Hock
Stifle
Knee
Cannon
Slope of Pastern
Cannon
Fetlock
Fetlock
Pastern
Coronet or Hoof head
Pastern
Foot
Foot

HORSE POINTS

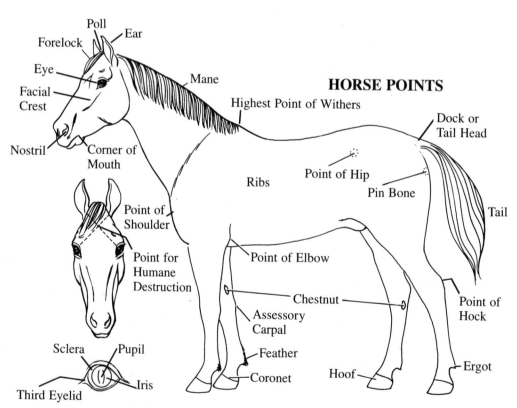

Poll
Ear
Forelock
Eye
Mane
Facial Crest
Highest Point of Withers
Dock or Tail Head
Nostril
Corner of Mouth
Ribs
Point of Hip
Pin Bone
Tail
Point of Shoulder
Point for Humane Destruction
Point of Elbow
Chestnut
Point of Hock
Assessory Carpal
Sclera
Pupil
Feather
Ergot
Third Eyelid
Iris
Coronet
Hoof

Fig. 5-1. External horse terms

Chapter 5

Terms, Points And Regions Of The Horse

THE BOOKS THEY SHOW
Edgar A. Guest

A certain rich man bought a book.
It had a most impressive look—
'Twas bound in leather, richly tooled
And penned by one most wisely schooled.
Full many a poor man passing by
Had seen it with an envious eye
And by his sigh made plainly known
His wish so rare this book to own.
To drain those pages shining bright
He would have read throughout the night.

A certain poor man stopped and found
The self-same volume paper bound
And gladly for this precious tome
Paid 50 cents and took it home.
Each night he sat and page by page
He drunk in the wisdom of the age
And made before he'd reached the end
The man who abridged it his friend,
Claimed the knowledge for his own
And by this book had wiser grown.

A friend beside the rich man's shelf
Exclaimed, "Why I've this same book myself.
Yours is a handsomer copy, though,
You've read it?" Exclaimed the rich man, "No.
Someday I may but now indeed
I find I haven't time to read."
And then he spoke one noble thought and said,
"I wish that knowledge could be bought like bread.
I can buy books but this I find.
Study alone improves the mind."

Oh you who read with eager eyes
The treasures that the rich man buys, know this
Though all men have of gold
Knowledge is neither bought nor sold.
Pages by fingers must be turned,
And knowledge by all men must be earned.
Oh you who read what prophets write
And sit with them throughout the night
Know more than they will ever know
Who never read the books they show.

There are thousands of terms that can be used to describe the various aspects of horse science and horsemanship. There are regional, breed, and type differences. In fact, there are so many areas and specialties that listing and learning the entire vocabulary is probably an impossibility.

Most of us oversimplify as we begin our career experience. Later, we tend to overspecialize. Intense specialization tends to alienate us from the less knowledgeable. Certainly, the terms must be learned. But success requires a balance be maintained.

Knowledge of the terms and traditions of the horse industry is respected, and can only be obtained by experience and study. Study of appropriate books and articles during a set aside time each day is a valuable habit. Both physical *and* intellectual effort are required to master this profession. Everyone must pay the same price for excellence.

A basic vocabulary is presented in this chapter. Learn these words. They may be used to describe or discuss a horse. Other words which pertain to the horse, its anatomy and the various operations of horseshoeing are described in the text. They may be readily found by referring to the index.

The more you learn to apply these words, the less you will be tempted to use offensive profane words. Someone has said, "Profanity is the effort of a feeble mind to express itself forcibly." A direct correlation has been found between a good vocabulary and the lack of profane expression. A horseshoeing account may be won or lost by your attention or lack of attention to vocabulary development.

Each Chapter introduces many terms that relate to the subject or special area being considered. These terms must be learned and built upon in order to progress. When development of terms is not sequential, reference is made to where the subject is discussed. There are many other fine books that go into detail on each of the subjects introduced in this textbook. Study as many as you can.

Sex, Age and Species

Mare—Sexually mature female horse, dam ("out of").

Stallion or Stud—Adult male horse, sire ("by"), entire (ungelded) sexually mature, also may be called horse.

Gelding—Male horse castrated or altered before developing secondary sex characteristics.

Stag—Male horse castrated after developing secondary sex characteristics.

Cryptorchid—Male horse with one or both testicles retained in the abdomen. Also called ridgling or original.

Filly—Immature female horse, (under 3 or 4 yr. of age).

Colt—Immature male horse, (under 3 or 4 yr. of age.).

Foal—A colt or filly before weaning from its mother (usually under 6 mo. of age).

Weanling—A colt or filly weaned from its mother (usually 6 mo. to 1 yr. of age).

Yearling—A colt or filly between 1 and 2 years of age.

Jack—Male donkey or ass. Mammoth jack is a large breed of asses.

Jenny or Jennet—Female donkey or ass.

Mule—Offspring or progeny of a jack and a mare.

Hinny—Offspring of a stallion and a jenny.

Mare mule—Female mule.

Horse mule—Castrated male mule.

Stud mule—Uncastrated male mule (mules are usually sterile).

Age—Determined by registration papers, breeders certificate, the eruption and wear of the teeth, the feel of the ribs, jaw or tail. One horse year is said to be equal 5 to 7 human years. Ageing by the teeth is covered in Chapter 7.

Size

Height—Measured in hands at the high point of the withers; one hand equals 4 inches.

Weight—Measured in pounds on a scale, approximate from heart girth.

Girth—Distance around body behind elbows and over withers; may be used as a reasonably accurate estimate of weight.

Hoof size—Corresponds to machine-made shoe size or steel length to cover hoof wall with a 3/4 inch web shoe.

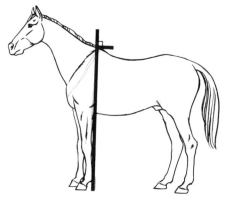

Fig. 5-2. Height of horses is measured in hands from the bottom of the hoof (not including the shoe) to the highest point of the withers. Each hand equals 4 inches.

HORSE HOOF

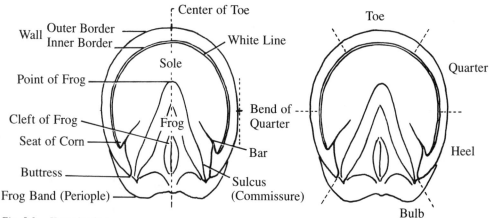

Fig. 5-3. Horse hoof terms.

Body Color

Appaloosa—Most are easily recognizable by their spots. However, they will always have: 1) mottled skin on muzzle and genitalia, 2) white sclera (ring around iris of eyes) and 3) striped hoofs.

Bay—The "points" (mane, tail, lower legs and feet, ear tips and muzzle) are black and the body some dilution of red.

Black— Rare. Uniform black hairs. Seen most commonly in Percheron, Walking Horse and Shetland pony breeds.

Brown—Body is brown to black and points may be black except muzzle and flanks are lighter brown.

Chestnut—The points are red or lighter and the body is varying shades of red. May have flaxen (white) mane and tail.

Sorrel—A light colored chestnut. Some say all but the liver or dark chestnut, others only the very light chestnut or orange.

Dun—Light colored body with black points and dorsal stripe. May have horizontal (called zebra) striping above the knee and hock. Darker dun is called red or claybank dun.

Buckskin—A type of dun. Light yellowish brown color with dorsal stripe.

Roan—Red or black hair mingled with white. Called strawberry or blue roan.

Gray—Born black or solid colored; become whiter as they get older. About 50 percent of Percherons and all Lipizzaners are gray. "Flea-bitten" gray (small red spots) is a variation of gray in Arabians. Dapple gray is an intermediate form between black and gray.

Grulla—Mouse color, gray or "blue" with black points, usually have dorsal and zebra stripes (See Dun).

Paint or Pinto—Piebald is black and white, skewbald is any other color (usually brown) and white. Tobiano has conventional face markings, white on back and all legs. Overo has bald face, often with blue eye(s), white on belly and legs solid colored.

Palomino—White mane and tail on golden yellow body. Will not breed true.

Cremello—Cream colored with blue eyes, may have white face markings; not true albinos since they do not have red eyes.

White—Psuedo-albinos have pink skin and pigmented eyes. True albinos have nonpigmented (red) eyes and are rarely born alive due to lethal genetic factors. Light gray horses have a dark skin.

Head Markings

Cowlicks, Whorls or Swirls—Hair patterns on the head and neck used for identification purposes by the Jockey Club.

Star—White in the middle of the forehead.

Stripe—White in the middle of the face.

Snip—White in the middle of the nose.

Blaze—White from forehead to nose area.

Bald—White including the nostrils and one or both eyes.

Leg Markings

Black—On a bay or dun horse.

Sorrel—Red to yellowish hairs.

Coronet—White above the hoof.

Pastern—One-half or all of pastern covered by white hair.

Fetlock or Ankle—White including the ankle.

Sock or Above Ankle—White above ankle.

Stocking—One-half, three-fourths and full covering of the cannon bone with white.

Grooming

Near Side—Left side.

Far or Off Side—Right side.

Curry—Rub hair coat with hard or pliable curry comb until dirt is loose and can be brushed off with a body brush.

Boot—To clip the long hair of the fetlock and lower leg.

Roach—To trim the mane short as in three-gaited and roping horses.

Clipping—Usually refers to cutting the hair in the ears and on the face. May refer to trimming body and leg hair.

Dock Tail—To cut or bob the tail to a length of about 6 inches as in Hackney and some Draft horses.

Cut and Set Tail—To cut the tendons on the underside of the tail and set it in a brace as in show Saddlebred and Walking Horses.

Pull Tail—To shorten or trim the tail by pulling the hairs one at a time as in Quarter Horses.

Hunter Braid—To braid the mane and tail for show in a way peculiar to the Hunter division.

TYPICAL HEAD MARKINGS WITH TERMS USED TO DESCRIBE THEM

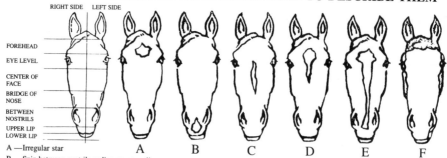

FOREHEAD
EYE LEVEL
CENTER OF FACE
BRIDGE OF NOSE
BETWEEN NOSTRILS
UPPER LIP
LOWER LIP

A —Irregular star
B —Snip between nostrils ending on upper lip
C —Narrow stripe starting between eyes and ending on bridge of nose
D —Star and connected narrow stripe ending in center of face
E —Star and connected stripe narrowing on bridge of nose, extending between nostrils and ending on upper lip
F —Bald face

TYPICAL LEG MARKINGS WITH TERMS USED TO DESCRIBE THEM

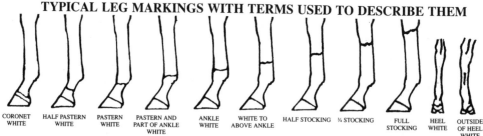

CORONET WHITE / HALF PASTERN WHITE / PASTERN WHITE / PASTERN AND PART OF ANKLE WHITE / ANKLE WHITE / WHITE TO ABOVE ANKLE / HALF STOCKING / ¾ STOCKING / FULL STOCKING / HEEL WHITE / OUTSIDE OF HEEL WHITE

Fig. 5-4. (A) Horse head and leg marking terms recognized by the American Horse Show Association. From Horse Show 47(4):16. (B) Horses may be positively identified by comparing chestnut size and form. Photo from Esi-Scan.

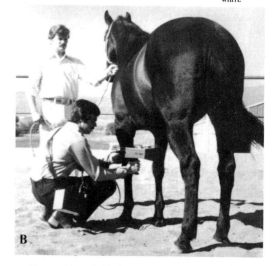

Aberdeen plait—To braid the top of the mane of draft horses with colored yarn.

Mud tie or French tie—To fold up and tie the tail of a draft horse.

Vices (Bad Habits)

Wood chewing—A common habit that begins because of boredom or mimicry of another horse with the vice.

Windsucking—Starts as horse swallows air instead of breathing normally. Progresses to cribbing.

Cribbing or Crib Biting—Horse sets upper incisor teeth against an object, arches its neck, pulls backward, and swallows large quantities of air.

Weaving—Swinging the head from side to side usually over a stall door or when tied.

Stall or Paddock Walking—Related to weaving nervousness, boredom.

Tongue Lolling—Throwing the head and dangling the tongue.

Pawing—Pawing usually with foot in one place in a stall.

Coprophagy—Eating manure; many horses do this naturally.

Biting—Biting the handler or shoer.

Striking—Kicking with the front feet.

Fighting—Aggressive action by a dominant horse on other horses.

Attacking—Aggressive action by a horse against persons or things.

Pulling Back—Pulls back when tied or led.

Kicking—Kicks people, other horses or walls, etc. with hind feet.

Breeding

Sire—Male or stallion, on the top side of a pedigree.

Dam—Female or mare, on the bottom side of a pedigree.

Purebred—Sire and dam of same breed.

Half-breed—Sire or dam not of the same breed.

Thoroughbred—A breed of horse.

Crossbred—Sire and dam of different breeds.

Cover—To breed.

Stallion Roll—A padded stick placed between the stallion and mare to prevent over penetration.

Stallion Ring—Plastic ring placed on penis behind glands to prevent erection and masturbation.

Stallion Cage, Support—A truss or support for an athletic stallion.

Breeding Hobbles—Placed on hind legs of mare to prevent kicking of stallion.

Breeding Season—Mare is seasonally polyestrus, April to October. Stallion is a continuous breeder but fertility is affected by season.

Estrus—Heat (sexual receptivity) period, 6 days average.

Diestrus—Non-heat (not sexually receptive) period, 15 days average.

Estrous Cycle—Sexual cycle including heat period and nonheat period, 21 days average.

Gestation Period—Time from conception to birth, 335 days (11 mo.) average.

Barren—Mare who will not conceive.

Speculum—Used by veterinarian to examine the cervix of a mare.

Open—Mare not carrying a foal.

Brood Mare—A mare used primarily to raise foals.

Foaling—The act of giving birth or parturition.

Stand at Stud—Advertise and accept mares to be bred to a stallion.

Stud—A farm or place where mares are bred, a stallion station. Also slang for stallion.

Hereditary Trait—Characteristic acquired from the genetic make-up of either or both parents at conception.

Congenital Trait—Characteristic acquired while developing in the womb during the gestation period.

Environmental Trait—Characteristic acquired after birth during growth.

Lactation—Mare's milk production, 30 pounds per day average.

Vital Signs

Temperature—Average 100 degrees F. (99.1 to 100.8 degrees F. range, influenced by age).

Pulse (Resting Heart Rate)—Average 44 beats per minute (23 to 70 range, influenced by age and fitness).

Respiration Rate (Resting)—Average 12 breaths per minute (8 to 16 range).

Urine—Average 5.5 quarts per day (3 to 9 range), deep yellow to brown color.

Feces—Average 40 pounds per day, brown to dark green well-formed balls. Defecates 8 to 9 times a day.

Horseshoeing

Often, words peculiar to the horseshoeing business have several meanings. The following words are defined as they are to be understood throughout this text:

Blacksmith—An iron worker, and in the past, frequently a horseshoer as well. In some parts of the country, it is still used to mean a horseshoer, probably because of the former close association of the two trades.

Farrier—A horseshoer, usually a specialist in horseshoeing only. Formerly, a person who cared for all aspects of a horse's health.

Plater—A race horse shoer, specifically a shoer of "flat track" or Thoroughbred and Quarter Horse running horses.

Cold Shoeing—Shoeing done with ready-made shoes where the shoes are shaped to fit the foot cold on the anvil without benefit of the forge.

Hot Shoeing—Shoeing done with a forge to heat and shape the shoes and trim the heels; often accompanied by hot fitting.

Hot Fitting—Often, but not always, done when hot shoeing; holding a hot shoe against the prepared bottom of the hoof until it scorches it sufficiently to indicate high spots of horn which need to be removed to make the surface of the hoof level. This fitting can be done cold by close observation but requires more skill.

"Cowboy" Shoeing—Shoeing done without fitting the shoe but simply cutting down the foot, shaping the shoe by opening or closing it, nailing the shoe on, and rasping the foot down to match the shoe. Excessive rasping of the lower border of wall producing a dubbed effect.

Balance—A condition which exists when the weight placed on each leg of the horse is distributed equally over the foot of that leg. A horse's foot is said to be in balance when viewed from the front or rear if the medial axis of the leg, pastern, and foot are in a straight line. The foot is said to be in balance when viewed from the side if the medial axis of the pastern coincides with the axis of the foot which is parallel to the hoof wall at the toe.

Normal or Physiological Shoeing—Shoeing of a normal foot taking into account the physiological movements of the foot so as to interfere in a minimal way with them. Balancing of the foot is considered of primary importance.

Corrective Shoeing—Shoeing to change the balance (fault of conformation) or way of going (fault of gait).

Pathological Shoeing—Shoeing to remedy a disease or injury of the foot or leg.

Specialized Shoeing—Shoeing a specific specialized breed or type of horse.

Anatomy

Hoof—The horny covering of the distal end of the horse's leg. (NOTE: The prefix horny may or may not be used when speaking of the external hoof structures.)

Foot—The hoof and all the structures contained within it. (NOTE: The terms hoof and foot are often used interchangeably.)

Leg—The portion of the limb of the horse below the knee or hock.

Digit—The portion of the leg of the horse below the fetlock.

Limb—The leg and the structures above it which join it to the trunk of the horse.

Axis (Axial)—The central line of the body or

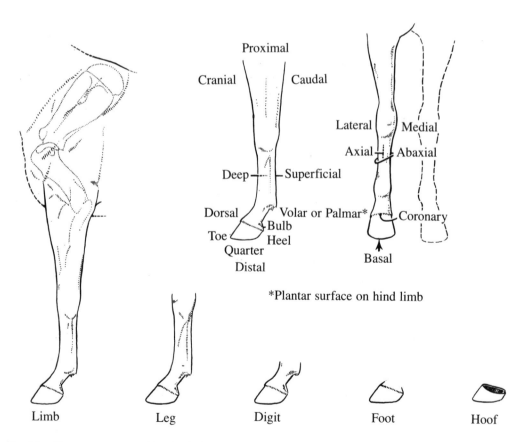

Fig. 5-5.   Horse anatomy terms. Drawing by L. Sadler.

any of its parts, on or close to the line about which the structure would rotate.

Abaxial—Away from the central axis of a structure.

Proximal—Close to the body or center of gravity.

Distal—Farther away from the body or center of gravity.

Medial—Inside, toward the center line of the body.

Lateral— Outside, away from the center line of the body.

Deep—Internal, close to the center of gravity.

Superficial—External, near to the skin.

Dorsal—Front surface of the legs.

Volar or Palmar—Rear surface of the foreleg below the knee.

Plantar—Rear surface of the hind leg below the hock.

Cranial—Front surface of the upper limb, nearest the head.

Caudal—Rear surface of the upper limb, nearest the tail.

Basal—Base or ground surface, part of hoof farthest from the coronary surface of the hoof at any given point.

Coronary—Coronet or hair surface, part of hoof farthest from the basal surface of the hoof at any given point.

Hoof Head—The enlargement where the hoof joins the digit at the coronary region and above.

Flex—To fold or decrease the angle of the bones of a joint.

Extend—To open or increase the angle of the bones of a joint.

The musculature of the horse is not covered in this text. Excellent illustrations of external muscles may be found in *An Atlas of Animal Anatomy for Artists* by W. Ellenberger, H. Baum and H. Dittrich, edited by L.S. Brown and published in 1956 by Dover of New York.

HORSE SKELETON

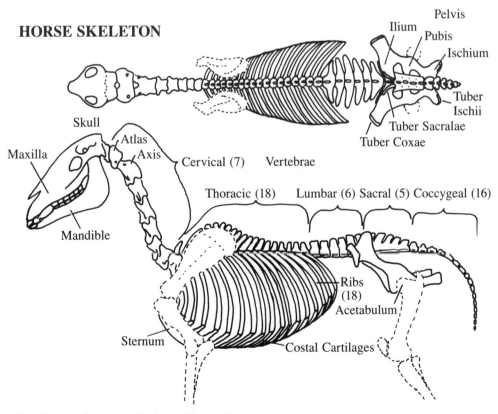

Fig. 5-6. Horse skeleton terms. Limbs are illustrated in Chapter 10.

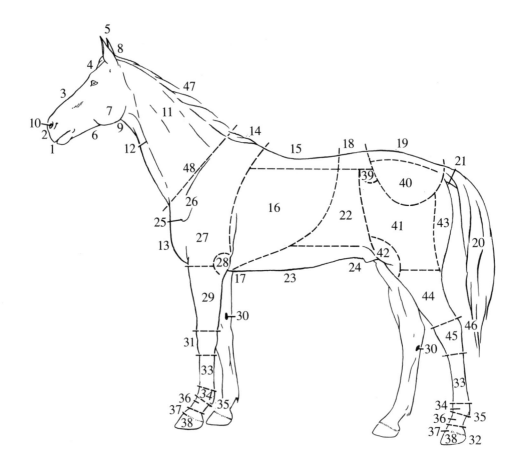

Fig. 5-7.   Horse external terms test. Drawing by L. Sadler.

1. Lips	19. Croup	37. Coronet (Coronary
2. Muzzle	20. Tail	band or hoof head)
3. Face	21. Dock	38. Hoof (Foot-hoof
4. Forehead	22. Flank	and its contents)
5. Ears	23. Belly	39. Point of the hip
6. Lower jaw	24. Sheath	40. Haunch
7. Cheek (Jowl)	25. Point of	41. Thigh
8. Poll	shoulder	42. Stifle
9. Throatlatch	26. Shoulder	43. Buttock (Pin bone-
10. Nostril	27. Arm	raised point)
11. Neck	28. Elbow	44. Gaskin
12. Jugular groove	29. Forearm	45. Hock
13. Breast (Chest-	30. Chestnut	46. Point of hock
between legs)	31. Knee	47. Mane (Crest-the
14. Withers	32. Heel	line of the mane
15. Back	33. Cannon	and forelock)
16. Ribs or Barrel	34. Fetlock	48. Slope of the
17. Girth	35. Ergot	shoulder
18. Loins	36. Pastern	

Chapter 6

Care and Management of the Horse

Many of today's pleasure horse owners have not had an opportunity to obtain the background or experience necessary to properly manage their horses. Lack of knowledge on the care of the horse may do as much damage as physical abuse.

This chapter provides you with information that can be tactfully supplied to the horse owner. Local offices of the Agricultural Extension Service (USDA) have many good publications that are free or of low cost which can be given to owners. Many feed companies also produce free informative literature. The references at the end of the chapter may be especially valuable as sources for more detailed information.

The horseshoer is usually respected as a source of professional information. To be worthy of respect and trust, you must know. Water cannot be drawn from a dry well. First, you must become a knowledgeable horseman. Then, you can help others get more enjoyment and value from their horses. If this is done purposefully and tactfully, the public will learn to rely on you. This will not only build and secure your business, but it will cause you to get more enjoyment from your work.

Selection

Selection is a key factor in determining success in the horse business. The fewer problems or predisposition to problems the horse has before it is purchased, the less it will have after purchase. It is wise to recommend a vet check or soundness examination of any horse to be purchased. The veterinarian should do this. But, the buyer may have such confidence in you that your opinion is asked. Horses that are bad to shoe usually get a poor recommendation! A procedure for conducting a soundness examination is given in Chapter 33.

Defects in the conformation of the legs and feet are pictured in Chapters 28 and 29. A discussion of other problems can be found in most of the books listed under References. Ageing horses by the teeth is covered in Chapter 7.

Be especially cautious when making predictions regarding a horse's future usefulness. A horse that would not be sound for use as a daily stressed runner may be ideal for an occasionally ridden pleasure horse. A horse is sold as sound for the use intended on the day he was examined. Usually, no other guarantee is expressed or implied.

A horse in good condition or fat is usually the safest buy. The fat horse can always be put on a diet and probably is an easy keeper. An easy keeper is one that requires little feed to maintain its condition. This characteristic is often associated with short-backed horses.

A horse that is in poor condition or thin may only need its teeth floated, worming and some of that wonder drug called feed. However, such horses may also have some invisible disease condition or be a hard keeper.

Feeding

Most novice horsemen underfeed or overfeed. Neglect is the most common cause of thin horses. Horse feeders should carefully look at their stock at each feeding. There is an old saying that fat looks good on a horse. And, the eye of the master fattens the stock. However, over nutrition is a most common nutritional disease. This can lead to serious complications such as founder if allowed to persist.

Each class or activity of horses requires a different quantity and quality of nutrients. Horses that are ridden intermittently may require no more than a maintenance diet. A horse is receiving a maintenance ration when, with minimum muscular activity and no requirement for growth or milk production, it neither gains nor loses weight. A balanced ration includes the optimum combination of nutrients to meet all the horse's needs within a particular class or for a particular activity.

Quantity of feed is independent of quality. One can feed a balanced ration (one with the correct combination or quality of nutrients), but not feed enough. The horse looks poor. One can also feed the correct quantity of nutrients, but not of the correct quality. The horse still looks poor.

The quantity of feed fed is a function of body weight and muscular activity or metabolic rate. A maintenance ration will weigh about 1½ percent of the horse's body weight (assuming 100% of the ration is dry matter). An active growing horse may consume 3 percent of his body weight in feed each day. Very few pleasure horses will ever need more than 2 percent of their body weight in feed per day. For a 1000 pound horse this amounts to about 20 pounds. Horse feeders should be encouraged to use a scale. They should weigh a few bales from each load of hay to aid in determining what fraction of a bale should be given to each horse at each feeding.

A horse's weight can be estimated using a weight tape available from most feed stores if a scale is not available. Bale and feed can weights may be determined by using a bathroom scale.

The quality of feed is not as easily determined. Horse feeding supplements have built a thriving business on the premise that "something" will always be missing from a ration. Hay quality can be accurately determined by sending a sample to a forage testing laboratory at most Land Grant colleges. Commercial feeds have an analysis on the tag. However, knowledge of average feeding values for several of the commonly used horse feeds is probably the best way to feed the correct quality. These values are compared to those requirements established for the horse by experimental research. Finally, the several ingredients are juggled to determine the combination which produces a balanced ration at the least cost.

Percentage of Total Digestible Nutrients (TDN) and Digestible Protein Contents of Dry Hay

Harvest Date	Grasses		Legumes	
	TDN	Protein	TDN	Protein
June 1	63	12.2	63	16.8
June 15	57	9.0	57	13.1
July 1	50	6.0	50	9.2
July 15	44	3.3	44	5.9

Percentage of Protein Content of Alfalfa and Timothy Hay at Different Stages of Maturity

Date	Alfalfa		Timothy	
	Stage	Protein	Stage	Protein
May 25	Vegetative	19	Vegetative	15
June 5	Bud	16	Boot	12
June 15	Early Flower	14	Early Head	10
June 20	Flower	11	Heading	9
July 5	Late Flower	8	Flower	6
July 25	Green Seed	5	Early Seed	3

When to Harvest Grasses and Legumes for Highest Quality

Crop	Stage of Maturity
Alfalfa	Full bud
Red clover	1/4 to 1/2 bloom
Birdsfoot trefoil	1/4 bloom
Smooth bromegrass	Early to medium head
Timothy	Early head
Orchardgrass	Boot to early head

Fig. 6-1. Hay quality is affected by the date of harvest as well as by weather and storage time. From Seaney (1975).

Hay usually makes up the majority of a ration because it is the least expensive per pound. Hay quality is dependent upon cutting date, curing conditions, storage time and forage species.

Generally, hay cut early in the plants' growth cycle is higher in protein and energy digestibility and lower in fiber and weed content. A few flowers in the bale indicate the best stage for harvesting legume hays such as alfalfa and clover. A few seed heads indicate the best stage for harvesting grass hays such as timothy or brome. Early cutting also prevents excessive weed development. Weeds are not as nutritious or as palatable as the cultivated forage plants. Traditionally, horsemen prefer the second cutting from a hay field because there are usually less weeds. Of course, the grower desires to achieve a balance so that tonnage per acre yield is at its highest without seriously affecting nutrient quality.

Ideally, hay should cure quickly without weather damage. Weather damage causes loss of palatability, carotene (Vitamin A activity) and protein quality. Moldy or very dusty hay should not be fed since it has been linked to respiratory (heaves) and reproductive (abortion) problems.

Storage times of over a year may seriously affect the quality of hay. The carotene level or Vitamin A activity associated with the green color of hay is nearly always affected. The protein and digestible energy may also be lowered.

The average crude protein content of grass hays is about 8 percent. The protein content of legumes is about 15 percent and is more digestible than that in grass. Thus, the species of hay is very important in determining the quality of a ration. The legume hays, when properly cut, cured and stored are ideal to maintain most classes of horses.

In summary, the quality of hay can be fairly accurately determined without analysis by examining the stage of growth of the hay plant, the percentage of weeds, the color, the smell and the species of the principal forage plants.

Hays are about 8 to 15 percent protein and about 50 percent total digestible nutrients (TDN). The digestible energy (DE) in a feed is a function of TDN. Grains are about 10 percent protein and 75 to 85 percent TDN. Small amounts (by weight) of grains which are 25 to 35 percent higher in energy value than hays will substitute for larger amounts of hays in the ration.

Grains are usually more constant in quality than hays. However, hull to kernel ratio can affect the quality of oats and moldy corn can produce mycotoxicosis. Grains should be fed by weight, not by volume. Similar weights produce similar energy values. Similar volumes will not since corn is much heavier per unit volume than oats.

Sweet feeds (those with molasses added) reduce dust and increase palatability. Protein, mineral and vitamin supplements are often mixed in sweet feeds. Most commercial horse feeds are marketed in this form. Sweet feeds may be pelleted to reduce waste, volume and dust.

Hays may also be pelleted with the same advantage as those for sweet feeds. However, poor quality roughage can be disguised in a pellet. Also, horses fed pelleted hay will have softer feces than those fed whole hay and they may develop vices due to boredom.

The factor of most concern for growing horses is protein. Horses do most of their growing in the first year of life. They reach 50 to 60 percent of their mature weight by 6 months of age. After 2 or 3 years they grow very little in height and skeletal structure.

The factor of most concern for mature working horses is energy. The protein requirement for horses does not increase when they work hard. However, the energy requirement may increase dramatically. Both energy and protein are of concern when feeding lactating and pregnant mares.

Feeding the correct level of protein is always of economic concern since it is usually the most expensive ingredient in the ration. Foals need rations which are 20 percent protein, weanlings 15 percent, yearlings 12 percent and mature horses 8 to 10 percent. Mares lactating or pregnant have a higher requirement (12%). A little excess protein probably doesn't harm the animal since the body automatically breaks down the extra protein molecules and metabolizes them as energy. The Nitrogen containing ammonia molecules are then eliminated in urine. However, protein is an expensive energy source.

The horse needs fresh clean water. Idle horses will drink from 5 to 10 gallons of water a day. A hard working horse on a hot day may drink

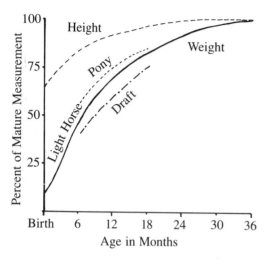

Fig. 6-2. Horses do most of their growing in the first year of life. From Ensminger (1977).

15 or more gallons of water. On cool days, water consumption will go down.

Trace mineralized salt should be provided free choice to horses. Mineral and vitamin supplement is unnecessary if a balanced ration is fed. However, calcium and phosphorus supplementation may be necessary in growing horses if grass hay is fed. Legume hay is adequate in calcium but may require phosphorus supplementation. This is usually taken care of by the addition of grain since it is naturally high in phosphorus. The ratio of calcium to phosphorous in the ration must be such that there is always more calcium than phosphorus.

Horses should be fed at least twice a day when confined. They should be fed at the same time each day. Changes in feed composition (e.g., species of hay) or form (e.g., hay or pellets) should be made gradually. Planning ahead prevents feed shortages and missed or erratic feedings. Adherence to the above rules prevents colic and other digestive upsets. Horses that are worked should have their grain ration reduced when they are rested to prevent azoturia.

Exercise

Ideally, the horse should be exercised every day. If the horse cannot be ridden or worked each day, then it should be allowed to exercise at will under pasture conditions. A minimum of one hour per day is recommended. A horse that is not exercised regularly is more prone to develop vices due to boredom. Horses that are kept confined in stalls should be warmed up and cooled off before and after forced exercise. Horses should be conditioned gradually to strenuous exercise.

Grooming

A healthy skin and shiny hair coat are stimulated by frequent brushing. Currying the hair with a rubber curry comb loosens dirt and stimulates blood circulation to the skin. A rubber oval or flexible plastic comb can be used over the bony prominences of the body and the legs. Use of steel curry combs is not recommended. The dandy or body brush should be flicked outward with the wrist as it is used in order to remove dirt from the hair coat.

Nutrient Requirements for Horses

Class or Horse	Daily Dry Matter Intake (% body wt.) (100% dry matter basis)	Crude Protein (% ration) (90% dry matter basis)	Digestible Energy (Mcal/lb. b.w.)	Calcium (% ration)	Phosphorus (% ration)	Vit. A Activity (IU/lb. b.w.)
Mature, maintenance	1.5	8.0	0.9	0.27	0.18	650
working	2.5	8.0	1.2	0.27	0.18	650
pregnancy	2.0	10.0	1.0	0.45	0.30	1400
lactation	3.0	12.0	1.2	0.45	0.30	1150
Yearling, 1 yr. old	2.0	12.0	1.2	0.50	0.35	800
Weanling, 6 mo. old	3.5	15.0	1.2	0.60	0.45	800
Foal, 3 mo. old	4.5	16.0	1.4	0.80	0.55	800

Fig. 6-3. Nutrient requirements change with age. Figures from National Research Council (1978).

EQUINE MALE GENITALS

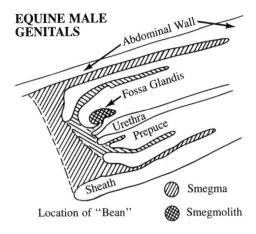

Smegma

Location of "Bean"   Smegmolith

Fig. 6-4. Location of the bean or smegmolith in the fossa glandis.

The genitals, especially the udder and sheath, should be cleaned as needed to remove smegma and other filth. Tender or sensitive horses can be coated with vasoline to loosen the smegma before washing is attempted. The sheath of geldings may become especially filthy. A smegmolith or bean often forms in the *fossa glandis* above the urethra. This must be periodically removed or it will cause pain to the horse and may cause straining or prevent urination.

The ears will occasionally be infested and irritated by ticks. The horse becomes extremely sensitive about his ears and head. This can be remedied by mixing some tick dust (Rotenone powder) with Furacin or vasoline and smearing it down deep inside the ear.

The mane and tail hairs should be separated, untangled and brushed before running a mane comb through them. Combing the hair from the bottom side prevents breaking of the top hairs. Manes and tails should be trimmed according to breed type and use.

Rinsing the horse's back with water after it has worked up a sweat on a hot day is appreciated by most horses. A sweat scraper squeezes the hair against the coat and removes water rapidly. A sponge may be used on the face. Towels or hair dryers can be used to dry a horse on cool days. Shampooing should not be done too often as important oils from the skin may be lost.

Care of the Feet

The hoofs should be washed and cleaned out with a hoof pick each time the horse is groomed. Picking out and inspecting the hoofs after a ride is also desirable. Foreign objects that may cause damage if left in the foot can be removed at this time. The most effective prevention for thrush is regular cleaning of the hoof.

Horse hoofs should be trimmed or shod about every six weeks. The ideal interval between shoeings is determined by the rate of growth and wear of the individual horse's hoofs. Use of the horse also influences shoeing interval. Precision gaits require constant attention to hoof balance, shoe weight and design.

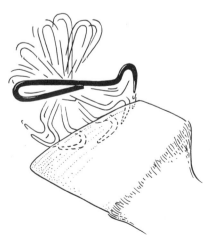

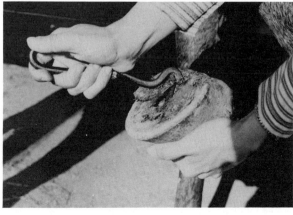

Fig. 6-5. Path of the hoof pick. Drawing by L. Sadler.

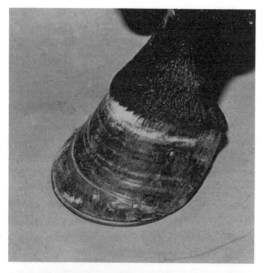
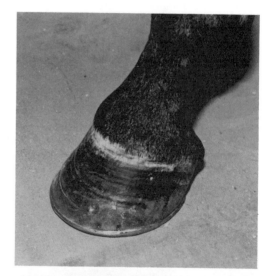
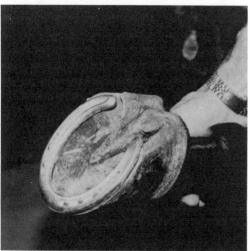
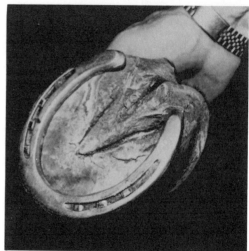
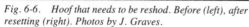

Fig. 6-6.   Hoof that needs to be reshod. Before (left), after resetting (right). Photos by J. Graves.

Conditions that indicate resetting or reshoeing is necessary:

1. The hoof is out of balance from heel to toe or from side to side.
2. The clinches are risen and the nails are loose.
3. Uneven wear or wearing through of the shoe.
4. Wall hanging over shoe at the heel (or toe if shoe slips back).
5. The shoe is loose or the wall is cracking due to excessive length.
6. The horse is stumbling or straining tendons due to excessive hoof length.

Dry hoofs can be prevented by routinely over flowing the water trough in the paddock or dry pasture. Hoofs of horses kept in stalls can be packed with wet clay overnight. The clay should be picked out in the morning. Hoofs can be protected in prolonged wet weather by application of oil base type hoof dressings.

Stabling

The horse will adapt very well to most weather conditions. Protection from rain, wind and snow is desirable but it does not have to be elaborate. Shade may be desirable during hot weather. A well-drained shed open on one side (usually the south) is adequate for inclement weather.

Good ventilation and dry bedding are most important if the horse is kept in a stall. Dirt floors composed of well-drained clay make ideal stall floors.

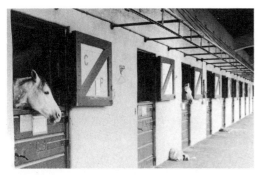

Fig. 6-7. Good ventilation and dry bedding are most important if the horse is kept in a stall. Photo by R. Rankin.

Several materials are popular for bedding stalls. Straw has been the most popular where available because of its high absorbency and comparatively low dust production. Straw absorbs nearly six times its weight, while wood shavings absorb only one third of their weight. Sawdust and sand are used where other materials are not available. A muzzle can be placed on a horse between feedings which prevents the horse from eating the bedding but allows it to drink. Black walnut shavings should never be used to bed horses due to the possibility of producing founder. Recently, shredded waste paper has been shown to be even more absorbent than straw and it is dustless, harmless, biodegradable and competes favorably in price.

Hay and grain storage should be kept in a secure area to avoid the possibility of over eating and founder. Fire protection is an important consideration in building design and location. Fresh water should be provided constantly.

Fences in corrals should be of lumber or pipe. Larger enclosures and pastures can be enclosed with tightly woven or V-mesh wire. Barbed wire should be avoided when possible. Probably more horses are crippled by barbed wire than any other factor. Barbless wire is available and when stretched tight is effective for containing horses.

Parasite Control

Horses are infested by four major types of internal parasites. Horses kept in confinement should be routinely wormed every 2 to 3 months for round worms (ascarids, strongyles and pin worms). Bots should be eliminated at least once a year one month after the last killing frost. Bot

eggs can be scraped or sanded off as a part of daily grooming.

Ideally, a fecal sample should be microscopically examined to determine the level of infestation before deciding to worm a horse. However, this is not always possible or practical. Studies have shown that after worming, parasite count drops to near zero, but after 2 months it is back to a very high level, often as high as preworming. This is due to the hardiness of the parasite eggs and rapid reinfestation.

Commercial wormers which can be mixed with the feed or given in paste form are as effective as tube wormers if the horse gets the recommended dose. Nearly all commercial wormers are 90 to 100 percent effective. Wormer base types should be alternated after two uses to prevent the parasites from building immunity.

Failure to worm regularly may result in irreparable damage to significant blood vessels and internal organs of the body. The most obvious result will be a poor haircoat and unthrifty condition.

Pasture rotation helps to reduce the parasite problem, but not significantly on an individual basis. This management practice helps the pasture and improves palatability more than it helps reduce the parasite infestation level in horses.

External parasites such as lice, mange, mites and ticks can be treated by dusting or spraying with appropriate insecticide. Once introduced

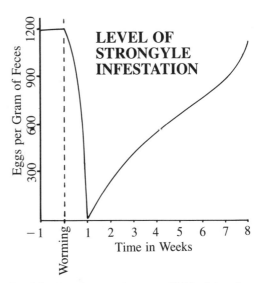

Fig. 6-8. Parasite counts increase to high levels in a short time.

into a group or stable of horses, they spread very rapidly. Ringworm can be treated by scrubbing with 7 percent iodine. It is transmittable to humans. Flies can be temporarily kept off the horse by various fly repellents. Fly traps and fly killers are in use at most stables. Improving sanitation practices can usually prevent some of the fly problem.

Disease Control

Horses should be current in their immunizations for Tetanus, Venezuelan Equine Encephalomyelitis (VEE), Eastern and Western Equine Encephalomyelitis (E & WEE). A vaccine is available that protects against all four diseases. Influenza (flu) and strangles (distemper) immunizations are also recommended for many horses. Give these several weeks before the horse is to be shown or worked. Some horses react to them. A blood test (Coggins) for detecting the presence of Equine Infectious Anemia (EIA) is required when transporting animals across state lines.

Immunization against Rhinopneumonitis, Brucellosis, Rabies, Leptospirosis or Anthrax may be required in endemic areas of disease. The veterinarian is the best judge in these matters.

Most of the Land Grant colleges in the various states have a Veterinary Medical Diagnostic Lab which can aid the veterinarian in the detection of poisoning or unusual diseases.

Knowing the normal vital signs on an individual horse can be a great help in recognizing a disease condition (See Chapter 33). First aid for commonly encountered conditions is discussed in Chapter 18.

Transportation

Horse owners need to break all their horses to travel in a trailer or truck. Most uses of horses require this, and owners are more likely to transport horses to be shod in a shop (your shop!) if they are trailer broke.

Feeding a young horse grain in the trailer is probably one of the safest ways of getting a horse to feel comfortable with the vehicle. Horses can be forced to load, but the result is usually traumatic for the horse and the trailer (and the loader!).

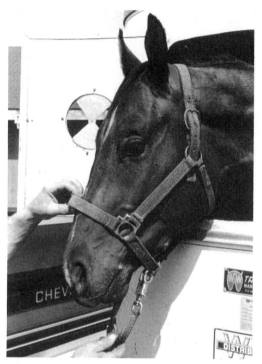

Fig. 6-9. *Horses should always be tied in trailers with panic snaps.*

Horses should also be taught to back slowly out of the trailer.

A horse should always be tied in the trailer and quick release or panic snaps should be used on trailer tie ropes. Broken necks or legs may result when the brakes are applied if horses are not tied and are allowed to travel in the wrong position. Young horses may even try to turn around and jump out of the trailer. Butt chains covered with rubber tubing should be used to keep horses off the tail gate. Partial partitions in two horse side by side trailers help a horse maintain its balance on corners.

Smooth driving (starts and stops) helps horses to enjoy the trailer ride. Feed makes it especially attractive. Short distance hauls with a familiar older horse will help a young horse get over any fear it may have of vehicles.

Horses traveling long distances should be let out at least every 4 hours to urinate, exercise and have a drink of water. Feed should be given frequently but in small amounts in transit.

Padding such as a head bumper, blanket, tail wrap, hock boots, shipping, calking, or bell boots are used by many horsemen to prevent injury and pulled shoes during shipment.

Breeding

Male horses should be gelded between one and two years of age. If they are kept for stallions they should not be used for breeding until they are at least 2 years of age. The stallion has a season of increased fertility corresponding to the mares, but he is a year-round breeder.

Fillies should not be bred until they are at least 3 to 4 years old. Mares have seasonally polyestrous reproductive cycles.

The mare's natural breeding season is in the late spring and summer. The mare completes an estrous cycle about every 21 days during the breeding season. Her reproductive system normally becomes dormant during the winter months. It goes through an erratic transition stage in the early spring and late fall. The mare's estrous cycle can be influenced by the use of artificial light and hormone injections. This is often done to move up the foaling date or treat reproductive cycle disorders.

The estrous or heat period lasts from 3 to 6 days and is a time of sexual receptivity and excitability. Trainers and horseshoers often experience difficulty with horses at this time. Mares are usually bred on every other day of a heat period when ovulation time cannot be determined.

The gestation period or length of pregnancy for a horse is an average of 336 days. Foals will weigh 80 to 120 pounds at birth. They must get the colostrum or first milk of the mare to give them antibodies against disease. The mare produces this colostrum for about 3 days. The foal gets antibody value from it for only about 2 days. Extra colostrum may be collected and stored in a freezer for use in saving an orphan foal.

Mares will come in heat about 9 days after foaling. They usually should not be bred during the first heat. Often, the uterus has not returned to its normal state and infection may be present. The second heat will follow the first or foaling heat by about 21 days. This is usually the best time to breed back the mare.

THE ESTROUS CYCLE OF THE MARE

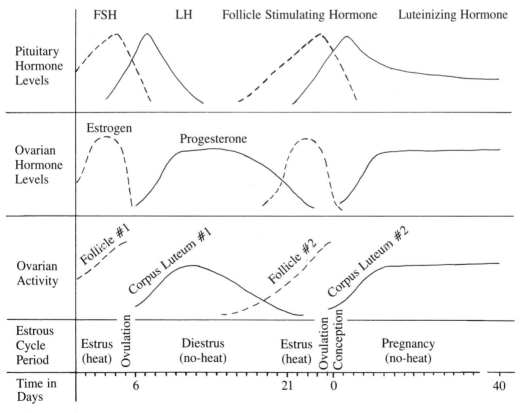

Fig. 6-10.   The estrous cycle of the mare.

The foal will nurse the mare for about 6 months or until she gets tired of it. Milk production reaches its peak at about 2 months and then declines sharply. Creep feeding (feed located in a place where the mare can't get it) can be started as soon as the foal will eat solid feed. This feed should have about 20 percent protein content. When the foal is weaned, it should be on full feed. Weanlings should get about 15 percent protein in their ration.

Weaning can be done from 3 to 6 months of age. The mare and foal should be separated for several days in safe places where they can't hear or see each other. If they are put where they can communicate, a very safe and impenetrable fence must be between them. They should be pastured separately for several weeks. Bringing them back together too soon may result in the disappointment of repeating the weaning process.

Horses usually live to be 25 or 30 years of age. They are most useful between the ages of 5 and 15 years. Many horses are not fully trained until they are 8 or 10 years of age. Few horses can stand consistent hard strenuous work before they are 5. Most will break down if subjected to heavy use at a young age.

References

Bello, T.R., S.D. Gaunt and B.J. Torbert. 1977. Critical evaluation of environmental control of bots (gasterophilus intestinalis) in horses. J. Equine Med. and Surgery. (Apr.):126.

Cunha, T.J. 1980. Horse Feeding and Nutrition. Academic Press, New York.

Drudge, J.H., E.T. Lyons and S.C. Tolliver. 1978. Critical and controlled tests and clinical trials with suspension and granule formulations of the anthelmintic, fenbendazole, in the horse. J. of Equine Med. and Surgery. (Jan.):22.

Ensminger, M.E. 1977. Horses and Horsemanship (5th ed.). Interstate, Danville, IL.

Evans, J.W. 1981. Horses. Freeman, San Francisco.

Harris, S.E. 1972. Horsemanship in Pictures. 5-H Acres School of Riding, Cortland, NY.

Harris, S.E. 1977. Grooming to Win. Charles Scribner's Sons, New York.

Hintz, H.F., J.P. Baker, R.M. Jordon, E.A. Ott, G.D. Potter, and L.M. Slade. 1978. Nutrient Requirements of Horses. NASNRC Publ., Washington, DC.

Schryver, H.F. and H.F. Hintz. 1975. Feeding Horses. Equine Research Bull. No. 1. New York State College of Agri.

Seaney, R.R. 1975. A Guide to Estimating Hay Quality. Cornell University. Ithaca, NY.

NOTES:

Chapter 7

Ageing Horses by the Teeth

Horseshoers are frequently called upon to age horses in conjunction with the shoeing job. Sometimes it is important to know the age of the horse when discussing the prognosis (probable result) of corrective or therapeutic shoeing. But more often it is a skill that is expected of a horseman by the public. Often, persons requesting you to age a horse have no knowledge of the process themselves. Occasionally, someone will want to test you to see how much of a horseman you are. Right or wrong, your future employment may be judged by your ability to perform this feat. All knowledgeable horsemen know how to age a horse by his teeth.

Type and Position of Teeth

There are two types of teeth. Bracydont teeth are short simple teeth. They stop growing after they erupt and are in use. They have a longer root than crown. They are found in carnivores (meat eaters) such as the dog and cat. The canine teeth and first premolars of the horse look somewhat like bracydont teeth.

Hippsodont teeth are long comparatively complex teeth. They continue to grow and push out as they wear. They have a high resistance to abrasion and create a grinding effect. The molars are especially efficient grinders. They have several vertical layers of hard enamel which project above the in-between layers of softer dentine. The surface of these teeth is continuously sharpened by wear. The temporary and permanent incisors, the temporary and permanent premolars, and the molars of the horse are examples

of Hippsodont teeth. This type of teeth is also found in ruminants such as the cow, sheep, and goat.

The horse's teeth are located in the upper (maxilla) and lower (mandible) arcades of the jaw in four areas. The incisors are located behind the lips and are for biting or shearing off plants. The canine (tusk, or bridle) teeth are present in males and only occasionally in females. The premolars and molars are used for grinding fibrous food. The first premolar is not constant in males or females and is like a small canine tooth in appearance. Hence, the name wolf tooth. It may be removed if it interferes with the bitting of a horse.

Horses, like humans, have two sets of teeth: temporary (deciduous, milk, or baby) and permanent. It is most important to distinguish between temporary and permanent teeth since a well grown 2 year old may be easily mistaken for an older horse. Permanent incisor teeth are larger, longer, darker (brown) in color and do

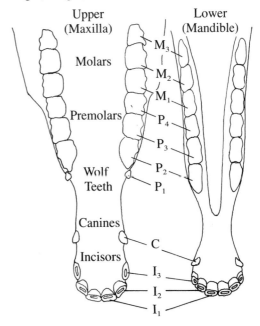

Fig. 7-2.   Upper and lower arcades of a mature male horse's jaw.

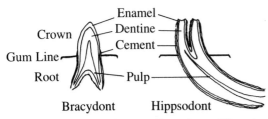

Fig. 7-1.   Mid-sagital section of bracydont and hippsodont incisor teeth.

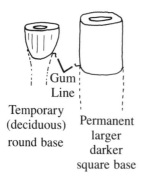

Fig. 7-3. *Temporary and permanent teeth differences.*

not have the narrow neck or shovel-shaped base joining the gum that temporary teeth do. In addition, recently erupted permanent horse incisor teeth have a deep infundibulum or cup in the occlusal (table) surface. Temporary horse incisor teeth are smaller, have a shallow cup, are whiter, and have five ridges in the labial (lip) surface of the tooth.

The horse nips off grass with the incisors and grinds food with the molars. As he grinds he moves his jaws from side to side. The horse can chew only on one side at a time and keeps the feed under his teeth with his tongue. Constant lateral motion helps keep the table surfaces of the molars level.

Tooth Shape

The shape of a permanent incisor tooth of the horse may be compared to a smashed and bent inverted cone. The cone is smashed at the top and bottom in opposite directions. The smashed bottom is bent away from and perpendicular to the widest part of the smashed top. The resulting shape resembles the incisor tooth of the horse.

A mid-sagital section of an incisor shows the depth of the cup, the position of the pulp (star) and the important parts of the tooth. Permanent incisor teeth continue to grow until the horse is 12 years old. After 12, they continue pushing and moving out of the gum to compensate for wear. The root end of the tooth is open while it is growing. At 5 years of age the incisor roots form and the teeth are 2½ to 3 inches long. At 25 years there is very little root holding the tooth in the gum and the teeth may be less than 1 inch long.

The change in shape and structure of the table surface of the incisor teeth is a principal means of estimating the age of the horse after the teeth erupt. If an incisor tooth were sawed into thin sections parallel to the gum line as it continued to grow and emerge, the appearance of the tooth sections would correspond to the table's appearance at the various ages of the horse.

A mid-sagital section of a molar shows the complicated nature of the enamel veins that produce sharp wavy ridged grinding surfaces. Permanent premolars and molars also develop roots at about 5 years and continue to grow and push out until 12 or 14 years of age. The angle and length of the molar teeth changes as the horse ages. The exposed sides of the teeth are continually built up by cement as they wear.

The canine teeth (tusks) of the horse erupt and usually stop growing within a year or so, instead of continually growing as they do in the boar. The canine or bridle teeth are more curved than the incisors and are usually present only in the male. However, a study of 8000 horses by Ellenberger quoted by Sisson and Grossman (1953) revealed that about 2 to 3 percent of mares have erupted canines in both jaws, 6 to 7 percent have them in the upper jaw, and 20 to 30 percent have

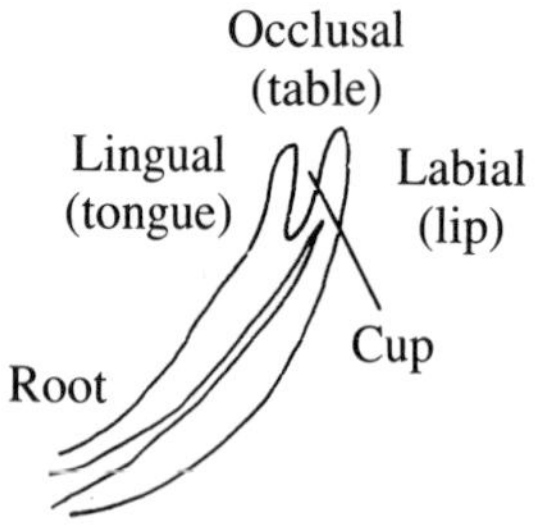

Fig. 7-4. *Surfaces of the teeth and tooth terms.*

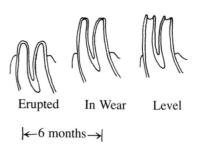

Fig. 7-5. *Definitions of tooth wear.*

them in the lower jaw. Many more mares have small unerupted canines which can be detected by a prominence of the gum. Deciduous canines occur in both sexes, but they do not erupt.

Eruption Time

Eruption time is the most accurate of the various methods used to detect the age of a horse by the teeth. Wear may be influenced by many factors, but eruption time is dependent only upon the horse's intrinsic growth pattern. These times must be memorized.

Temporary (deciduous, baby, or milk) incisor teeth follow an easy to remember pattern. The central incisors erupt at approximately 8 days, the intermediates at 8 weeks and the corners at 8 months. Temporary canine teeth do not erupt.

Permanent incisor teeth replace the shedding temporary central incisors at 2½ years, the in-

	I_1	I_2	I_3	C
Temporary erupt	8 da.	8 wk.	8 mo.	
Permanent erupt	2½ yr.	3½ yr.	4½ yr.	4-5 yr.

Fig. 7-6. Eruption times of incisor teeth. Temporary canines (if any) are present at birth.

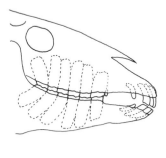

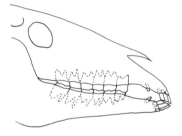

Fig. 7-7. Comparison of tooth roots of a young and aged horse.

termediates at 3½ years and the corners at 4½ years. Permanent canine teeth (usually in male only) erupt at 4 to 5 years of age.

The eruption of the molar teeth is not frequently used to estimate age due to the difficulty in visualizing their activity. However, their eruption is very predictable and is important to understand when diagnosing bitting and chewing problems.

No molars are present when the foal is born. The temporary premolar teeth are present at birth or erupt in the first 2 weeks of life.

The inconstant first permanent premolars or wolf teeth (when they are present) erupt at 5 to 6 months. These usually appear only in the upper jaw and are usually less than ¼ inch in length. They are often shed at 2½ years when the temporary premolars behind them are replaced by permanent teeth. Wolf teeth rarely erupt in the lower jaw.

The second (first full size) permanent premolar teeth erupt at 2½ years. They push the temporary molar or cap out until it falls out. The shed teeth or caps will sometimes be found in the feed manger. The permanent premolars of the lower jaw may erupt as much as 6 months earlier than those of the upper jaw. The premolars and molars of the lower jaw are two-thirds the width of those of the upper jaw.

The third permanent premolar erupts at 3 years and the fourth at 4 years. The horse may be shedding caps for a period of 2 years. Sometimes caps may be troublesome if they do not let go all at once and become twisted in the mouth. They can be easily extracted when they are recognized as the problem.

The molar teeth are not present or even developed at birth. The horse's jaw must lengthen to provide room for them to erupt. The perma-

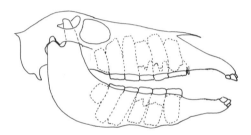

Fig. 7-8. Check teeth exposed on a 2½ year old horse. Note deciduous premolars or caps.

	P₁	P₂	P₃	P₄	M₁	M₂	M₃
Temporary erupt			–birth to 2 wk.–				
Permanent erupt	5-6 mo.	2½ yr.	2½-3 yr.	3½-4 yr.	6-12 mo.	2-2½ yr.	3½-4½ yr.

Fig. 7-9. Eruption times of cheek teeth. Molar teeth are present at birth. Note that cheek teeth (P_2 to M_3) erupt in or near years corresponding to their number. The lower teeth may erupt as much as six months earlier than the upper ones. Eruption times given are ranges compiled from various authoritative works.

nent premolar and molar teeth each have two roots, except the third molar which usually has three. The first molar teeth erupt at 9 to 12 months, the second at 2 years and the third at 3½ to 4 years.

While the premolars and molars are erupting, the roots of the teeth may swell and be noticeable on the lower jaw. These swellings will usually recede by themselves. If they do not, and the animal goes off feed, an abscess may be present. Abscessed teeth may have to be removed. This is done under general anesthesia. The teeth are literally punched out from above or below the mouth through a hole drilled in the sinus and jawbone.

Sharp Teeth

The rows of cheek teeth in the lower arcade are closer together than those of the upper arcade. If the horse ideally grinds his food by moving the jaws from side to side, the teeth will wear relatively flat.

However, the domesticated horse frequently

develops a condition known as sharp teeth or shear mouth. This must be corrected before the horse damages his tongue or cheeks. Pain in this area will cause the horse to go off feed, lose weight, and/or throw his head when being ridden.

The problem can easily be remedied by a process known as floating. A float is a small piece of fine cut rasp or coarse file attached to a handle. Floating may be done without a speculum. Care must be taken not to cut the tongue or cheeks by uncontrolled strokes. The purpose is not to level the teeth, but rather to remove the sharp edges. Special care must be taken when caps are present since they can easily be knocked loose.

Some horseshoers float teeth as a sideline to their shoeing business. The Author does not recommend this. However, you should recognize the need for it and advise the owner to call the veterinarian. This is one way to insure a good working relationship with your local veterinarian.

Age Estimation by Wear

After the teeth have erupted, estimation of age by determining the degree of incisor tooth wear is less accurate. Comparison of the following criteria to the mouths of thousands of horses of known ages has produced an average standard. It represents the mean of a bell-shaped curve and should only be referred to as an estimation.

Variations in genetic makeup, climate, soil type, nutrition and habits influence tooth wear. The coarseness of the diet, the percentage of silica, flourine, calcium, and other minerals are

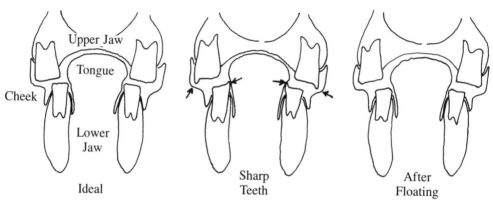

Cheek · Upper Jaw · Tongue · Lower Jaw · Ideal · Sharp Teeth · After Floating

Fig. 7-10. Sharp teeth and their treatment.

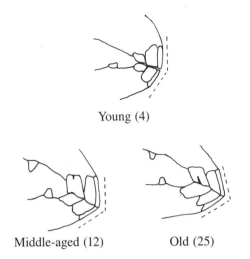

Young (4)

Middle-aged (12)   Old (25)

Fig. 7-11. Incisor tooth profile is a general indicator of age.

especially important. The habits or vices of wood chewing and cribbing also create premature wear on the incisors.

Characteristics of the lower incisor teeth which may be observed due to wear and compensating growth are the cup, star and table shape. The hook or notch and Galvayne groove on upper corner incisor teeth are less reliable indicators but may be used to strengthen the age estimate. The profile and curvature of the teeth in the jaw are only general indicators of a young or old horse.

The **profile** or angulation of the teeth will indicate the general age of the horse. The angle of the bite is nearly perpendicular when the animal is young. It becomes more acutely angulated as the horse ages. This simple check may be observed at a distance when the horse smacks his lips or yawns.

The **curvature** of the lower incisor teeth is a general indicator of age. The surface of the incisors is seen as a half circle in a young horse and a straight line in an old one. The teeth diverge from the median plane in a young horse and converge from it in an old one.

The **cup** is a valuable indicator of wear between the ages of 5 and 8 years in the lower incisors. It is less reliable, but sometimes used, to estimate age from 9 to 12 years in the upper incisors. The upper incisors lose their cups after the lower incisors and without as much regularity. After the cup disappears, the enamel spot or cement filled enamel remains until the mid-teens (age 13 to 16 yr.).

Occasionally, a horse may be seen that has been bishoped. This involves drilling and staining or burning holes in the incisors to fool inexperienced horsemen. It is easily detected by comparing to table shape and observing that the phony cups have no enamel rings.

The **star** or dental star is the remnant of the closed distal end of the pulp cavity. It first appears as a dark yellow line in the dentine of the central incisor at the age of 8 years. The star (line) appears in the intermediate incisors at 9 years and the corners at 10 years. The star has moved to the center of the lower incisors by the age of 13. The dental stars become round, dark and distinct in the lower incisors at 15 years.

The incisor **table shape** changes according to age. The chewing surface changes from horizontal to vertical when viewed by parting the lips. The central incisor tooth table is horizontal at eruption, becomes round at 9 years, triangular at 14 years and biangular or vertical at 18 years.

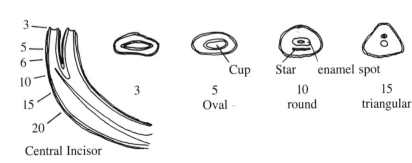

Central Incisor

Fig. 7-12. The cup depth, dental star position and tooth table shape change with age.

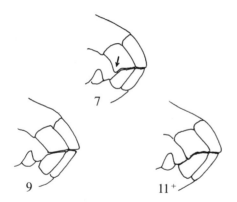

Fig. 7-13. The hook comes at 7, is gone at 9 and back at 11.

The **hook** on the upper corner incisors is unreliable by itself but may be used to strengthen an estimate. The hook appears at 7 years, may disappear by 9 years and be back again at 11 years. It may be present until 17 or 18 years. About 60 percent of a group of 1,208 horses studied by Weekenstroo (cited by Habel, 1975) had a hook on one or both corner incisors from age 8 to 18 years.

The **Galvayne groove** is less reliable than other indicators but may be the only means of estimating the age of an older horse. It also may strengthen an estimate in the teen years. The Galvayne groove appears at the gum line of the upper corner incisor at about 10 years, is halfway down at 15 years, and all the way down at 20 years. The groove emerges from the gum and can be seen in the bottom half of the tooth at 25 years and disappears at about 30 years.

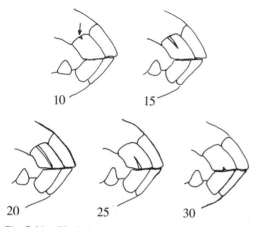

Fig. 7-14. The Galvayne groove comes at 10 and is gone at 30. It is about the only means of estimating the age of an older horse.

Estimation Procedure

Age estimates should always be cautiously phrased. The horse should be disturbed as little as possible to get the information needed. Parting the lips may be all that is necessary on young horses. Grasping the tongue and holding it to the side may be necessary for an extended look on older animals. Molar examination may be done by running the hand up in the mouth from the side and shoving the tongue between the teeth on the opposite side to be examined. A mechanical speculum to force the mouth open need rarely, if ever, be used by anyone other than a veterinarian.

Eruption and leveling of the teeth should always be given more weight than the signs of wear. Some consideration should be given to the condition and background of the horse. A long mane or tail, a sunken depression above the eye, and graying hair around the eye are signs of old age. The time of year may help in rounding off age estimates on young horses. Most horses are born in the spring. Diagrams and descriptions of teeth of each age may be obtained from several of the references listed.

Steps in ageing a horse:
1. Is it *young or old*? Look at the profile and jaw curvature as the lips are parted. Note the eyes (wrinkles, depression, and hair color), and mane or tail length. Size may fool you.
2. Are the incisors *temporary or permanent*? This may be determined with only the lips parted.
3. Are *canine teeth* present? They probably won't be if it's a female, but they should be if it is a male over 5 years.
4. Are the teeth *erupting, level* or *in wear*? It is important to be exact under 5 years.
5. Are *cups* present? A 1 or 2 year old may be mistaken for a 5 year old.
6. What is the shape and position of the *star*? Distinguish between star (soft and depressed) and enamel spot (hard and elevated).
7. What is the *table shape*? Oblong—1 to 7 years, round—9 to 11 years, triangular—14 to 17 years, biangular (oval)—18 years and older.
8. Are *hooks* present? Check both sides.
9. Is the *Galvayne groove* present? Check both sides.
10. Guess! Phrase your estimate cautiously. For example: "This horse appears to be ___years of age by its teeth."

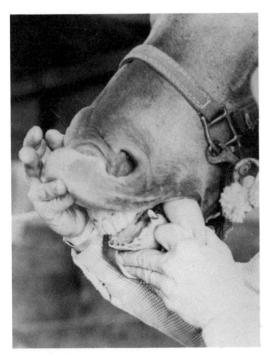

Lower Jaw	I_1	I_2	I_3
Temporary erupt	8 da.	8 wk.	8 mo.
Permanent erupt	2½ yr.	3½ yr.	4½ yr.
Permanent level	3	4	5 (full mouth)
Cup gone	6	7	8
Dental star appears	8	9	10
Dental star centers	13	13	13
Dental star round	15	15	15
Enamel spot disappears	16	16	16
Table round (diam. equal)	9	10	11
Table triangular	15	16	17
Table biangular (oval)	18	19	20
Upper Jaw			
Cup gone	9	10	11
Hook or Notch			7, 11 to 18 yr.
Galvayne's groove			10 to 30 yr.

Fig. 7-16. Summary of eruption, wear and other age estimation indicators. Times are averages compiled from various authoritative works.

Fig. 7-15. Parting the lips and holding the tongue to view the teeth.

References

A.A.E.P. 1966. Official Guide for Determining the Age of the Horse. American Association of Equine Practitioners, Golden, CO.

Goody, P.C. 1976. Horse Anatomy. J. A. Allen, London.

Goubaux, A. and G. Barrier. 1892. The Exterior of the Horse (translation by S.J.J. Harger). J.B. Lippincott, Philadelphia.

Habel, R. E. 1975. Applied Veterinary Anatomy. R.E. Habel, Ithaca, NY.

Nickel, R., A. Schummer, E. Seiferle, and W. O. Sack. 1973. The Viscera of the Domestic Mammals. Springer, New York.

McMullan, W.C. 1971. How old is he? The Southwestern Veterinarian. Spring: 213.

Pope, G. W. 1936. Determining the Age of Farm Animals by Their Teeth. USDA, Washington, DC.

Sack, W.O. and R.E. Habel. 1977. Rooney's Guide to the Dissection of the Horse. Veterinary Textbooks, Ithaca, NY.

Sisson, S. and J.D. Grossman. 1953. The Anatomy of the Domestic Animals. W. B. Saunders Co., Philadelphia.

Siegmund, O.H. (Ed.).1979. The Merck Veterinary Manual (5th ed.). Merck and Co., Inc., Rahway, NJ.

NOTES:

Chapter 8

Horse Handling and Shoeing Positions

Horseshoeing is one of the few businesses where one can literally be "kicked out of business." It is dangerous work. It is hard work. A potential horseshoer must understand something about horses and their nature, and have some experience handling them.

Skill Must Be Developed

Effective horse handling is a skill which successful horseshoers must develop. This skill can only be developed by experience. There is no other way to gain "horse sense" than to be around and work with horses. Some people pick this skill up faster than others, but they all acquire it the same way. Those who have highly developed the skill of horse handling can "feel how the horse feels," and sense his next move almost before the horse does. Such a sense is very advantageous for a horseshoer to possess, especially when handling horses of questionable character.

Horse Sense

A potential horseshoer must have a liking for horses and be unafraid of them. Horses can sense to a great degree how a person feels toward them and they react to this feeling. They can often tell if a person doesn't like them and/or is afraid of them. Horses generally feel more secure and react favorably when confidence and concern for their welfare is "expressed" by the person working around them.

Much of the "sensing" horses experience is through touch. Horses can sense by touch when a person is angry, tense, scared, confident, firm, determined, patient or in a general sense, his attitude, and they react to this sensation.

Some sensing is by sight. A horse can detect fear or confidence in the way one approaches and moves about him. The dress of a person may also be associated with a former good or bad experience. Quick movement is frightening to most horses.

Some sensing is by smell. Horses often smell the horseshoer and his tools to determine their acceptability. Some horses associate particular odors with pain, such as those that are frightened by the smell of alcohol because of its association with a needle.

The sense of hearing is also a factor. The tone of voice of the horseshoer is especially noticed by horses. Noisy distractions such as loud music or motorcycles can cause difficulty when shoeing a horse. Tapping of the anvil, nail or shoe bothers some horses.

Master Yourself

Working with horses effectively requires a great deal of self-control. Since the attitude and reaction of the horseshoer so strongly influences the actions of the horse, it follows that the man must learn to control himself in order to control the horse. The proverb, *"Master yourself and you can master anything,"* seems to be very true, for if the horseshoer can control his attitudes and action, then the control of the horse becomes very simple. This fact is one of the basic fundamental laws of horse training and should give all potential horseshoers an incentive to improve themselves.

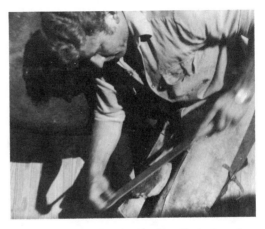

Fig. 8-1. Horseshoers must develop effective horse handling skills.

65

A feeling of mutual respect must be developed between man and horse. The horse must learn to trust the horseshoer, and the horseshoer must provide every chance for this relationship to develop. This type of relationship is initiated by the man and is learned by the horse through association. It often takes some time as well as patience to create a favorable situation.

In 1878, a prominent horse trainer named Magner (1888) wrote a summary of the above principles and discussed the traits necessary for effective horse handling in the following paragraph:

…We see that certain elements are necessary (for horse training)—coolness, firmness, steadiness of purpose, energy, and perseverance. We have brought all these qualities into exercise. We have cultivated and strengthened them in ourselves. We have seen the importance of not showing fear, and the harm of anger, hastiness, revenge, etc., with the importance of keeping uppermost, feelings of kindness, forbearance, etc. Thus, when we proceed on right principles, according to the real laws of the case,

we are all the time cultivating the better side and restraining the worst side of our nature. We must, in a word, have the keenest discernment, the broadest and soundest judgment, the truest courage, the most persistent perseverance and patience, and the highest instincts of benevolence and kindness. In this spirit, viewing the subject any way we will, it incites with strongest incentives to self-improvement, thereby offering the most frequent suggestions and repetitions of motives for the cultivation of all our highest and best powers.

Problems in Handling Horses

There are at least three major problem areas which must be understood when dealing with horses:

1. Horses are stronger than horseshoers. It is true it is advantageous to be strong when working with horses, but even a strong man is outweighed and "outstouted" by most horses. Matched muscle for muscle, the horse will almost always win. A horseshoer must learn techniques which put the horse in the position of "working against himself." In this manner, the horse will use his own strength to defeat himself.
2. Horses cannot reason in the sense that people can. Horses have limits of learning which are based on their experience. Their learning is limited to association of action with input from the senses previously discussed. They must learn and "unlearn" things by association.
3. Horses cannot understand language. They must be shown and taught, not just told. Horses must be shown and taught in a way that they can comprehend and then associate a specific action with a command. The pitch and tone of the voice must be repeated exactly to achieve consistent results and are much more important than the spoken word.

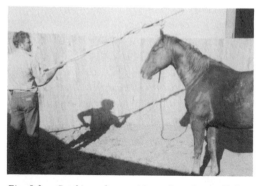

Fig. 8-2. Catching a horse with a pole and rope (Jeffery method).

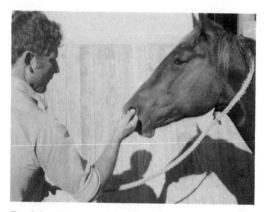

Fig. 8-3. Horses can sense and react to a person's attitude.

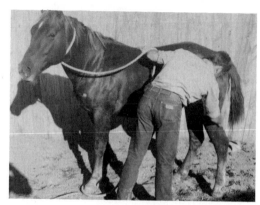

Fig. 8-4. Changing horse behavior requires special skill.

An understanding of the principles of horse handling allows a horseshoer to predict and even "sense" a horse's reaction to a given situation and helps him to deal with it. Once a horse is conditioned to do a certain thing, good or bad, he will do it over and over until the association with the action is changed in order to neutralize or counteract the impression. It is necessary for horseshoers, therefore, to get experience with horses, study the degree to which it is possible to change their behavior, and learn and practice the most effective means of changing their behavior for the better.

Catching

As a rule, horseowners should be encouraged to catch their horses for the horseshoer. However, if the horses to be shod have been left in a small enclosure for the horseshoer to catch, the following procedure may be helpful:

1. Place the midpoint of the lead rope over your left arm and unbuckle the head strap. Take hold of the buckle and strap in your left hand, holding them such that you can release the strap and still have hold of the buckle.
2. "Corner" the horse.
3. Approach the horse slowly but deliberately from the left side.

4. Reach out with your right hand and rub the horse gently on the neck and pass your hand over the neck in an area about midway from the shoulders to the head.
5. Pass the halter under the neck with your left hand and receive the head strap with your right hand. Now you have caught the horse.
6. Move the halter forward up the neck with both hands, lower the halter so the nose band will pass over the nose, and then pull the nose band up over the nose.
7. Buckle the halter with the rope still remaining looped over the left arm.
8. Take hold of the lead rope near the halter with the right hand and hold the rest of the rope in the left hand.

Roping a horse should be considered only as a last resort. It is usually not a good idea even if you have practiced and are confident. A frightened horse may injure itself.

Observation

Make it a habit to observe a horse move before and after it is caught and determine if it shows any signs of lameness, tendency toward faulty leg or foot conformation, limb interference, or "spookiness." If any of these conditions is present, advise the owner or whoever is responsible

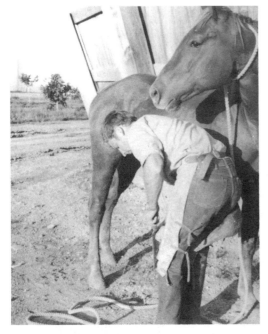

Fig. 8-5. A horse will usually stand quietly when a shoer has gained its confidence.

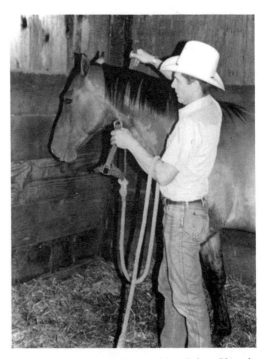

Fig. 8-6. Catching the horse with a halter. Photo by J. Graves.

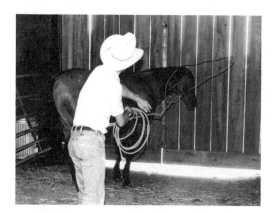

Fig. 8-7. Catching a reluctant horse by roping is a difficult skill to master. Also, it may cause the horse to be frightened and injure itself.

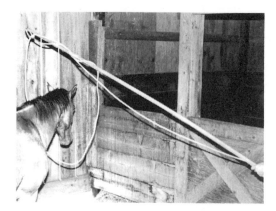

Fig. 8-8. Placing the catch rope on a pole is a preferred method.

before commencing work on the horse. Such a policy will prevent disagreement and dispute later if the above conditions become apparent. Other important factors to observe are covered in Chapter 17.

Working Place

Choose a safe place to work which is free from "wire traps" and "spooks" of all types. The ideal place is usually an area far away from the center of activity at the stable but one that is familiar to the horse; a place where he could not hurt himself or damage any property if he "blows up." Ideally, it should be level, dry, protected from the elements, easily accessible from your horseshoeing outfit and with room enough to work comfortably and safely.

Holding

Whenever possible have the owner, or someone who is familiar with the horse, hold the horse. Many horses won't stand well when tied up, especially when away from familiar surroundings. The holder should be instructed to stand on the *same* side of the horse as the horseshoer is working. The holder is then in a position to pull the hind feet of the horse away from the shoer in case of trouble.

Tying

When it is not possible to work with a capable holder, the horse must be tied. A strong halter and tie rope should be a part of every horse-

shoer's equipment. Nylon halters and ropes are preferable to leather because of their durability and strength. If the horse must be tied, tie it to a safe and immovable object properly and securely with a halter and rope that *won't break*. Tie a knot that will hold but can be easily released. Knots that are pulled tight by a struggling horse can be loosened with a pair of pliers.

Crosstying is wise where practical. Crosstying is done by snapping two ropes to the halter, one on each side, and tying them about 8 to 12 feet apart. This method of tying allows you more room to work in front of the horse and prevents most horses from pulling back.

Hoof Handling

A horseshoer must learn how to handle horses' hoofs. Hoof handling is the "hard work" of shoeing horses. Learning how to handle hoofs and assume the shoeing position safely and comfortably saves time, work, and energy. The result is greater profit and more satisfaction from your work. Hoof handling skill should be thoroughly studied and practiced on a gentle horse until it becomes part of you. A horseshoer's degree of mastery of this skill determines to a great degree his success in the profession.

The techniques demonstrated here should be learned by all potential horseshoers. They are safe and effective. As you gain more experience, other methods that save time may become apparent. Adopt them when you feel confident in doing so.

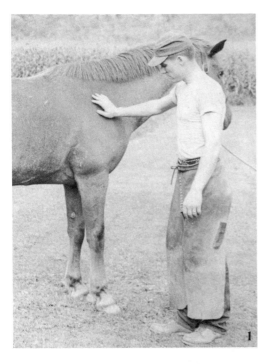

Raising and Positioning a Front Foot

Steps in raising and positioning a front foot:

1. Approach the horse slowly from near his head. Rub him on the neck and pat him before trying to pick up a foot. This helps him to know you are there, and it helps you to determine his reaction to you.
2. Facing the rear of the horse, place the hand closest to the horse on his shoulder and run your other hand down his leg and grasp it in the pastern area.
3. Push against the horse's shoulder. As he shifts his weight to the opposite foot, "fold up" the leg.

    At this point, the lateral balance of the foot should be checked and the amount to be trimmed from each heel noted.

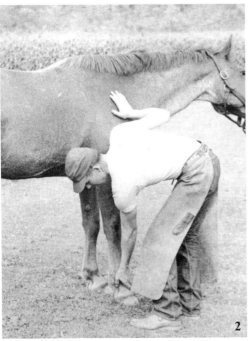

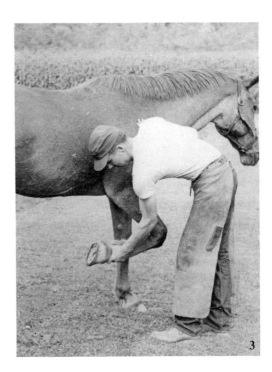

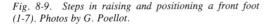

Fig. 8-9. Steps in raising and positioning a front foot (1-7). Photos by G. Poellot.

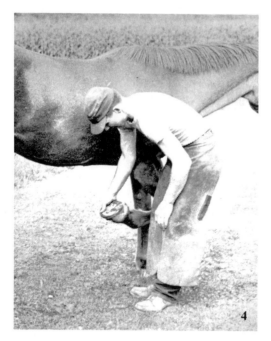

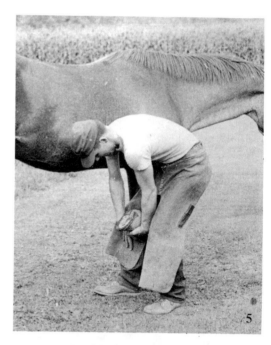

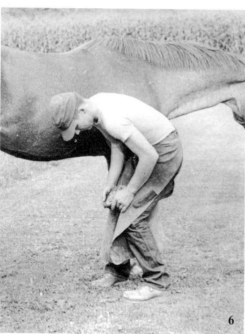

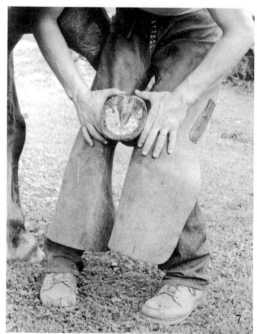

4. Bring your hand from the shoulder to the toe of the foot.
5. Step forward with the leg nearest the horse and pass the leg between your legs, grasping the foot with one hand while positioning your apron with the other.
6. Grasping the foot with both hands, position it on your knees so that it is comfortable for you and not cramping the horse.

7. Turn your toes in and heels out and crouch slightly. This will force your knees together and make it possible for you to hold the foot securely with a minimum of muscular effort. Learn to relax when the horse is relaxed and exert pressure when the horse resists. This position and movement must become natural to you.

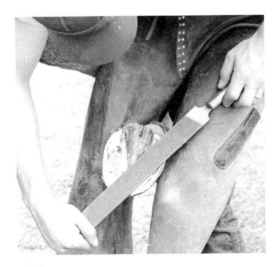

Fig. 8-10. *Leveling a positioned front foot with a hoof rasp.*

Taking a Front Foot Forward

Most horseshoers take the front foot forward to finish the clinching, remove flares or shape a deformed foot. The forward position allows a shoer to obtain a better view of what he is doing and to do a smoother job in the shaping and finishing operations. However, holding the foot in the forward position can be an awkward and dangerous practice if done incorrectly.

Some shoers use "foot stands" for working on the feet in a forward position. Even if you choose to use one, practice this position until it becomes natural to you. A foot stand may not always be available or practical to use.

Steps in taking a front foot forward:
1. Remove the foot from between your legs and bring it to the hanging or "home" position with your hand nearest the horse holding the toe of the foot.
2. Take a step backward and turn with your back toward the horse's head. Your feet should be in line with the horse's body. Place the foot between your knees and in such a position that it forms a "V" with the ground. Note that the arm nearest the horse is over his leg and holds it against your body as you work on it. Turning your toes in helps to force your knees against the foot as you crouch slightly to work.
3. After work is completed on the outside of the foot, move back to home position.

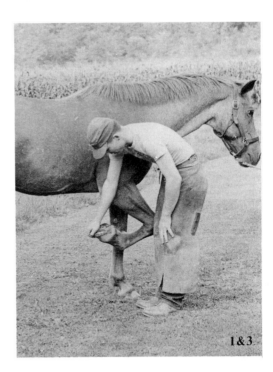

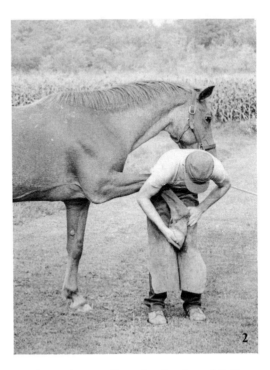

Fig. 8-11. *Steps in taking a front foot forward (1-4).*

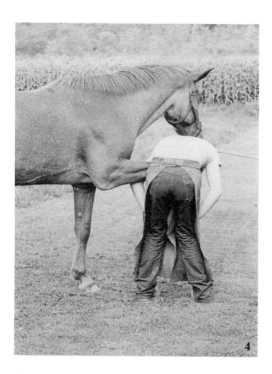

4. Take a step backwards and turn with your back away from the horse's head and place your feet in line with the horse's body. Place the hoof between your knees. Again, the foot should form a "V" with the ground.

It is recommended that you trim corresponding pairs of feet, i.e., both fronts and then both hinds, in succession. This practice makes it easier for you to balance pairs by comparison. It is easier to remember what you did to the opposite foot and thus make both feet the same. It is also easier to fit shoes in pairs.

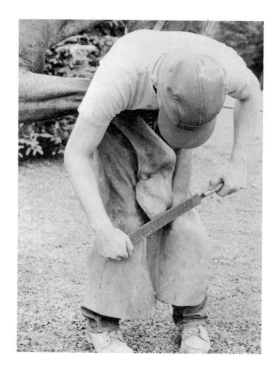

Fig. 8-12. Removing a flare on the outside of a front foot in the forward position.

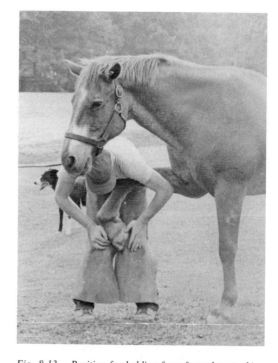

Fig. 8-13. Position for holding front foot when working on its inside surface.

Raising and Positioning a Hind Foot

Steps in raising and positioning a hind foot:
1. Starting from near the shoulder, slide your hand toward the rear of the horse and place it on the point of his hip.
2. Starting high on the hip, run your other hand down the back of the hind leg to a point just above the fetlock.
3. Push against the horse's hip and at the same time raise the leg by pulling it toward you.
4. Step forward and under the hind leg with your leg nearest the horse.

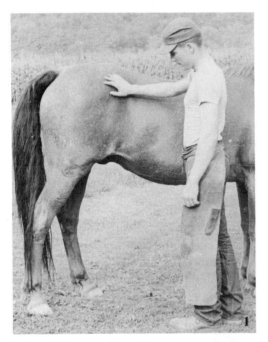 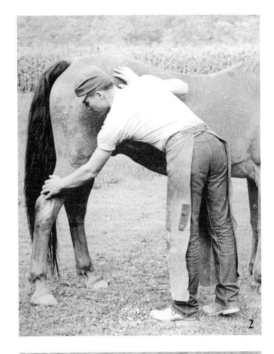

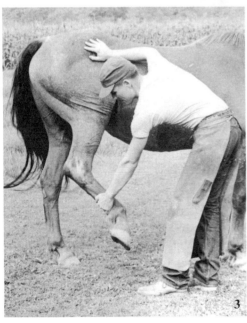 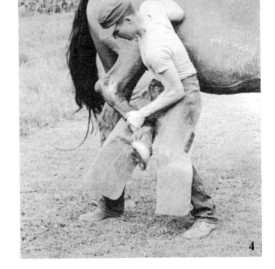

Fig. 8-14. Steps in raising and positioning a hind foot (1-7).

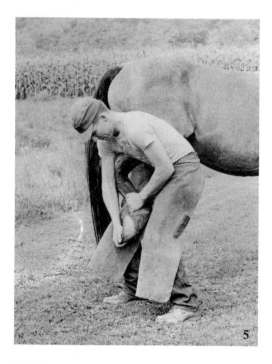

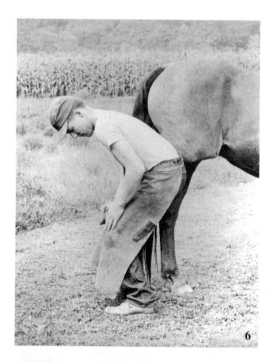

5. Bring your hand from the hip and grasp the toe of the foot.
6. Place the foot upon your knees. Note that the cannon bone is nearly perpendicular with the ground.

   The foot should be sighted while in this position to determine the amount to be cut from each heel. This is done by straightening the upper part of your body and sighting down the leg and over the foot.
7. Turn your toes in and heels out and slightly crouch. Note that the knees are slightly apart giving lateral support to the foot and that the foot rests mostly on the outside knee and inside thigh.

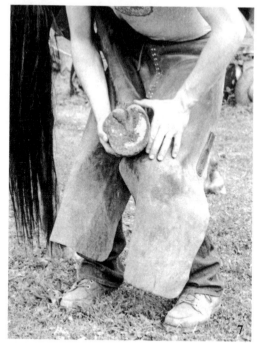

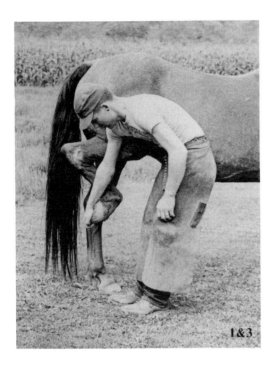

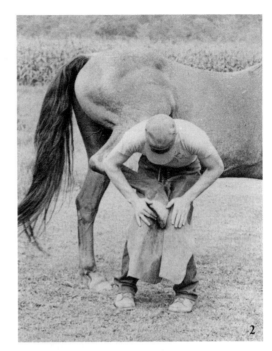

Taking a Hind Foot Forward

Steps in taking a hind foot forward:

1. Grasp the foot with your hand nearest the horse and step back. This is the hanging or "home" position for the hind leg. If you happen to "cramp" a horse or for some other reason he wants to move around, grabbing hold of the toe and returning the leg to this position will often make it easier for you to control the action of that leg. This is particularly true with young horses.

2. Step backward and under the horse with your back facing the horse's body. Line your feet up with the horse's body and place the foot between your knees so that it forms a "V" with the ground. Turn your toes in. Note the position of the arm over the horse's leg. This helps to hold the foot against your leg.

3. After work is completed on the outside of the foot, return to the home position.

4. Step backward and turn your back away from the horse. Place your feet so that they are nearly in line with the horse's body. Again the foot forms a "V" with the ground. Your arm nearest the horse is placed over the leg and holds the horse's leg against you in a

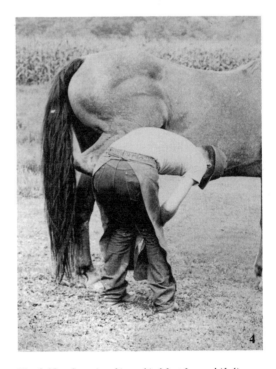

Fig. 8-15. *Steps in taking a hind foot forward (1-4).*

secure position. The position of your arm is especially important when finishing the inside of a hind foot. This demonstrated position allows you to have both your hands free to operate your tools. This position is considered by most horseshoers to be the most difficult. Master this position.

Experience in handling horses in general and picking up and holding their hoofs in position for shoeing is necessary before learning to trim or shoe them. Gentle, well-trained horses should be sought for this practice.

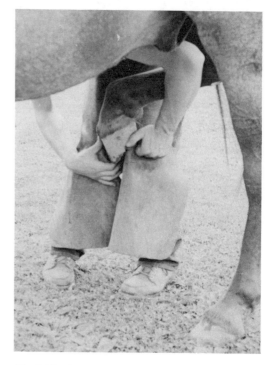

Fig. 8-16. Position for holding a hind foot when working on its inside surface.

References

Costin, R. and D. Butler. The Jeffery method of horse handling for horseshoeing. Amer. Farrier's J. 5(1):8.

Dyer, R. 1979. Proper shoeing positions. Amer. Farrier's J. 5(1):10.

Ives, H.S. 1968. John Rarey rules for training horses. Hoof and Horns. (June):22.

Magner, D. 1875. The New System of Educating Horses (11th ed.). The Courier Co., Buffalo, NY.

Magner, D. 1888. The Art of Taming and Educating the Horse. Review and Herald Publ., Battle Creek, MI.

Magner, D. 1899. ABC Guide to Sensible Horseshoeing. The Werner Co., Akron, OH.

Magner, D. 1909. Standard Horse and Stock Book (Part I). The Saalfield Publ. Co., Akron, OH.

Thorpe, T.B. 1861. Rarey, the horsetamer. Harper's. 22(131):615.

Wright, M. 1973. The Jeffery Method of Horse Handling. Dyamberin, Armidale, N.S.W., AUSTRALIA.

NOTES:

Chapter 9

Horse Training and Restraint

More than a few of the horses a beginning horseshoer is called upon to shoe are not gentle and well-mannered. Often it is necessary for a horseshoer to "train" or "retrain" the horses so that they can be safely and properly shod. Experienced horseshoers should "charge accordingly" for this service. Owners should be encouraged to train and work with their horses prior to asking a horseshoer to work on them. Horses which need training for trimming or shoeing can be divided into three major categories:

1. Foals.
2. Horses which have never been handled or shod before.
3. Spoiled or malicious horses which have been handled improperly.

The principles for handling these three groups of animals are usually quite different, and each case must be handled individually and according to the situation involved.

Foals are best handled for trimming calmly and quickly.

Young horses can be taught best firmly and slowly.

Spoiled horses are handled best with restraint measures and attention diversion devices.

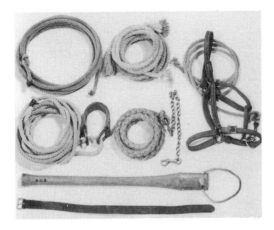

Fig. 9-1. Horse training equipment. (1) catch rope, (2) nylon tie ropes, (3) halter, (4) leg rope and pastern collar, (5) lead chain, (6) twitch, (7) leg strap. Photo by G. Poellot.

Confidence and self-control must always be present in the horseshoer. Practice and experience are the best teachers. One should proceed with the intent of getting the "drop" on the animal so as not to provide a chance for him to disobey. An experienced helper is a valuable asset when trimming or shoeing horses in these categories.

Equipment

The following equipment is useful when training horses for shoeing:

1. *Catch rope* (3/8 in. to 7/16 in. x 35 ft. treated nylon). A catch rope can be used to catch young foals or elusive spoiled or unbroken horses in a corral, make a war bridle, or tie down a horse when good help is available. A catch rope requires practice and judgment in its use to be of value. A catch rope hung from a long pole may be used to catch horses in a corral when roping skills have not been developed.
2. *Tie ropes* (1/2 in. to 5/8 in. x 14 ft., soft cotton or nylon). Tie ropes can be used to tie up a horse that pulls back, pick up a hind foot, hold back a tied-up hind foot for shoeing, or tie front and hind legs together on the same side when a horse is thrown for shoeing. Use only nylon for tying horses that pull back.
3. *Halter*. A leather or nylon halter is necessary for use with a lead chain, and is easiest to use when a person is available to hold the horse to be shod. A nylon halter is preferred when it is necessary to tie up the horse.
4. *Leg rope and pastern collar* (1/2 in. to 3/4 in. x 25 ft. cotton). A leg rope can be used to make a scotch hobble to tie up a hind leg for shoeing, or when tying a horse down. A leather pastern collar protects the pastern from being rope burned. Collars can be made from leather or a short cinch.
5. *Lead chain*. A lead chain (also called a lip chain or stud shank) can be used under the lip, over the horse's nose, or in his mouth to aid in controlling him and focusing his attention on his head rather than on his feet.
6. *Twitch*. A twitch can be used on the nose, lower lip, or ear for the same purpose as a lead chain. Horses differ in their response to the twitch and other restraint measures.

7. *Leg strap*. A leg strap can be used to hold up a front foot for shoeing. A stirrup leather from an English saddle, nylon hobbles or two heavy nylon dog collars buckled together make a good front leg strap.

There are many other variations of these devices which employ the same basic principles. A variation or combination of these devices, in the hands of a skillful horseman, will work to "train" almost any horse for shoeing. Those horses that cannot be handled with these simple devices should be given a tranquilizer or sedative by a veterinarian before attempting to shoe the animal. However, this should be done only if the animal is "untrainable."

Knots

A horseshoer should learn how to tie all of the basic knots taught in the Boy Scout Handbook or other good knot manual. Especially important are: the bowline, the slipknot, the halter or horse hitch, the clove hitch, the honda knot, and two half hitches. Knowledge of these knots

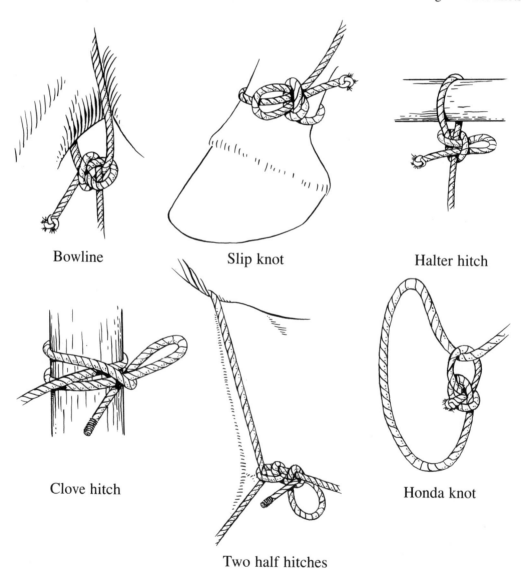

Bowline   Slip knot   Halter hitch

Clove hitch   Honda knot

Two half hitches

Fig. 9-2. *Useful knots for horse handling. Drawings by L. Sadler.*

is especially necessary when working with untrained or spoiled horses.

Handling Foals

Foals often present a problem since they are usually not halter broken or gentle when they are trimmed for the first time, and they are understandably frightened by the presence of a horseshoer.

Foals can be easily handled and trimmed in a corner with a competent holder(s). One effective way to catch a foal is to crowd him into a corner with the mare, who is usually easily caught. Catch the foal by passing an arm in front of him and one in back of him. Avoid grabbing the skin or flank. Then slip your hands around the foal's neck with the halter in hand. Pull the halter up over the foal's nose and fasten it. Now lead the mare away a few steps and trim the foal in the corner he was caught in. If stalls are available, place the mare in the stall adjacent to the one in which the foal is being trimmed. A stall with a smooth, tightly woven wire screen separating the two is even more desirable.

The area where the foal is caught and trimmed should be free from wire and other dangerous objects. Foals will usually struggle and may throw themselves the first time or two that they are handled. A padded stall is very desirable when

a lot of foals are to be trimmed or broken to lead. A padded head bonnet is available to go under the halter strap for situations where wall padding is unavailable.

A foal, or any unbroken horse, will react to pulling on his head by pulling back or rearing and throwing himself. Always pull to the side, never straight away. If the foal must be led some distance, use a rope forming a loop over his withers and around and above the hocks. He can be pulled with this rope and guided by the halter.

The front feet of foals are usually much harder to handle and trim than the hind. Give the foal a chance to get used to you by trimming the hind feet first. Place the foal's nose in the corner and have the holder stand on the same side you are working. The object is to prevent the foal from going forward and turning the corner. The natural reaction of most horses when their back feet are being worked on is to go forward and kick back. The position of your holder should prevent this.

Pick up the hind leg and crowd him to the wall with the hand you have on the hip. Move into position and hold the foal against the wall with your body weight until you feel him relax. Then let him stand straight up on his own while you work. Work as quickly as possible. Be gentle but firm. Speak softly. Bodily force him to obey. Be patient and teach him that "it isn't that bad." The impression a foal gets the first time it's handled will shape its attitude toward future trimming and shoeing experiences.

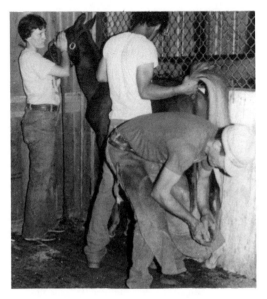

Fig. 9-3. Position for handling a foal's hind foot. Photos by J. Graves.

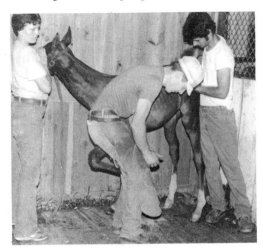

Fig. 9-4. Position for handling a foal's front foot.

After work on one hind foot is completed, have the holder change sides and move the foal's hindquarters against the other wall of the corner, while keeping his head stationary in the corner. Trim that hind foot.

Now "swap ends" on the foal and place his hindquarters in the corner and crowd him against one wall. The holder should stand to the outside against the foal and prevent him from coming out or going forward. The natural reaction to having the front feet worked on is to go back or up. Pick up the front foot and lean against the foal. Place the foot between your legs and begin trimming. Work rapidly and allow him to relax and stand up straight as soon as he will.

A foal which continually rears must be dealt with patiently and may have to be trimmed "one-handed." One hand holds the foot while the other operates the tools. Time is usually the biggest limiting factor in forcing the horseshoer to do this. A third person can help by holding the foals hindquarters against the wall. This prevents the foal from backing out of the corner.

Again, change sides, keeping the hindquarters in the corner. Push the foal over against the other wall and repeat the process.

Most foals respond very well to this procedure. There are few that cannot be trimmed in this manner.

Young Unbroken Horses

"Broncs" or unbroken horses need to be broken or trained to stand for trimming or shoeing. It is usually best if the owner does this or has it done before he calls the horseshoer. However, you will find this is not always done, especially when working with neglected and "pet" horses. A horse that has been regularly handled and trimmed since it was a foal will be easy to handle and will stand readily for shoeing.

If it is necessary for you to break the horse to shoe, you should probably charge for it. The horse should be caught, roped if necessary, and taught to lead and stand for shoeing. Some horseshoers prefer to perform this service free of charge for their steady customers. They realize it will pay dividends in making the horse easier to shoe later on.

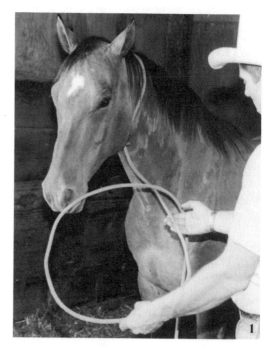

Fig. 9-5.   Steps in applying the come along (1-4).

The Come Along

A "green" or unbroken horse can be taught to lead, load in a trailer or stand for shoeing with a variation of the cowboy's war bridle or "come along." This bridle is applied using the same rope that was used to catch the horse. This technique should not be used on horses being trained with a hackamore. They will try to back up instead of coming forward.

Steps in applying the come along:
1. Face the horse. Hold the rope in your left hand with your palm down. Your right hand should be below the left and palm up on the rope. Rotate the wrist of your left hand counterclockwise as you lift and fold the rope over itself with the right hand. The rope should form a backwards figure 6 as you face the horse.
2. Grasp the right side of the loop of the backwards 6 with your right hand. Reach through the loop with your left hand and grasp the rope hanging in the loop. Pull it toward you and through the loop with your left hand. Now you are holding the nose piece in your left hand and the poll piece in your right hand.
3. Place the nose piece on the nose and the poll piece behind the ears on the poll. To do this, stand on the left side of the head and raise your right hand, bringing the bridle up. Place

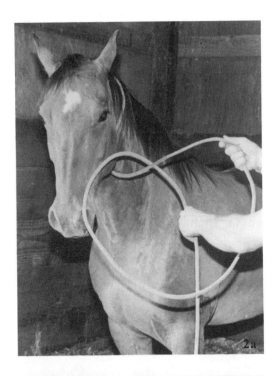

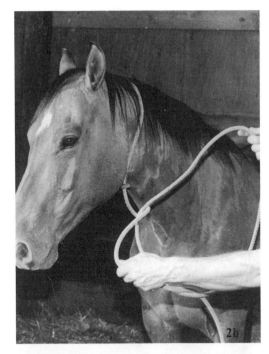

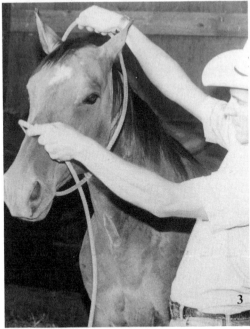

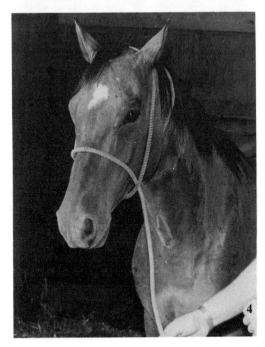

the nose piece in your left hand on the horse's face between the eyes and nostrils. Continue to bring your right hand up and then back placing the poll piece first over the right ear and then over the left.

4. Adjust and tighten the head and nose pieces until the poll piece is directly behind the ears and the nose piece is just below the facial crest. The bridle must be snug and adjusted properly to work effectively.

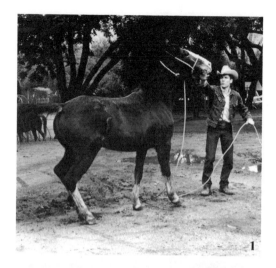

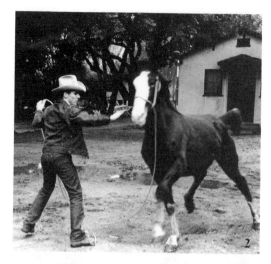

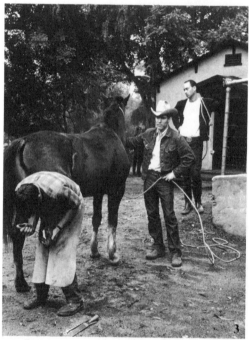

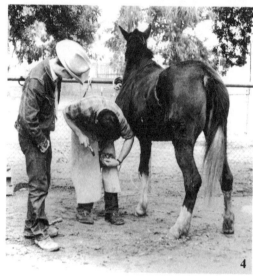

Fig. 9-6. Using the come along. Pull the "bridle" tight; walk up to the horse and release the pressure (1). The horse will soon come to your outstretched hand (2)...and stand for trimming(3)...and shoeing (4). Photos by R. Rankin.

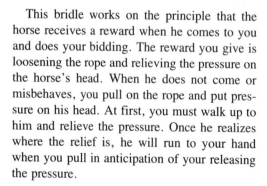

This bridle works on the principle that the horse receives a reward when he comes to you and does your bidding. The reward you give is loosening the rope and relieving the pressure on the horse's head. When he does not come or misbehaves, you pull on the rope and put pressure on his head. At first, you must walk up to him and relieve the pressure. Once he realizes where the relief is, he will run to your hand when you pull in anticipation of your releasing the pressure.

The come along usually will work wonders by instilling confidence in the horse's mind concerning you and your ability to help rather than hurt him. Many green or ignorant, untrained horses will stand perfectly still and allow you to shoe them after such a treatment because of the acquired confidence they have in you.

Methods of restraint that are normally used on spoiled or malicious horses are frequently used on young green horses when time and conditions don't permit slow, patient training. The choice is determined by the conditions encountered and the individual animal. Often several techniques must be tried before one is found which works well.

Spoiled or Malicious Horses

Spoiled horses, especially those that are fractious (dangerous), require some type of restraint which prevents them from injuring the horseshoer and themselves. Some horses are very difficult to shoe with any type of restraint. A few are nearly impossible without some type of stock to hold them or drug to anesthetize them. They should quickly find their way to the sale yard.

Restraint methods operate on two principles. One is that the item applied bothers the horse more than what you are doing. It, therefore, will concentrate its attention on what "hurts" most. The twitch and lip chain or stud shank work on this principle.

Other types of restraint methods operate on the principle that the horse will get tired quicker and the horseshoer will stay "sound" longer if the horse works against himself when restrained. The powerful limbs of the horse are put in po-

sition where they can't do any damage. The horse also learns that he cannot win and must yield to your will. Tying up a hind leg with a foot rope or scotch hobble is one method which uses this principle. Another is tying up one front leg with a leg strap or rope. And still another, the most drastic of the restraint measures (without stocks or drugs), is tying a horse down. In many cases, these types of restraints are also useful aids when training young unbroken horses.

Twitch

The twitch is very useful for restraining some types of horses. It seems to work best on "cold-blooded" horses. These are horses that are not easily excited. They are usually stubborn and dull in temperament.

The twitch is most commonly applied on the upper lip or nose. However, it can be applied on the lower lip or the ear. One place may be effective in distracting his attention where another will not.

The twitch must be properly adjusted to be useful. If it is too loose, it will not work; if it is too tight, it will shut off the circulation and the area will soon become numb and the restraint will no longer work.

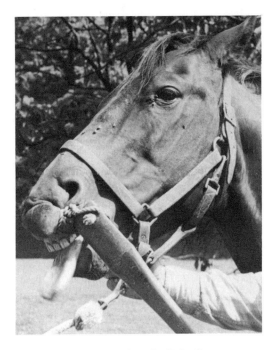

Fig. 9-7. Nose twitch. Photos by G. Poellot.

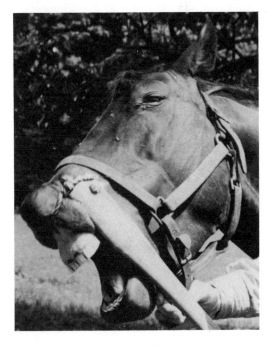

Fig. 9-8. Nose twitch—too tight.

Care must be taken to always twist the twitch away from the gums when applying it to the lips and back against the neck when applying it to the ear. The Author prefers a homemade twitch with a long handle and nylon rope nose band to the commercial short-handled chain type.

Lead Chain

The lead chain or stud shank is usually very effective for restraining "hot-blooded" horses. Horses which are very excitable, high-strung, and nervous will usually stand much better with a lip chain than a twitch.

The chain can be applied over the nose, placed in the mouth, or put under the upper lip on the gums above the teeth. What works on one horse may not work on another. The mere presence of the chain will discourage some horses from acting up, especially spoiled horses who have felt one before.

To put on the chain, rest it on your middle and ring fingers. Fold the lip back with the pointer and thumb and little finger. Pull the chain up snug between the upper lip and gum.

The lead chain should be used with judgment and self-control. It can be very destructive in the hands of an angry person. Only sufficient pressure should be applied in order to discourage the bad behavior of the horse. Pressure should be applied at critical times and released when the horse stands. Some horses like to play with the chain in their mouth with their tongue. Well-broken horses that are spoiled about shoeing will often behave with a chain in their mouth. They associate it with a bit and control.

Scotch Hobble

A scotch hobble, or side line as it is sometimes called, can be used to partially immobilize the hind legs for shoeing. It works equally well on unbroken and spoiled horses. Many horse breakers use the scotch hobble to break horses to shoe. A scotch hobble with a pastern collar is especially desirable. It prevents the horse's pastern from being burned during the struggle of putting the hobble on. Note how the horse is in a position to work against himself when he struggles after the hobble is on. Many horses will give up and stand for shoeing after they have struggled with a leg tied up.

NOTE: When working alone, it may be necessary to tie a horse up to put the scotch hobble on. However, it is most important that a horse be untied when using a scotch hobble and that the ground and area around is clear and safe. Horses often move around and fall when strug-

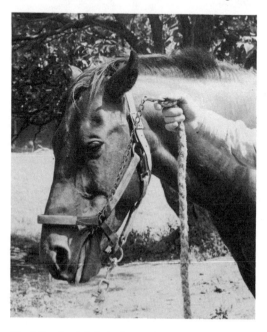

Fig. 9-9. Lead chain in the mouth.

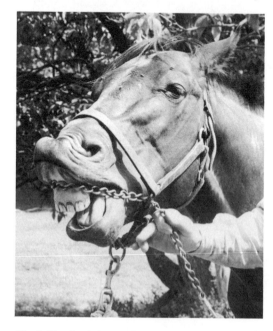

Fig. 9-10. Lead chain under the upper lip.

gling to free themselves from this restraint the first time they experience it. A solid board or tightly woven wire corral or arena is ideal. If none is available, work in a clear area and control the horse's movement with its halter rope.

Steps in putting on a scotch hobble with a pastern collar:

1. Pass the leg rope around the neck. Tie a bowline knot over the shoulder. A braided-in snap and adjustable ring is easier and provides a faster release.
2. Run the long end of the rope through one ring of the pastern collar from the outside to the inside and run the end of the rope back through the neck loop. Secure the end of the rope to the neck loop with an overhand knot.

3. Stand behind the horse and let the ropes sag and rest on the ground. If the rope is too short, snap a lead line, or other short piece of rope, on the free end of the collar. This allows you to stand out of range of the hind feet while putting on the rope.
4. Move the horse or in some way encourage him to step over the ropes with his hind leg. Draw the ropes up between the horse's hind legs. If the horse seems especially bothered by the presence of the ropes, continue to gently move them back and forth until the horse calms down and stands fairly still.
5. Bring the lead rope and collar to the side staying out of range of the hind feet.
6. Untie the overhand knot on the neck loop and pass the end of the rope through the open ring of the pastern collar from the inside to the outside.
7. Run the end of the rope up under the neck collar. Pull the slack out of the rope keeping the ropes above the hock.

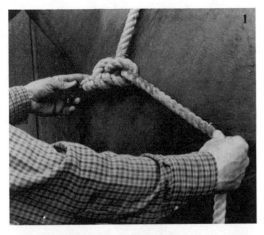

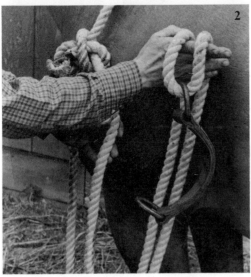

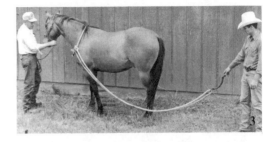

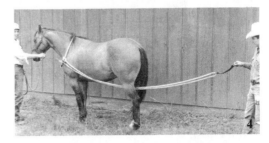

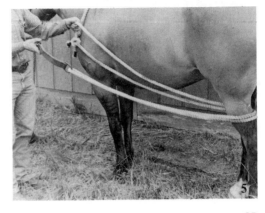

Fig. 9-11.   Steps in applying a scotch hobble with a pastern collar (1-12). Photos by J. Graves.

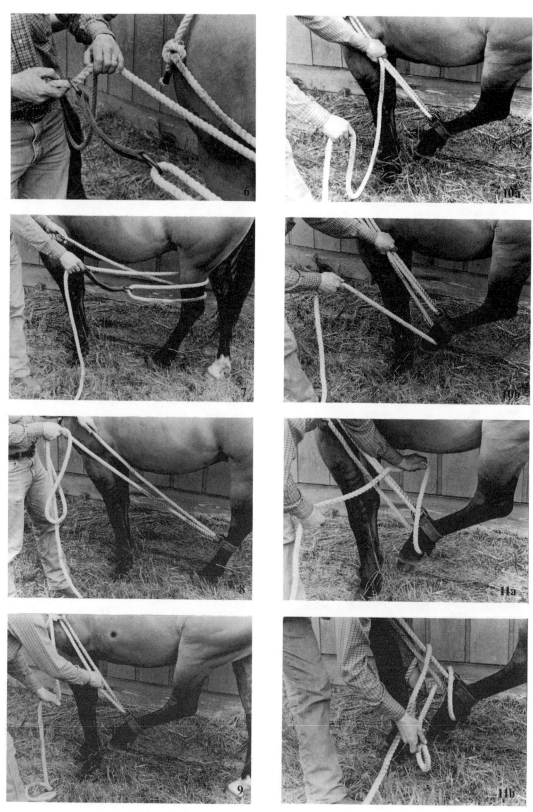

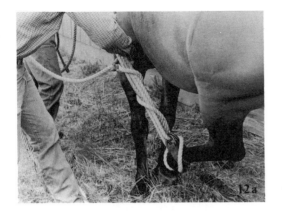 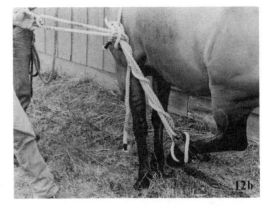

8. Hold up on the ropes as you let the pastern collar slide down the leg until it rests above the pastern. The horse may try to kick it off at this point. Keep the slack out of the ropes to prevent the collar from being kicked off.

9. Pull the free end of the rope against the neck rope to raise the leg. At first, the leg should be raised about a foot off the ground. The horse will struggle and get tired. Later, it may be tied up only enough to prevent kicking, allowing the horse to rest its foot on the ground when it is not raised for shoeing.

10. When the leg is at the desired height, clamp the ropes (3) with the hand closest to the horse and loop the end of the rope from below up around the pastern.

11. Pass a loop above the ropes around the leg. Pull the loop toward you, give it a half twist and place it over the foot. The rope should be above and below the collar. This prevents the collar from slipping off when the horse struggles.

12. Wrap the remaining rope around the other three lines several times before tying it to the neck loop with a half hitch and slip knot. This wrapping back prevents the horse from stepping in the ropes or catching the horseshoer in them during a struggle. Pull the leg to the side and encourage the horse to resist. Shoeing may commence when the horse will let its leg hang resting against the ropes and stand relaxed on three legs.

Fig. 9-12. Steps in applying a scotch hobble without a pastern collar (from 1-12).

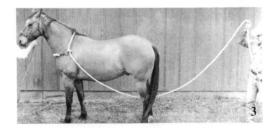

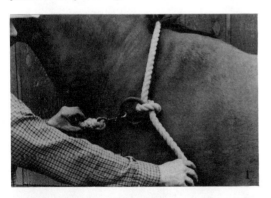

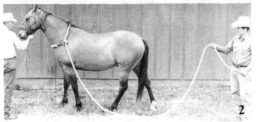

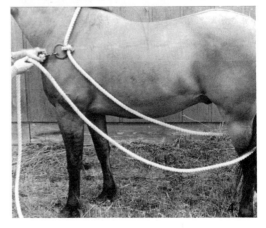

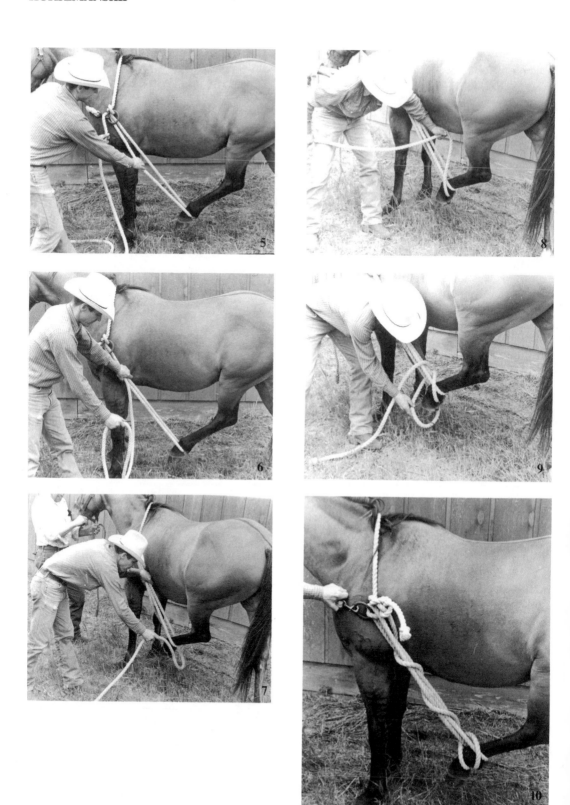

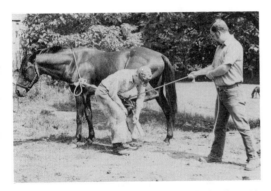

Fig. 9-13. Position for working on a hind foot tied up with a scotch hobble. Photo by G. Poellot.

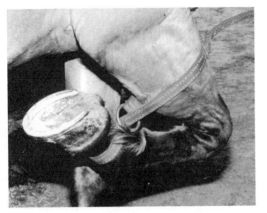

Fig. 9-14. Front leg tied up using a hobble strap. Photos by J. Graves.

Front Leg Strap

A leg strap is useful when a horse will not hold his front foot up for trimming or shoeing. A stirrup leather from an English saddle, nylon hobbles or two heavy nylon dog collars buckled together make a good front leg strap. A leg strap is especially good to use when nailing, to prevent a rough horse from dragging a freshly-driven nail through your leg before it can be turned or wrung off.

Leg straps must be put on high up the forearm and next to the foot. They must be tight. Once the horse discovers he can't take the foot at will and gives up, the strap can be removed. Many horses will give up in a very short time. The leg strap should not be left on for more than a few minutes at a time. Circulation might be impaired if the leg is left overflexed for very long.

Another type of front leg restraint can be made with a long rope tied to the pastern with a slip knot, and then passed over the withers and around

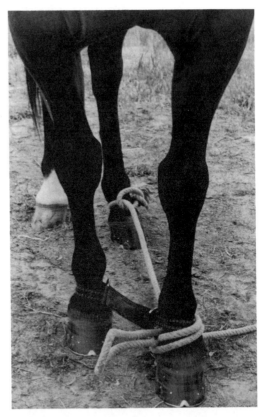

Fig. 9-15. Front legs hobbled with one hind leg tied to a front leg. This is useful in training horses that won't stand when a hind foot is raised. Apply this only in a clear area where the ground is soft.

the barrel of the horse. The end is tied around the pastern with a clove hitch. Still another can be made by lashing a rope around the pastern and forearm. The leather or nylon strap is a preferable method in most cases, especially when working alone.

Tying a Horse Down

There are several ways to throw a horse and tie it down to immobilize it sufficiently to permit shoeing. All of them require experienced help and are potentially dangerous to the horse and horseshoer. There are exceptions, but as a rule, the Author does not recommend any of them.

Throwing a horse and tying it down should always be considered a last resort and an undesirable solution. Try every way to shoe a horse standing up. If a bad horse must be shod, the horse should be tranquilized or immobilized by a veterinarian. Even then, it is safest to restrain the feet securely before commencing work.

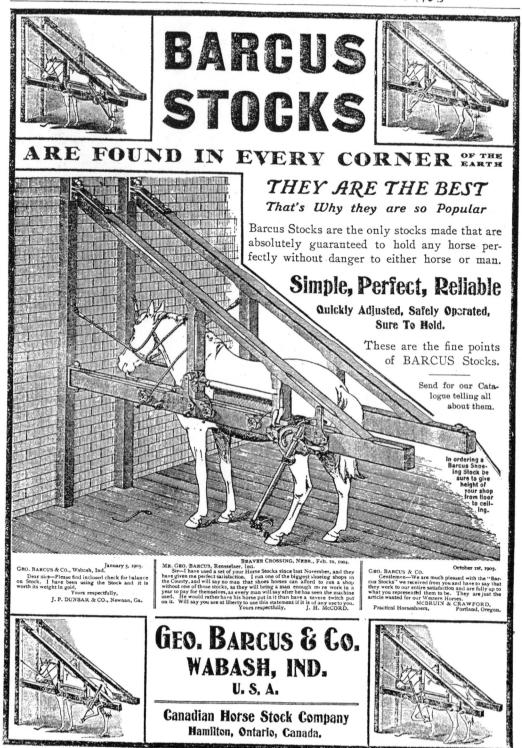

Fig. 9-16. An old ad for the popular Barcus shoeing stocks.
From The American Blacksmith, *Feb., 1905.*

References

Banner, S. 1973. Handling your horse for the shoer. The Western Horseman. (Aug.):70.

Barcus, G. 1905. Barcus Stocks. American Ironsmith. (Feb.):14.

Boy Scouts of America. 1979. Fieldbook. Boy Scouts of America, North Brunswick, NJ.

Eaton, E.O. 1967. Making Knots and Hitches with Rope. Cornell 4-H Club Bull. No. 88. N.Y. State College of Agri.

Fowler, M.E. 1978. Restraint and Handling of Wild and Domestic Animals. Iowa State University Press, Ames.

Freeman, J. 1968. Discipline when and how. The Western Horseman. (Nov.):94.

Leahy, J.R. and P. Barrow. 1953. Restraint of Animals (2nd ed.). Cornell Campus Store, Ithaca, NY.

Mackenzie, S. 1980. The leg restriction theory. The Western Horseman. (Apr.):12.

Magner, D. 1888. The Art of Taming and Educating the Horse. Review and Herald Publishing House, Battle Creek, MI.

Magner, D. 1899. ABC Guide to Sensible Horseshoeing. The Werner Co., Akron, OH.

McCalmont, J.R. 1959. Rope on the Farm. U.S.D.A. Bull. No. 2130.

Miller, R.W. 1975. Western Horse Behavior and Training. Doubleday and Co., Inc., Garden City, NY.

Nelson, B. 1980. Restraining horses. The Western Horseman. (Oct.):89.

Plymouth Cordage Co. 1946. Useful Knots and How to Tie Them.

Sabin, S.W. 1971. Catching and Leading Horses. Cornell 4-H Member's Guide M-4-19. N.Y. State College of Agri.

Sabin, S.W. 1971. Haltering and Tying Horses. Cornell 4-H Member's Guide M-4-17. N.Y. State College of Agri.

Spencer, D. 1967. Horse Breaking. The Western Horseman, Colorado Springs, CO.

Staff. 1966. Lanham Riley's method of haltering. The Western Horseman. (Jan):26.

Stambaugh, V.G. 1923. Breaking and Training Colts. U.S.D.A. Bull. No. 1368.

Ward, F.E. 1958. The Cowboy at Work. Hastings House, New York.

Wiseman, R.F. 1974. The Complete Horseshoeing Guide (2nd ed.). Univ. of Oklahoma Press, Norman.

NOTES:

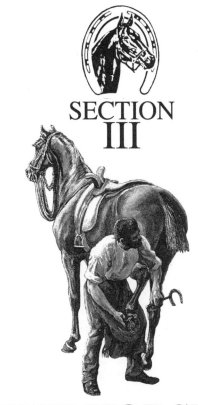

SECTION
III

THE HORSE'S
FOOT

Chapter 10

Bones And Joints

The Foot

The horse's foot is defined as the hoof and its contents. The structures of the foot may be divided into hoof, sensitive, elastic, tendon, ligament, bone and joint structures. The foot is the foundation of the horse. Each foot is uniquely designed to support weight, absorb shock, resist wear, replenish itself, provide traction, conduct moisture and assist in pumping venous blood. The foot must be healthy to operate at peak efficiency. It must be protected by proper care to remain sound. "No Foot, No Horse."

Need for Anatomy Study

Horseshoers need to have a working knowledge of the structure (anatomy) and function (physiology) of the horse's foot. Competent mechanics don't try to overhaul engines unless they know what the parts are and their functions. Horseshoers need to know the workings of the mechanism they overhaul even more so than mechanics. The foot is a *living* structure. Horseshoers perform surgery each time they shoe a horse. Veterinarians learn anatomy and physiology before they learn surgery.

Horseshoers must know where the structures of the foot are in relation to each other in order

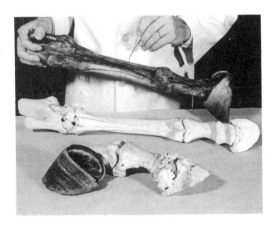

Fig. 10-1. Horseshoers should know as much about the anatomy of the foot and lower leg as a veterinarian. Photo by L. Sadler.

to safely remove horn from a normal or distorted foot, drive nails into it, or change weight distribution over a foot. Knowledge of structure and function is essential when shoeing lame horses. Horseshoers should be as familiar with the anatomy and physiology of the horse's foot as veterinarians.

Joseph Coleman, in his book *Pathological Horse Shoeing* published in 1876, said:

It is the duty of every horseshoer who aspires to superiority to acquire a correct, if not profound knowledge of the nature and functions of the structures he is called upon to operate, in order that:

1. He might then more intelligently cooperate with the owner of the horse or the veterinarian having a case in his charge.

2. He may justly be entitled to the confidence of his employer who may not be able to give any special instructions in the matter.

3. He may be able to distinguish between healthy and unhealthy conditions.

Commence your study of foot anatomy and physiology with these things in mind. Once you understand the anatomy, i.e., the character and position of the structures of the leg and foot and their relationship to each other, horseshoeing becomes simply a matter of applying "common sense" principles to create a desirable change by trimming or shoeing the hoof.

Learning the proper names of anatomical structures is an important part of anatomy study. It is very advantageous for a horseshoer to be able to talk to a veterinarian in scientific terms when discussing a lameness, foot disease, or shoeing problem. A knowledge of scientific terms as well as the common terms allows one to read veterinary literature with less difficulty and greater understanding. The opportunities for learning more about your profession are thereby increased. The Author has chosen to use the common terms wherever possible, since these are the terms most horsemen use. In some cases, however, only the scientific name will adequately describe the structure or condition.

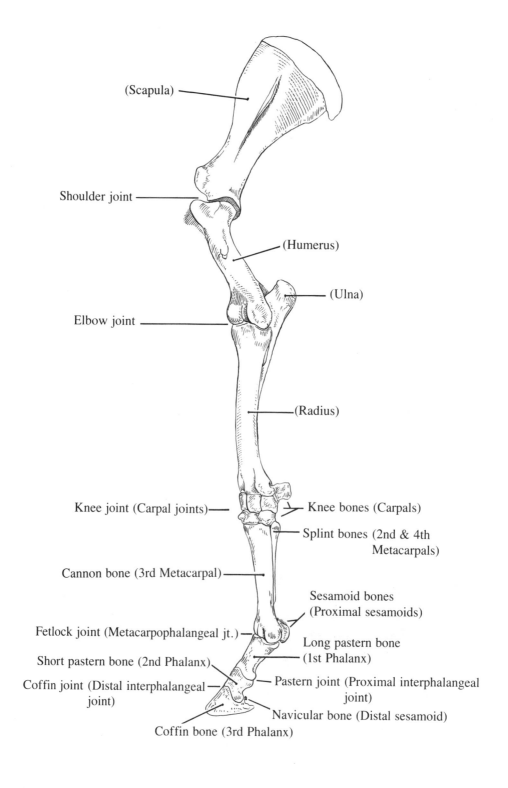

(Scapula)

Shoulder joint

(Humerus)

(Ulna)

Elbow joint

(Radius)

Knee joint (Carpal joints)

Knee bones (Carpals)

Splint bones (2nd & 4th Metacarpals)

Cannon bone (3rd Metacarpal)

Sesamoid bones (Proximal sesamoids)

Fetlock joint (Metacarpophalangeal jt.)

Long pastern bone (1st Phalanx)

Short pastern bone (2nd Phalanx)

Coffin joint (Distal interphalangeal joint)

Pastern joint (Proximal interphalangeal joint)

Navicular bone (Distal sesamoid)

Coffin bone (3rd Phalanx)

Fig. 10-2. Front limb bones and joints. Drawings by L. Sadler.

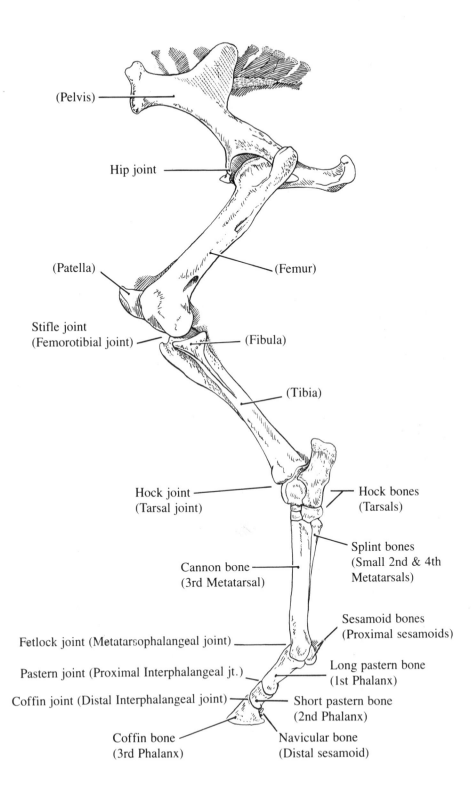

(Pelvis)

Hip joint

(Patella)

(Femur)

Stifle joint
(Femorotibial joint)

(Fibula)

(Tibia)

Hock joint
(Tarsal joint)

Hock bones
(Tarsals)

Splint bones
(Small 2nd & 4th
Metatarsals)

Cannon bone
(3rd Metatarsal)

Sesamoid bones
(Proximal sesamoids)

Fetlock joint (Metatarsophalangeal joint)

Long pastern bone
(1st Phalanx)

Pastern joint (Proximal Interphalangeal jt.)

Coffin joint (Distal Interphalangeal joint)

Short pastern bone
(2nd Phalanx)

Coffin bone
(3rd Phalanx)

Navicular bone
(Distal sesamoid)

Fig. 10-3. Hind limb bones and joints.

Differences Between Front and Hind Limbs

The horse has four limbs—one on each corner; two front and two hind. The front limbs carry about 60 percent of the horse's weight, the hind about 40 percent. The center of gravity of a horse is about 6 inches above and 6 inches behind its elbow. The front limbs mainly have a supporting function and "push down" when the horse moves. The hind limbs have more of a driving function and the horse "pushes off" them when moving.

The upper portion of the front and hind limbs have an entirely different structure from the knee end of the cannon bone up, but are essentially the same from that point down to the coffin bone. The common names are the same for the bones below the knee and hock joint. The scientific names are the same below the fetlock joint.

Other less obvious differences between a front and hind leg are the fact that a hind leg has a longer and thicker cannon bone, a larger lateral splint bone, and a more upright pastern bone than the front leg. A hind leg also has a more oval hoof and a more concave sole than the front leg.

Characteristics Common to All Bones of the Leg

Bone is not static. It is constantly remodeling itself in response to pressure from conformation, conditioning and diet. Unequal pressures or stresses on the bone column result in unequal growth and strength. It is essential that uniform weight bearing on the limb bones be achieved through regular trimming and shoeing of the hoof. Bone remodeling may take a natural and desirable form to strengthen a stressed area. Or, it may be unnatural and undesirable. Trauma may cause an increase in circulation and osteophyte (bony growth) formation. Pressure may cause a decrease in circulation and rarefaction (degeneration) of bone.

All bones of the leg have a fibrous sheath covering which surrounds and protects them called the periosteum. If this "bone skin" becomes torn, irritated, or bruised, periostitis or exostosis (bony growth projecting from the bone) is the result.

Exostosis is a result of the deposit of calcium and phosphorus by the body in an effort to strengthen the injured and consequently weakened area. This process is hastened by inflammation and the resulting increased circulation in the area. An exostosis usually appears as a hard lump on the leg. A horse may or may not be lame when an exostosis is present. Various common names have been given to these bony growths to identify their location.

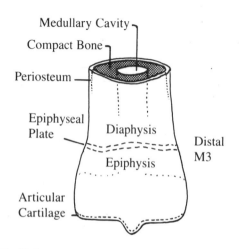

Fig. 10-4. Bone Terms.

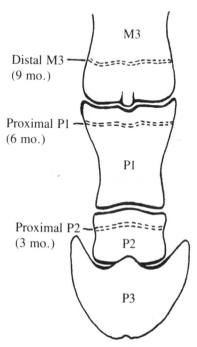

Fig. 10-5. Epiphyseal bone growth plates of the lower limb and approximate closure times.

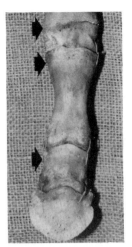
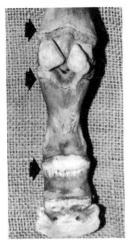

Fig. 10-6. Front and rear view of front leg bones of a young horse. Arrows point to epiphyseal plates. Photos by J. Graves.

A place where bone growth is generated is called a physis. Bones have a diaphysial region in the shaft of the bone and epiphyseal region on the ends of the bone. A physis is influenced by endogenous and exogenous factors. Endogenous factors are from within the body such as genetic makeup and hormones. Exogenous factors are from outside the body such as diet or trimming.

All long bones of the young horse's leg have an epiphyseal cartilage plate near their ends. These areas proliferate bone cells and cause the bone to grow in length. The growth pattern of the leg can be affected by the distribution of weight on the cartilage. Trimming or the lack of it may affect the straightness of the limbs up until the time the epiphyseal plates close.

Epiphysitis may be caused by uneven weight distribution on the plates or an unbalanced diet. Excess feeding of high grain rations to hasten growth of young animals supplies an excess of phosphorus and a deficiency of calcium. This causes an epiphysitis that may be reversible if the ration is improved when the condition first occurs.

The legs of very young foals may be straightened by a process called epiphyseal stapling. One side of the cartilage plate is prevented from moving and the other is allowed to grow at the normal rate until the leg is straight. The staple(s) is then removed. The maturity of race and per-

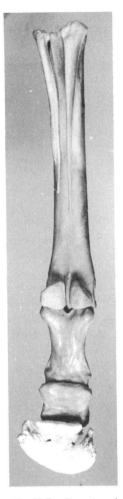
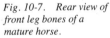

Fig. 10-7. Rear view of front leg bones of a mature horse.

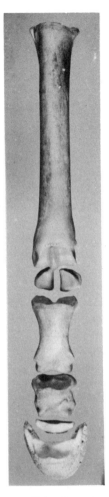

Fig. 10-8. Front view of hind leg bones of a mature horse.

formance horses may be determined by radiographs (x-ray pictures) of the epiphyseal line(s).

Epiphyseal closure times for the lower limb bones have a wide range but the following averages should be memorized:

Proximal Short Pastern bone (P2)	3 mo.
Proximal Long Pastern bone (P1)	6 mo.
Distal Cannon bone (M3)	9 mo.
Distal Tibia	8 mo.
Distal Radius	24 mo.

Cannon Bone

The cannon bone is located just below the knee and has the bones of the knee bearing on it.

The front cannon bone is oval-shaped and flat

in front. The hind cannon bone is thicker and longer than the front one. It is somewhat rounded in shape and slightly pointed in front.

The function of the cannon bone is to support and bear weight. It is subjected to a terrific amount of stress. No man-made structure of similar proportion could withstand the force placed on it at speed.

The cannon bone is remodeled by the body according to the stress that is placed upon it. This condition is very noticeable when viewing a cross section of the bone. Usually, the inside of the bone is thickest. However, a crooked leg or foot could cause the outside of the bone to be thicker. The inside or medial joint surface of the distal end of the cannon bone is always the widest.

The cannon bone also functions as a lever. The relationship between the length of the cannon and the length of the pastern bones has been shown to affect the speed of horses. A relatively short cannon in relation to a long pastern seems to be the most desirable combination in terms of creating leverage for speed and reducing concussion to the upper legs.

The symptoms of shin buck (bucked shins or shin splints) are the result of irritated or torn periosteum on the front of the cannon bone. These are usually associated with a hairline fracture of the cannon bone. It is due to poor conditioning coupled with overexertion.

Splint Bones (2)

The splint bones are located on either side and in back of the cannon bone. Their upper ends form part of the bearing surface of the knee. When the foal is born, the splint bones are not attached to the cannon bone by bone but by ligaments (interosseous ligaments). The splint bones usually fuse naturally to the cannon bone by the time the horse reaches the age of six.

The splint bones are shaped like long drawn-out triangles or icicles and have small nodules on the pointed ends. Occasionally, the distal ends of these bones are fractured.

The function of the splint bones is to protect the tendons and ligaments and especially the blood vessels and nerves which pass down the back of the leg. They also provide a greater bearing surface for weight by supporting a portion of the carpal bones of the knee joint. They are necessary, not vestigial.

The inside splint bone usually bears more weight than the outside splint bone. The inside splint bone supports a portion of two of the carpal bones of the knee while the outside bone only supports a portion of one. An inside bone can be easily distinguished because it has two

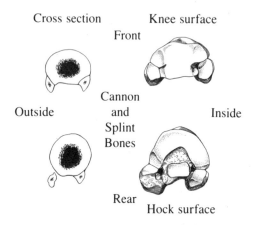

Fig. 10-9. Cross-section of front and hind cannon bones compared to knee and hock joint surfaces of front and hind cannon and splint bones. Drawing by L. Sadler.

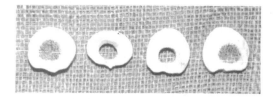

Fig. 10-10. Cross-section of cannon bones showing the effect of unequal weight distribution. Photos by J. Graves.

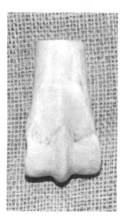
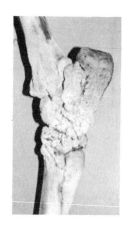

Fig. 10-11. Distal end of the cannon bone showing the larger medial surface (left) and extensive exostosis in a hock joint (right).

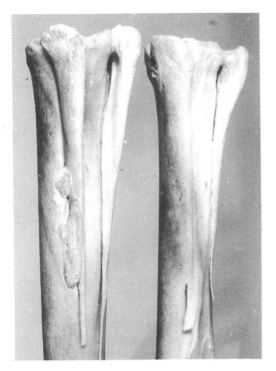

Fig. 10-12. "Splint" from a young horse (left) and naturally fused splint and cannon bone from an older horse (right). Photo by G. Poellot.

facets or bearing surfaces and an outside bone has but one. The increased stress on the inside bone is a contributing factor in causing the appearance of "splints" to be more common on the inside of the leg. The outside splint bone of the hind leg is much larger than the inside one.

"Splints" are hard bumps formed by an exostosis between the splint bone and the cannon bone. The irritation of the periosteum caused by the movement of the splint bone against the cannon bone due to the sprain or rupture of the interosseous ligament causes a periostitis which results in an exostosis on the bone in the damaged area. If the irritation remains, the bony growth will continue to enlarge until the irritation ceases or the exostosis immobilizes the irritation. Once splints are "set" or quit growing they are usually considered blemishes.

Sesamoid Bones (2)

The sesamoid bones are located at the back of the fetlock joint next to the cannon bone.

The sesamoids are shaped like small pyramids. They are held in place by many ligaments.

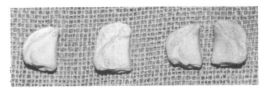

Fig. 10-13. Normal sesamoid bone (far left) and bones showing sesamoiditis (right). Photos by J. Graves.

Occasionally one of the ligaments is torn. This is commonly called a "popped" sesamoid. An inflammation of these bones is called sesamoiditis. Sometimes, these small bones fracture as a result of a heavy blow or severe strain.

The function of the sesamoid bones is to act as a fulcrum for the ligaments and tendons which support and move the leg. The sesamoids also create a larger surface for rotation of the fetlock joint and thereby strengthen the position of the cannon bone in the joint. They may be compared to the bridge on a stringed instrument. There is a great deal of strain on them.

Long Pastern Bone

The long pastern bone is located between the fetlock joint and the pastern joint.

It is shaped somewhat like the cannon bone but is much shorter, usually about one-third the length of the cannon on an ideally proportioned horse.

The function of the pastern is to increase the flexibility of the fetlock joint and thereby reduce concussion. The length, flexibility, and angle or slope of the pasterns strongly influence the smoothness of a horse's gait. The angle and

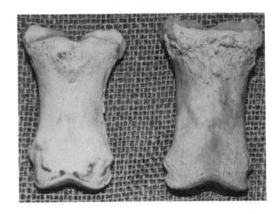

Fig. 10-14. Normal Long pastern bone (left) and bone showing an osselet (right).

flexibility of the shoulder and arm also determine smoothness of gait. A few degrees difference in angle may make a great difference in the desirability of the gait.

Horses with relatively long pasterns and short cannons are more desirable as speed horses because of the possibility of increased leverage this structure creates. However, very long and very sloping pasterns are an undesirable weakness which increases the probability of occurrence of bowed tendons and other unsoundness.

Exostosis of the proximal end of the long pastern bone (on the front of the fetlock joint) is called an osselet. Osselets are most often caused by trauma produced during hyperextension of the fetlock joint.

Fractures of long pastern bones are called screw driver fractures. Most of them go through the groove in the proximal end of the bone. It appears that the bone was pried apart by the ridge on the distal end of the cannon bone.

Short Pastern Bone

The short pastern bone is located between the long pastern bone and the coffin bone and is one of the bones which makes up the coffin joint in the foot. Approximately one-half of the short pastern bone is encased within the hoof.

The short pastern bone is nearly cube-shaped. The shape of its ends are rounded in such a manner that they allow the foot to twist or move from side-to-side in order to adjust to uneven ground. The short pastern bone may fracture if violently twisted. This occasionally happens in the hind feet of cutting and reining horses.

Exostosis located on either the short or long pastern bone, and not involving a joint, is called false ringbone. It is usually caused by a severe blow to the affected area. High ringbone is located around the pastern joint. Low ringbone is

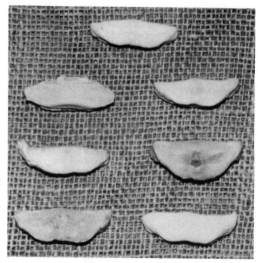

Fig. 10-16. Navicular bones. Normal (top) and various types of exostosis and rarefaction.

located around the coffin joint. Ringbone is also referred to as interarticular (between the joints) and periarticular (around the joints).

Navicular Bone

The navicular bone is located between and underneath the short pastern and coffin bone. It is part of the coffin joint.

The navicular bone acts as a fulcrum for the deep flexor tendon which passes directly under it and attaches to the semilunar crest of the coffin bone.

The navicular bone is somewhat boat-shaped and comparatively very thin. Its blood supply is quite limited and subject to ischemia due to blood vessel constriction.

The location of the navicular bone makes it very susceptible to injury. Not only is it compressed by the pastern against the taut deep flexor tendon during movement, but it is easily bruised and occasionally punctured because of its position over the center of the bottom of the hoof.

This bone may suffer from osteophyte formation as a result of concussion or rarefaction as a result of compression. Problems in this area are called navicular disease.

Coffin Bone

The coffin bone is completely encased within the hoof or "box" of horn. It has no epiphysis and ossifies from the center.

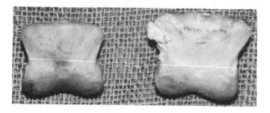

Fig. 10-15. Normal short pastern bone (left) and bone showing high ringbone (right).

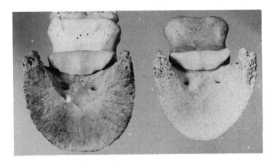

Fig. 10-17. The shape of the hoof is determined by the shape of the coffin bone. Front foot (left), hind foot (right). Photo by G. Poellot.

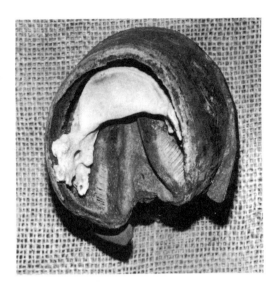

Fig. 10-19. Coffin bone in hoof showing ossification of the lateral cartilages or sidebone.

The shape of the hoof is determined by the shape of the coffin bone. As a rule, the front feet have rounded, flattened, and wide coffin bones; the hind feet have pointed, comparatively steep, and narrow coffin bones. The round front foot encourages the horse to breakover in the center of the toe. The narrow hind foot allows the horse to turn with ease from side to side.

The shape of the last one-third of the hoof in the heel region is not determined by the coffin bone since the lateral cartilages attach to the "wings" of the coffin bone and extend into the heel area. Ossified lateral cartilages are called side bones.

A principal function of the coffin bone is to provide for the attachment and protection of blood vessels and nerves. The circulating blood forms a "hydraulic cushion" between the bone and hoof during the weight bearing phase of locomotion. The coffin bone is extremely porous and thus it is very fragile and subject to fracture.

The coffin bone is also the point of attachment for the tendons that move the lower leg. The main (common or long) extensor tendon has its principal insertion in the extensor process of the coffin bone. The deep flexor tendon has its insertion in the semilunar crest of the coffin bone.

The coffin bone may become irritated due to unequal weight bearing, pressure or trauma and develop pedal osteitis. The coffin bone (especially the front) naturally has a slight notch ("toe stay") in the toe. This is filled with horn and is thought to prevent twisting of the bone in the hoof. However, hammered down clips, close nails or infection may cause abnormal notching or pedal osteitis that can be seen in radiographs.

Characteristics Common to All Joints of the Leg

The function of joints is to bear weight and allow for movement. The general structure of all of the joints of the horse's leg is quite similar. The joints are enclosed by the capsular ligament and are bound together by various ligaments. A joint capsule may be thought of as a balloon full of grease between two bones.

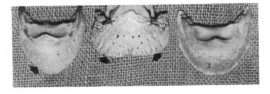

Fig. 10-18. Normal coffin bone (right) and bones showing pedal osteitis (left). Note deformities at arrows. Photos by J. Graves.

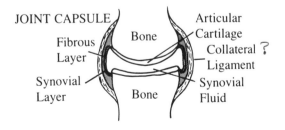

Fig. 10-20. Simple hinge joint showing the capsular ligament.

The interior of the capsular ligament or side of the joint capsule forms the synovial membrane which produces the "joint oil" called synovial fluid. The joint capsule is filled with this fluid and it lubricates the articular cartilages on the ends of the bones and thus decreases friction between articulating bone surfaces. The natural reaction of the synovial membrane is to increase the production of synovial fluid when the joint is injured and inflamed. The general term for this condition is arthritis.

Normally, the articular cartilages are smooth and slippery. There is less friction between them than ice sliding on ice. However, the articular surfaces may become eroded. This process may be caused by excess body weight, unequal weight distribution, abnormal movements or gait, trauma, excessive corticosteriod injections and degenerative joint disease. Eventually the joint surfaces may become dry and ankylosis (fusing of a joint) takes place.

Synovial fluid is made up of a dialysate of blood plasma and a mucopolysaccharide called hyaluronic acid. The viscosity (resistance to flow) of joint fluid increases exponentially with an increasing concentration of hyaluronic acid. Synovial oil also lubricates tendon bursas and tendon sheaths.

There are three kinds of joints in the limbs. The fetlock is an example of a ginglymus or hinge joint. It moves in two directions only. The coffin and knee (carpus) are examples of arthrodial or plane joints. The hip and shoulder joints are examples of enarthrodial or ball and socket joints.

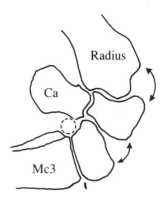

Fig. 10-22. Knee flexion. The most distal joint does not open.

Knee Joint

The knee or carpus is actually made up of seven bones and three joints. It is composed of two rows of bones. There are usually seven bones present. Rarely there are eight. The horse's knee corresponds in structure to the wrist of man. The "true" knee of the horse is the stifle joint.

The radius (large bone of the forearm) articulates with the radial, intermediate, ulnar, and accessory carpals to form the radiocarpal joint. The accessory carpal is a large sesamoid bone located at the back of the joint. It does not bear weight. The other three carpal bones of the upper row bear weight.

The intercarpal joint is formed between the two rows of carpals. The radial, intermediate, and ulnar carpals of the upper row articulate with the second, third and fourth carpals of the bottom row.

The carpometacarpal joint is formed between the first (when present), second, third and fourth

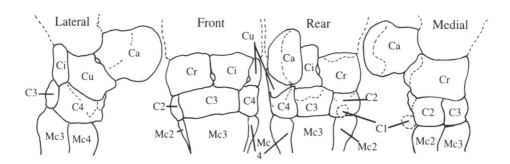

Fig. 10-21. Knee joint. Lateral, front, rear, and medial views.

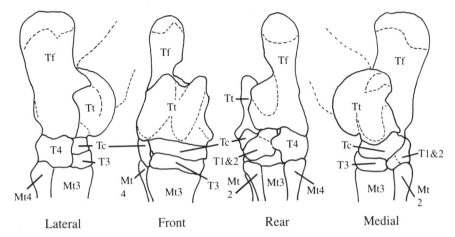

Fig. 10-23. Hock joint. Lateral, front, rear, and medial views.

| Lateral | Front | Rear | Medial |

carpals and the cannon bone (large or third metacarpal) and the splint bones (small or second and fourth metacarpals). This joint does not open. It communicates (has fluid in common) with the intercarpal joint.

The first carpal bone is a small round bone located on the inside (behind) of the carpal joint when it is present. It is absent in all but a few horses and does not bear any weight.

The carpal bones move in several directions when weight is placed upon them. As a group, they compress and bounce back each time a load is placed on and removed from them. This, combined with the hydraulic shock absorbing qualities of the synovial fluid of the joint, makes the normal knee very efficient in reducing shock.

Race horses and other performance horses are subject to frequent knee injuries. Slab fractures occur on the front of the knee. They are most common in calf-kneed horses. Carpitis or "popped" knee can develop into a sizable exostosis, sometimes called knee spavin.

Hock Joint

The hock or tarsus of the hind leg corresponds in position to the knee of the front leg of the horse. The hock is similar in structure and positional function to the ankle joint of man. It is located between the tibia and the cannon and splint bones.

The hock is composed of six bones. The tibial tarsal bone articulates with the tibia and the fibular tarsal bone. This is the main articulation

of the hock. It is slanted to allow the upper leg to go out and around the barrel of the horse.

The fibular tarsal or calcaneus is the long bone which forms the outside and point of the hock. It forms a groove on the inside of the hock that acts as a fulcrum and track for the deep flexor tendon. The point of the fibular tarsal bone acts as a lever arm for the attachment of the powerful muscles of the gaskin. The superficial flexor tendon also attaches here.

A "false" (inconstant) bursa under the skin may cover the portion of the superficial flexor tendon which passes over and attaches to the tip of this bone when capped hock is present.

A ligament which runs from the tip of the fibular tarsal to the outside splint bone is called the plantar ligament. Curb is the name given to the sprain of this ligament.

The central tarsal is located beneath the tibial tarsal and fibular tarsal bones. Bone spavin (ex-

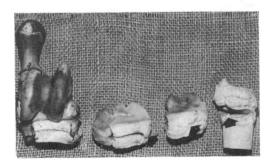

Fig. 10-24. Normal hock joint (left) with bone spavins indicated by arrows. Photos by J. Graves.

ostosis in the hock) rarely occurs in this area but is considered very bad when it does.

The central tarsal bone articulates with the third tarsal, the fused first and second tarsals (inside and back) and the fourth tarsal (on outside). Spavin is common at this level on the inside of the hock. The central tarsal may be fused to the others in some spavin cases.

The third tarsal, the first and second tarsal, and the fourth tarsal articulate with the cannon bone (third metatarsal) and splint bones (second and fourth metatarsals). Spavin also occurs in this area, especially between the third tarsal and the cannon bone.

The movement of the bones in the hock joint is much more limited than that of the knee but the angle of partial flexion of the joint prevents severe concussion except in animals which are post-legged (very straight) or sickle-hocked (very crooked).

The general name for exostosis in the hock is bone (jack) spavin. Distention of the hock joint capsule is called bog spavin. Distention of the deep flexor tendon sheath at the hock is called a thoroughpin. Hard stopping and fast working horses are susceptible to these conditions.

NOTE: Horseshoeing of a corrective or therapeutic nature has little direct effect on the knee or hock of the horse but is often useful when applied in combination with veterinary medical treatment. (See Chapters 35 and 36.)

Fetlock Joint

The fetlock joint is located between and forms an angle with the cannon bone and the long pastern bone. The cannon bone, the two sesamoid bones, and the long pastern bone make up the joint.

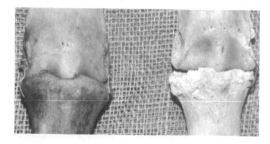

Fig. 10-25. The fetlock can move in two directions only. Normal fetlock joint (left), an osselet on the front of the fetlock joint (right).

The fetlock is a true or perfect hinge joint. It moves in two directions only. It is supported by many ligaments, the largest of which is the suspensory ligament. The tongue and groove arrangement of this joint prevents twisting of the lower leg and stabilizes the foot in motion. It also limits any change that can be made to the upper limb by hoof manipulation.

The function of the fetlock is to absorb shock and bear weight. The fetlock joint is subjected to great stress at high speed. Slow motion pictures reveal that the fetlock nearly touches the ground when the horse is fatigued during the latter part of a race. This kind of stress often causes a sprain of one of the ligaments in this area. However, a "springy" fetlock is very desirable for riding comfort and contributes to the soundness of the horse.

An exostosis which develops in the dorsal fetlock area is called an osselet. Distention of the fetlock joint capsule is called articular windpuff or articular windgall.

Pastern Joint

The pastern joint is located between the long and short pastern bones.

The pastern joint is an imperfect hinge joint since it moves in two directions mainly but does have a slight degree of movement from side-to-side. This joint is not as flexible as the coffin joint. In fact, it can be considered immovable in a biomechanical model.

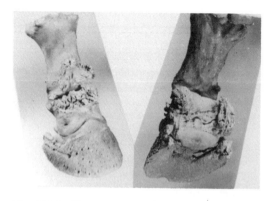

Fig. 10-26. The pastern joint has very limited motion. High ringbone at the pastern joint (left).

Fig. 10-27. The coffin joint is located within the hoof. Extensive exostosis of the coffin joint including low ringbone, pedal osteitis and navicular disease (right).

The function of the pastern joint is to absorb shock and adjust to uneven terrain and twisting movements of the horse's feet. The limited movement and position of this joint make it susceptible to sprains and joint lamenesses. Exostosis in the area of the pastern joint is called high ringbone.

Coffin Joint

The coffin joint is located within the hoof between the short pastern and coffin bones. The navicular bone also makes up part of this joint.

The coffin joint is a very flexible imperfect hinge joint and as such allows considerable side-to-side movement. This makes it possible for the horse to stand and move comfortably on uneven ground.

Another function of the coffin joint is to absorb concussion. The position of the navicular bone makes it possible for a great deal of concussion from the short pastern bone to be transferred to it and its suspensory ligament and therefore away from the fragile coffin bone. The navicular bone also functions as a fulcrum to aid the deep flexor in flexing the extended leg.

Exostosis in the coffin joint is called low ringbone. Often the navicular bone becomes affected. Navicular disease usually begins as a bursitis in the navicular bursa between the deep flexor tendon and navicular bone. However, in its late stages, it may involve the other bones of the joint. Likewise, advanced cases of low ringbone may involve the navicular bone.

References

Adams, O.R. 1974. Lameness in Horses (3rd ed.). Lea and Febiger, Philadelphia.

Bradley, O.C. and T. Grahame. 1946. The Topographical Anatomy of the Limbs of the Horse (2nd ed.). W. Green and Son, Ltd., Edinburgh, SCOTLAND.

Coleman, J.B. 1876. Pathological Horse-Shoeing. Coleman and Fish, Chicago.

Frandson, R.D. 1974. Anatomy and Physiology of Farm Animals (2nd ed.). Lea and Febiger, Philadelphia.

Gillette, E.L., D.E. Thrall and J.L. Lebel. 1977. Carlson's Veterinary Radiology (3rd ed.). Lea and Febiger, Philadelphia.

Hoover, R. 1965. Farrier Science. Hoover, San Luis Obispo, CA.

Rooney, J.R. 1974. The Lame Horse. A.J. Barnes and Co., Cranbury, NJ.

Sisson, S. and J.D. Grossman. 1953. The Anatomy of the Domestic Animals (4th ed.). Saunders, Philadelphia.

NOTES:

THE HORSE'S FOOT

Chapter 11

Tendons and Ligaments

Characteristics of Tendons and Ligaments

Tendons and ligaments are made of strong, cord-like fibers and are either cable or sheetlike in shape. Tendons connect muscles to bones, glide in lubricated sheaths and are totally inelastic. The function of tendons is mainly movement of the body. Ligaments connect bones to bones and generally are more elastic than tendons. The function of ligaments is mainly support of the body and its parts.

There are no functional muscles below the knee or hock of the horse, so the long tendons allow the muscles of the upper leg to move the foot and leg by "remote control." The origin of a tendon is proximal where the muscle mass attaches to bone. The insertion is distal where the tendon attaches to the bone(s) that moves.

Tendons "bow" when the tendon tears or ruptures. In severe cases, the tendon sheath and ligament attachments of the tendon sheath also rupture. When tendons are strained, stretched or ruptured, the chances for complete recovery without hampering scar tissue are very low.

Ligaments may be torn or sprained. A "sprain" usually refers to a condition where the ligaments are stretched or torn but the bones are not dislocated (luxated). The word "strain" is usually used to describe excessive stretching or rupturing of muscles and/or tendons.

Bursae are small, lubricating, sac-like cushions containing synovial fluid which are located between the two opposing surfaces of a bone prominence and a tendon. When a bursa be-

comes injured and inflamed, the condition is called bursitis. Navicular bursitis, a form of navicular disease, is an inflammation of the bursa between the deep flexor tendon and the navicular bone. A "false" bursa or bruise under the skin (subcutaneous) is formed in the capped elbow (shoe boil) and capped hock conditions.

Synovial sheaths lubricate and protect tendons when they must travel long distances over a bone or other tendons or ligaments. The synovial sheath is a closed synovial fluid-filled sac around a tendon. An inflammation of a synovial sheath is called synovitis (also tenosynovitis, vaginitis, and peritendinitis). Tendinous windpuff, at the fetlock joint, is a common mild synovitis. If both the tendon and the synovial sheath are involved, it is called tendosynovitis. The synovial sheath of the superficial flexor tendon is involved in most cases of bowed tendon(s).

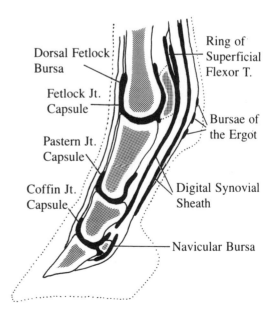

Fig. 11-2.   Bursae and tendon sheaths of the lower leg.

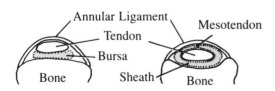

Fig. 11-1.   Cross-section of a bursa and a tendon sheath.

109

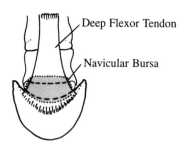

Fig. 11-3. The navicular bursa in relation to the deep flexor tendon viewed from the bottom.

Deep Flexor Tendon

The deep (digital) flexor tendon attaches to the semilunar crest of the coffin bone and folds (flexes) the leg as the deep flexor muscles contract and pull the tendon over the fulcrum points formed by the navicular and sesamoid bones. The deep flexor muscle mass is the largest of the flexor tendons and is formed by several muscles in both the front and hind leg.

The navicular bursa is located between the deep flexor and the navicular bone.

Superficial Flexor Tendon

The superficial (digital) flexor tendon passes down the back of the leg and divides (bifurcates) below the fetlock and attaches to the bottom end of the long pastern and the upper end of the short pastern bone at the pastern joint. It passes over and forms a ring or collar around the deep flexor tendon at the sesamoids. The sesamoid bones act as a fulcrum to assist the tendons in their flexing action.

The superficial flexor of the hind leg functions mainly as a ligament in the "stay apparatus" of the limb (See Chapter 12). The flexor tendon runs through the center of a small muscle mass from the back of the femur and attaches to the point of the hock. Below the hock there is no muscular effect on the tendon. It acts entirely as a ligament.

The superficial flexor tendon of the front leg frequently develops tendinitis or bowed tendon in race horses. The hind legs are rarely affected. Traditionally, one-fourth of all horses retired from racing have been afflicted with bowed tendon(s).

Main Extensor Tendon

The common (digital) extensor tendon of the front leg is essentially the same below the knee as the long (digital) extensor of the hind leg is below the hock. It passes down over the front and slightly to the leg's outside and attaches to the long pastern, short pastern, and coffin bone. The widest point of attachment is on the extensor process of the coffin bone. The main extensor tendon is joined on each side of the pastern by branches of the suspensory ligament. The main extensor extends the leg.

Lateral Extensor Tendon

The lateral extensor assists the common extensor in extending the front leg and the long extensor in extending the hind leg. The lateral (digital) extensor tendon is anatomically different in the front and the hind legs of the horse.

The lateral extensor tendon of the front leg normally runs separately but parallel to the common extensor. It is attached (inserted) on the upper end of the outside surface of the long pastern bone just below the fetlock joint.

The lateral extensor tendon of the hind leg is variable but usually joins the long extensor tendon just below the hock. In some cases, it may form an insertion on the long pastern bone as it does in the front leg.

The portion of the lateral extensor tendon of the hind leg(s) which passes over the hock is sometimes surgically removed from horses afflicted with the stringhalt condition.

Check Ligaments

There are three check ligaments which function to prevent excessive muscle strain by overextension of the flexors and to assist the suspensory and other ligaments to form the stay apparatus of the limbs. Check ligaments are really part of tendons.

The **radial check ligament** is located above the knee and connects the superficial flexor tendon to the radius about one-third of the way up the bone from the proximal carpal joint.

The **subcarpal check ligament** is located below the knee and connects the deep flexor tendon to the carpal bones at the bottom of the knee. It is the thickest and most pronounced of the check

Front Leg

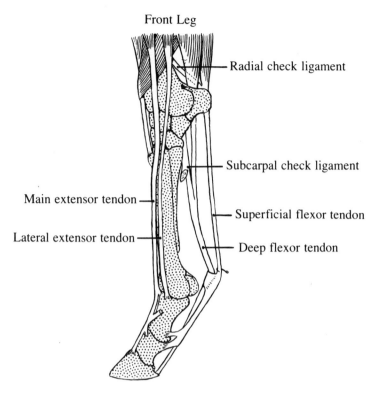

Radial check ligament

Subcarpal check ligament

Main extensor tendon

Superficial flexor tendon

Lateral extensor tendon

Deep flexor tendon

Fig. 11-4. Tendons and check ligaments of the front leg.
Drawings by L. Sadler.

Outside views

Hind Leg

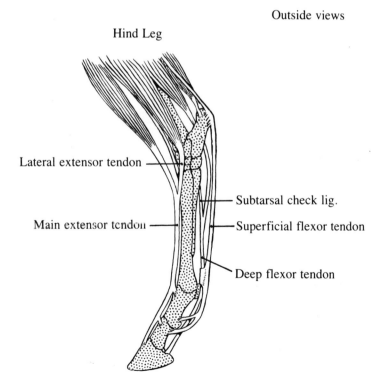

Lateral extensor tendon

Subtarsal check lig.

Main extensor tendon

Superficial flexor tendon

Deep flexor tendon

Fig. 11-5. Tendons and check ligaments of the hind leg.

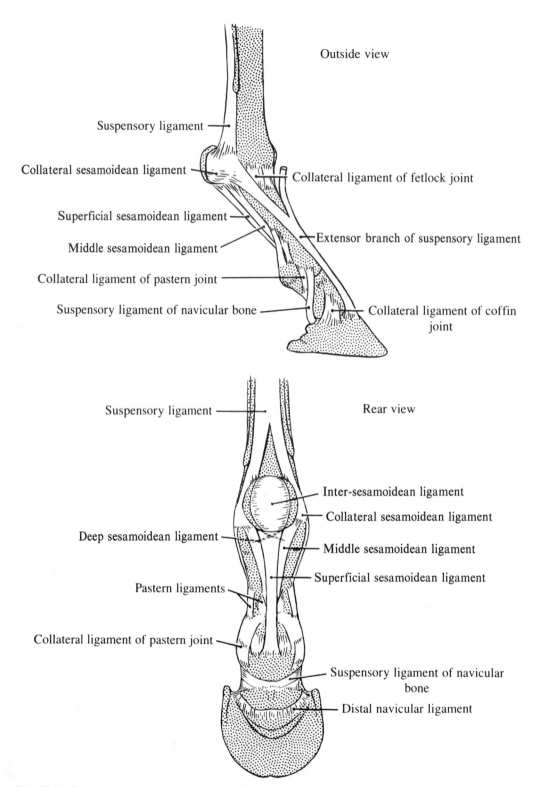

Fig. 11-6. Suspensory, sesamoidean and pastern liga-
ments of the lower right leg. The annular ligaments and
tendons have been removed.

ligaments. It is most frequently sprained in hunters and jumpers. Occasionally, it is injured in draft horses used in pulling contests.

The **subtarsal check ligament** is located below the hock and connects the deep flexor tendon of the hind leg to the tarsal bones at the bottom of the hock joint. It is the thinnest of the check ligaments and is occasionally absent in horses. It is usually not present in mules.

There is no check ligament on the superficial flexor tendon in the hind leg. The tendon of the superficial flexor passes over and attaches to the point of the hock and connects to the back of the femur above the stifle joint. It has very little muscle mass and so mainly functions in its entirety as a part of the stay apparatus of the hind limb.

Check ligaments are rarely sprained except in cases of bad tendon bows and heavy draft (pulling).

Suspensory Ligament

The suspensory ligament is the largest ligament in the leg. It originates from its main attachment at the upper end of the cannon bone. The wide flattened oval-shaped ligament runs down the back of the cannon bone and divides (bifurcates) just above the nodules on the ends of the splint bones. Each branch then divides again, and portions join to the sides and top of the sesamoid bones. The largest portion of each of the divided branches attaches to the top of each sesamoid, and the smaller portions pass forward and down to join the common or long extensor tendon at about the level of the pastern joint.

The main function of the suspensory ligament is to support and prevent "oversettling" (hyperextension) of the fetlock. It relieves stress from the flexor tendons. The suspensory ligament absorbs concussion and gives impulsion to flexor tendon movements. The sesamoid ligaments are a vital part of the functioning of the suspensory ligament. The suspensory and the sesamoidean ligaments are important components of the stay apparatus of the limb. The stay apparatus allows the animal to rest his limb muscles or "sleep" while standing.

The suspensory ligament possesses some elasticity. It is composed of mainly tendinous fibrous tissue; however, it also contains a variable amount of striped muscular tissue, especially visible in foals and yearlings. The suspensory is sometimes called the interosseous muscle or tendon.

The suspensory ligament is not sprained as often as tendons are bowed. A sprain or rupture of the suspensory ligament varies in degree of severity. In the hind leg it is often called "breaking down" or "run down." It usually occurs above the fetlock, however, it can occur below the sesamoids or at the knee. Sprains of the suspensory ligament often involve the sesamoid bones since they are so strongly attached to the ligament. Common causes of sprains are fatigue (usually from lack of conditioning when racing), and uneven ground surface when traveling at speed.

Sesamoidean Ligaments

There are many sesamoidean ligaments. They join the sesamoid and pastern bones. The sesamoidean ligaments support the sesamoid bones and aid in supporting the fetlock joint.

The **superficial sesamoidean ligament** is the largest of the sesamoidean ligaments and may be considered a continuation of the suspensory ligament. It vertically connects the bottom surface of the sesamoid bones to the fibrocartilage of the rear upper third of the short pastern bone. The superficial sesamoidean ligament is primarily responsible for the rigidity of the pastern joint. This ligament is sometimes called the straight or Y ligament due to its shape.

The **middle sesamoidean ligament** lies beneath the superficial. It vertically joins the bottom of the sesamoid bones to a wide surface area of the long pastern bone. This ligament is sometimes called the oblique or V ligament due to its shape.

The **deep sesamoidean ligaments** lie beneath the middle. They obliquely join the adjacent lower corners of the sesamoid bones to the upper edge of the long pastern bone. They cannot be palpated and can only be seen if the fetlock joint is opened. These ligaments are sometimes called cruciate or X ligaments due to their shape.

The **short sesamoidean ligaments** join the outer lower borders of the sesamoid bones to the upper edge of the long pastern bone. They are not visible unless the joint is opened and are of little consequence.

The **collateral sesamoidean ligaments** horizontally join and stabilize the sesamoids to the distal end of the cannon and the proximal end of the long pastern bones.

The **inter-sesamoidean ligament** horizontally joins the sesamoid bones and forms a groove for the flexor tendons to glide in. This ligament is very thick and strong.

Sesamoidean ligaments are sprained when a horse overextends or twists the fetlock and often accompany a sprained suspensory ligament. A sprain of any of these ligaments is commonly called a "popped" sesamoid. This is usually the result of fatigue and an uneven track surface.

Pastern Ligaments

The pastern ligaments support the pastern joint along with the superficial sesamoidean ligaments on the back of the pastern joint. There are two pairs of them. Those nearer the center of the bone are called axial. Those farthest away from the center are called abaxial. The pastern ligaments are occasionally sprained and inflamed.

Annular Ligaments

Annular ligaments are fibrous sheets or bands which pass around the circumference of a bone or joint and hold a tendon(s) in place. There are three below the knee and hock on each leg. They are the *volar* (front leg) or *plantar* (hind leg) sometimes called palmar, *proximal digital*, and *distal digital annular ligaments*.

The volar or plantar (palmar) annular ligament holds the flexor tendons in the sesamoid groove at the fetlock joint. A portion of the volar annular ligament may be severed or surgically removed in an operation for bowed tendon(s) in order to allow the scar tissue of a "low bow" to move without constriction.

Capsular Ligaments

Capsular ligaments are those which surround a joint. The inner layer of these ligaments produces the synovial or joint fluid. The outer layer is fibrous and contains the fluid in the joint. Puncture of the capsular ligament can produce a dry joint and ankylosis (fusing of joint). Excessive strain on the joint can produce a distention of the capsular ligament, which is commonly called windpuff (articular) at the fetlock, and bog spavin at the hock.

Collateral Ligaments

Collateral ligaments are flat cord-like ligaments on the sides of joints which bind the bones of the leg together. Those in the pastern and foot area are sometimes sprained as a result of working a fatigued horse on uneven ground or trimming the foot out of balance.

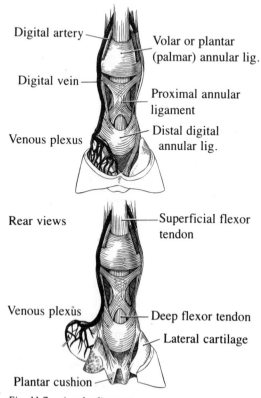

Digital artery
Digital vein
Venous plexus
Volar or plantar (palmar) annular lig.
Proximal annular ligament
Distal digital annular lig.

Rear views
Venous plexus
Superficial flexor tendon
Deep flexor tendon
Lateral cartilage
Plantar cushion

Fig. 11-7. Annular ligaments.

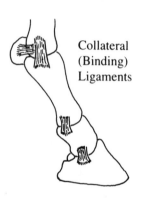

Collateral (Binding) Ligaments

Fig. 11-8. Collateral ligaments.

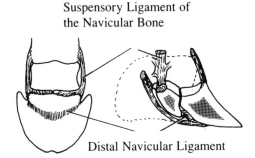

Suspensory Ligament of
the Navicular Bone

Distal Navicular Ligament

Fig. 11-9. Navicular ligaments.

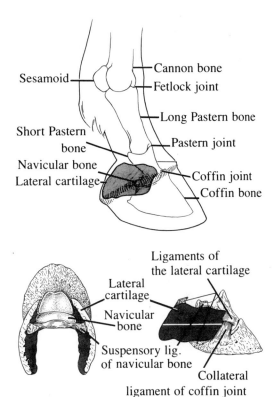

Sesamoid
Cannon bone
Fetlock joint
Long Pastern bone
Short Pastern bone
Pastern joint
Navicular bone
Lateral cartilage
Coffin joint
Coffin bone

Ligaments of
the lateral cartilage
Lateral cartilage
Navicular bone
Suspensory lig.
of navicular bone
Collateral
ligament of coffin joint

Fig. 11-10. Position and ligaments of the lateral cartilages. Drawing by L. Sadler.

Navicular Ligaments

The navicular ligaments suspend and support the navicular bone.

The **suspensory ligament of the navicular bone** is in the form of a strong sling which supports weight and absorbs concussion. It originates from the sides of the long pastern bone just above the pastern joint and inserts on the sides and top edge of the navicular bone.

The **distal navicular ligament** is a short broad ligament which fastens the bottom edge of the navicular bone to the edge of the coffin joint surface above and in back of the semilunar crest on the bottom of the coffin bone.

Ligaments of the Lateral Cartilages

The lateral cartilages are joined to the pastern, navicular, and coffin bones by numerous small ligaments. They support and contain the lateral cartilages by helping to "equalize" concussion forces.

Plantar Ligament

The plantar ligament is a very strong flat band which covers the outside portion of the rear (plantar) surface of the hock. It runs from the point of the hock on the fibular tarsal bone down to the fourth tarsal bone and the large upper end of the outside splint bone. A sprain or tearing of the middle of this ligament results in a swelling known as curb. The swelling can be seen approximately a hand's width below the point of the hock.

Interosseous Ligaments of the Splint Bones

The interosseous ligaments of the splint bones join the splint bones to the cannon bone in a young horse. They often become sprained or torn in young horses. An exostosis at the site of the sprain is called a splint. The interosseous ligaments may naturally turn to bone (ossify) in older horses.

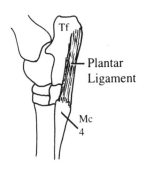

Tf
Plantar
Ligament
Mc
4

Fig. 11-11. Plantar ligament of the hind limb.

115

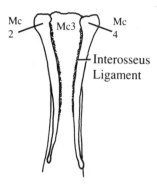

Fig. 11-12. Interosseus ligaments of the splint bones.

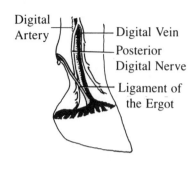

Fig. 11-13. Ligament of the ergot.

Ligament of the Ergot

The ligament of the ergot runs from the ergot down to the pastern joint. It is very superficial and may be joined to the skin. It crosses the vein, artery and posterior digital nerve. It may be mistaken for the nerve by the veterinary surgeon during a nerving operation.

References

Popesko, P. 1977. Atlas of Topographical Anatomy of the Domestic Animals (2nd ed.). Saunders, Philadelphia.

Sisson, S. and J.D. Grossman. 1953. Anatomy of the Domestic Animals (4th ed.). Saunders, Philadelphia.

Sack, W.O. and R.E. Habel. 1977. Rooney's Guide to the Dissection of the Horse. Veterinary Textbooks, Ithaca, NY.

NOTES:

Chapter 12

Foot Biomechanics

The horse's body is engineered for athletic activity. The form and angles of the body provide maximum mechanical advantage for efficient movement and concussion absorption. The complex foot has a very unique design and performs weight supporting, concussion reducing, blood pumping and nonslipping functions.

The Stay Apparatus

The stay apparatus makes it possible for the horse to remain standing for extended periods of time with minimum muscular activity. It is often said that horses can sleep standing up. However, even though minimal muscular energy is expended to support its heavy weight when standing, the horse gets a more complete rest when it lays down in deep sleep.

The stay apparatus is a series of ligamentous structures that prevent the overflexion or extension of the joints of the limb. The structures of the stay apparatus are essentially the same from the knee and hock down. The elbow joint of the front limb has a unique design with collateral ligaments eccentrically placed forward from the

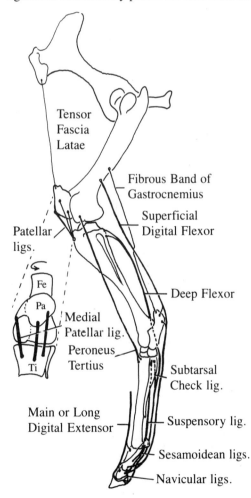

Fig. 12-1. Front limb stay apparatus (lateral aspect).

Fig. 12-2. Hind limb stay apparatus (lateral aspect).

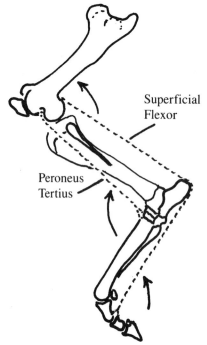

Superficial
Flexor

Peroneus
Tertius

Fig. 12-3. Hind limb reciprocal apparatus.

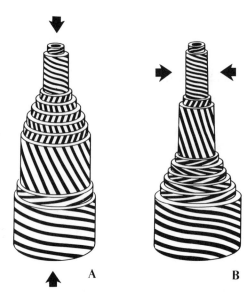

A   B

Fig. 12-4. Hoof tubules resist vertical compression (A) and horizontal flexion (B). Drawing by D. Leach (after Nickel).

center of rotation. The ulna forms a stop on the back of the joint. A slight muscle tonus in the triceps and brachiocephalicus muscles locks the elbow joint.

The hind limb has a special variation called the reciprocal apparatus. It makes possible the synchronized flexion and extension of the joints in the hind limb or a rigid locking of the bone column in the standing position. Control of the entire limb is influenced by stifle joint position. A slight muscle tonus in the tensor fasciae latae muscle of the hind limb keeps the patella locked over the medial ridge of the trochlea of the femur. Thus, both front and hind limb can be locked rigid with minimal conscious muscular effort.

Structures of the stay apparatus may be sprained in cases where fatigue removes the dampening action of muscles and the tendons and ligaments take the full impact of repeated concussion.

Weight Supporting Structures

The hoof is designed to bear weight. The hoof tubules have a spiral columnar structure that makes them resist compression and flexion. The conical shape of the hoof provides a strong structural support.

The laminar attachment of hoof to bone suspends the skeleton and weight of the body from the hoof wall. The laminae redirect the forces acting on them and dissipate the concussion coming up from the ground and down from the body. The primary and secondary laminae increase the surface area for dissipating concussion as much as 30 times. These unique structures increase the surface of attachment from several square inches to several square feet. The area of laminar attachment has been calculated to be from 8 to 10 square feet (Fleming, 1872). The rear third of the hoof is attached to the lateral cartilages.

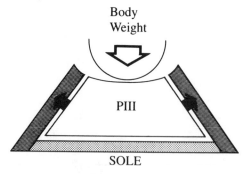

Body
Weight

PIII

SOLE

Fig. 12-5. The laminar attachment suspends the skeleton from the hoof wall over a large surface area created by the laminae. Drawing by D. Leach.

The sole is normally arched and can support some weight. However, its function is primarily protective. The frog may support weight at the heels if the wall and bars are weak or sink into soft ground.

Concussion Reducing Structures

The angle or slope of the shoulder and pastern is especially important in determining the amount of concussion that can be absorbed by the limb. A sloping shoulder and pastern not only create less and absorb more concussion than straighter ones, but they make a smoother riding horse. The elasticity of the suspensory and sesamoidean ligaments also relates to the concussion absorption qualities of the fetlock joint.

The elasticity and movement of the wall absorbs some degree of concussion. The sole descends or flattens slightly to absorb concussion. The white line absorbs concussion as the wall moves out and the sole flattens. The laminae of the foot diminish concussion to the coffin bone as they transfer weight and redirect forces between the hoof and skeleton.

The frog in its normal state absorbs concussion from two directions. The frog acts as a

rubber shock absorber of concussion force from the ground. It also acts as a stop and redirects concussion force coming down from the pastern laterally through the plantar cushion to the lateral cartilages and hoof. When there is no frog pressure (contact with the ground), the plantar cushion "draws" the lateral cartilages in as it descends under compression from the pastern bones. This may produce contracted heels.

Nearly all of the structures of the horse's foot are elastic or springy to some degree. The lateral cartilages, the plantar cushion, and the coronary cushion are classified as elastic structures. Elastic structures are highly elastic, and have as their primary purpose the reduction of concussion. They cause the hoof to expand and contract at the heels. They not only act as shock absorbers, but also function as "pumps" and "valves" to assist in circulating the blood.

The **lateral cartilages** are wing-like structures attached to the sides (wings) of the coffin bone. Approximately one-half of the lateral cartilage is within the hoof and one-half protrudes above the coronet. The cartilages of the forefeet are usually thicker and more extensive than those of the hind.

The lateral cartilages are normally composed of highly elastic hyaline and fibrous cartilage. They are in a position to reduce concussion because of their location between the wall and plantar cushion. This position allows the rear

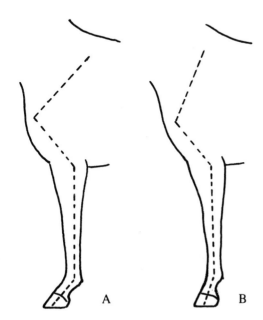

Fig. 12-6. Concussion is absorbed more efficiently by a sloping shoulder and pastern (A) than a steep shoulder and pastern (B).

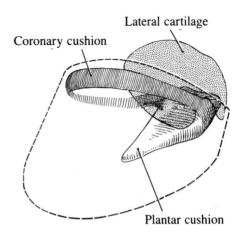

Fig. 12-7. The relationship of the coronary cushion, plantar or digital cushion and lateral cartilage. Drawing by L. Sadler.

third of the wall to expand and contract slightly since it is attached by the laminae to the elastic lateral cartilages rather than the rigid coffin bone.

One or both lateral cartilages may ossify and lose its (their) elasticity in horses that have conformation faults and are subject to excessive concussion. This condition is commonly called sidebone(s).

The **plantar** or **digital cushion** is a wedge-shaped structure with a fibro-fatty composition. It is very elastic and has few blood vessels and nerves.

The plantar cushion is located in a "wedged-in" position between the lateral cartilages on the sides, the deep flexor tendon and overlying short pastern and navicular bones on the top, and the frog and frog stay or spine on the bottom and rear. When it is compressed by the pastern bones and frog, it absorbs shock, cushions the bones, and is divided by the frog stay or spine so that it is forced outward and obliquely upward against the lateral cartilages with near equal intensity.

The **coronary cushion** is the elastic portion of the coronary band. This fibro-fatty cushion is covered by the sensitive portion of the coronary band which produces and nourishes the wall of the hoof. The coronary cushion is thickest at its center where it covers the extensor process and attaches to the common extensor tendon, and

thinnest at the quarters where it attaches to the lateral cartilages. Then it widens out and thickens to form the base of the bulbs of the heel where it blends in with the plantar cushion. Thus, the form of the coronary cushion causes the variation in thickness of the hoof wall.

The coronary cushion contributes to the reduction and transfer of concussion between the hoof wall and the coffin bone and other internal foot parts.

The Blood Pumping Mechanism of the Foot

Blood is necessary for growth, normal functioning, and repair of injured or worn-out tissues. Blood is pumped by the heart through arteries to the foot and is assisted in its return to the heart by a "pumping mechanism" in the foot. This mechanism must be present due to the position of the foot in relation to the heart. There are no muscles in the lower leg or foot, as we find in other parts of the body, to aid in returning the venous blood to the heart.

Located on both sides of each of the lateral cartilages and in the sensitive structures of the foot are large venous plexuses. Each venous plexus is made up of an extensive network of veins. The compression of these veins by the plantar cushion against the lateral cartilages or

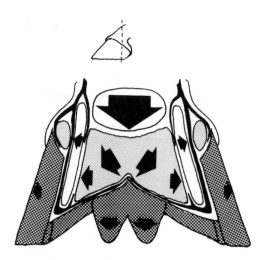

Fig. 12-8. *The coronary cushion, digital cushion, lateral cartilages and frog absorb concussion during weight bearing. Veins are also compressed and blood is pumped out of the foot at this time.*

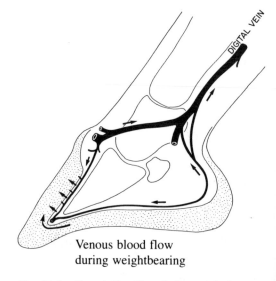

Venous blood flow during weightbearing

Fig. 12-9. *Venous bloodflow during weight bearing. Drawing by D. Leach.*

the coffin bone (and lateral cartilages) against the hoof acts as a "pump" to force the blood up the leg and back to the heart.

Blood is prevented from returning to the foot by valves in the veins of the leg. Compression of the plexuses also acts as a "valve" to contain blood in the vessels of the foot below the plexuses. This produces a "hydraulic cushion" that further dissipates concussion and protects the fragile coffin bone.

This valve action also creates a fluid pressure which causes the blood to exit up the leg and the plexuses to fill when the foot is raised and the compressed veins open. Each time the foot bears weight, the veins are compressed. Each time the foot is raised, the veins open and blood is pushed in by the arterial pulse and gravity.

Nonslipping Design

The hoof functions in a nonslipping manner due to its shape, consistency, and motion. The sole is concave and as such acts as a suction cup against the ground. The frog is wedge-shaped and serves to hold the foot as it lands on soft ground. It is also of a rubbery consistency and thus creates traction on harder ground. The sharp-angled toe of the hoof cuts and digs into the ground as it breaks over and thereby reduces the possibility of slipping. Wide front hoofs provide lateral stability. Narrow hind hoofs allow for lateral breakover and maneuverability when making sharp turns.

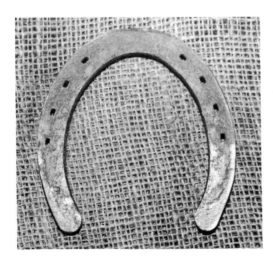

Fig. 12-10. Hoof heel movements are revealed by examination of the foot surface of a worn shoe. Photo by J. Graves.

Hoof Strength and Elasticity

Hoof yield strength and elasticity have been measured by use of an Instron compression machine (Butler, 1976 and Leach, 1980). Apparently, these qualities of hoof are very constant. Changes in diet, mineral assay, color or growth rate of hoofs do not seem to change hoof strength or elasticity. However, moisture content has been shown to significantly affect the hoof's biomechanical properties. Extremely dry (less than 19% moisture) or extremely wet (more than 30% moisture) hoof walls are weak and subject to failure from compression or shearing forces. The average compression yield strength of the measured hoof walls was 146 mNm^2 (megaNewtons per square meter). The tangent modulus of elasticity just prior to failure was 3.716 mNm^2 (Butler, 1976).

Hoof Movements

Examination of the foot surface of a shoe that has been worn for several weeks by an active horse will demonstrate the location and amount of movement in the ground surface of the hoof.

The movements of the hoof and concussion forces have been studied by various scientists for more than 100 years. A composite summary of their discoveries reveals numerous movements of the various hoof parts.

Physiological Shoeing

Shoeing should be applied so as to least interfere with the functions of the foot. Some have called this physiological shoeing. Corrective or therapeutic shoeing may necessitate the violation of some physiological principles for a short period of time:

1. The wall must be kept reduced to its proper proportions if balanced natural wear does not occur.
2. Changes in hoof angle of more than a few degrees should not be made all at once, except in special cases, due to the possibility of injury to ligaments and tendons. Changes in lateral balance should not be made in mature horses except as a last resort to prevent limb interference.
3. The frog should be trimmed as little as good hygiene will allow. Ideally the frog should be about level with the ground surface of the wall at the heels.

4. The heels of the wall should not be trimmed below the ground surface of the frog for shoeing unless: a large frog and thick shoe warrant it, the proper angle of the hoof can be maintained, and there exists no danger of corns being produced by such a practice.

5. The bars should be trimmed level with the wall at the heels. They should be trimmed flush with the sole where they project above it in order to avoid the accidental breaking or cracking of the portion of the bar which doesn't normally bear weight. The heel of

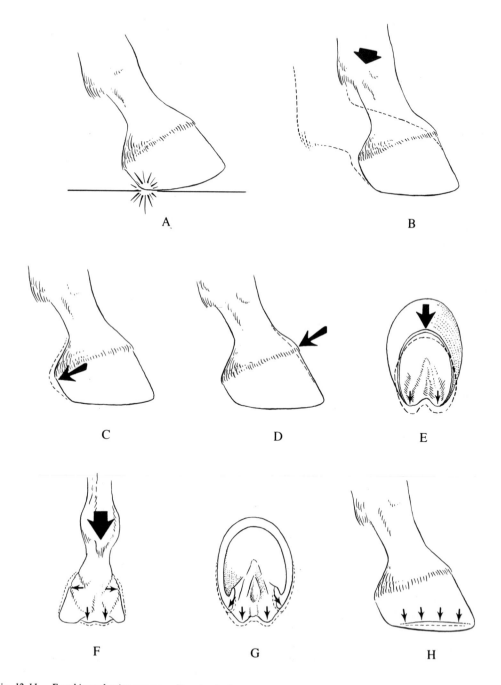

Fig. 12-11. *Foot biomechanics summary. Drawing by L. Sadler.*

the shoe should bear weight from the bar at the heel. The bars should not be cut back to the buttress (often called "opening the heels") as this destroys their supporting and weight-bearing function.

6. The sole should be trimmed only enough to cosmetically remove the flaking off (exfoliating) or "dead" material. The full "live" (unexfoliated) thickness of the sole is needed to protect the underlying structures of the foot. The outer edge of the sole should not bear weight. A horse trimmed to go barefoot should be left with a little more wall than normal to prevent the need for excessive trimming or "concaving" the sole at its junction with the wall. Shoes, especially those for the "flatter" front feet, should be concaved on the inner foot surface web to prevent sole pressure.

7. The exterior surface of the wall should be left intact except in cases of severe distortion (flaring or wry hoofs) where "sculpturing" is necessary to create a balanced stance or gait. In cases where attention is needed and rasping must be done, it may be necessary to add water and a "hoof dressing" to prevent evaporation of hoof moisture. The application of a hoof dressing is normally not necessary or advisable unless the exterior of the wall is rasped excessively or the animal is to be exposed to a very moist environment for an extended period of time.

8. The shoe should be made to accurately fit the outline of the balanced and shaped hoof wall. "Expansion" (fitting the shoe slightly wider than the outside border of the hoof from the last nail hole back to the heel) at the heels of the shoe will allow for the natural elasticity and movement of the hoof at the heels.

9. The pattern of the shoe should be the lightest and simplest possible to provide the protection, traction, wear or other service needed for the interval between shoeings.

10. The shoe should have a level bearing surface and rest on the wall. Shoes can be leveled and fit cold, but more skill is required to match the shoe to the foot. Hot fitting should be done when clips or rocker-toes need to be seated into the wall.

11. The heels of the shoe should be long enough to cover the buttresses, but not long enough to be easily stepped on. The bulbs of sloping heeled feet should be protected by longer than normal heels when feasible.

12. The shoe should be secured with as few and as small a size nail as possible to retain the shoe on the hoof for the interval between shoeings. Nails should not be driven higher than is necessary to avoid old nail holes and to hold the shoes on for the interval between shoeings. Ideally, the nails would be driven only slightly higher than the distance the wall will grow down in the interval between shoeings.

References

Adams, O.R. 1974. Lameness in Horses (3rd ed.). Lea and Febiger, Philadelphia.

Armistead, W.W. 1955. Horseshoeing (Part I and II). The Southwestern Vet. 3(3 and 4):224; 324.

Butler, K.D. 1976. The Effect of Feed Intake and Gelatin Supplementation on the Growth and Quality of the Equine Hoof. Ph.D. Thesis, Cornell Univ., Ithaca, NY.

Butler, D. 1982. The sensitive structures of the horse's foot. Amer. Farriers' J. 8(6):383.

Dollar, J.A.W. 1898. A Handbook of Horseshoeing. William R. Jenkins Co., New York.

Evans, J.W. 1981. Horses. W.H. Freeman and Co., San Francisco.

Fischer, A. 1927. Der Fuss des Pferdes. M. and H. Schaper. Hannover, GERMANY.

Fleming, G. 1871. Observations on the anatomy and physiology of the horse's foot. The Vet. 44:142.

Fleming, G. 1872. Observations on the anatomy and physiology of the horse's foot. The Vet. 45:1.

Kirby, E. and D. Leach. 1982. Ingenious engineering. Equus. 56:34.

Knezevic, P. 1962. Clinical study of contracted hoof and the principles of ungulography in horses. Wien. tierarztl. Mschr. 49:777.

Knezevic, P. 1963. Measurement of expansion of the hoof in horses and cattle. Proc. World Vet. Congr. 17(2):1367.

Lambert, F. 1966. The role of moisture in the physiology of the hoof of the harness horse. Vet. Med./S.A.C. 61:342.

Leach, D.H. 1980. The Structure and Function of the Equine Hoof Wall. Ph.D. Thesis. Univ. of Saskatchewan. Saskatoon, Sask., CANADA.

Lungwitz, A. 1891. The changes in the form of the horse's hoof under the action of the body-weight. J. of Comp. Path. and Ther. 4(3):191.

Rooney, J.R. 1969. Biomechanics of Lameness in Horses. Williams and Wilkins, Baltimore.

Rooney, J.R. 1970. Autopsy of the Horse. Williams and Wilkins, Baltimore.

Rooney, J.R. 1974. The Lame Horse. A.S. Barnes and Co., Inc., Cranbury, NJ.

Sack, W.O. and R.E. Habel. 1977. Rooney's Guide to the Dissection of the Horse. Veterinary Textbooks, Ithaca, NY.

Smith, F. 1921. A Manual of Veterinary Physiology (5th ed.). Alex Eger, Chicago.

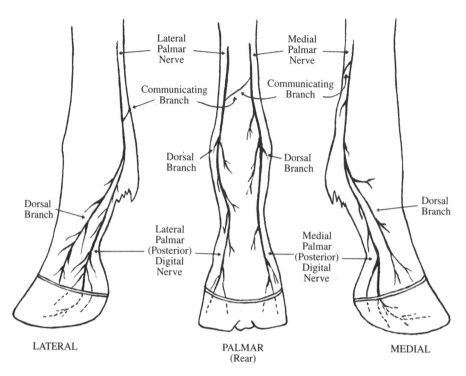

Fig. 13-1. *The major sensory nerves of the horse's leg. Modified from Sack and Habel (1977).*

▨ Medial palmar (posterior) digital nerve

▨ Lateral palmar (posterior) digital nerve

▨ Medial dorsal branch of digital nerve

▨ Lateral dorsal branch of digital nerve

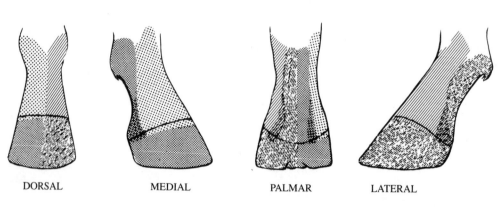

Fig. 13-2. *Sensory nerve endings in the equine digit. Modified from Sack (1975).*

Chapter 13

Sensitive Structures

Characteristics of Sensitive Structures

The sensitive structures of the horse's foot are called sensitive because they contain so many nerve endings and blood vessels that any injury to them causes pain and bleeding. Sensitive structures are located under every part of the horny hoof. Each hoof structure has a corresponding sensitive structure. An understanding of the location, structure, and function of the sensitive structures or coriums is an important prerequisite to successful diagnosis and shoeing or treating of many of the diseases of the hoof and foot.

The sensitive structures are innervated by the digital nerves. Nerves are the wiring of the body. Visible nerves are actually bundles of parallel fibers enclosed in sheaths like insulated wires. Nerve fibers are different from wires in that they have the ability to carry an electrical impulse their entire length without a reduction in electrical energy.

Motor nerves carry electrical impulses or signals that cause muscles to contract and move the body. The horse has no motor nerves below the knee or hock. However, motor nerves are activated by a reflex arc through sensory nerves to the spinal cord when pain is experienced in the foot. Sensory nerves inform the body of changes in temperature, pressure or trauma. Environmental changes are detected by nerve endings beneath the skin and hoof. Changes in temperature, pressure or trauma are detected by nerve endings in the coriums under the hoof. Apparently, nerve endings do not extend into the hoof. Sensation from the hoof is suppressed since the hoof is relatively thicker than the skin and an effective insulator. Also, there is a great deal of difference in each individual horse's tolerance to pain.

Anesthetics are substances which block the passage of nerve impulses. Nerve blocks are local anesthetics which are commonly used to desensitize a specific region. Blocks may be used as diagnostic aids. Nerving is performed by removing sections of the lateral and medial palmar (posterior) digital nerves. This removes sensation from the heel, frog, sole, lower laminar and navicular regions of the foot. The dorsal branches of the digital nerve supply sensation to the coronary band around the hoof and the upper portions of the sensitive laminae. There is much variation in the topography of the nerve branches in the horse's foot (Sack, 1975).

The sensitive structures are supplied with blood by the digital arteries. Arteries are thick-walled and round. They carry bright red oxygenated blood from the heart to the capillaries. Arteries have a pulse which may be easily felt by lightly pressing the artery against a sesamoid bone. A stronger than usual pulse indicates inflammation is present in the foot. Capillaries are the small vessels that exchange nutrients from the blood with the tissues. Much of the tissue of the sensitive structures is composed of capillaries. Veins are thin-walled and collapsible. They carry dark red deoxygenated blood back to the heart. Valves are present in large veins to help direct the flow of blood toward the heart. There are many more veins than arteries in the foot. The veins of the foot form plexuses. These are networks of interlaced blood vessels. They are drained by the digital veins.

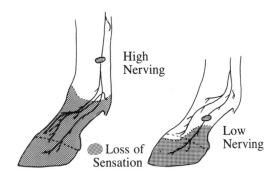

Fig. 13-3. The effect of high and low nerving.

125

The thin-walled venous vessels of the sensitive structures are compressed between the horny hoof and the coffin bone as the foot bears weight. When the veins of the venous plexus on either side of the lateral cartilages are open, blood is pumped into the venous plexuses by this compression. As the veins of these venous plexuses adjacent to the lateral cartilages are constricted, and finally closed by additional weight and pressure, the blood which is in them is pumped up the leg. The blood remaining in the veins of the sensitive structures is locked in the foot at

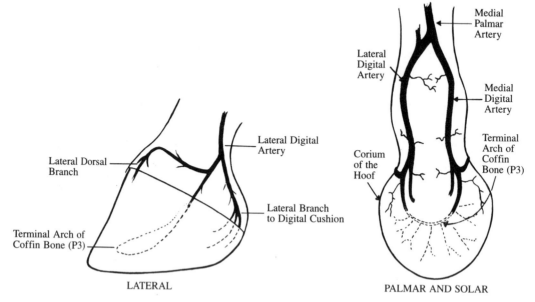

Fig. 13-4. Major arteries of the equine digit. Modified from Sack and Habel (1977).

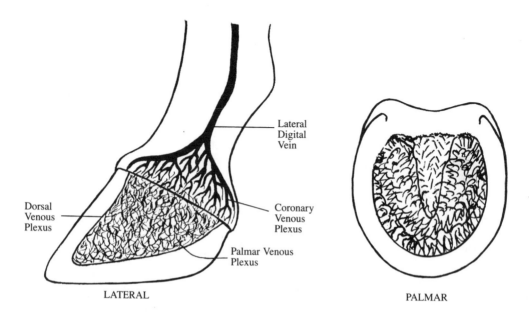

Fig. 13-5. Major veins of the equine digit. Modified from Sack and Habel (1977).

126

this point and forms a hydraulic cushion between the coffin bone and the horny wall. This cushion protects the fragile coffin bone from the effects of concussion.

Lymph vessels are also present in the sensitive structures, especially the laminae, where a lymph vessel is said to exist in the attached edge of each of the primary sensitive laminae. A large lymph vessel plexus is located at the base of the plantar cushion under the frog. The sensitive structures nourish the horny hoof and contribute to the moisture balance in the hoof by supplying internal moisture from circulating lymph and blood plasma.

The relationship of the sensitive structures to the hoof structures is much like that of the dermis to the epidermis of the skin. The sensitive structures nourish the horny structures and allow them to grow. This process is similar to the scaling off (desquamation) of the epithelial cells of the

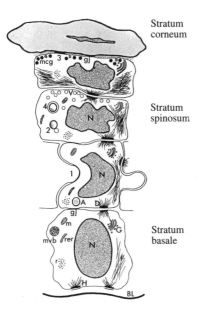

Fig. 13-6. Diagram of the ultrastructural changes occurring in the keratinization of hoof wall in the stratum germinativum: (A) annular gap junction; (BL) basal lamina; (D) desmosome; (F) tonofilaments; (G) Golgi complex; (H) hemidesmosomes; (N) nucleus; (V) aggregation of empty appearing vesicles in cytoplasm; (gj) gap junction; (m) mitochondria; (mcg) membrane-coating granules; (mvb) multivesicular bodies; (r) ribosomes; (rer) rough endoplasmic reticulum; (l) invagination from one cell into another, involving area of gap junction attachment; (2) annular gap junction abutted by lysosome-like vesicle; (3) type 3 junction; (4) degenerating annular gap junction within single membrane. Drawing by D. Leach.

skin by the dermis. The difference is that the cells of the hoof are hardened and turned to horn (keratinized) at a transitional zone (keratogenous zone) between the horn-producing layer of cells (stratum germinativum) and the horny hoof. The hoof grows as a result of cell division by the cells in the stratum germinativum. It can be thought of as the outer or "growth" layer of the sensitive structures. The newly-formed cells are keratinized and pushed toward the ground to produce the hard and tough horny hoof.

The sensitive laminae on the outer surface of the coffin bone performs an additional function of suspension and weightbearing. Its attachment to the horny laminae of the wall suspends and supports nearly the entire weight of the horse at a point during the support phase of the stride.

The sensitive structures are classified according to microscopic differences and the horny structure of the hoof that each produces and nourishes. Five areas are classified as separately recognizable sensitive structures which produce and nourish the indicated corresponding horn structures of the hoof. These are: Coronary Band—Hoof Wall, Perioplic Ring—Periople, Sensitive Laminae—White Line, Sensitive Sole—Horny Sole, Sensitive Frog—Horny Frog.

Sensitive Coronary Band

The sensitive coronary band is located around the upper border of the hoof under its junction with the skin. (The term coronary band can be confusing in that it is sometimes used in place of coronet and may be meant to indicate the periople, the perioplic ring, and the coronary cushion in addition to the sensitive coronary band.)

The sensitive coronary band functions as the primary growth and nutritional source for the bulk of the hoof wall. The function of the hoof wall and bars is to bear weight. The portion of the coronary band which turns back on itself at the heels to produce the bars of the wall is not clearly distinguishable from the sensitive frog. The horn-producing layer of cells (stratum germinativum) on and between the papillae of the coronary band "produces" the hoof wall (stratum medium) and the horny laminae (stratum lamellatum).

The outer layer of the coronary band is composed of very small papillae which are well supplied with numerous microscopic blood vessels. This area resembles velvet in appearance. Each of these papillae fits into a funnel-like cavity in the center of a spiral, multi-layered horn tubule of the hoof wall. Three types of hoof cells are produced on and between the papillae of the outer layer of the sensitive coronary band. They are tubular horn, intertubular horn and intratubular horn.

Tubular horn is produced by the sides of the coronary papillae. They form the multi-layered horn tubules of the wall. Tubular horn is primarily responsible for the vertical and horizontal elasticity and rigidity of the hoof wall.

Intertubular horn is produced by the areas between the papillae. It is a tightly-packed "cement-like" substance that holds the tubules together. The outer intertubular horn cells contain the pigment which gives color to the hoof. Those next to the white line and those which make up the horny laminae have no pigment.

The intratubular horn is produced by the tips of the papillae and fills the hollow centers of the horn tubules. It is a loosely-packed "pith-like"

substance thought to be primarily responsible for moisture conduction and regulation in the hoof. Intertubular horn also conducts moisture, but to a minor degree. The moisture content of healthy hoof wall is about 25 percent.

The hoof wall grows downward at the rate of about 1/4 to 3/8 inch per month. Since the average hoof is 3 to 4 inches in length at the toe, the horse could be said to grow a "new" hoof every year. A severe injury to the sensitive coronary band will cause defective wall horn to be produced at that point. Variations in climate, nutrition, metabolism and health will cause "growth rings" to be produced on the hoof wall. Close observation of the hoofs can reveal 12 months of information about the horse.

Perioplic Ring

The perioplic ring is a narrow ring which is located just above the coronary band and next to the hair line of the coronet. The horn-producing cell layer (stratum germinativum) of its nearly microscopic papillae produces the periople. The periople normally extends about 3/4 to 1 inch down the wall from the coronet, except at the heel where it blends in with the frog.

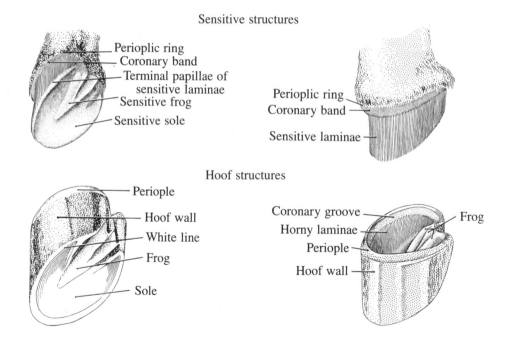

Sensitive structures

Perioplic ring
Coronary band
Terminal papillae of sensitive laminae
Sensitive frog
Sensitive sole

Perioplic ring
Coronary band
Sensitive laminae

Hoof structures

Periople
Hoof wall
White line
Frog
Sole

Coronary groove
Horny laminae
Periople
Hoof wall
Frog

Fig. 13-7. The position and relationship of the sensitive structures to the hoof structures. Drawings by L. Sadler.

The periople protects the sensitive coronary band at the junction of the skin and hoof. It is very tough and has about the same consistency as the horny frog. The underside of the periople flakes off and is carried down as the hoof wall grows out to produce the hoof varnish (stratum tectorium). The hoof varnish is a very thin layer of cells. Often it is naturally absent. Or, it may be partially present at varying distances from the ground surface of the hoof.

Sensitive Laminae

The sensitive laminae is engorged with blood vessels and has the largest area of the sensitive structures. It lies between the hoof wall and the coffin bone. The sensitive laminae covers the coffin bone's outer surface, the outside bottom half of the lateral cartilages and turns inward at the heels to form the sensitive laminae of the bars.

The sensitive laminae or lamina "leaves" interlock (interdigitate) with the horny laminae of the wall. One is the mirror image of the other. The entire inner surface of the hoof wall is lined with horny laminae. Since the sensitive laminae are attached to the coffin bone, the horse is literally "suspended" from the wall by this union of the laminae leaves. This interlocking system allows the hoof wall and horny laminae to grow downward from the coronary band at about 1/4 to 3/8 inch per month while maintaining its strength of attachment with the sensitive laminae on the coffin bone. The union of the two is so firm that they can only be separated with difficulty. This attachment is damaged when a horse has the disease known as founder (laminitis).

There are approximately 600 primary laminae. These are easily visible with the naked eye. On each of the primary laminae there are about 100 microscopic secondary laminae which run parallel to the primary laminae. A cross section of the laminae viewed under a microscope reveals that the secondary laminae are arranged perpendicular on the primary laminae. They appear like feathers or leaves. This unique laminar arrangement provides the horse with a tremendous surface area (about 60,000 attachments) over which to distribute its weight.

A mature saddle horse has a surface area of attachment of hoof to bone of about 8 square feet for each foot. This amounts to a weight distribution of about 4 ounces per square inch of attachment, when the horse supports his weight on one foot during the support phase of a stride. There would be several hundred pounds per square inch placed on the bone if it were united to the hoof by a simple attachment. This feature is an important factor contributing to the soundness of the horse.

The bottom ends of the leaves of the sensitive laminae are covered with small terminal papillae. The horn-producing layer of cells (stratum germinativum) of these terminal papillae produces a tubular interlaminar horn which is much like that of the sole. (The terminal papillae could be considered a continuation of the sensitive sole.) The combination of this horn and the horny laminae (stratum lamellatum) of the wall make up the white line (zona lamellatum).

The white line is actually somewhat yellow in color. It is normally about 1/8 inch wide. The part of the wall (stratum medium) visible adjacent to the white line from the ground surface is actually white since it has no pigment. It forms an irregular line around the hoof. It is especially noticeable in dark-footed horses. However, this area of the wall can be readily distinguished from the yellow "white line" by the presence of the ends of the horny laminae.

The outside of this laminated white line is the guide line for placing horseshoe nails to be driven into the hoof. The white line also serves as a "buffer zone" between the slight physiological movements of the sole and wall.

Sensitive Sole

The sensitive sole covers the crescent-shaped bottom of the coffin bone. It is composed of small, short papillae much like those of the coronary band. The sensitive sole nourishes the horn-producing layer of cells (stratum germinativum) that produces the horny sole.

The horny sole is composed of horn tubules which vary in length. The sole is unique in that it scales or sloughs off (exfoliates) and does not normally maintain itself at a thickness greater than that of the wall (about 3/8 in. at the toe and 1/4 in. or more at the heel in an average saddle horse foot). A horse that retains the sole is said to have a false or retained sole.

The sole is normally thickest at its junction with the wall at the toe. The sole usually grows at about the same rate as the wall but it wears away much faster due to exfoliation and its softer texture. The moisture content of a healthy horny sole is about 33 percent.

The sensitive sole is easily bruised, especially when the sole is pared thin. Rocky, uneven or extremely hard ground increases the possibility of sole injury. Bruises may occur anywhere on the sole. Chronic sole bruises appear as red spots or "strawberries." The most common location for bruises is in the area commonly referred to as the seat of corn. Bruises in this area are called corns. They are often caused by neglect of regular shoeing. Some horses have naturally thin soles. Leather or plastic pads between the hoof and shoe may be applied to protect thin or bruised soles.

The function of the sole is to protect the sensitive parts above it. The sole is not designed to efficiently support weight, as can be seen from the discussion on the sensitive laminae. It, therefore, should not be subject to constant pressure from a shoe or the ground. The sole's concave shape prevents this from occurring in the natural state on hard ground. The concave shape of the sole also provides the horse increased traction over softer surfaces. The sole of the hind foot is naturally more concave than that of the front. This design provides the driving part of the body with the most traction.

Sensitive Frog

The sensitive frog covers the portion of the plantar cushion which projects beneath the coffin bone. It is composed of very small, short papillae much like those of the perioplic ring and could be considered a continuation of it. The sensitive frog nourishes the horn-producing layer of cells (stratum germinativum) that produces the horny frog.

The horny frog and periople are different from the other hoof structures in that the tubular and intertubular horn produced is not completely turned into hard horn (keratinized or cornified) and thus is more elastic.

The horn tubules of the frog are also different in that they are slightly bent. Coiled fat secreting or "sweat" glands originating in the plantar

cushion pass through the sensitive frog into the cleft area of the frog. The greasy fluid which they secrete, in addition to the normally high (about 50%) moisture content of the frog, helps to maintain the pliable and elastic condition of the horny frog.

A healthy frog is normally the consistency of a new rubber eraser. The consistency of the frog is often a good indication of hoof health. The frog serves as a shock absorber, traction device, and circulation aid due to its special position and consistency. Dryness, overtrimming, atrophy due to lack of pressure, uncleanliness, and neglect may bring about an unhealthy and diseased condition of the frog.

A frog which is untrimmed will usually shed at least twice and sometimes several times a year. However, due to natural wear and the trimming of loose, ragged portions of thrushy areas, this is rarely observed except on neglected horses.

The sensitive structures provide nourishment, growth and nervous sensation to the hoof. Each portion of the hoof has a corresponding corium to provide these functions.

References

Emery, L., J. Miller, and N. Van Hoosen. 1977. Horseshoeing Theory and Hoof Care. Lea and Febiger, Philadelphia.

Leach, D.H. 1980. The Structure and Function of the Equine Hoof Wall. Ph.D. Thesis, Univ. of Saskatchewan, Saskatoon, Sask., CANADA.

Lungwitz, A. and J.W. Adams. 1913. A Textbook of Horseshoeing (11th ed. reprint). Oregon State University Press, Corvallis.

Mishra, P.C. and D.H. Leach. 1983. Electron microscopic study of the veins of the dermal lamellae of the equine hoof wall. Equine Vet. J. 15(1):14.

Mishra, P.C. and D.H. Leach. 1983. Extrinsic and intrinsic veins of the equine hoof wall. J. Anat. 136(3):543.

Nickel, R. 1939. Microstudy of tubules and horn (translation by L.F. Gray). Dtsch. Tierarztl. Mschr. 47:521.

Sack, W.O. 1975. Nerve distribution in the metacarpus and front digit of the horse. J.A.V.M.A. 167(4):298.

Sack, W.O. and R.E. Habel. 1977. Rooney's Guide to the Dissection of the Horse. Veterinary Textbooks, Ithaca, NY.

Sisson, S. and J.D. Grossman. 1953. The Anatomy of Domestic Animals (4th ed.). W.B. Saunders Co., Philadelphia.

Smith, F. 1921. A Manual of Veterinary Physiology (5th ed.). Alex Eger, Chicago.

Trautmann, A. and J. Fiebiger. 1952. Fundamentals of the Histology of Domestic Animals (translation by R.E. Habel). Comstock Publ. Assn., Ithaca, NY.

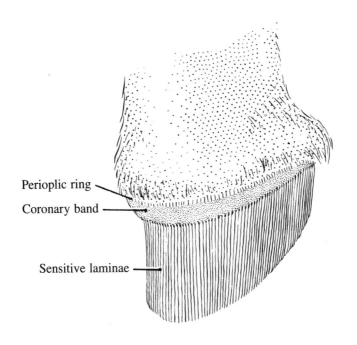

Perioplic ring

Coronary band

Sensitive laminae

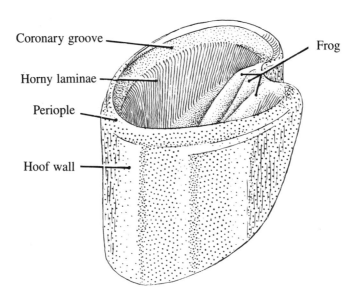

Coronary groove

Horny laminae

Periople

Hoof wall

Frog

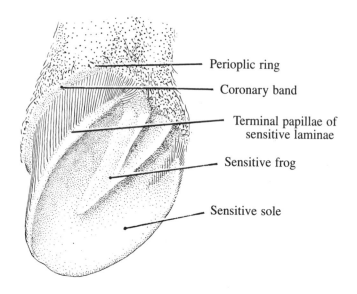

Perioplic ring

Coronary band

Terminal papillae of sensitive laminae

Sensitive frog

Sensitive sole

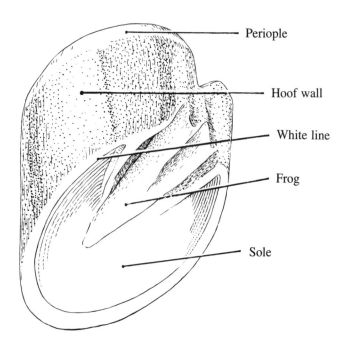

Periople

Hoof wall

White line

Frog

Sole

Chapter 14

Hoof Structures

The Hoof

The horse's hoof may be divided into five regions: the wall, the sole, the frog, the periople (including the bulbs) and the white line. The hoof grows as a result of cell division in the outer horn-producing cell layer (stratum germinativum) of the sensitive structures. This process may be affected by many factors or seriously disrupted by disease as in the case of founder (laminitis). In such cases a distorted hoof is often produced.

The hoof wall is of primary concern. It bears most of the horse's weight, is the most subject to wear and trauma, and is that portion of the hoof which can be seen when the horse is standing.

The wall is related to the papillae of the sensitive coronary band and the laminae of the sensitive laminae. Horn tubules are formed around each of the papillae. Intertubular horn is formed between the papillae and intratubular horn is formed at the tip of each of the papillae. The thick, laminated sides of the horn tubules are

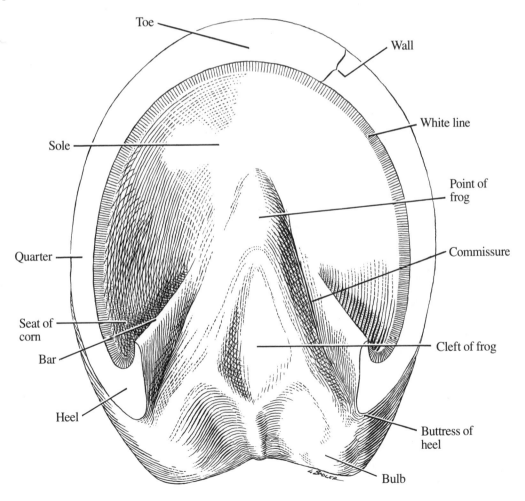

Fig 14-1.   The parts of the hoof. Drawing by L. Sadler.

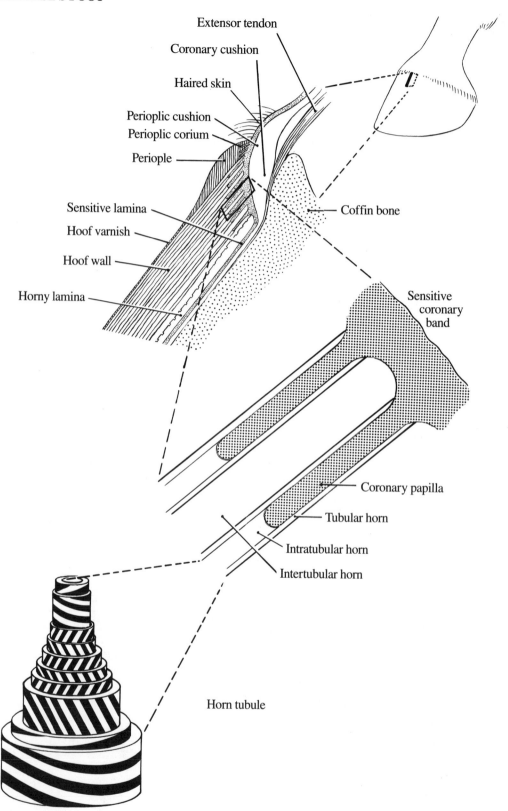

Fig. 14-2. The papillae of the coronary band and horn tubules of the hoof wall. Drawing by L. Sadler.

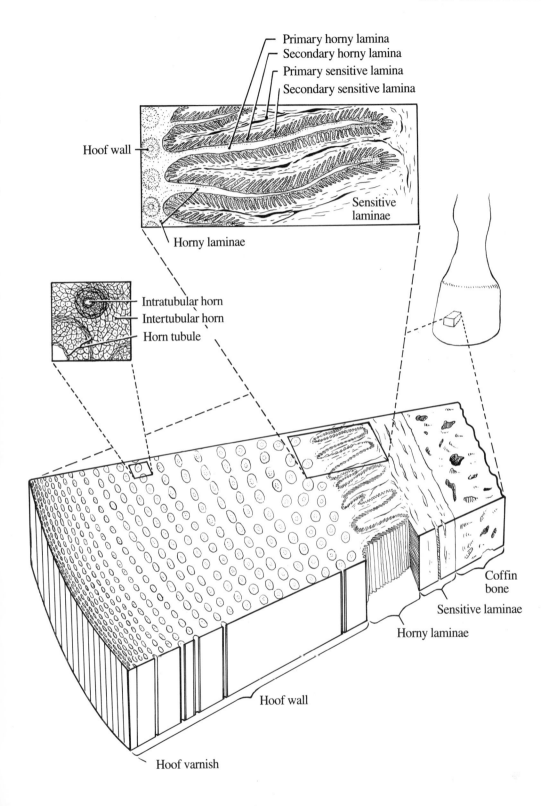

Primary horny lamina
Secondary horny lamina
Primary sensitive lamina
Secondary sensitive lamina

Hoof wall

Sensitive
laminae

Horny laminae

Intratubular horn
Intertubular horn
Horn tubule

Coffin
bone

Sensitive laminae

Horny laminae

Hoof wall

Hoof varnish

Fig. 14-3. The interlocking of the sensitive and horny lam-
inae showing the relative size of the horn tubules of the hoof
wall. Drawing by L. Sadler.

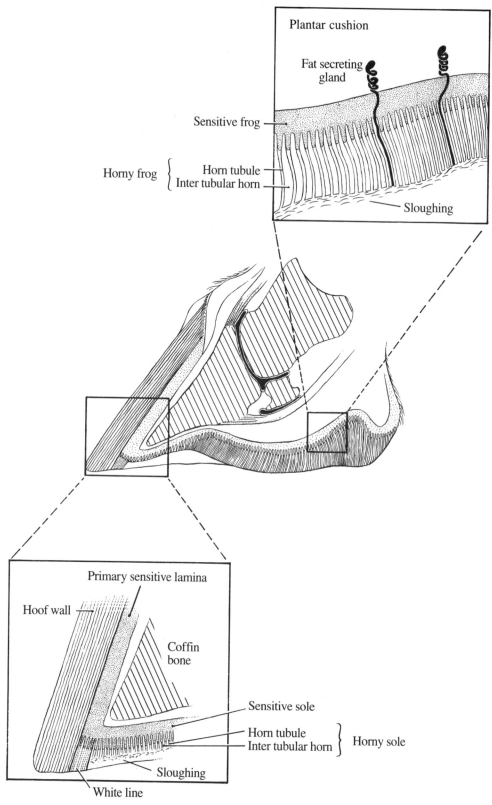

Plantar cushion

Fat secreting gland

Sensitive frog

Horny frog {
Horn tubule
Inter tubular horn

Sloughing

Primary sensitive lamina

Hoof wall

Coffin bone

Sensitive sole

Horn tubule
Inter tubular horn } Horny sole

Sloughing

White line

Fig. 14-4. The sensitive and horny structures of the white line, sole and frog. Drawing by L. Sadler.

primarily responsible for the hoof's strength, elasticity and resistance to wear. Each tubule has the ability to bend or flex slightly (somewhat like a leaf spring) and to compress slightly (somewhat like a coil spring). Each tubule is filled with cells which absorb and conduct water. The function of hoof tubules can be compared to the damper action of a hydraulic shock absorber located within a coil spring (somewhat like the suspension system on the front end of a car).

The inside surface of the wall is composed of horny laminae leaves which interlock (interdigitate) with the leaves of the sensitive laminae (somewhat like the network formed by the teeth of meshed gears). Such an arrangement permits the hoof to grow downward (distally) and yet remain attached to the coffin bone. The attachment may be compared to a velcro fastener.

The thickness and consistency of the sole is important since it protects the coffin bone from injury and fracture due to sharp projections and the uneven surfaces encountered by the horse. The frog's consistency and shape make it effective (in its normal state) as an anticoncussion and nonslipping device. At varying times (usually twice a year) the frog sheds. Often the horse's feet are tender shortly thereafter.

Hoof Growth

The rate of hoof growth is one of the most important considerations in the hoof's physiology. Rapidly growing hoofs are usually of higher quality and easier to keep properly shod than slower growing hoofs.

Factors said to affect hoof growth are: nutrition, climate, level of exercise, level of metabolism, peripheral blood flow, physical condition, parasitism, weight distribution or pressure on the hoof, wear, age, sex, hormones (especially thyroid), part of hoof, soil quality (as it affects forage nutrients and hoof wear), neurectomy, irritation or massage of the sensitive structures, color, shape and angle, front or hind, moisture content, season of the year, temperature (body and environmental), hereditary factors, congenital factors and trimming interval.

Only a few of the above factors have been shown to have any effect on horse hoof growth in scientifically controlled experiments. These

are age, season, irritation or injury of sensitive structures, front or hind, neurectomy and nutrition. Exercise, wear, sex, and temperature have been shown to have an effect on hoof, claw and nail growth in other species.

The following average growth rates of hoof wall (in mm per day) compared to those of claw and nail horn have been reported by the respective investigators for the various species. Note the differences between breeds as well as species.

Rat	0.102	mm per day	(Godwin, 1959)
Man	0.100		(Babcock, 1955)
	0.105		(Clark, 1971)
	0.110		(Bean, 1963)
Sheep	0.187	(Merino)	(Wheeler, 1966)
	0.144	(Southdown)	(Wheeler, et al., 1972)
Cow	0.142	(Ayrshire)	(Prentice, 1973)
	0.155		(Knezevic, 1959)
Horse	0.287		(Knezevic, 1959)
	0.278		(Adams, 1917)
	0.208		(Reeks, 1925)
Horse Foal	0.506	(Standardbred)	(Butler, 1976)
Pony Weanling		(Shetland)	
	0.384	Ad libitum feed	(Butler, 1976)
	0.254	Restricted intake	(Butler, 1976)
Horse Yearling	0.405	(Quarter Horse and Thoroughbred)	(Richardson, 1978)
Horse Two Yr.	0.243	(Quarter Horse)	(Shannon and Butler, 1979)
Horse Three Yr.	0.238	(Quarter Horse)	(Shannon and Butler, 1979)
Horse Aged	0.227	(Quarter Horse)	(Shannon and Butler, 1979)

Hoof growth rate seems to be highly correlated to heart rate. Young animals have a heart rate at least twice as fast as that of older animals. Similarly, young horses have a faster hoof growth rate than older horses. Hoof growth rate decreases as the horse's age increases. The hoofs of horses under 1 year grow about twice as fast as those of horses over 12 years of age. Well conditioned horses usually have a slower heart rate at rest than idle animals, but it appears that the exercise they receive to attain this condition is enough to offset any prolonged effect the slower heart rate when idle may have on hoof growth.

Summary of the Effect of Age on Horse Hoof Growth Rate

	(mm per day)	(mm per mo.)	(in. per mo.)
Foals	0.5	15.0	0.60
Yearlings	0.4	12.0	0.50
Mature	0.3	9.0	0.33
Aged	0.2	6.0	0.25

Hoof growth rate is significantly faster during the spring season of the year. It may be influenced by climate. Average hoof growth rate for all horses is about 10 millimeters (0.40 in.) per month or 3/8 inch.

Stimulation of the sensitive structures by strong counter irritant, vesicant (blister), or massage are thought to increase hoof growth. However, experiments indicate that products commonly applied by horsemen do not create any significant difference in hoof growth rate (Scott and Butler, 1980). Systemic fever or injury of the sensitive structures does result in rapid hoof growth. A hoof growth measurement of 19 millimeters (0.75 in.) per month was made in a case of accidental tearing off of a pony's foot by Jackson (1969).

As early as 1852, it was discovered that neurectomy hastened hoof growth. Several experiments reported in the 1870's by Fleming and a limited number of recent observations had similar results.

Hind hoofs grow approximately 12 percent faster than front hoofs in foals and approximately 7 percent faster in weanlings. The difference between front and hind hoof growth rate diminishes as age increases until there is little, if any, difference between front and hind hoof growth rate in yearlings. Experiments with older animals have shown that the front hoofs grow 6 percent faster than hinds. The change in body weight distribution upon the hoofs as an animal matures may explain these observations. It is known that the part of the hoof bearing the most weight will grow the least. Uneven hoof growth caused by unequal weight distribution causes distortion (flares) and shearing (cracks).

Hoof size has no effect on hoof growth rate, except as size is a function of age.

A number of nutritional factors are said to influence hoof growth, including various nutritional supplements. There is no evidence that gelatin or any other of the commonly used additives have a positive effect on hoof growth rate. Thus far, level of intake is the only nutritional factor that has been experimentally shown to have a highly significant effect. Adequate to over intake (*ad libitum*) of a ration balanced to meet the needs of the class of horse being fed encourages maximum hoof growth. However, caution must be advised since founder is a prime danger of over nutrition in mature horses.

Hoof Moisture

Hoof moisture balance has a direct effect on hoof quality and physiology.

There is constant evaporation taking place from the hoof. Moisture must be replaced regularly to compensate for this loss in order to maintain an ideal moisture balance. Systemic water is transferred from the extensive blood and lymph supply of the sensitive structures to adjacent horn cells, and they, in turn, transfer it to other horn cells. In this way, moisture can be "circulated" throughout the horny structures of the foot. Exercise has a positive effect on the moisture circulation process.

Environmental water is conducted throughout the hoof in a similar manner. A balance of the two sources of moisture is probably maintained through the principle of osmosis. When one source is insufficient for one reason or another, the other is more heavily depended upon by the animal.

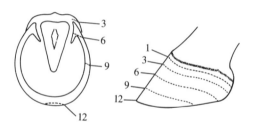

Fig. 14-5. Age of the hoof wall in months.

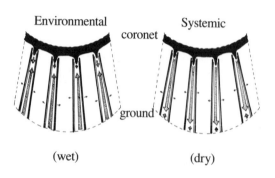

Fig. 14-6. Hoof moisture balance. Size of arrows indicates the relative influence of source on hoof moisture content.

Capillary attraction (capillarity) is also an important factor in moisture conduction up and down hoof horn tubule centers.

Moisture retention is aided and evaporation loss is prevented by the anatomy of the rigid, closely spaced, flattened horn tubules in the external portion of the wall and by the periople of the coronet. The so-called hoof varnish, which flakes off from the underside of the periople and is carried down as the hoof wall grows out, may also assist in retaining hoof moisture. However, since it is a very thin layer of cells, it is usually worn off and absent from at least the lower half of the wall. The contribution that hoof varnish makes to the prevention of evaporation from the hoof is therefore very insignificant.

The ground surface portions of the horny sole and frog dry and harden and are retained longer when environmental moisture is low.

Different portions of the hoof have different moisture contents. The wall is approximately 25 percent water, the sole 33 percent and the frog 50 percent. (Exact figures usually indicate the sole is slightly higher and the frog somewhat less than these approximations, and are variable depending on the horse's systemic and environmental conditions.) Variations in moisture content among and within hoof parts influence several of the important qualities of hoof horn, including elasticity and hardness. The frog is the most elastic, and the wall is the least. The wall increases in elasticity from toe to heel. The young thin wall of the heel is more elastic than the older thick wall at the toe.

Age of the horse has an effect on moisture content of hoof parts. The wall increases about 3 percent, the sole remains the same, and the frog decreases over 10 percent in moisture content as the horse gets older (Miyaki, et al., 1974).

The moisture content of the wall does not vary, on the average, more than 2 percent from the coronary to the sole borders of the hoof. Hind hoofs only contain approximately 0.05 percent more moisture than front hoofs. Water is nature's hoof conditioner. It is the only preparation which has been shown to have a positive effect on maintaining hoof moisture balance.

Factors which encourage an ideal hoof moisture balance are: ground water that horses can periodically stand in (such as that purposely ov-erflowed around the water trough), daily packing saturated clay in the bottom of the hoof, antiseptic hoof packing under a pad and shoe, washing the hoofs each time they are regularly picked out, and in some cases, applying hoof dressing after moisture is added to the hoof. In the rare circumstance where too much environmental moisture is consistently present, the addition of rosin to a grease or oil base hoof dressing has been recommended. Clips are especially helpful in holding shoes on soft hoofs.

Factors which interfere with hoof moisture absorption and circulation are: stabling in sand lots, stabling in deep manure and urine salts, careless and excessive rasping of the sides of the hoof, turpentine and most commercial hoof dressings.

Hoof quality may relate more to the hoof's ability to regulate the moisture content than anything else. As the moisture content in the hoof wall decreases, the hoof becomes harder and tougher. Younger horses have softer hoof walls than older horses. There is a variation in the moisture content of young and old wall in the same hoof. This contributes to its biomechanics since the young wall of the heel and top is more flexible than the old wall of the toe and bottom.

Hoof Composition

There have been many studies to determine the chemical composition of hoofs. Moisture content is usually treated separately since it is so critical in maintaining hoof integrity.

Hoof carbon content has been shown to be 21 percent, hydrogen 7 percent, and oxygen 20 percent.

Hoof nitrogen content has averaged around 17 percent. Some of the nitrogen in a horse's hoof (perhaps 10%) is nonprotein nitrogen (NPN). The protein content of hoof is very high and approaches 95 percent. Carbon, hydrogen, oxygen and nitrogen make up amino acids. Hoof protein or keratin is 18 percent cystine and 0.7 percent methionine (Larsson, et al., 1956).

Sulfur content is closely related to protein content since amino acids are joined into protein molecules by sulfur bonds. The hoof contains 2 to 4 percent sulfur. The nitrogen and sulfur content of the wall is at least 1 percent higher in the wall than the other parts of the hoof.

Hoof fat content has been shown to range between 1 and 4 percent.

Hoof ash (total mineral) content has varied between 0.5 and 1.5 percent.

Specific mineral content is measured in ppm (parts per million). Horse hoof has been reported to be 326.5 ppm calcium, 227.5 sodium, 225.0 potassium, 181.5 phosphorus, 142.5 and 125.0 zinc, 68.5 magnesium, 14.0 iron, and 12.0 copper. Other substances reported in hoof were silica, cobalt and chlorine.

Mineral levels in the hoofs are affected by age, diet, and part of hoof. For example, older animals have less sodium but more potassium in their hoofs. Animals with a limited feed intake had higher zinc levels in the hoofs. The wall is higher in zinc than the other hoof parts. The frog is significantly higher in potassium, magnesium and calcium and lower in zinc than the other hoof parts. The relative amounts of the minerals in the various hoof parts is fairly constant.

Selenium is a mineral that is required in small amounts (0.5 ppm) and toxic in larger amounts (5 or more ppm). When the animal gets a toxic dose from hay or pasture, its mane and tail hair may fall out and its hoofs may slough. "Alkalied" horses are usually lame. They may be reclaimed by changing the diet and protecting the foot.

Vitamin A is necessary for the growth and development of normal hoofs. Horses deficient in vitamin A produce a characteristically poor hoof wall in which the tubules will not hold together. The hoofs may slough in later stages. Feeding green feed usually prevents this condition. Dry range or brown poorly cured and/or stored hay may cause a deficiency of vitamin A in the ration.

Pigmentation (color) of the hoof does not affect its compression yield strength. The average compression yield strength of hoof in one study was 146 mN/m² (mega Newtons per square meter) or 21,150 psi (pounds per square inch). This gives hoof a modulus of elasticity of 3.722 mN/m² or 538 psi (Butler, 1976). There is no significant difference in moisture content or hoof hardness between white and black feet on the same horse. However, there appear to be differences in hoof strength between horses. A few breeds, when selecting for preferred color patterns, have apparently selected for hoofs of poor quality. There is an old saying about horses with white hoofs:

> One white foot, buy him;
> Two white feet, try him;
> Three white feet, deny him;
> Four white feet and a white nose—
> Take off his hide and feed him to the crows.

Hoof Size and Shape

A hoof proportional to body size allows an ideal distribution of body weight over the laminar surface area of the foot, prevents the overcompression of the sensitive and bony structures and allows the normal expansion of the hoof during movement.

There has been a trend, especially in a few breeds, to select for small feet for aesthetic purposes. Hoof size in horses is apparently highly heritable since it correlates with bone growth. Recent research indicates that the hoof continues to increase in size until the age of six.

Hoof size is influenced by nutrition. A recent study revealed an 82 percent increase in hoof sole border area of weanling ponies fed an *ad*

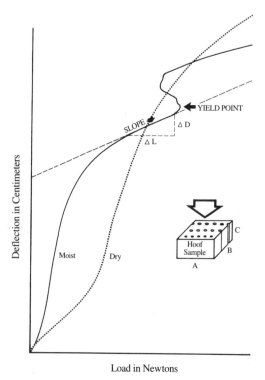

Fig. 14-7. The modulus of elasticity of the average hoof. From Butler and Hintz (1977).

libitum intake as opposed to those fed a limited intake of the same balanced ration. Optimum nutrition encourages maximum bone and also hoof size development. Hoof size proportionate to body size encourages soundness.

Many experiments have been done which demonstrate the change in the shape of the hoof when it strikes the ground. The foot travels through the air with tremendous velocity, accelerating to as much as 60 mph and then strikes with a force of several times the horse's body weight, depending on the gait and speed the horse is traveling (Dalin, *et al.*, 1973). While under load, each part of the hoof changes shape. These minor hoof movements absorb shock and have been measured with intricate electronic apparatus (Knezevic, 1962). The understanding of these movements is essential when administering any type of corrective shoeing. Consideration of the hoof's function and motion has been called physiological horseshoeing (See Chapter 12.).

Hoof size and shape can be influenced by shoeing. Confining the hoof in a smaller than ideal size shoe and/or raising the foot unnaturally high off the ground may restrict hoof sole area

and prevent the natural spreading (expansion) of the hoof. A wry or twisted hoof can be altered to a normal shape by repeated rasping and close fitting of a shoe. This may or may not be desirable depending on what it does to the balance of the foot and leg.

Hoof Shoeing

Consideration of the hoof's function and movements when shoeing has been called physiological horseshoeing.

The lightest shoes which are proportional to the weight and work of the animal should be used. Heavier horses require heavier shoes. Shoes should last for the period between shoeings. One way to get light shoes to give longer service is to add borium (tungsten carbide particles in a mild steel filler) to the rim of the shoe. A way to get more sole protection from a shoe and still retain lightness is to use handmade shoes with a wide web and minimum thickness such as 1/4 inch x 3/4 inch. Borium may also be used on these shoes. In addition to preventing wear, borium also provides traction. It is especially effective on slick, rocky surfaces and highways. Toe or side clips are often used in conjunction with borium since they reduce the strain on the nails created by traction producing projections.

Normally, very little sole or frog should be removed with the hoof knife during the shoeing process. Nipping the hoof wall and rasping the hoof level into a balanced position is sufficient on most horses. This is especially important on flat-soled animals. Turpentine is sometimes used to toughen thin-soled hoofs. Horses which have

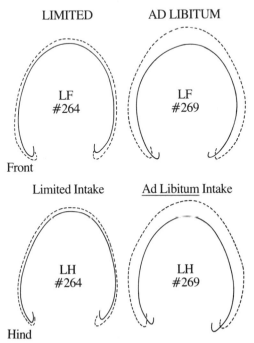

Fig. 14-8. Hoof size comparison of weanling ponies fed limited and ad libitum *(free choice) amounts of a balanced ration. Solid line is April measurement, dotted line is September measurement (5 months growth). Measurements were made on freshly trimmed hoofs. From Butler (1976).*

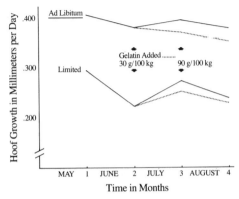

Fig. 14-9. Hoof growth in ponies fed gelatin supplement at two levels. From Butler and Hintz (1977).

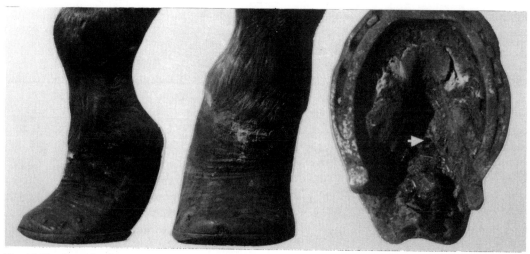

Fig. 14-10. *Excess hoof normally deforms the wall, flakes from the sole and sheds from the frog. Arrow is pointing to hole penetrating the sensitive structures resulting from untreated thrush.*

a tendency to be "tender-footed" should be padded. The inner foot surface of the shoe should be concaved away from the sole to prevent pressure as the hoof moves.

As a rule, shoes should be fit with sufficient expansion at the heels to allow for the physiological movements of the foot. However, when the horse is to be traveling over excessively muddy or rocky areas it is often wise to omit this practice in order to prevent shoes from being prematurely loosened and lost. Of course, shoes fit close must be reset frequently to prevent corns.

Extended or spooned heels may be a desirable addition to shoes if the horse is to travel over rocky terrain which may damage the bulbs (sloping heeled horses are especially susceptible). They give the horse added protection to a potentially tender area of the foot.

NOTES:

References

Adams, J.W. 1917. Diseases of the foot. Practitioners Short Course in Veterinary Medicine. Iowa State University, Ames. 2:234.

Babcock, M.J. 1955. Methods for measuring fingernail growth rates in nutritional studies. J. Nutr. 55:323.

Bean, W.B. 1963. Nail growth—a twenty year study. Arch. Internal Med. 111:476.

Berge, E. and J. Bruggemann. 1938. Notes about the sulphur content and its distribution in the healthy and unhealthy hoof horn of horses. Arch. Tierhk. 72:445.

Butler, K.D. 1976. The Effect of Feed Intake and Gelatin Supplementation on the Growth and Quality of the Equine Hoof. Ph.D. Thesis, Cornell University, Ithaca, NY.

Butler, K.D. and H.F. Hintz. 1977. Effect of level of intake and gelatin supplementation on growth and quality of hoofs of ponies. J. Animal Sci. 44:257.

Clark, W.E. 1971. The Tissues of the Body (6th ed.). Clarendon, Oxford.

Dalin, G., S. Drevemo, I. Fredricson, K. Jonsson and G. Nilsson. 1973. Ergonomic aspects of locomotor asymmetry in Standardbred horses trotting through turns. ACTA Vet. Scand. Suppl. 44, Stockholm.

Dinger, J.E., E.E. Goodwin and E.C. Leffel. 1976. Factors affecting hardness of the equine hoof wall. Paper #2212, Maryland Agricultural Experiment Station.

Fleming, G. 1871. Observations on the anatomy and physiology of the horse's foot. The Vet. 44:142.

Godwin, K.O. 1961. Skin hair and nail in protein malnutrition. World Rev. Nutr. Diet. 3:103.

Gramatzki, H. 1938. Ein Beitrag zur chemischen Zusammensetzung des Hufhorns. Inaug. Diss., Berlin.

Howell, C.E., G.H. Hart and N.R. Ittner. 1941. Vitamin A deficiency in horses. Amer. J. Vet. Res. 2(2):60.

Jackson, L.L. 1969. Regrowth of the equine hoof following traumatic removal. Iowa State Vet. 31:44.

Kaplan, J.S. and J.D. McCall. 1978. Researchers hoof it at the University of Maryland. Quarter Horse J. 30:248.

Knezevic, P. 1959. Study of effect on hoof growth and quality by various hoof salves. Wien. Tierarztl. Mschr. 46:70.

Knezevic, P. 1962. Clinical study of contracted hoof and the principles of ungulography in horses (translated by W.O. Sack). Wien. Tierarztl. Mschr. 49:777, 869, 944.

Larsson, B., N. Obel and B. Aberg. 1956. On the biochemistry of keritinization in the matrix of the horse's hoof in normal conditions and in laminitis. Nord. Vet. Med. 8:761.

Leach, D.H. 1980. The Structure and Function of the Equine Hoof Wall. Ph.D. Thesis, Univ. of Saskatchewan, Saskatoon, Sask., CANADA.

Miyaki, H., T. Ohnishi, and T. Yamamoto. 1974. Measurement of water contents of hoof wall, sole and frog in horses. Exp. Rpt. (Japanese) Eq. Hlth. Lab. 11:15.

Nitsche, H. 1937. Sulphur and nitrogen in the urine, hair and hooves of the draught horse. Nutr. Rev. 7:988.

Prentice, D.E. 1973. Growth rate and wear rates of hoof horn in Ayrshire cattle. Res. Vet. Sci. 14:285.

Reeks, H.C. 1925. Diseases of the Horse's Foot (2nd ed.). Alex Eger, Chicago.

Richardson, G.L. 1978. Influence of Protein Quality on Growth, Development, Hoof Growth and Hoof Quality in Yearling Foals. M.S. Thesis. Univ. of Florida, Gainesville.

Scott, J.M.B. and K.D. Butler, 1980. Effect of several externally applied irritants on hoof growth. Amer. Farrier's J. 6(4):148.

Shannon, R.O. and K.D. Butler. 1979. Influence of age, season and hoof location on equine hoof growth. Amer. Farrier's J. 5(2):44.

Smith, F. 1887. The chemistry of the hoof of the horse. Vet. J. 25:313.

Smith, F. 1921. The foot. A Manual of Veterinary Physiology. Alex Eger, Chicago.

Sutton, B. and D. Butler, 1980. Selenium toxicity in horses. Amer. Farrier's J. 6(2):44.

Weiser, W., M. Stockl, H. Walch, and G. Brenner. 1965. The distributions of sodium, potassium, calcium, phosphorus, magnesium, copper, and zinc in horses' hoofs. Archiv. Exp. Vet. Med. 19:927.

Wheeler, J.L. 1966. Hoof growth, a possible index of nutrition in grazing animals. Proc. Australian Soc. Anim. Prod. 6:350.

Wheeler, J.L., J.W. Bennett, and J.C.D. Hutchinson. 1972. Effect of ambient temperature and day length on hoof growth in sheep. J. Agr. Sci. 79:91.

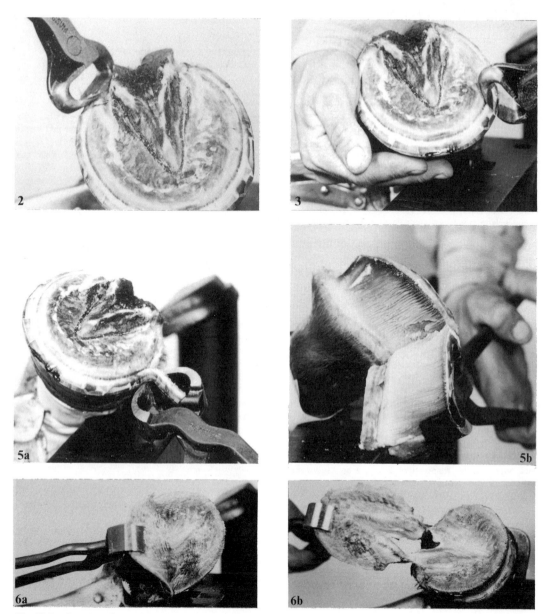

Fig. 15-1. Steps in making a simple dissection of the horse's foot (From 1-14). Photos by G. Poellot.

Chapter 15

Foot Dissection

Dissection Necessary to Understand Anatomical Relationships

Horseshoers should be as familiar with the anatomy and physiology of the horse's foot as veterinarians. Horseshoers must know where the structures of the foot are in relation to each other in order to safely remove horn from a normal or distorted foot, drive nails into it, or change weight distribution over a foot. Knowledge of structure and function is essential when treating and shoeing to correct diseased or lame horses.

There is no better way to become familiar with and obtain a working knowledge of foot anatomy than by dissection and study of each structure. Dissection is also valuable when studying the physiology of the foot. Every student of horseshoeing should perform several dissections of the foot.

Specimens Readily Obtainable

Most large cities have a pet food plant or a carcass removal service where horse legs removed at the knee or hock can be obtained for anatomy study and trimming and shoeing practice. Extra legs can be stored in an old freezer in plastic bags. Clamps can be built, which hold legs for shoeing practice that are removed at the fetlock, to make better use of storage space. Formalin-fixed specimens injected with latex should be used for more detailed dissections such as the one described by Sack and Habel (1977).

Study and Understand the Specimen

Dissection is best practiced under the supervision of a skilled teacher. It is helpful to have preserved, pre-dissected and labeled specimens or prepared models available to aid you in locating and identifying important structures.

Each structure and its function has been discussed in detail in the previous Chapters. Identify each structure and review its function. The dissection will start from the outside and proceed inward; the study of each structure started with the bones and proceeded outward to the hoof.

Dissection of the Horse's Foot

Steps in making a simple dissection of the horse's foot:

1. Secure the dead leg in a bench vise and trim the hoof as you would for a normal shoeing job.
2. Trim down the wall, with the nippers perpendicular to its outer face, until blood can be seen in the area of the white line all the way around from the toe to the heels. Note the distance to blood from ground surface of the sole of a hoof prepared for shoeing.
3. Trim the buttresses away with the nippers by cutting out a piece of the heel portion of the wall from the white line at the buttresses to the bulbs.
4. Make a cut with the nippers at the heel separating the wall from the sole and the sensitive laminae at the heel.
5. Insert the pull offs at the heel on the wall. Pull around against the wall and peel it off. Fresh specimens are very difficult to separate. Dead feet which have been unrefrigerated for several days come apart easily. Note the interlocking nature of the sensitive and horny laminae. Examine the papillae of the sensitive coronary band and perioplic ring. Cut (section) the wall parallel and perpendicular to the horn tubules and note its relative elasticity and thickness of the quarters, heels and toe. Observe the relative size and spacing of the horn tubules under a magnifying glass.
6. Insert the pull offs under the sole at the toe and peel it back. The entire horny sole and frog should separate from the sensitive sole and frog. Note the shape of the sensitive sole and frog and their relationship to the corresponding horny structures. Examine the papillae of the sensitive sole and frog. Section the sole and frog and note the thickness of each. Seeing these structures and their relationship to each other aids one in developing judgment and feel for how much horn can be safely trimmed from the various regions of the hoof.

7. Skin the leg. Carefully separate the skin from the hoof at the hair line. Preserve and observe the venous plexuses on the outside of the lateral cartilages. Note that the main arteries, veins and nerves supplying the foot run together on both sides of the pastern and arteries and nerves disappear under the wings of the lateral cartilages.

8. Scrape the sensitive laminae and the coronary band off and from around the lateral cartilage(s). Note the abundance of blood vessels in the sensitive structures.

9. Remove the lateral cartilage(s) being careful to cut close to it (them) with the knife so as not to destroy the venous plexus(es) directly under it (them). Demonstrate the blood pumping mechanism of the foot by pressing the pastern down on the plantar cushion and noting the movement of blood through the venous plexus(es). The pumping and valve action of the elastic structures and the venous plexuses is essential to keep the blood circulating through the foot and to create a hydraulic cushion that protects the coffin bone in the hoof.

10. Remove the plantar cushion by making a deep and angled cut the full length of the commissures of the foot and another one separating the upper surface of the cushion from its attachments. Note the absence of blood vessels in the body of the plantar cushion and its fibro-fatty composition. Observe its qualities of cushioning and elasticity.

11. Separate the tendons by cutting the volar or plantar, proximal and distal annular ligaments in half on the back of the fetlock and pastern and severing the ring which joins the tendons at the fetlock. Note the points of attachment (insertion) of the tendons and the action they have on the foot.

12. Remove the tendons by cutting and scraping them away from the bone at their point(s) of attachment (insertion). Note the point(s) and extent of attachment. Study the relationship of the deep flexor to the superficial flexor tendon. Examine the position and extent of the navicular bursa between the deep flexor tendon and the navicular bone.

13. Compare the flexibility of the pastern and coffin joints. Note that the pastern joint is comparatively rigid due to the presence of the superficial sesamoidean and pastern ligaments. Cut apart the coffin joint by pushing a boning knife into the coffin joint at a 45 degree angle to the bone column cutting the joint capsule and collateral ligaments. Note the capsular ligament (joint capsule) which holds the slippery lubricating fluid (synovial fluid) between the surfaces of the joint. The gliding joint surface helps the horse to adjust to uneven terrain as he places weight on the leg. Note the strong collateral ligaments and suspensory ligament of the navicular bone at the sides of the pastern and coffin joint.

14. Cut apart the rest of the coffin joint and note the ligaments of the navicular bone. Study the location of the navicular bone in relation to the sides and bottom of the hoof. Knowledge of its location and relative size is essential when testing for navicular disease. Note how light and porous the coffin bone is. The hoof must be strong and healthy to protect it.

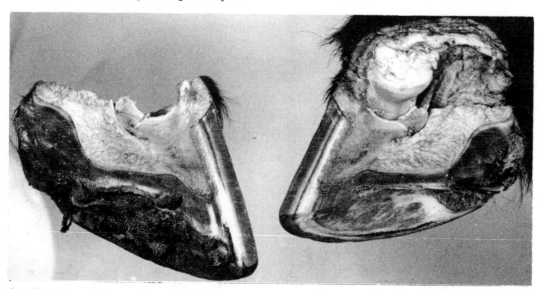

Fig. 15-2. Foot sawed in half. Left—untrimmed. Right—trimmed.

Several structures can be best observed by sawing a dead foot in half. This also gives one a different perspective on the parts and functions of the foot.

Steps in sawing apart a dead foot:

1. Secure a dead foot in a vise and saw it in half with a cross cut saw. A band saw works better, if available. Frozen specimens are easier to saw than fresh specimens. Note the position of the navicular bone and the bursa between it and the deep flexor tendon. The thickness of the wall and sole can be compared. The untrimmed sole is usually about the same thickness as the wall that it joins. The relationship of the sensitive structures to the horny structures can also be studied.
2. Make another cut parallel to the horn tubules and perpendicular to the outside surface of the hoof wall in the midquarter region. The line should be about two-thirds of the way to the buttress from the center of the toe. The blood vessels forming the plexuses can be easily seen and their action studied in a specimen cut in this manner.

Models

Models of the various systems or structures of the leg and foot are very useful for anatomy and physiology study. The prepared specimens can be studied at will and eliminate the necessity of acquiring fresh tissue for each period of study. The experience of dissecting and preparing a specimen also helps one to picture the structures and their relationship to each other.

Models of the bones of the leg and foot are handy for personal study and client education. You should make several. Simmer a skinned dead leg covered with water until all the soft tissue falls off the bones. This usually takes about 24 hours. Separate out the bones and wash them with a high detergent soap. Scrub them with a wire brush. The bones should then be soaked in a strong cleaning solution for several days. Next, let the bones dry a week or so. A fan helps speed up the process. You may want to mount them on a wood or metal stand after fastening them together with glue or wire.

Models to show tendons or ligaments should be dissected, soaked in formaldehyde or other preservative, and dried in position. Soft tissue and hoof models are harder to preserve but can also be dried after treatment with formaldehyde or alcohol. Specimens must be protected from bugs and kept dry to prevent mildew. Prepared specimens are available commercially from biological supply houses[1].

[1]*Carolina Biological Supply Co., Burlington, NC.*

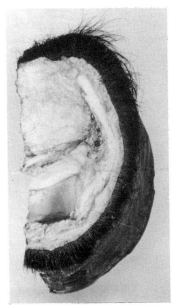

Fig. 15-3. View from above (proximal) of foot sawed in half and cut off just above the coronary band.

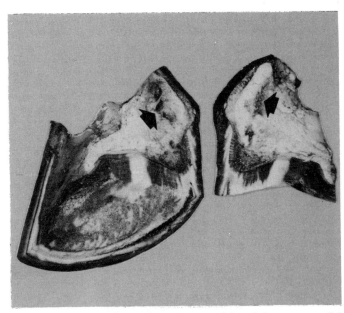

Fig. 15-4. Half of foot sawed through the quarter parallel to the horn tubules to demonstrate the venous plexuses surrounding the lateral cartilage (arrows).

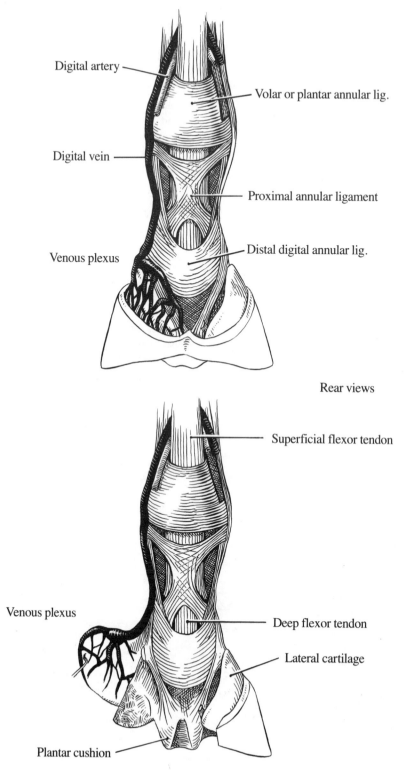

Digital artery

Volar or plantar annular lig.

Digital vein

Proximal annular ligament

Distal digital annular lig.

Venous plexus

Rear views

Superficial flexor tendon

Venous plexus

Deep flexor tendon

Lateral cartilage

Plantar cushion

Fig. 15-5. Rear (volar or plantar) view of superficial structures of the digit after the skin and facia are removed. Drawing by L. Sadler.

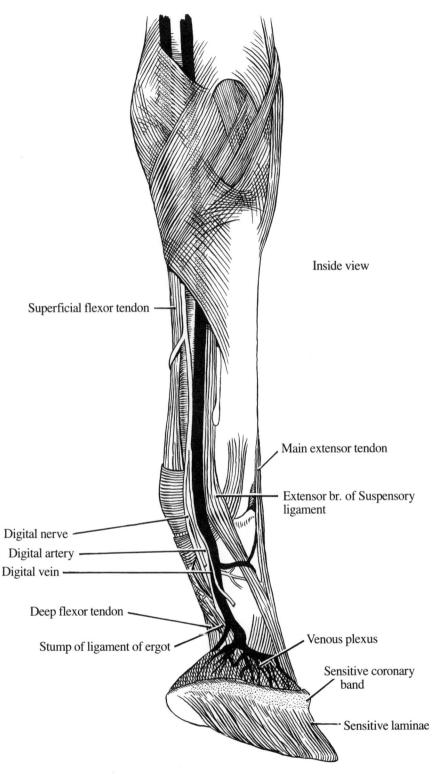

Inside view

Superficial flexor tendon —

Main extensor tendon

Extensor br. of Suspensory
ligament

Digital nerve —
Digital artery —
Digital vein —

Deep flexor tendon —

Stump of ligament of ergot —

Venous plexus

Sensitive coronary
band

Sensitive laminae

*Fig. 15-6. Inside (medial) view of superficial structures
of the horse's leg after the hoof and skin are removed.
Drawing by L. Sadler.*

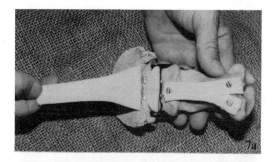

References

Ellenberger, W., H. Baum and H. Dittrich. 1956. An Atlas of Animal Anatomy for Artists. Dover Publ., New York.

Habel, R.E. 1975. Applied Veterinary Anatomy. R.E. Habel, Ithaca, NY.

King, J.M., D.C. Dodd and M.E. Newson. Gross Necropsy Technique for Animals. J.E. King, Ithaca, NY.

Rooney, J.R. 1970. Autopsy of the Horse. Williams and Wilkins Co., Baltimore.

Sack, W.O. and R.E. Habel. 1977. Rooney's Guide to the Dissection of the Horse. Veterinary Textbooks, Ithaca, NY.

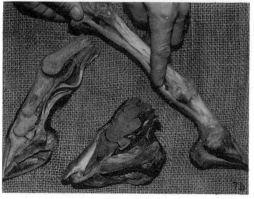

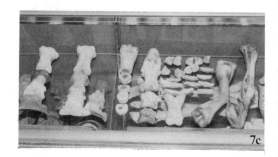

Fig. 15-7. Specimen models are handy for personal study and client education. Photo by J. Graves.

NOTES:

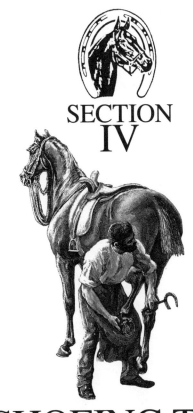

SECTION
IV

SHOEING THE STRAIGHT AND SOUND PLEASURE HORSE

Chapter 16

Horseshoeing Tools and Skills

Henry Ward Beecher said "A tool is but the extension of a man's hand."

A fine tool in the hands of a skilled craftsman can be so much an extension of a man's hand that the resulting workmanship almost seems to have flowed directly from the body of the artisan into the work.

Personal tools made by blacksmiths are as distinguishable and distinctive as a man's signature. Favorite tool patterns and trade secrets have been handed down from generation to generation through the apprentice system.

The balance and "feel" of a fine tool is an unexplainable quality recognized instantly by a craftsman. Horseshoers not only need tools that will allow them to do quality work, but they also want tools which save them time and effort. Even though fine quality horseshoeing tools are available commercially, many horseshoers make a few of their own tools.

Fine tools are a good investment. Tools can be obtained from most suppliers. Centaur Forge, Ltd.[1], is the largest distributor of blacksmithing and horseshoeing supplies in America.

Apron

A leather horseshoeing apron is designed to protect the horseshoer's legs from driven nails before they are finished and cutting tools which may slip off the foot while he is working on it.

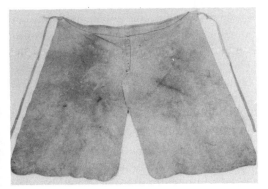

Fig. 16-1. Apron. Photos by G. Poellot.

[1]*Centaur Forge, Ltd., Burlington, WI.*

Aprons also protect clothes from being burned by scale from hot iron. The open-legged style may be removed quickly if a nail gets caught in it. Many are made double thickness. Some horseshoers sew a knife pocket on their aprons to carry and protect their knives when fitting and trimming without a tool box. Aprons are sometimes called shoeing chaps.

Hoof Pick

A hoof pick is used for cleaning out the bottom of a horse's foot. An excellent hoof pick can be made from an old pitchfork tine.

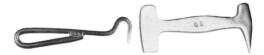

Fig. 16-2. Hoof pick. *Fig. 16-3. Clinch cutter.*
Photos by McLain.

Clinch Cutter

A clinch cutter, or buffer as it is sometimes called, consists of two parts, the blade and the point. The blade, preferably an inch wide, is used to cut or to raise clinches. It is placed under the clinch and struck with the driving hammer. The point is used to punch nails and broken stubs out of the hoof. It can be used to raise the head of a nail from the crease of a shoe sufficiently to enable the pinchers to grasp the nail head for removal. The pointed end can also double as a hoof pick. Some horseshoers make these from discarded rasps or leaf springs obtained from junk cars.

Pull Off

Pull offs or pinchers are used to remove shoes, nail stubs and improperly driven nails. They can be used to turn the clinches. Some types of pull offs can also be used as nail cutters and others can be used as shoe spreaders. Pull offs have knobs on the ends of the handles to make them distinguishable at a glance (or touch) from nippers.

153

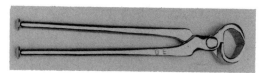

Fig. 16-4. Pull off.

Hoof Nipper

Hoof nippers are used to remove the surplus growth of the wall. They should be used only for this purpose; *never on nails*. Several sizes are available: 14 and 15 inch nippers are most commonly used on saddle and draft horses, 12 inch on show, race horses and foals. A light race track nipper with 14 inch handles is also available.[2]

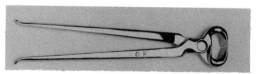

Fig. 16-5. Hoof nipper.

Hoof Knife

A hoof knife is used to pare away the dead sole from the hoof, to remove ragged parts from the frog, to relieve pressure on corns and cracks, and to remove foreign bodies from the foot. The wide-bladed, 2½ to 3 inch knife is the most commonly used. Short, narrow-bladed knives have their primary use in therapeutic work, such as locating infection in the foot. Hoof knives are available in right-handed and left-handed styles.

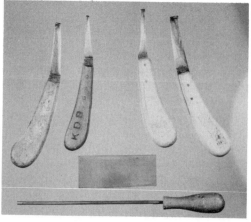

Fig. 16-6. Hoof knives, sharpening file and slipstone. Photo by G. Poellot.

[2]GE Forge and Tool Works, Arroyo Grande, CA.

A fine-cut round file, such as is used to sharpen chain saws, is excellent for rough sharpening hoof knives. A tapered flat slipstone is useful for finishing blades to a sharp edge.

Double-edged knives are available but have not found wide popularity among horseshoers. Most horseshoers like to push and steady the hoof knife with the thumb of their opposite hand. This can't be done with a double-edged knife.

Sole Knife

A sole knife is used to remove dead sole from hard, dry hoofs. It is held in one hand and struck with the driving hammer. Sole knives can be bought commercially or made from rasps or leaf springs.

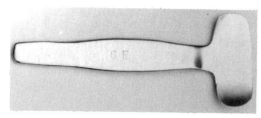

Fig. 16-7. Sole knife. Photo by McLain.

Rasp

A rasp is used to make a level bearing surface after the hoof has been trimmed with the nippers and to shape a distorted or flaring foot. After it becomes too dull to be effective for hoof preparation, it is used for a clinching-up or finishing rasp. As a finishing rasp, it is used to make clinches all the same length, to remove the burr under each clinch, to smooth the clinches after they are turned, and to finish the hoof. The same rasp is then used as a hot-rasp until it is worn out to finish heels on shoes after they are cut. The 14 inch double extra-thin tanged rasp (Plater's Special) is the most popular. One side is coarse for rapid removal of horn. The other side is fine for finishing work.

Rasps can be resharpened if they are not used for metal filing. A rasp may be cleaned with a

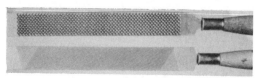

Fig. 16-8. Rasp. Photos by G. Poellot.

wire brush periodically to remove mud and manure. Hardened mud and hoof particles may be removed from a rasp with a horseshoe nail.

Finishing File

A 14 inch flat file is used by some horseshoers to smooth the clinches and the rasped areas of the foot. A mill bastard-cut flat file is the most popular for finishing work.

Fig. 16-9. Finishing file.

Hoof Gauge, Divider and Rule

A hoof gauge, divider and rule are used for determining the exact hoof angle and toe length so that a corresponding pair of feet can be trimmed the same length and angle. They are not widely used on saddle horses except for corrective shoeing.

Hoof gauges or protractors are used extensively on show and racing horses, where the hoof angle and toe length influence gait, way of going, and stride arc. Some gauges are read from the bottom of the foot and others from the side.

A metal rule mounted on the tool box is a useful aid for setting and reading the divider. A small measuring tape is useful for measuring toe length from the coronary border of the wall to the ground, as is required on show horses.

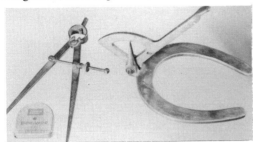

Fig. 16-10. Hoof gauge and divider.

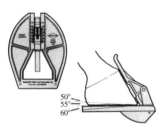

Fig. 16-11. Spring loaded hoof gauge. Drawing by Diamond.

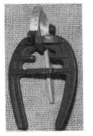

Fig. 16-12. Ward and Story hoof gauge. Photo by J. Graves.

Driving Hammer

A driving hammer, sometimes called the shoeing hammer, is used to drive horseshoe nails and to turn over or wring off (twist) nails after they have been driven to the proper height. The weights generally used are a 10 ounce on race horses, a 12 to 14 ounce on saddle horses, and a 16 ounce on show and draft horses. A 6 ounce hammer is available[3] for race horse shoeing.

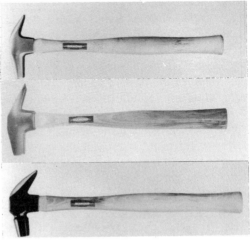

Fig. 16-13. Types of driving hammers. (Top) 10 oz., (middle) 14 oz., (bottom) 16 oz. Photos by Diamond.

Clinch Block

A clinch block is used to turn the clinches. Many shoers use just a block of steel, such as a fender block (body tool). Some use their pull offs as a clinching block. Numerous styles of blocks are available.

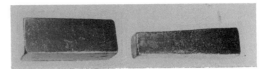

Fig. 16-14. Clinching blocks. Photo by G. Poellot.

Nail Cutter

Nail cutters or nail nippers are used to cut off clinched, turned-over, or wrung-off nails to an equal length. Many horseshoers rasp the clinched nails to the same length with the smooth side of a rasp. The nail cutter is also used when removing nails from worn shoes being prepared to be reset.

[3]*Thoro'bred Racing Plate Co., Inc., Anaheim, CA.*

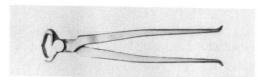

Fig. 16-15. Nail cutter. Photo by G E Forge and Tool Works.

Clincher

Clinchers, clinching tongs, or alligators are used to draw down the clinches. They were designed for use on horses bothered by hammer and block clinching. Clinchers are of two general types: saddle horse clinchers, and gooseneck clinchers. Saddle horse clinchers are designed for use on No. 5 nails and up. The goosenecks are designed for use on the smaller nails driven in racing plates and pony shoes. The farrier's clincher is a type of gooseneck clincher. Draft horse clinchers are heavier and have the teeth farther apart than saddle horse clinchers.

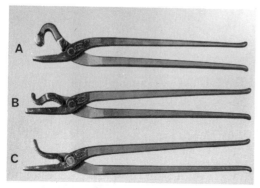

Fig. 16-16. Types of clinchers. (A) farrier's clincher, (B) gooseneck clincher, (C) saddle horse clincher. Photo by G. Poellot.

Crease Nail Puller

A crease nail puller is designed for easy removal of driven nails from creased shoes.

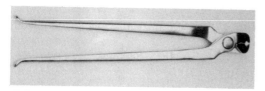

Fig. 16-17. Crease nail puller. Photos by McLain.

Shoe Spreader

A shoe spreader is designed to spread a shoe slightly at the heels after it has been nailed on. Some beginners find the use of this tool an easy way to give a shoe expansion at the heels. The use of this tool is not recommended on feet with thin "shelly" walls.

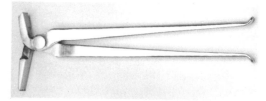

Fig. 16-18. Shoe spreader.

Hoof Tester

A hoof tester is used to determine the location of a painful area in the foot of a lame horse. It is more specific than tapping the hoof with a hammer. A hoof tester may be used to locate bruised or punctured areas of the foot, or to diagnose foot bone diseases or injuries. To test for a foot problem, place the end of one jaw on the suspected area, and the other on the outside of the wall, and exert pressure in that area by closing the handles. The reaction of the horse to the pressure in that area is the basis for the diagnosis of lameness. A sound hoof should be compared to the lame one to determine an individual horse's response to pain. See Chapter 33.

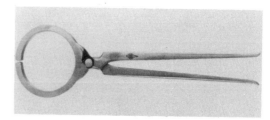

Fig. 16-19. Hoof tester. Photo by G E Forge and Tool Works.

Shoeing Box

There are nearly as many types of shoeing boxes as there are horseshoers. A box should be difficult to tip over, make the tools readily accessible, and be light in weight so that it can be easily moved from foot to foot. Only those tools regularly used on the foot should be carried in

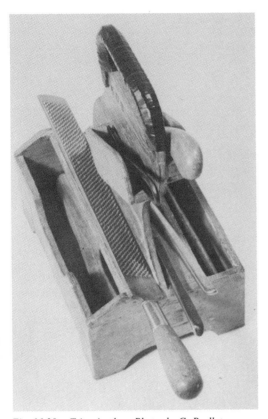

Fig. 16-20.   Trimming box. Photos by G. Poellot.

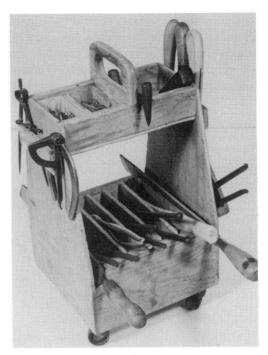

Fig. 16-22.   Shop shoeing box.

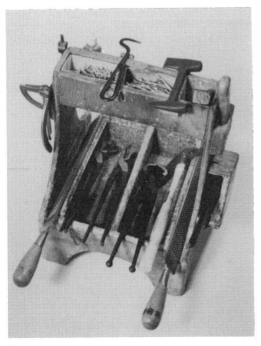

Fig. 16-21.   Shoeing box.

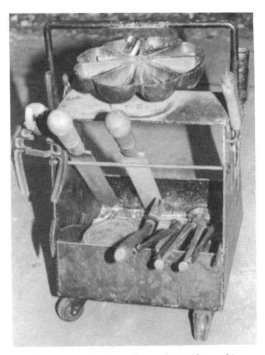

Fig. 16-23.   An aluminum shoeing box with a multi-compartment nail tray. Photo by J. Graves.

the shoeing box. Others may be added as needed. Boxes can be made from light plywood and covered with fiberglass or they can be made from welded or cast aluminum. An aluminum box with a multi-compartment rotating nail tray is available for shoeing show horses[4].

Summary of Tools and Equipment Needed for Horseshoeing

An anvil, shaping hammer, and pritchel are also necessary to shoe a horse with machine-made cold shoes. These tools will be discussed along with forging tools in Chapter 23.

Many tools and supplies will be needed to begin the business of horseshoeing. The following list may be used as a guide.

In Tool Box

Apron	Rasp(s) w/Handle (14 in. Extra Thin)
Hoof Pick	Hoof Gauge, Dividers and Rule
Clinch Cutter	Driving Hammer (10 to 14 oz.)
Pull Offs	Clinch Block
Hoof Nippers	Clinchers
Hoof Knife (Right or Left Handed)	Crease Nail Puller
Sole Knife	Chalk

At Anvil Stand

Rounding Hammer (2 to 2½ lb.)	Straight Hardy
Tongs	Nail Cutters
Stamp(s)	Heavy Wire Brush
Pritchel(s)	Bob Punch
Shoe Fitting Tongs or Pritchel	Assorted Punches
Creaser	Assorted Tongs
Old Rasp	Assorted Hammers
Half-Round Hardy	Other Specialized Tools for Each Type of Horse

In Truck or Shop

Forge—Coal or Gas Fired	Hoof Tester
Anvil	Wire Brush
Anvil Stand	File(s)
Vise	Sharpening Stone
Water Bucket	Chalk
Fire Tools (Shovel and Poker)	Oxy-Acetylene Welder with Welding, Borium and Brazing Rods

For Horse

Halter	Rope—25 ft. cotton (1/2 to 3/4 in.)
Lip Chain	Leg Strap and Hobbles
Twitch	Rope(s)—14 ft. Nylon (1/2 to 3/4 in.)

Supplies

Coal or Gas Supply	Pads—Leather and Plastic, Corrective Wedges
Assorted Shoes and Nails	Packing for Pads (Pine Tar and Oakum or Forshner's)
Assorted Steel Bar Stock	First Aid Medicines (Iodine—7%, Furacin, Ichthammol—20%)

References

Bealer, A.W. 1976. The Art of Blacksmithing (2nd ed.). Funk and Wagnalls, New York.

Peih, W.S. 1983. Blacksmiths' and Horseshoers' Supply Catalog. Centaur Forge, Ltd., Burlington, WI.

Slone, E. 1964. A Museum of Early American Tools. Ballantine Books, New York.

Watson, A.A. 1968. The Village Blacksmith. Thomas Y. Crowell Co., New York.

[4]Scott M. Colson Shop, Jackson, MS.

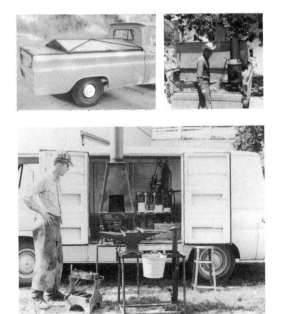

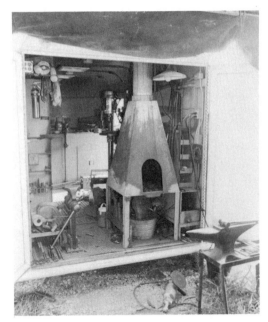

Fig. 16-24. Completely outfitted mobil shoeing shops. Photos by G. Poellot and J. Graves.

NOTES:

Shoeing Record Card

Owner _____ Address _____ Phone _____

Name of Horse _____ Year Foaled _____ Color and Marking _____

| DATE | FRONT FEET | | | | HIND FEET | | | | REMARKS | Chg. | Pd. |
	Angle	Length	Type of Shoe	N/R	Angle	Length	Type of Shoe	N/R			

Fig. 17-1. *Shoeing Record Card. Type of Shoe column is for size and style of shoe. N/R column indicates new or reset shoes. Remarks column can contain such information as behavior of the horse, oddities of the feet, call back time. Chg. column is price of the job; Pd. column is record of payment.*

Chapter 17

Trimming

Preliminary Examination

The inspection of the horse prior to trimming or shoeing is called preliminary examination. Experienced shoers develop a "feel" for the preliminary examination and rely on all their senses to determine the condition of the horse and its feet. A thorough examination is necessary when lameness is suspected.

Records on each horse are often useful in conducting a preliminary examination, especially for show horses which are regularly shod and often require special shoeing. Shoeing records can be kept in a card file or notebook. Appointments can be scheduled and billing can be monitored with such a card.

Follow a definite step-by-step procedure to be sure that nothing is overlooked. *You cannot "start over" once the foot is trimmed!*

1. Observe the horse in *motion* as he is being brought to you and note any signs of *lameness* or *limb interference*. Lameness and faults of gait are more easily detected when the horse is trotting directly away from or directly toward you. Any abnormality should be reported to the owner before any attempt is made to correct it.

2. Observe the *overall conformation* of the horse as he is tied up or held for you. Is it likely to predispose him to any faults of gait or unsoundness? For example, a long-legged shortbacked horse is likely to forge with his first set of shoes if his conformation is not taken into consideration when shoeing.

3. Observe the *position of each foot axis* from the front and the side when the horse is standing squarely on his feet. Is the axis of each leg and foot straight or broken? Is the foot balanced, i.e., is the axis broken in, broken out, sloping or stumpy, etc.? If it is not straight, is the deviation due to wear, growth of the hoof, or a conformation problem? Where and how much must each foot be trimmed to put it in balance?

4. Note unusual *deformities* or *characteristics* of the *feet* and *legs*. For example, do the feet appear to be dry, brittle, and cracking? Compare the size of corresponding feet. Are they the same? If not, trim all that is possible off the largest one. Then the smaller one can be trimmed (or built-up) to match it.

5. Pick up *each foot*. Clean it out with the hoof pick, and examine it before starting to shoe the horse. Run your hand down the leg and quickly examine it as you pick up each foot. This may save time and grief, especially on lame horses with special problems. Note the position of the wear on the shoes or feet, the style of the shoes, and the condition of the shoes and feet. This procedure also gives you some indication of the horse's temperament.

6. Question the *owner*:
   1. How does the horse usually stand for shoeing? Has the horse any bad habits?
   2. How long has it been since the horse was last trimmed or shod?
   3. What will the horse be used for and how hard will it be worked? Would you prefer new shoes?
   4. Has the horse ever been lame or interfered (hit himself)?
   5. Do you have any preference as to style of shoe?
   6. Do you understand how much the job will cost? How do you plan to pay?

Visualizing the Ideal

Visualize in your mind a balanced well-shod hoof. You may form this image as you describe to the owner the differences that shoeing an unbalanced and distorted hoof will make in the horse's stance and ability to perform. Begin with the end in mind. Let the visualized ideal guide your hands to create that which your mind imagines. Joseph Gamgee (1871) said we must sculpture the true foot from a mass of deformity:

> There is a common saying, that in shoeing, "the shoe should be made to fit the foot, and not the foot to fit the shoe." This hackneyed adage, when closely examined, amounts to nonsense. The horse-shoer, if he be an artist worthy of the art, is required to know the foot, so that he can, to the greatest possible exactness and extent, economize its want of substance and energy; he must, like the sculptor with his clay or marble, bring out the true figure from a mass

of deformity. That the over-reduced and weak hoofs are the most numerous, is granted; but I have seen numerous bad cases of deformity and lameness due to excess of horn in the wrong places.

Frequency of Trimming

Trimming, for shoeing or to go barefoot, should be done regularly and as often as necessary to meet the needs of the animal or the owner. The time period between trimmings cannot be arbitrarily set at six weeks, although that is about the average time for many horses. This time period can vary from two weeks to two months depending on:

1. Growth and changes in the horse's hoof.
2. How important it is for the hoof length, angle, and balance to remain the same.
3. The wear on the shoe or hoof.
4. Seasonal, use, or medicinal changes.
5. The owner's preference.

Cleaning the Hoof

If the feet are covered with mud, either wet or dry, it should be removed before raising the foot for shoeing. Wet mud can be removed readily by wiping the feet with an old burlap sack or towel. Dry mud which is caked on the foot can be scraped off with the edge of an old rasp.

Encourage horse owners to do this before asking the horseshoer to work on the feet.

The hoof pick is used to clean out the bottom of the foot. The dull edge of the hoof knife or the end of a handle on the hoof nippers may also be used for this purpose.

Follow these steps for fast, efficient cleaning:

1. Insert the point of the hoof pick between the end of the heels or buttress of the foot and the frog. While pulling the pick toward the toe with one hand, push down carefully and force it to the bottom of the commissure (sulcus) with the other hand.
2. Repeat this process on the other commissure.
3. Place the pick at the inside of one heel of the shoe or wall and pull it around in a circular motion following the inside border of the shoe or wall.

The combination of these three motions should clean all of the foreign material from the bottom of the foot. However, if any remains, scrape it off with the edge of the hoof pick.

Treat thrush infection if present. Put medication on after you finish working on the foot to avoid staining your hands and tools. Thrush treatment is covered in Chapter 18.

Removing the Worn Shoe

Worn shoes, if present, must be removed before trimming the hoof. Shoes which have been

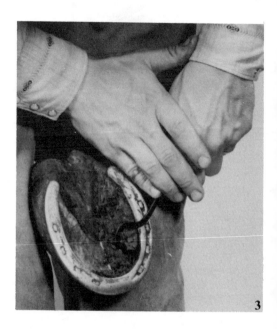

Fig. 17-2. Steps in cleaning the hoof (1-3). Photos by G. Poellot.

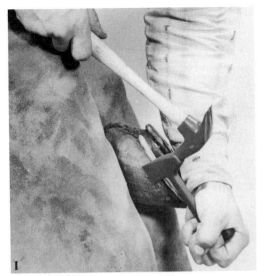
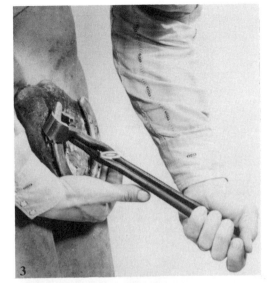
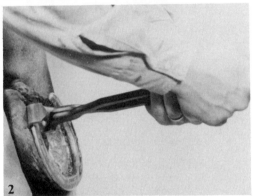
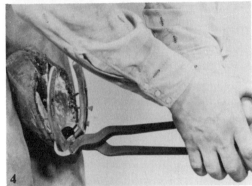

Fig. 17-3. Steps in removing the worn shoes (1-4).

on for some time (so that the old nail holes in the wall will be trimmed away) and are loose can be pulled without cutting the clinches. Some horseshoers rasp off the clinches, especially when working on sensitive-footed horses. The clinches must be removed before pulling the shoe in order to prevent the wall from breaking away as the shoe is pulled. The clinch cutter is designed for this purpose.

Steps in removing the worn shoes:
1. Open or cut the clinches by striking the clinch cutter with the driving hammer. Start the clinch cutter at a steep angle to the wall. Then, hold the clinch cutter as flat as possible against the wall to avoid cutting the wall along with the nails.
2. Insert the jaws of the pull offs under one heel of the shoe.
3. Close the handles and pull down toward the toe and in toward the center of the foot. Support the toe with your knees. When hard

pulling is necessary, support the toe with one hand in order to avoid injury to the joints of the lower leg.
4. The pull offs should be gradually worked toward the toe on first one branch of the shoe and then the other until the shoe works loose from the foot.
5. Discard the shoe where the horse will not step on it if he moves around. Many horseshoers throw the pulled shoes in their shoeing box temporarily to keep them from being under foot.

Trimming the Hoof

Steps in trimming the hoof:
1. Note the conformation of the foot. Sight the foot and check for lateral balance. Hold the foot naturally at the fetlock and position your head directly above the foot. Decide how much is to come off *before* starting to trim. A homemade T-square is useful as an aid for visualizing the relationship of the

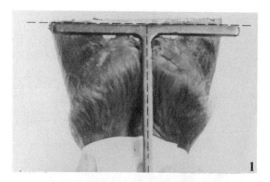

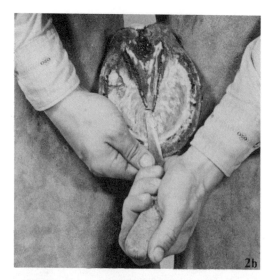

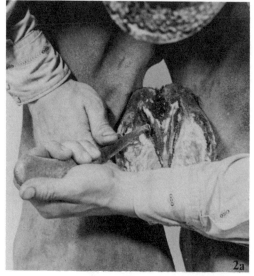

Fig. 17-4. Steps in trimming the hoof—shaping the sole (1-2).

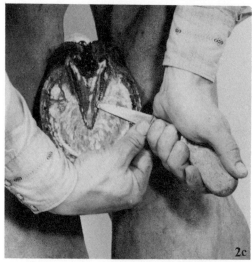

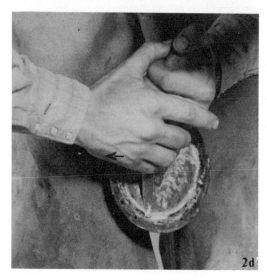

axis of the bones to the ground surface of the hoof. It is especially valuable for teaching beginners how to sight a foot.

2. Pare away and shape the "dead" sole with the hoof knife. Use your thumb to support the knife and to help guide it. Remember that the front foot has a naturally flat sole, while the sole of the hind foot is naturally concave. Trim the bars of the hoof level with the trimmed sole at the same time. Long thick bars may need to be trimmed with the nippers before trimming the wall. The bars need to be trimmed flush with the sole so they will not be broken or torn and cause injury to the foot if the horse steps on a rock.

If the dead sole is extremely hard, use a sole knife. The sole knife is guided by one hand while it is struck with the driving hammer. It should always be used to chip or shave the sole off and never be driven deeply.

Judging the amount to trim off the feet is often a problem for beginners. A rule which

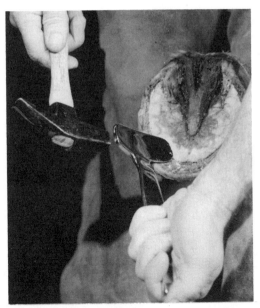

Fig. 17-5. Sole knife in use.

"Trimming or shoeing short," as this is called, is not as popular among trail riders and others who ride in rough country as it is with race or show horse fanciers. Horses that are to be used on rocky terrain or ridden on roads should be trimmed without removing any sole. The wall should be trimmed level with the dead sole. This sole serves as a protection to the foot until it is worn away and replaced by new growth.

Horses which are stabled should have the dead sole removed from their feet for hygienic purposes since they do not naturally wear it away. The object is to trim the sole without making it look like it has been trimmed.

3. Trim the ragged edges and loose pieces from the frog. This must be done to prevent thrush. Dirt and filth will become trapped in these ragged areas and thus provide an ideal medium for the anaerobic thrush organism to thrive. A properly-shaped frog also facilitates regular hoof cleaning with a hoof pick. Again, when the horse is to be used on rocky terrain, do not trim the frog unless it is diseased.

4. Open the nippers and place the inside cutting edge on the sole that has been trimmed in the previous step. They are now in position to start to trim the wall at the toe. Hold the nippers in such a way that an imaginary line bisecting the open handles will be perpendicular to the proposed bearing surface of the foot.

5. Close the handles of the nippers toward the imaginary line bisecting the handles.

6. Rotate the cutting head of the inside jaw to the right or left about one-half its width

works well on dead feet used for instructional purposes, but may not be applicable to the feet of some horses because of their conformation, is to trim the sole *at the toe* down to glossy or "live" material. Turn the knife around with the handle up to do this. This flat spot at the toe forms a seat for the nippers to rest on. This facilitates making a level cut at the proper depth with the nippers. Dead sole is dull and flaky, while live sole is glossy and smooth. There is about ⅜ inch to ¼ inch of live sole covering the sensitive sole of the average saddle horse.

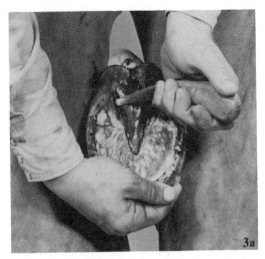

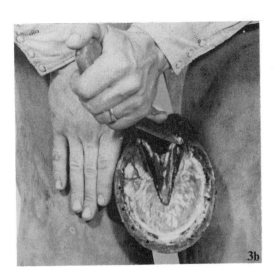

Fig. 17-6. Steps in trimming the hoof—shaping the frog (3).

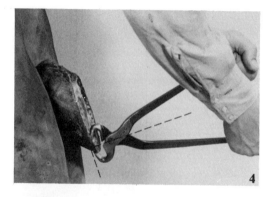

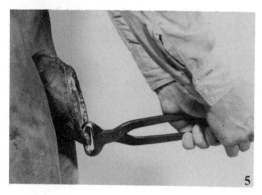

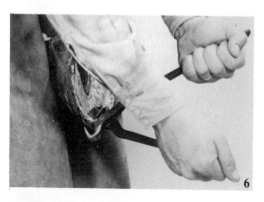

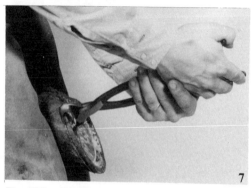

Fig. 17-7. *Steps in trimming the hoof—nipping the wall (4-9).*

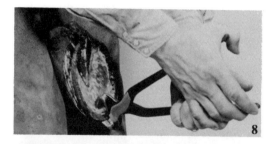

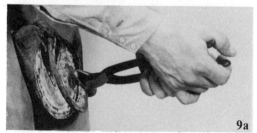

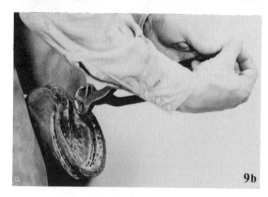

and make another cut. This allows for some overlap and provides a guide for the next cut.

7. Continue cutting back toward the heel, constantly keeping in mind at what depth you want to terminate with at the heel. Be careful not to cut too deep in the quarters of the foot, as this is easily done due to the shape of the sole in this area.

8. Upon reaching the end of the heel, return the nippers to the toe and place them in the guide you have already made for yourself.

9. Cut back toward the desired depth you wish to come out on this heel.

The Author has found the above procedure very effective in teaching beginners how to cut a hoof level and at the proper depth. The above explained method is also very useful when working on a foot that needs corrective trimming since it facilitates the process of cutting each side of the hoof to a different depth.

Some horseshoers start at one heel and continue around the hoof to the other heel. Others cut from each heel toward the toe.

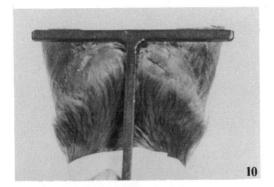

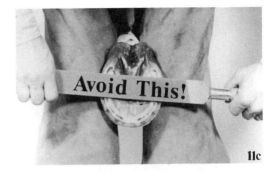

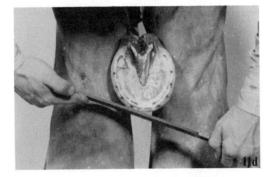

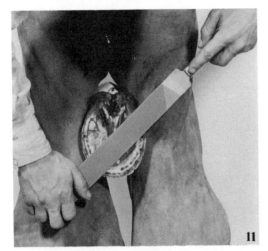

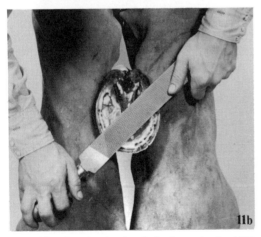

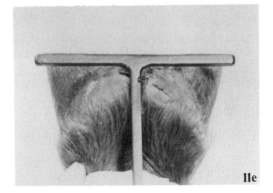

Fig. 17-8. Steps in trimming the hoof—rasping level (10-11).

10. Sight the foot to determine which side needs to be rasped the most.
11. Level the hoof with the coarse side of the rasp. Use the fine side of the rasp to finish the job and thus create a level bearing surface for the shoe. Sight the foot as often as

it is necessary to determine when it is level and balanced. Use the T-square only until you can visualize the ideal.

Rasp from heel to toe and from toe to heel so that rounding of the hoof and lowering of the quarters does not occur. Hold the rasp against the hoof, making contact at heel and toe, and let it slide over the foot in a downward, sweeping motion. On the other half of the hoof, run the rasp in a similar manner, only with the sweeping motion being made upward instead of downward. Avoid pushing hard on the rasp. This usually causes a rounding of the hoof wall and makes proper shoe fitting difficult.

It will be noted that a right-handed or a left-handed person always rasps a hoof in the same direction (i.e., counterclockwise

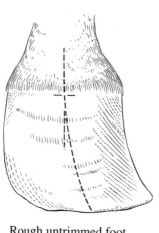

Rough untrimmed foot

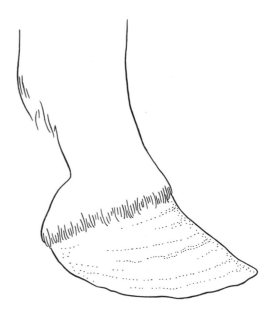

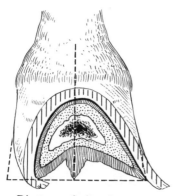

Diagram of trimming

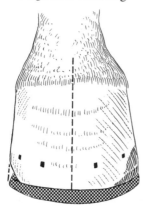

Trimmed & shod

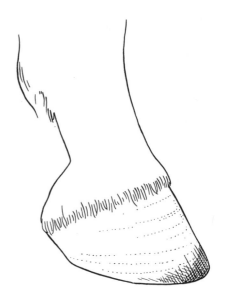

Fig. 17-9.   Principles of shaping the hoof.

or clockwise). If one puts more pressure on one side than the other, the hoof will not be level. Careful rasping in the above-described manner prevents this. Rasping from side-to-side causes unlevelness from toe to heel, as well as from side to side, and therefore should not be done.

Reduce the sharp edge of the level hoof wall by lightly running the fine side of the rasp around it.

12. Open your calipers to the length of the trimmed foot at mid-toe. Push your thumbnail against the hoof's upper edge at mid-toe and adjust the calipers from your thumb to the ground edge of the hoof. Place the calipers on the opposite untrimmed foot in the same place and scribe a line on the center of the toe. Make your nipper cut just below this line. Rasp until you reach the line and the angle of the opposite foot.

Shaping the Hoof

If the shape of the hoof is normal, the shoe may be fit to it at this point. However, if it is not, it will be necessary to take the foot into the forward position and remove any outward distortions (called flares or wings) of the wall that may be present. Visualize how the foot should look. Let this vision guide your hands as you shape the foot.

Two rules that can be useful guides (but are by no means absolute) when working on distorted and out-of-balance feet are:

1. Trim the foot no more than ¼ in. out-of-balance at a trimming. There is a possibility of injuring the joints, ligaments, or tendons of the leg if too drastic a change in foot position is made over a short period of time.
2. Remove no more than one-half the thickness of the wall at a trimming when trying to correct a distorted or flared hoof. Weakening the wall more than this may cause further distortion of the hoof and will not allow nails to be driven safely into the foot.

Steps in shaping a hoof:
1. Observe the level foot on the ground and note the degree of flaring.
2. Sight the foot and note the degree of flaring. A straight edge held on the side of the hoof may be useful in determining the degree of distortion.
3. In severely distorted cases, hold the nippers at a 45 degree angle and cut the sharp edge of the wall back to one-half of its thickness. This gives you a line on the ground surface of the hoof to rasp down to and reduces the amount of wall to be removed with the rasp.

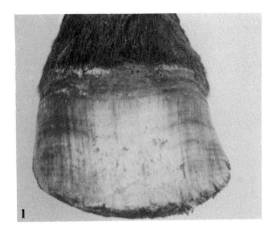
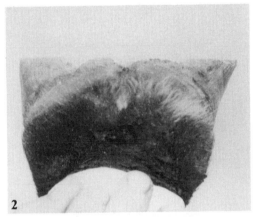
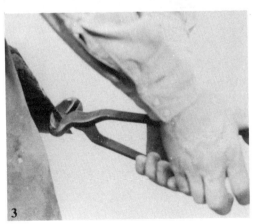

Fig. 17-10. *Steps in shaping a hoof (1-6).*

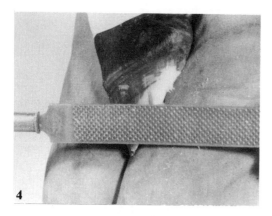

4

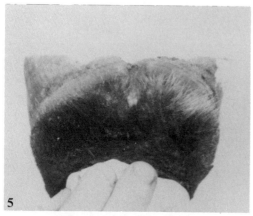

5

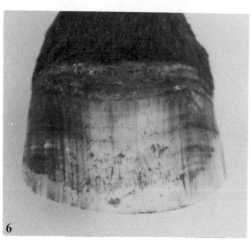

6

4. Rasp to the mark and blend the rasped area into the slope of the undistorted upper part of the wall.
5. Sight the foot and check the slope of the wall at the quarters.
6. Check the hoof in the standing position.

See Chapter 27 for further explanation of trimming and shoeing crooked, unbalanced, and out-of-shape feet.

When the feet are balanced, level, shaped, and corresponding pairs coincide, the horse is ready for shoes.

Trimming to Go Barefoot

A barefoot horse that is to be ridden extensively, or is to be kept on an abrasive surface, should not be trimmed as short as one which is stabled.

If the horse is to go barefoot, the outer edge of the wall should be rounded to prevent chipping and cracking. The wall should be well-rounded to one-half of its thickness all the way around. On feet with thick walls, this operation can be speeded up by holding the hoof nippers at a 45 degree angle to the ground surface and clipping off the sharp edge of the hoof. It is then a simple matter to round the hoof with the fine side of the rasp.

Rounding the hoof wall with the rasp can be done rapidly and smoothly by following these three steps:

1. Rasp (or trim with the nippers) from one side around to the other at a 45 degree angle to one-half the thickness of the ground surface of the wall.
2. Rasp at a larger angle next to the wall around the line that was formed from Step 1.
3. Rasp lightly around and against the wall to remove the line that was formed in Step 2.

References

Gamgee, J. 1871. A Treatise on Horseshoeing and Lameness. Longmens, Green and Co., London.

Lungwitz, A. and J.W. Adams. 1966. A Textbook of Horseshoeing. Oregon State University, Corvallis.

War Department. 1941. The Horseshoer. United States Government Printing Office, Washington, D.C.

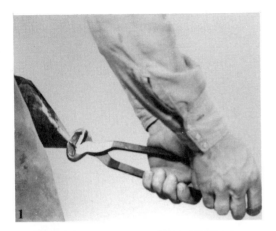

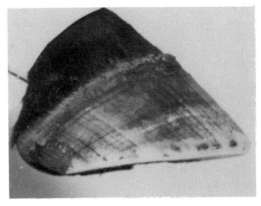

Fig. 17-12.   Completed foot trimmed to go barefoot.

NOTES:

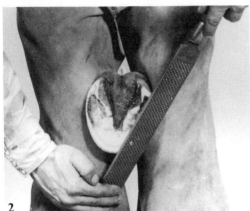

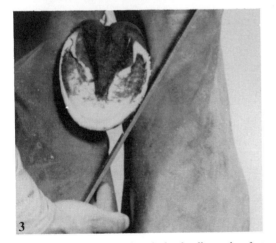

Fig. 17-11.   Steps in rounding the hoof wall to go barefoot (1-3).

Chapter 18

First Aid

First aid implies immediate treatment of an abnormal condition. This may be routinely necessary for commonly encountered hoof conditions. It may be occasionally necessary for serious accidents.

Horseshoeing is a potentially dangerous activity. The horse or the horseshoer may be accidentally injured. Preparation involves gaining general knowledge of conditions including recognition and treatment of diseases discussed in Chapters 6 and 33. Proper preparation also includes providing for possible emergency situations with a first aid kit.

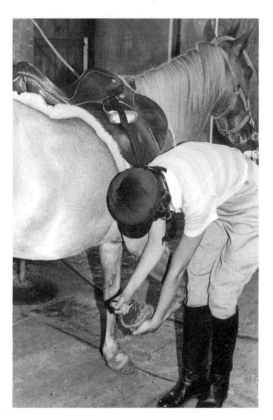

Fig. 18-1. Cleaning the foot regularly is good preventative medicine. Photo by J. Graves.

First Aid Kits

A first aid kit for the **horse** could include:

Cotton roll—used on the end of the hoof pick to clean pus and debris from recesses in the hoof. Also used to hold foot dressing in place.

Gauze roll and telfa pads—used to stop bleeding and hold dressing in place.

Adhesive tape (1 in. roll)—used to hold gauze in place.

Elastic bandage (1½ in. to 3 in. wide)—used for strains and sprains.

Furacin dressing (nitrofurazone)—antibiotic salve used under bandage on the foot.

Iodine (7%)—used for thrush treatment or deep foot wounds.

Kopertox (copper sulfate)—used for thrush treatment, soaked in cotton under pad.

Turpentine—used to toughen a soft, overflexible sole. May be used with iodine crystals as a dramatic thrush treatment.

Sulfa-urea cream—used to treat mild cases of grease heel (scratches).

Ichthammol (20% black salve)—used to poultice abscesses.

Searcher or Thin bladed knife—used to create drainage for abscesses.

Insect repellent—used to keep a horse quiet when shoeing.

Pine tar and oakum—used for packing under pads.

Peat moss hoof packing—used for packing under pads.

Syringe and blunt needle—used for irrigating a deep wound in the foot.

Hydrogen Peroxide—used to irrigate wounds and abscesses before dressing.

Epsom salts—used for soaking an abscessed foot.

Heavy bucket—used to soak the foot in.

A first aid kit for the **horseshoer** could include:

Band-aids—for minor self-inflicted wounds.

Neosporin ointment—for application to wounds.

Burn spray or ointment—for burns.

Gauze roll, telfa gauze pads and adhesive tape—for larger wounds.

Elastic support wrap (Ace bandage)—for sprains.

Insect repellent—to keep flys and mosquitoes away.

Needle and tweezers—for removing splinters.

Eye wash—for rinsing out foreign particles.

Soap and towels—for washing wounds and wiping off sweat

Water jug with cold water—to revive the spent shoer.

Tetanus immunization should be maintained at recommended intervals in both horse and man.

Safety First

Most accidents can be prevented. Unskilled horse and tool handling cause many accidents. Skill development requires practice and time. Carelessness is also a primary cause of accidents. Correct hand position is most critical when using the knife and nailing. Concentration will

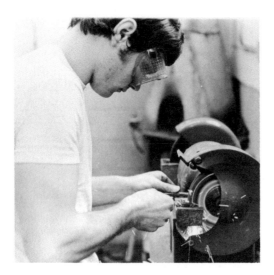

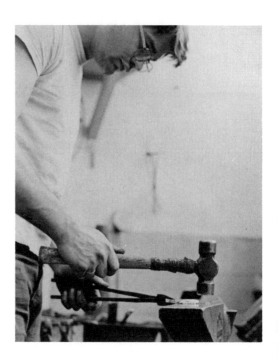

Fig. 18-2. Protective eye covering should always be worn when using power equipment (left) and when working at the forge (right).

be rewarded by the consistent and safe production of precision work.

Proper clothing is important to the safety of the shoer. Boots should be high enough to give ankle support and protect from sparks. Steel-toed boots are desirable to prevent smashed toes. Long sleeved shirts and long legged pants protect from hot scale and sparks. However, most shoers learn to work in a tee shirt during the summer months and tolerate the inevitable scale burns on their arms. Eye glasses or eye protection of some kind is essential when working at the anvil. Some shoers wear cotton or leather gloves, but most learn to work with their hands unprotected. A hat should be worn to protect the hair from sparks. A few shoers wear a helmet for head protection. A leather apron should always be worn when working around the fire and horse. Rings and watchbands are dangerous when worn during nailing. Current tetanus immunization is a necessity.

A proper work area is important to the safety of the horse. Choose a safe place to work which is free from "traps" and "spooks" of all types. The ideal place is usually an area far away from the center of activity at the stable but one that is familiar to the horse; a place where he could not hurt himself or damage any property if he "blows up." Ideally, it should be level, dry,

protected from the elements, easily accessible from your horseshoeing rig, with room enough to work comfortably and safely.

Whenever possible have the owner, or someone who is familiar with the horse, hold the horse. Many horses won't stand well when tied up, especially when away from familiar surroundings. The holder should be instructed to stand on the same side of the horse as the horseshoer is working. The holder is then in a position to pull the hind feet of the horse away from the shoer in case of trouble.

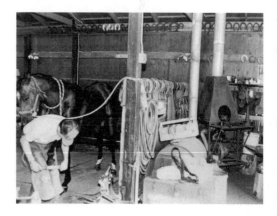

Fig. 18-3. Shop tools and fire work area should be separated from the horse. Photo by J. Graves.

When it is not possible to work with a capable holder, the horse must be tied. A strong halter and tie rope should be a part of every horse-shoer's equipment. Nylon or cotton halters and ropes are preferable to leather because of their durability and strength. If the horse must be tied, tie it to a safe and immovable object properly and securely with a halter and rope that *won't break*. Tie a knot that will hold but can be easily released. Do not tie to a wire fence.

Cross-tying is wise where practical. Cross-tying is done by snapping two ropes to the halter, one on each side, and tying them about 8 to 12 feet apart. This method of tying allows you more room to work in front of the horse and prevents most horses from pulling back.

There is a proper tool for each job. Shoers should be totally familiar with their tools and keep them sharp. Dull tools produce awkward workmanship which may cause accidents.

Commonly Encountered Conditions Requiring First Aid

Neglected feet including overgrown hoofs, thrush, loose and worn out shoes are regularly encountered. Owners need to be reminded of their responsibilities to the horse. In many cases the owner needs to be taught how to properly take care of the animal. This must be done tactfully. Nevertheless, it must be done.

If a set time period between shoeings will not suffice, then recognizable guidelines including toe-length, angle and shoe wear must be used.

A reduction of more than one-half the shoe's thickness by wear is a reasonable indicator of the need for new shoes, when tightness, toe-length and angle are not significant factors. Indicators that a reset is necessary are listed in Chapter 6.

Thrush is a common disease of the foot caused by a bacteria (*Spherophorus necrophorus* or *Fusobacterium necrophorum*) which can live only in an anaerobic, or no air, environment. Most manure and dirt contains this organism. If allowed to pack into the foot and remain for very long, the bacteria will attack the hoof. The presence of thrush can be determined from the foul-smelling odor it produces and the "cheesy" appearance of the frog. Regular cleaning of the hoof prevents thrush from getting started by allowing air to reach the exposed area. Once the disease is present, several therapeutic procedures are advisable:

1. Trim and shape the frog with the hoof knife so that all diseased tissue that can be safely removed is cut away.
2. Scrub the frog and sulcus area (commissures) with an old tooth brush or similar instrument and soap and water.
3. Rinse the foot and allow it to dry completely.
4. Apply 7 percent iodine, Kopertox or similar drying germicidal preparation.
5. Follow up with a routine *daily* hoof *cleaning* and *care* program. If the frog is badly deteriorated, the washing program should be continued daily until a marked improvement is noted. Scientists have discovered that once this organism has been established in an anaerobic condition, it will continue to grow in an aerobic (exposed to air) environment for about three days.

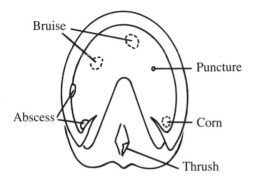
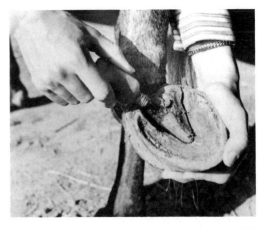

Fig. 18-4. Neglected feet often require some form of first aid. (Left) Location of common foot ailments, (right) treating a mild case of thrush with 7% iodine.

6. In some advanced cases, packing the hoof with medication and shoeing with a pad may be necessary to treat and protect the affected area. (See "Procedure for Applying a Pad.")

7. *Horse owners should be encouraged to clean the bottom of the foot regularly (daily if possible) in order to prevent thrush.* Filthy stabling conditions that encourage the disease should be corrected.

Thrush can easily be distinguished from a shed frog. The process of shedding is a natural thing and may occur two or three times a year.

Flares or lateral distortions of the hoof are frequently present on neglected feet. The procedure for dealing with them is covered in Chapter 17, under "Shaping the Hoof."

Hoof Cracks may be superficial due to hoof dryness or deep due to serious trauma. Relieve pressure from the area that tends to move. Avoid driving nails directly into cracks causing further splitting. The principles of patching hoof cracks are covered in Chapter 34.

Dry Hoofs can be treated with water. Often the water trough can be overflowed creating a muddy area to keep the horse's feet moist. If this is not possible without creating a filthy condition (as in a stall), the foot can be packed with wet mud and covered with a piece of waxed paper each day. This is routinely done in many racing stables.

Wet Hoofs tend to spread and flare excessively. The amount of moisture entering the hoof may be reduced by adding bees wax or rosin to any oil or tar base hoof dressing (Lungwitz and Adams, 1913).

Bruises of the sole appear as so-called "strawberries". They may be due to rocks, hard mud balls or ice pressing on the sole of the hoof. Treatment consists of relieving pressure by removing the cause and padding the hoof with leather or plastic between the shoe and hoof. Sometimes, severe bruises turn into abscesses.

Corns are a specific type of bruise. They occur within the angle of the wall at the heel. This area between the wall and bar is frequently called the seat of corn. Leaving the shoes on too long is a common cause. Shoes fit too short, unlevel shoes, contracted heels, heels cut too low, and heel calks may cause corns. Lowering the sole in the seat of corn area lower than the hoof wall and bars may be sufficient. A bar shoe placing pressure on the frog and removing pressure from the seat of corn is required in serious cases. Most corns appear as red spots and are the dry type. Infected (suppurating) corns are very serious and should be treated like abscesses.

Abscesses are infections of the sensitive tissue of the hoof. They are often called gravels or pus pockets. They may be the result of puncture wounds, or the trapping of anaerobic bacteria by the natural expansion and contraction of the hoof. Abscesses will also develop where necrotic tissue is present, e.g., severe bruises or laminitis. It is best to contact a veterinarian when working on an abscess. The horse may need a tetanus shot and systemic medication which a horseshoer cannot give. The veterinarian may want to dig the abscess out or he may want to supervise while you dig it out.

After the tracts of the abscess are rinsed out with a germicide, it is usually advisable to pack the hole with a poultice such as Ichthammol and germicidal materials such as Furacin. A shoe with a removable plate or bar which protects the sore area and holds in medication is often used. Good drainage is important in treating abscesses. However, the horse's recovery time to usefulness is usually faster with a small hole.

An abscess that cannot be completely drained from the sole should be soaked in an Epsom salts solution. It may take several soakings over a period of several days for these types of abscesses to drain and relieve pressure from the sensitive structures of the foot. The foot should be bandaged or otherwise protected between soakings.

A pad should be applied to hold in medication and prevent dirt and foreign material from entering the wound. (See "Procedure for Applying a Pad".) Commercial or home made slip-on boots make daily care possible in the stabled horse. A method for making a simple pad foot cover for frequently changed dressings has been described by Bill Miller (1979). He recommended nailing a pad on at the toe as a shoe. Then, the rear portion of the pad is taped up against the foot. The dressing can easily be changed each day. A section of truck inner tube may also be used to cover and protect the foot. It may be fastened around the pastern.

Sole or Frog Puncture Wounds resulting from nails, staples or other sharp objects should

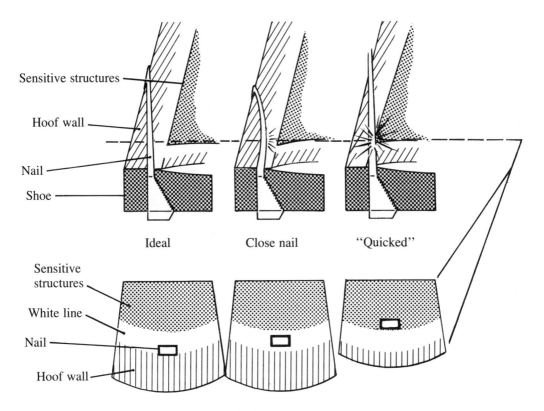

Sensitive structures

Hoof wall

Nail

Shoe

Ideal   Close nail   "Quicked"

Sensitive structures

White line

Nail

Hoof wall

Fig. 18-5. Quicking is a serious accident requiring first aid. Drawing by L. Sadler.

be handled according to their seriousness. Those objects that have pierced the sensitive structures should be removed and the wound(s) disinfected. The owner should be advised of the need for current tetanus immunization. Abscesses should be treated as described.

Dermatitis of various types may be observed when shoeing. These include scratches or grease heel, ringworm, mange and tick infestation. Your primary responsibility is to inform the owner about them and avoid spreading them to other horses (or yourself).

Serious Accidents Requiring First Aid

Quicking (also called pricking, or nailing) refers to penetration of the sensitive structures of the foot by a nail. Usually the horse will jerk and let you know of your error if you chance to accidentally quick him. However, this may not always be the case. You may note a difference in sound as you drive the nail or you may note blood around where it enters or leaves the foot. Occasionally the nail may be just "close" to the

sensitive structures and the resulting pressure causes the horse to be lame later.

The following things should be done if you "quick" or "close nail" a horse:
1. Remove the nail.
2. Do not redrive the nail in that nail hole in the foot.
3. Pour 7 percent Iodine or other suitable germicidal agent into the entrance and exit hole (if there is one) made by the nail. Antibiotic in a plastic syringe designed for mastitis works well.
4. Suggest to the owner that the horse obtain current tetanus immunization.

Sole or Frog Puncture with the nippers or hoof knife may occur during the trimming process. This is embarrassing and indicates incompetence. However, accidents may occur even when you are careful. Occasionally, the horse will step on a nail, shoe clip, or tool while being shod. Usually, the wound will stop bleeding in a short time. Cotton can be placed over the wound to absorb the blood. A germicidal medication such as Furacin should be placed in and around the wound and held in place by a pad.

Minor injuries need no more attention than disinfection with 7 percent iodine. The shoe should be concaved or seated out away from the injured area when wounds occur near or in the region of the white line. Current tetanus immunization is essential in these cases. Most of these accidents heal with no complications. A few will abscess and require special treatment.

Skin wounds resulting from slippage of a dull knife or carelessness should be treated and wrapped. An elastic wrap should always be used around the limb to avoid the possibility of circulation constriction. An excellent description of wound treatment and lower leg wrapping has been given by Matthew MacKay-Smith (1977 and 1978).

Imbalance resulting from overtrimming one area of the hoof can be corrected with leather or plastic wedges. Corrective shoeing wedges or heel lifts made of polyurethane plastic are available in several degrees of thickness.[1] These are ideal when one heel is overtrimmed. Leather wedges can be made from pad scraps. Degree pads may be used when both heels need correction. A reversed degree pad will correct the angle of an overtrimmed toe. Sole pressure can be corrected by concaving the shoe on a hoof with rounded walls. A previously dubbed toe can be corrected by fitting the shoe full and even with the lines of the upper part of the hoof. Special nail hole punching may be required.

[1]Multi-Chem, Studio City, CA.

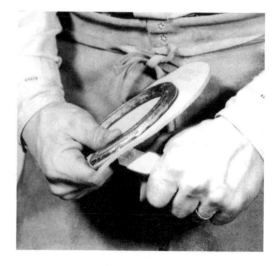

Fig. 18-7. Trimming a light leather pad with a knife to fit the shoe.

Procedure for Applying a Pad

1. Trim and shape the foot.
2. Shape the shoe to the outline of the hoof. Allow for the thickness of the pad by making the shoe slightly larger than the foot when using a thick pad, especially when using more than one pad. Extend the shoe over the toe approximately the width of the thickness of the number of pads and over the border of the quarters on each side about the width of one-half the thickness of the pads.

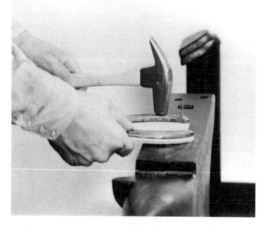

Fig. 18-6. Securing a light leather pad to a light shoe with copper rivets. Photos by G. Poellot.

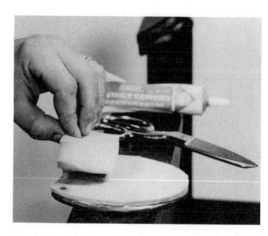

Fig. 18-8. Gluing a piece of foam rubber to the foot surface of the pad.

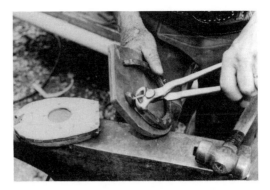

Fig. 18-11. *Securing a heavy pad to a weighted shoe with steel rivets (nails). Photos by J. Graves.*

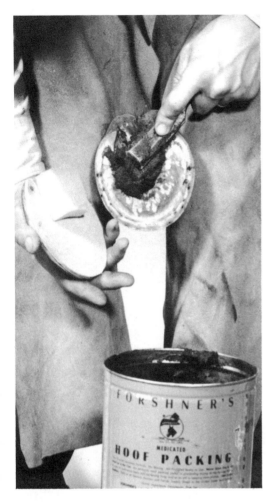

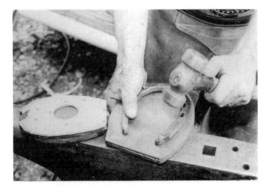

Fig. 18-12. *Rivet using the rounded head of the hammer.*

Fig. 18-9. *Packing the foot with hoof packing.*

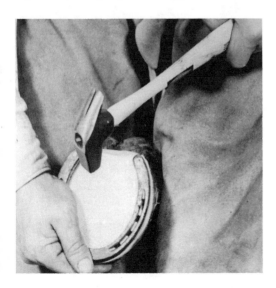

3. Secure the pad to the shoe. Light shoes should be drilled and the pad riveted at the heels. This procedure discourages a light shoe from spreading and the pad from working loose. Pads on heavy shoes can be temporarily held in place for trimming and fitting by nails driven one-half way through the center nail holes of the shoe and bent down toward the middle of the shoe on both ends. The bent nails can then be pulled out and discarded once the shoe is secured on the hoof.

4. Trim the pad with a sharp knife or Duval pad cutter[2] to fit the shoe. If plastic pads are used, it is easier to trace and cut each pad individually. However, when several pads are stacked and nailed together, they can be cut easiest on a band saw. A saber saw or hoof nippers work well for single thicknesses of the tougher materials. Scissors work well for cutting felt or thin foam rubber for race horses.

5. Shape the pad to the shoe with a hoof rasp and taper it to match the slope of the hoof. This is not necessary, but it makes accurate nailing easier.

Fig. 18-10. *Setting the shoe and pad and nailing them on.*

[2]*The Shoeing Shop, Yucaipa, CA*

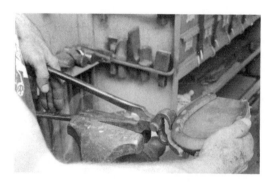

Fig. 18-13. Trimming a heavy pad to fit the shoe with nippers held in a vise.

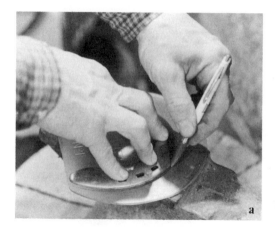

6. Cut a piece of foam rubber the width of the distance between the buttresses of the foot and glue it to the foot surface of the pad. This will compress into the commissures of the foot and prevent the hoof packing from escaping and dirt from entering the bottom of the foot.

7. Pack the prepared foot with hoof packing. Such packing is necessary under a pad, even if the hoof is not to be medicated, to prevent pathogenic anaerobic bacterial growth. Pine tar and oakum can be used instead of commercial medicated peat moss packing. Step 6 is unnecessary when using oakum.

8. Set the shoe and pad in place, allowing for the thickness of the pad if it has not already been shaped, and nail them on.

9. Rasp the overhanging portions of the pad(s) flush with the shoe and wall.

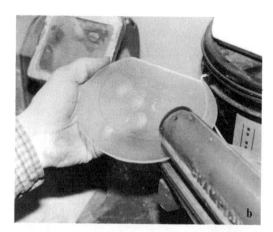

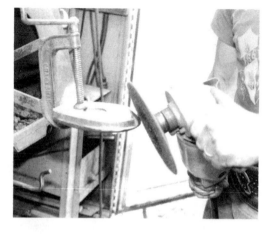

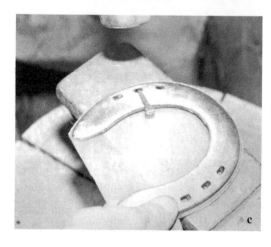

Fig. 18-14. Grinding the edges of the pad to conform to the circumference of the shoe and hoof.

Fig. 18-15. Steps in fitting a light plastic pad to the shoe and foot of a chronically foundered horse: (a) trace the shoe, (b) cut out the pad with a pad cutter, (c) nail the pad to the shoe by driving nails half-way in and bending them over (d) to hold the pad securely in place, (e) pack the foot, (f) nail on the shoe, (g) remove the bent nails, (h) rasp the hoof and pad down to the shoe (i) for a smoothly finished job.

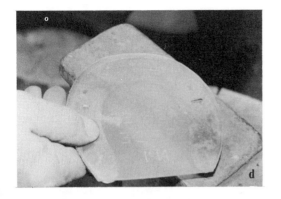

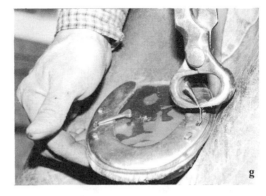

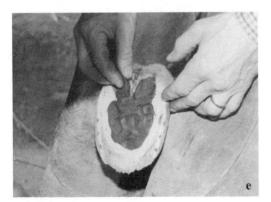

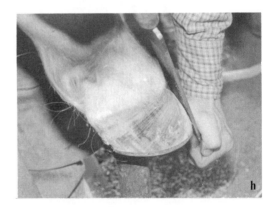

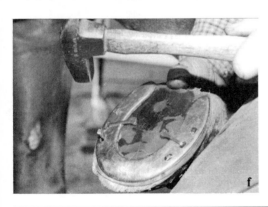

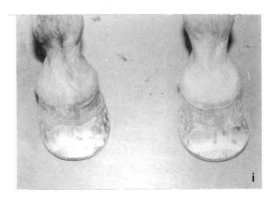

References

Beeman, M. and P. Close, 1971. First aid for horses—part 1. The Western Horseman. 36(9):38.

Beeman, M. and P. Close. 1971. First aid for horses—part 2. The Western Horseman. 36(10):62.

Brighoff, C. 1981. Is your horse trimmed right? Practical Horseman. 9(4):55.

Denning, C.H. 1975. First Aid for Horses. Wilshire Book Co., No. Hollywood, CA.

Jones, W.E. 1972. Basic First Aid for Horses. Caballus, Fort Collins, CO.

Lieberman, B. 1978. The diseased hoof. Equus. 4:34.

Lieberman, B. 1981. Lame the day after shoeing? Equus. 40:33.

Lungwitz, A. and J.W. Adams. 1913. A Textbook of Horseshoeing (Reprint 1966). Oregon State University Press, Corvallis.

McGuire, B. Horse Health Primer. Cornell University, Ithaca, NY.

MacKay-Smith, M. 1977. Taking the mystery out of wound care. Equus. 4:51.

McKibbin, L.S. and A. Sugerman. 1977. Horse Owner's Handbook. W.B. Saunders Co., Philadelphia.

Miller, B. 1979. Hot tip. Amer. Farriers' J. 5(3):93.

Miller, R.M. 1979. Don't overtreat that wound. Western Horseman. 44(1):72.

War Office General Staff. 1908. Animal Management. H.M. Stationery Office, London.

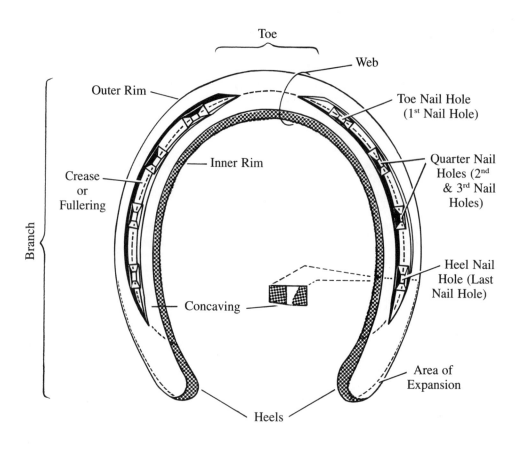

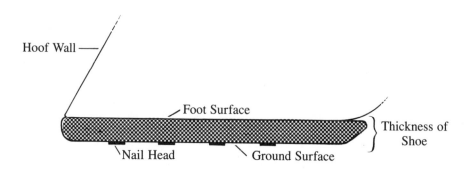

Fig. 19-1. The parts of the horseshoe. Drawing by L. Sadler.

Chapter 19

Selecting, Shaping and Fitting Cold Shoes

Use of the Horseshoe

Horseshoes are unnecessary under ideal conditions where the growth of the hoof equals or exceeds the wear on the hoof. The feet of a horse that is allowed to go barefoot must be trimmed as often as growth exceeds wear to maintain the proper functioning of the foot.

The use of the horseshoe is at best a necessary evil. No matter how applied, it prevents the normal functioning of the foot. However, a properly made and fit horseshoe applied to a properly

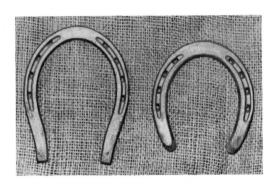

Fig. 19-2. Keg shoes. (Left) hot or long-heeled shoe, (right) cold (ready-made) short-heeled shoe. Photos by J. Graves.

prepared hoof does very little damage to the foot. The aim of "physiological horseshoeing" is to minimize the harmful effects of the horseshoe, and to take advantage of its useful effects.

The horseshoe is a beneficial tool to:
1. Protect the horse's foot from excessive wear and resulting tenderness when its continuous use is necessary.
2. Provide traction when necessary for safety and/or speed on slippery surfaces.
3. Correct or influence the stance and/or gait of the horse.
4. Correct or improve "abnormal" and pathological conditions of the feet and legs.

Terms

The parts of the shoe should be related to the parts of the hoof. Study the parts of the hoof, the parts of a machine-made shoe and differences in front and hind hoofs.

A **keg** shoe is another name for a machine-made shoe. A **hot** shoe is a long-heeled machine-made shoe. A **cold** shoe or **ready-made** shoe is a short-heeled machine-made shoe.

Hot shaping refers to shaping and cutting the heels of a shoe heated in a forge. **Cold shaping**

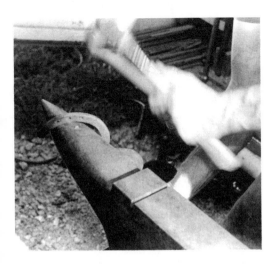
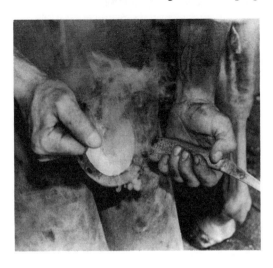

Fig. 19-3. Hot shaping (left) and hot fitting (right) sometimes called "hot shoeing".

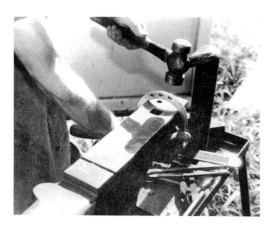 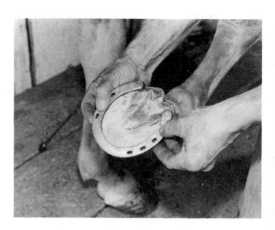

Fig. 19-4. Cold shaping (left) and cold fitting (right) sometimes called "cold shoeing".

refers to shaping (and occasionally cutting the heels) of a shoe without the use of heat.

Hot fitting refers to placing a level hot shoe momentarily against the hoof to scorch high places and seat clips. When properly done, there is no danger to the horse and a perfect union between hoof and shoe is easily obtained. **Cold fitting** refers to leveling the hoof and shoe and creating a union between them without the use of heat. Great skill is required to obtain a proper cold fit.

Hot shoers are those who use a forge and hot fit their shoes. **Cold shoers** are those who do not use a forge and cold fit their shoes. Most modern horseshoers use a combination of both **hot shoeing** and **cold shoeing** depending on the individual needs of their customers' horses.

A **pair** of horseshoes consists of two **front** or two **hind** shoes for the same horse. A **set** of horseshoes is four shoes: a pair of fronts and a pair of hinds for the same horse. When a horse is shod with **new shoes** all'round he has on a new set of shoes. Horses are **reset** when shoes which are on the horse and not worn more than halfway through are taken off, cleaned up, and nailed back on the trimmed hoof. New shoes or resets are nearly always put on in a pair or a set and not one here and one there. Differences in the weight of the shoes or length of hoof on opposite feet can throw the horse out of balance and adversely affect his gait.

Cowboy Shoes

A number of years ago, manufacturers of hot or long-heeled shoes developed a short-heeled pattern for use where a forge was not practical. At first they were used by the military and then by ranchers, packers and outfitters. These so-called cold shoes had the same size designation as hot shoes and were referred to by the manufacturer as "cowboy" shoes.

Cowboy shoes were made in a compromise pattern rather than a front and hind pattern as hot shoes had been. Thus, front and hind shoes were made with the same web width and weight. Formerly, front shoes were made wider (and heavier) than hind shoes to provide more sole protection. The nail holes in cowboy shoes were roughly punched and had to be opened with a pritchel. The nail holes were spaced far apart around the shoe and placed close to the outside

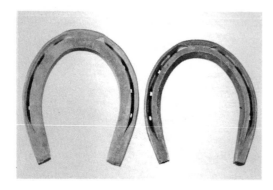

Fig. 19-5. Cowboy shoes. Photo by G. Poellot.

184

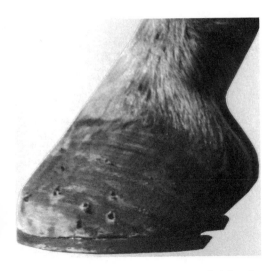

Fig. 19-6. Unskilled cold shoeing often called "cowboy shoeing".

edge. Secure nailing required dubbing (rasping the outside wall) of the hoof. The heels were square-cut and unfinished. There was a large difference between each size. The heel nail holes were placed in the last one-third of the branch of the shoe to help secure the shoe in rough terrain. However, nails in this position also inhibited normal heel expansion of the hoof.

These characteristics made it difficult for even an experienced person to do a good shoeing job. Thus, when cowboy shoes were put in the hands of a poor workman, "cowboy shoeing" was the result. Cowboy shoeing has given cold shoeing a bad name.

Cold Shoes

The modern cold or "ready-made" shoe is a modification of the cowboy shoe. It has become very popular in America within the last few years. These shoes are usually manufactured in a compromise pattern (may be adapted to front or hind feet); have the nail holes open (require no pritcheling); have the nail holes graduated from toe to heel (to correspond to the thickness of the wall); and have the heels cut and rounded (finished). In addition, ready-made shoes are sized in "half-sizes", with only a ¼ inch difference in each heel. However, the last nail hole is still located behind the widest part of the hoof and therefore prevents natural hoof expansion. Also, the nail holes are punched perpendicular

to the shoe instead of corresponding to the slope of the hoof.

Some companies make shoes in front and hind patterns, make the front shoes concaved and wider-webbed than the hinds and offer a great variety of shoe patterns, styles and weights.

Modern cold shoes save the shoer time and work, make more accurate cold fitting possible and require less iron working skill to shoe a horse. However, hoof working skill is most important.

Cold Shoeing

Cold Shoeing has been discriminated against by particular horse owners. Cold shaping and fitting have been said to be inferior to hot fitting. Invariably poor quality work is due to incompetent workmen and not the type of shoeing. A person with few tools and very little training can shoe a horse using the cold process. Cowboy shoes made quality cold shoeing difficult. Ready-made shoes have made excellence possible. A properly shaped, leveled and fit modern cold shoe does not harm the foot of a horse with a normal foot.

In America, most beginners learn shoeing using the cold fitting process. As they increase in skill, they learn the more complicated and demanding techniques of iron work. This way foot work is stressed from the very beginning.

The majority of the horses in the U.S. are pleasure horses. Most pleasure horses are shod with machine-made cold shoes. However, the various elite breed/types of the horse world require special knowledge and skill in foot work and especially iron work that must be gained by experience.

The principal advantage to cold shoeing is speed. Time is money. Another advantage is that it takes less skill to be able to do the work. However, it takes a lot of skill to be able to do it well. Skill development requires effective teaching, practice and experience over time.

The disadvantages of cold shoeing include: public prejudice in many areas, limited to a few types of shoeing, limited to fitting "normal" shaped hoofs, corrective work often limited to hoof trimming, large shoe inventory required and iron working skill need not be developed and therefore may be absent or lost.

Shoe Selection

Horseshoes are selected considering three criteria: manufacturer, pattern or style, and size.

Selection of horseshoe *manufacturer* is influenced by:
1. The price of the shoes.
2. The ease of obtaining the shoes.
3. The preference of the horseshoer.
4. The preference of the owner.
5. The sizes and style variations manufactured.

Selection of horseshoe *pattern or style* is influenced by:
1. The type of work the horse does.
2. The terrain the horse is worked on.
3. The integrity of the horse's foot.
4. The size and weight of the horse.
5. The variety of ground surface patterns available.

Selection of horseshoe *size* is influenced by:
1. The length of the heels (should just cover the buttresses of a sound foot).

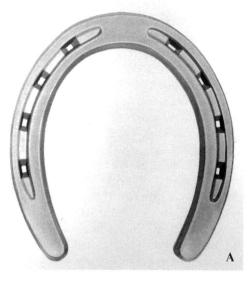
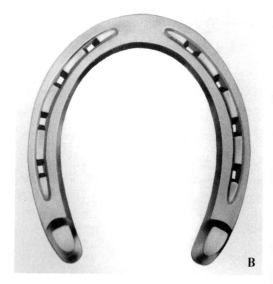
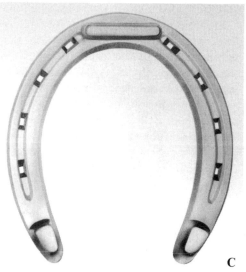
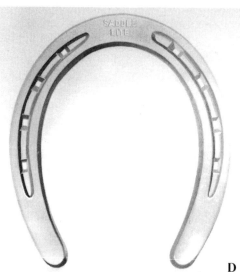

Fig. 19-7. Modern ready-made or "cold shoes". Plain bronco shoe (A), heeled only bronco shoe (B), toe and heeled bronco shoe (C), and saddle-lite shoe (D). Photos by Diamond.

Comparison of cold shoe sizes.

Inches of Steel	10½	11	11½	12	12½	13	13½	14	14½
Cowboy Shoes									
Phoenix (U.S.)	00	0	1			2		3	
Ready-Made Shoes									
Plain Diamond (U.S.)	000	00	0	1		2		3	
Saddlelite Diamond (U.S.)	00	0	1		2				
Baker (English)	3	4	5	6		7		8	
Hyatt (U.S.)	4	5	6	7		8	9		
Multi-Product (Japanese)	3	4	5	6		7	8		9
Pioneer (U.S.)	00	0	½	1	1½	2	2½		

Fig. 19-8. Comparison of cold shoe sizes.

2. The position of the heel nail hole (should not be farther back than the widest part or bend in the quarter of the hoof).
3. The web or width (should cover the wall and protect the wall and sole junction. Ideally, the web should be twice the thickness of the wall).
4. The weight or thickness of the shoe (should be as light as possible to prevent fatigue, but sufficient to last for the interval between shoeings).
5. The nail hole size (should accommodate a nail that is the proper size for the foot. Ideally, the smallest nail that can be driven to a secure height is preferred).
6. The nail hole position (should be the width of the wall from the outside edge of the shoe all along the branch of the shoe).

NOTE: Frequently, several of the above factors have to be compromised when using machine-made shoes. However, the length of heels should *not* be compromised as the horse's soundness and/or the rider's safety may be jeopardized.

Cold shoes are sized differently than the sizing pattern of hot shoes or cowboy shoes. Sizes of some of currently popular cold (ready-made) shoe manufacturers are different and should be compared.

Ready-made Shoe Disadvantages

Keg shoes have the distinct disadvantage of having the nail holes in a fixed position punched perpendicular to the shoe. Some makes of shoes are punched fine (close to the outside edge) and a few are punched coarse (toward the inside edge). Nail hole position must be taken into consideration when fitting a shoe. Ideal location is practically impossible to achieve in a machine-made shoe due to hoof variations. Most hoofs, even when properly fit with keg shoes, require rasping on their lower border. This is a serious disadvantage of keg shoes since a portion of the weight-bearing surface of the hoof is removed.

Nails should be driven into the outer border of the white line. If nails are driven inside the white line, "quicking" or penetration of the sensitive structures of the foot may result. If nails are driven outside the white line, the wall usually breaks or splits the height of the nail. This may result in a cast or thrown shoe.

Cold Shoe Patterns

A shoe pattern or style is a feature of the ground surface that makes it unique for a special purpose or terrain. The foot surface is usually flat. Most all machine-made (cold or hot pattern) saddle horseshoes are made from mild steel. A few types are made from high-carbon steel. They wear longer but are harder to shape.

A flat shoe with nail holes in it is referred to as a plate, slick, countersunk or stamped shoe.

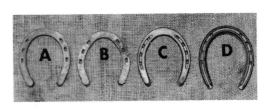

Fig. 19-9. Popular cold shoe patterns. Countersunk front and hind (A and B), creased compromise (C), and rim compromise pattern (D). Photo by J. Graves.

187

A flat shoe with a groove or crease in each branch is called a creased (or, in some cases, a plain) shoe.

A flat shoe with a groove or crease all the way around is called a rim, fullered or full-swedge shoe. The crease fills with dirt and provides more traction. Light shoes of this type are called training plates. A shoe with a crease all the way around and with a higher inside rim is called a polo or turf shoe. A shoe with a crease all the way around and with a higher outside rim is called a rim or barrel racing shoe.

A shoe with heel calks is called a heeled shoe. A shoe with toe and heel calks is called a toe and heeled shoe. In some areas, sharper screw or drive calks (corks, never-slips or studs) are used in place of heel calks.

Rubber shoes are used on horses ridden or driven on city streets.

Horseshoe borium may be added to shoes after they are shaped. Its application is covered in Chapter 43.

A shoe with a sloping inside border tapering to a sharp edge on the foot surface is called a concave, self-cleaning, mud or snow shoe. This pattern may be incorporated into any horseshoe style.

Shoes for donkeys and mules are designed to correspond to the unique foot shape of these animals.

Small pony shoes and large draft horse shoes represent the opposite extremes in machine-made shoe sizes.

Weighted shoes for gaited pleasure horses, thin aluminum shoes for race horses and thick aluminum shoes for jumpers are also manufactured in ready-made cold fitting patterns.

Marking the Shoes

Shoes should be marked to correspond to the foot they are being shaped for in a consistent and identifiable manner. The Author uses the following pattern for cold shoes:

Left front shoe—center punch mark on the inside of the ground surface web of the *outside* branch (right side with toe up) between third and fourth nail holes, (or the heel nail hole and the next nail hole, if the shoe has less than eight nail holes).

Right front shoe—center punch mark on *outside* branch (left side with toe up) between third and fourth nail holes.

Left hind shoe—center punch mark on *outside* branch (right side with toe up) at the heel end of the crease (or about 1 in. from the end of the heel, if the shoe has less than eight nail holes).

Right hind shoe—center punch mark on *outside* branch (left side with toe up) at the end of the crease.

Cold Shaping Principles

Cold shaping is done without benefit of the forge or tongs. The shoe is held in the hand and the anvil is used as a fulcrum to shape the shoe. Except for extremely drastic changes in light shoes and regular shaping of heavy shoes, most shaping of ready-made shoes can be done cold. The advantage of cold shaping is speed.

Cold shaping does not directly affect the quality of a shoeing job. However, a precise fit is sometimes difficult to obtain without heat. Too often, shoers will give up and accept a poor quality fit because of the hard work involved in controlled cold shaping.

Cold shaping can be very difficult, even on light shoes, without an understanding of the basic principles of the use of the anvil and hammer to change the shape of a shoe. One of the best ways to learn these principles is to practice general shaping of shoes cold.

First, practice shaping a front shoe from a machine-made compromise pattern. Then, make

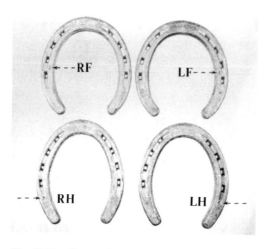

Fig. 19-10. Shoe marking pattern. Photo by G. Poellot.

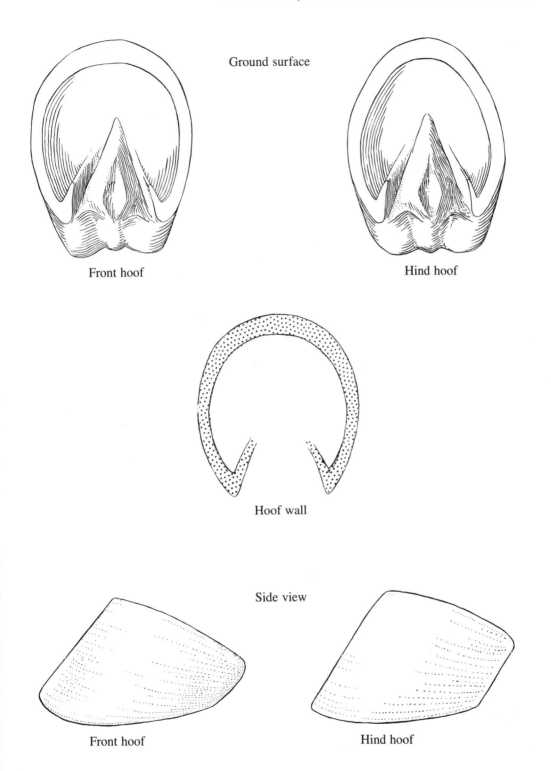

Ground surface

Front hoof

Hind hoof

Hoof wall

Side view

Front hoof

Hind hoof

Fig. 19-11. *Visualize the shape of the hoof wall as you are shaping shoes. Drawing by L. Sadler.*

a front into a hind, and then a hind into a front pattern. Next, shape a shoe to an odd-shaped shoe or pattern of the same size. Finally, practice shaping and fitting to trimmed feet.

Each time you shape a shoe, strive to make a minimum number of trips back and forth from the horse to the anvil. Measure the width of the hoof and mark it with chalk on the edge of your anvil to use as a reference when shaping the shoe. Try to *visualize the shape of the hoof wall* as you are working on the shoe at the anvil. This will help you shape and fit the shoe accurately and rapidly. Remember—skill equals accuracy *plus* speed.

Also practice applying only a *few hard* blows to the shoe between the nail holes each time you shape it in order to avoid mangling it. It takes less effort to do the work this way and makes a nicer looking finished job.

Rest the shoe solidly on the anvil so it won't sting your hand when hit. Hold the shoe rather loosely and allow it to bounce when hit. Let the hammer and the anvil do the work. Hold your hand away from where the hammer is striking. Always start at the toe of the shoe and proceed shaping toward the heels. This is especially important when making major alterations. Often major cold alterations of the shoe make it nec-

essary to hammer the shoe radically out of shape at one point in the process to get the required bend in the shoe. This fact is very confusing to beginners. However, the end result is the same as if it were done hot.

Scott Simpson (1983) has written an excellent book on cold shaping principles. He has given names to the common hoof shapes and teaches a system of shaping cold shoes for each one.

Note the general differences in the shape of a front and hind hoof:

The outside border of the wall of a *front* hoof is round and full at the toe, relatively straight through the quarters, and turned in sharply for the last inch or so at the heels.

The outside border of the wall of a *hind* foot is more pointed and narrow at the toe, rounded through the quarters, and almost straight at the heels.

Cold Shaping Front Shoes

1. **To Flatten or Round the Toe:** Place the toe of the shoe over the horn of the anvil. The space between the shoe and anvil, and hence its position on the horn, should be governed by how much you want to flatten the toe and/ or open the shoe. Strike on the center of the toe.

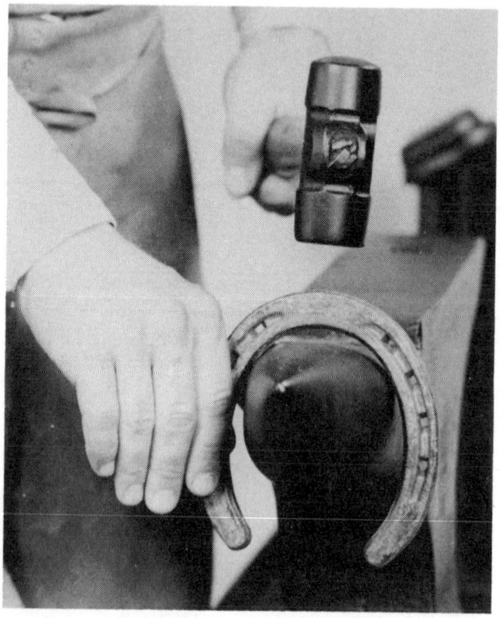

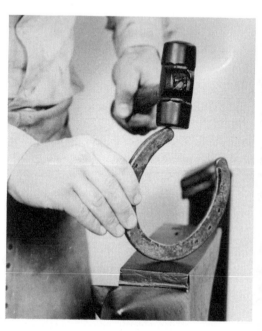

Fig. 19-12. *To flatten or round the toe. Photos by G. Poellot.*

Fig. 19-13. *To bring the branches in and round the fore quarter.*

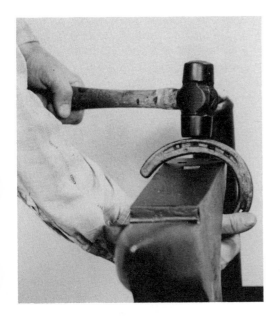

Fig. 19-14. To straighten the quarter.

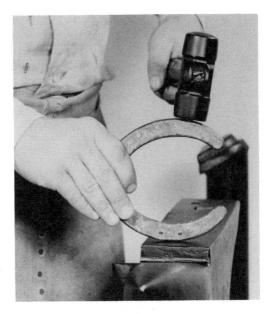

Fig. 19-16. To close the shoe.

2. **To Bring the Branches in and Round the Fore Quarter:** Place the toe of the shoe on the face of the anvil with the branches up and hit one branch at a time.

3. **To Straighten the Quarter:** Place the branch of the shoe over the heel of the anvil and strike in the center of the place where the shoe is too full or rounded.

4. **To Turn in the Heels:** Place the heel of the shoe over the horn of the anvil (or heel) and hammer on the heel as you pull the shoe

around under the horn. The hammer must strike only slightly toward you from the fulcrum point on the horn to avoid causing the shoe to jump out of your hand when struck.

5. **To Close the Shoe:** Place the shoe on the anvil by holding it at the toe and letting the branches face away from you. Strike the branch of the shoe.

6. **To Open the Shoe:** Place the shoe over the edge of the anvil and strike the toe.

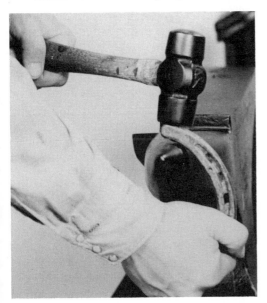

Fig. 19-15. To turn in the heels.

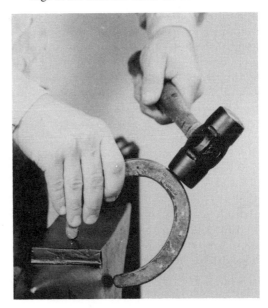

Fig. 19-17. To open the shoe.

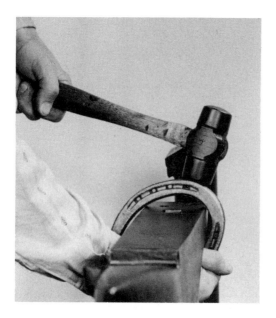

Fig. 19-18. To point or narrow the toe.

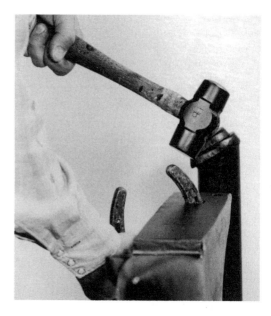

Fig. 19-19. To round the quarter.

Cold Shaping Hind Shoes

1. **To Point or Narrow the Toe:** Place the shoe over the heel of the anvil with the upper branch rotated as far toward you as the shoe size and the heel of your anvil will allow. Strike over and as close to the farthest corner of the heel of the anvil from you as possible.

This action will straighten the branch at that point. Turn the shoe over and repeat on the other branch. Close the shoe to about its correct width. This operation must be practiced in order to determine the exact position to place the shoe to get the desired amount of "point" in the toe.

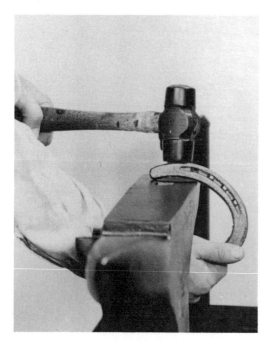

Fig. 19-20. To straighten the heel.

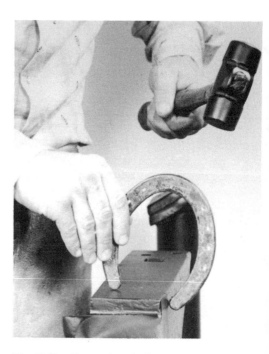

Fig. 19-21. To extend one heel.

2. **To Round the Quarter:** Place it over the horn (or heel) of the anvil, with the midpoint of the area to be rounded over the horn (or edge of the heel), and proceed as in turning in the heels of a front shoe. An easier way, when working a cold shoe, is to push the heel of the shoe up through the hardy hole of the anvil, and rest the center point of the desired bend against the fulcrum point of the hole. Strike the end of the heel of the shoe. This method is also effective for turning in the heels of the front shoe.

3. **To Straighten the Heel:** Place the shoe over the heel of the anvil with the inside edge of the heel of the shoe resting on the face. Strike near the heel of the shoe until the desired bend is obtained.

   Occasionally, it is necessary to extend one heel of a hind shoe, i.e., change the position of the center of the toe of the shoe due to the shape of the foot. This can be done cold on small light shoes, although it is usually thought of as an operation that must be done hot.

4. **To Extend One Heel:** Place the shoe over the face and body of the anvil as if you were going to open the shoe and shift the side which you want to be longer down over the base. Hit the side of the toe to force that branch down and extend it. Then finish by pointing the toe of the shoe over the heel of the anvil. This operation can also be done by opening the shoe and placing the entire short branch up through the hardy hole. However, this method is not as desirable due to the sharp corners that often result in the shoe.

Leveling the Cold Shoe

Cold Shaping usually warps shoes out of level. It is a good idea to roughly level a shoe as you shape it. This makes the shaping process easier and prevents the shoe from opening during the leveling process.

Steps in leveling a shaped cold shoe:

1. Place the shoe on the anvil face with the foot surface up. Try to get as much of the shoe on the anvil as possible. The easiest way to do this is to hold one heel in your hand and place the other heel on the edge of the anvil face nearest you. Then rotate the shoe until the toe comes to the edge of the anvil face away from you.

2. Strike overlapping blows slightly inclined toward the inner edge on the inside half of the web starting from one side of the toe and progressing around to the opposite branch to a point about 1½ inches from the heel.

3. Rotate the shoe and treat the foot surface of the other branch similarly.

4. Turn the shoe over so that the ground surface is up. Apply overlapping blows slightly inclined toward the outside edge on the outside half of the web, starting from one side of the toe and progressing around to the opposite branch to a point about 1½ inches from the heel. Strike flat overlapping blows on the entire branch from this point back to the heel. (The last 1½ in. must be flat so that the heels of the foot will have a flat surface on which they can easily "expand" when the horse places weight on the foot.)

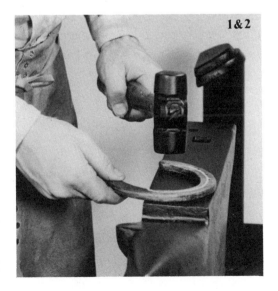

1 & 2

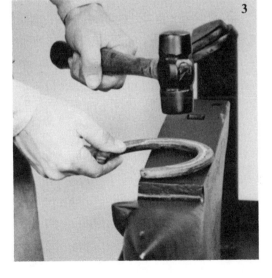

3

Fig. 19-22. Steps in leveling a cold shoe (1-5).

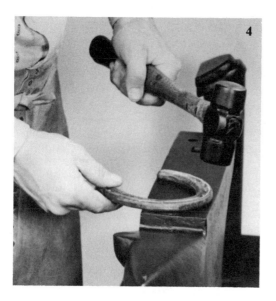

4

5. Rotate the shoe and treat the ground surface of the other branch similarly.
6. Sight the shoe to see that it is level. Cradle it in your hand and sight over the foot surface from the heels to the toe and across the heels to be sure they are level with each other. To double check, rotate the shoe and sight over the branches from the side.
7. If the shoe is not level, note the high points and place the shoe on the anvil in such a way that they can be hit with the hammer and flattened. Then resight the shoe.

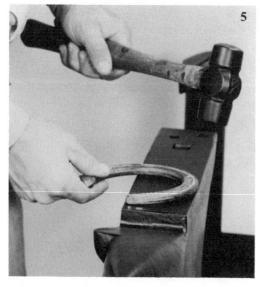

5

Expansion in the Heels

Most saddle horses should be shod to allow for the natural expansion of the heels of the foot. However, some horses should not be shod with the heels wider than the wall of the hoof. These include horses which pull shoes readily, paw the ground, or work in muddy conditions, etc.

The shoe should follow the outline of the trimmed and shaped hoof wall exactly from one bend in the quarter around the toe to the opposite bend in the quarter. Starting from zero at the last or heel nail hole, there should be about 1/16 inch of the shoe extending laterally from the outline of the wall at the heel. This "expansion" in the shoe allows for the lateral movement of the heels of the foot as weight is placed on them.

Expansion can be put in the shoe rather easily by holding the shoe over the heel of the anvil with the heel on the edge of the face closest to you, and striking a glancing blow toward you.

Final Fitting

Things to check when making a final fitting:
1. Ideally, the outer half of the ground surface of the shoe and the wall of the foot should fit tightly against each other. In cases where this is not possible, such as feet with chipped-out walls, try to obtain a solid three-point landing on the toe and heels. The shoe should not rock from side-to-side or from toe-to-heel. A shoe that rocks may cause the nails to work loose.
2. The heels of the shoe should fit flat against the heels of the foot. This condition can be quickly checked by tilting the foot forward and sighting under the heels of the shoe as it rests on the hoof. An eased or sprung heel may result in cast shoes or may cause corns.
3. The inner half of the foot surface of the shoe and the sole of the foot should not touch each other. This may be achieved by the concavity of the sole or shoe or both. Sole pressure may produce bruising of sensitive tissue and lameness.
4. The heels of the shoe should be long enough to cover the buttresses but short enough that the shoe cannot be easily stepped on and pulled off. Short heels cause corns, long heels may cause shoe boils, injuries and cast shoes.
5. The nail holes in the shoe should be open and conform to the head and shank of the size of the nail to be used. The nail holes should be

positioned over the outer border of the white line. Small nails in the proper position make a secure shoe with minimum damage to the hoof.

6. The shoe should be shaped to fit the outer border of the hoof with allowance for hoof expansion at the heels. Corns may be produced by a tight-heeled shoe left too long.

References

Canfield, D.M. 1968. Elements of Farrier Science. Enderes Tool Co., Inc., Albert Lea, MN.

Holtby, M.E. 1967. In defense of the cold shoe. The Western Horseman. (Feb.):53.

Kreider, J. Cold Horseshoeing. 4H Horse Project. USDA.

Lindholm, O.W. 1966. Hot and cold shoeing. The Western Horseman. (Aug.):128.

Simpson, J.S. 1983. The Mechanics of Horseshoeing Simplified. Scott Simpson, Walla Walla, WA.

NOTES:

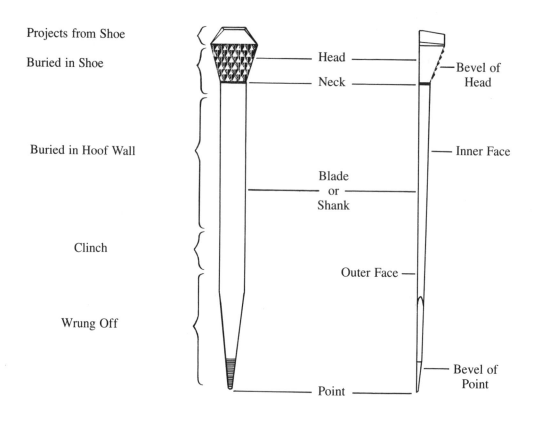

Projects from Shoe

Buried in Shoe

Buried in Hoof Wall

Clinch

Wrung Off

Head

Neck

Blade
or
Shank

Bevel of
Head

Inner Face

Outer Face

Point

Bevel of
Point

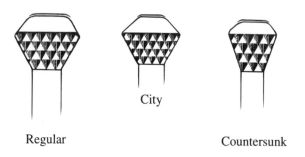

Regular

City

Countersunk

Fig. 20-1. The parts of the horseshoe nail. Drawing by L. Sadler.

Chapter 20

Nailing and Finishing

After a hoof has been trimmed, a shoe is prepared and nailed to the foot. A machine-made shoe must be properly selected, shaped and fit to the trimmed hoof. A handmade shoe must be turned, punched and fit. The shoe must be attached with nails that fit correctly in the nail holes of the shoe and are the proper size for the foot.

Horseshoe Nail Sizes

Horseshoe nails are especially designed for fastening the shoe to the foot. They are made from a uniformly high-quality steel in a shape that makes them hard enough to drive into the hoof, yet soft enough that they can be easily bent and wrung (twisted) or cut off.

There are many sizes and several head types of horseshoe nails available to supply the needs of the various horseshoeing situations. The smallest size nail which will securely fasten the shoe to the foot for the required length of time should always be used. More structural strength is retained in a thin hoof wall when small nails are used. The shoes usually stay on these feet longer than when large nails are used. Clips should be drawn on shoes rather than using larger-sized nails when increased security is desirable. However, thick walled horses are more securely shod with the larger nails appropriate for heavier shoes.

Nails are numbered in half sizes from No. 3 ½ to No. 4½ and in full sizes from No. 5 to No. 12 and No. 16. There is about ⅛ inch difference in length between each size. There are also differences in thickness. No. 3½ nails are used to nail on aluminum racing plates. No. 4 and No. 4½ are used to nail on steel training plates and other light shoes. No. 5 and No. 6 nails are used to nail on saddle horse shoes. No. 8 nails are used to nail on most draft horse and many gaited horse shoes. No. 7 and No. 9 are intermediate sizes that are not commonly used. No. 10, 12, and 16 nails are used to fasten heavy shoes to the extended hoofs of gaited and walking horses.

Horseshoe Nail Head Styles

Capewell (American-made) horseshoe nails come in four head styles: regular, city, special and countersunk. Variations of head styles make it possible to fit the various depths and shapes of nail holes in machine-made shoes. A proper fit will leave ¼₆ inch of the nail head projecting from the shoe. The checked pattern or face with the nail trademark on the beveled side of the nail head should be buried in the shoe. Only the smooth part of the nail head above the bevel should project from the shoe. If the nail head goes too deep in the hole, the shoe is impossible to clinch tight and will become loose and lost. The projecting head is needed to block the nails and to resist the bottom jaw of the clinchers. If a nail head projects from the shoe beyond this point, it will wear off prematurely and cause the shoe to loosen and be lost.

Generally the city head nail will fit the smaller sizes of American-made shoes. The regular head nail is useful for resets when the nail holes have been enlarged by wear. It may also be used on larger shoes when a smaller nail is needed due to the condition of the hoof wall. Special head nails come only in size No. 5. They are useful for extra light shoes and thin walled hoofs. Countersunk head nails are used mostly for handmade shoes and foreign-made horseshoes.

Mustad (Swedish-made) are also made in regular, city and countersunk (E) head styles. In addition, they make an ASVC racing head which is similar to a city head in the smaller sizes (No. 3 to No. 4), but more like the special head in the larger sizes (No. 4½ to No. 6). Mustad also makes a rib or ice nail. This provides a temporary means of sharp shoeing a horse in the winter months.

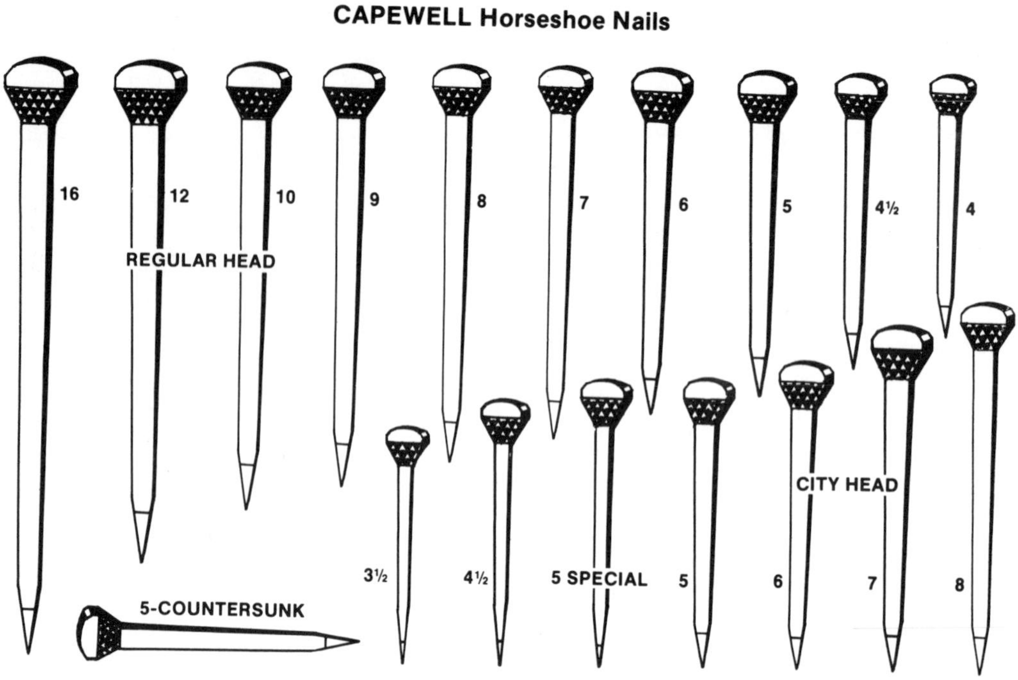

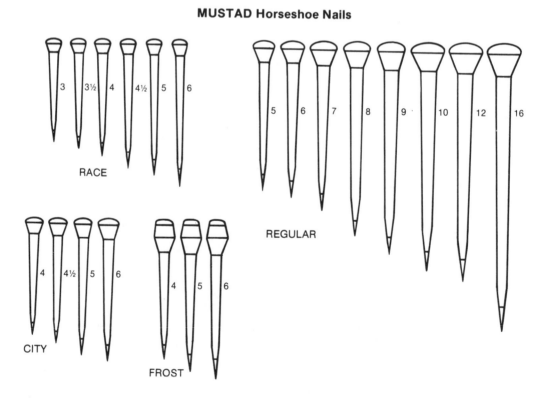

CAPEWELL Horseshoe Nails

16   12   10   9   8   7   6   5   4½   4

REGULAR HEAD

CITY HEAD

5-COUNTERSUNK

3½   4½   5 SPECIAL   5   6   7   8

Fig. 20-2.   Capewell horse nail sizes and styles.

MUSTAD Horseshoe Nails

3   3½   4   4½   5   6

RACE

5   6   7   8   9   10   12   16

REGULAR

4   4½   5   6

CITY

4   5   6

FROST

Fig. 20-3.   Mustad nail sizes and styles.

Nailing on the Shoe

Nailing the shoe on the hoof worries beginners more than anything else about horseshoeing. They are concerned, and rightly so, about hurting the horse when driving the nails, and injuring themselves if the horse jerks after the nails project from the hoof. Nailing technique affects the quality of the shoeing job as much as any one thing.

Beginners should practice driving nails at a chalk line drawn on dead feet (or on live horses) until they are able to get them to come out on the line every time. Don't be afraid to use the line until you perfect your technique.

Steps in nailing on a shoe:
1. Draw a chalk line along both sides of the hoof at the height that you want the nails to come out. For the average saddle horse with a sound hoof, this should be about ¾ to 1 inch above the shoe.

   The horse's hoof grows an average of ⅜ inch per month. If nails are driven ¾ inch into the hoof, in two months the nail holes will have grown down and will not be in the way at the next shoeing. Ideally, the more often a horse is shod, the lower the nails should be driven. (Race horses are shod about twice as often as saddle horses. The small nails are driven about half as high as a larger nail would be on a comparable saddle horse hoof.) However, it may be necessary to drive nails higher than ¾ inch when the wall is weak or chipped and broken away in the quarters or to bypass old nail holes. Normally, nails must be driven at

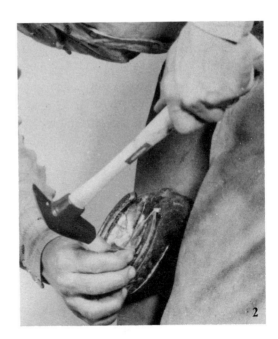

2

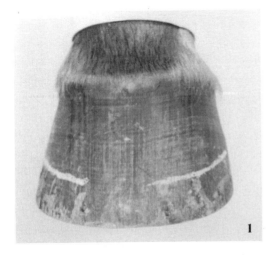

1

Fig. 20-4. Steps in nailing on a shoe (1-11). Photos by G. Poellot.

least ⅜ inch above old nail holes to provide solid attachment for shoes.

Nails can be driven in old nail holes if necessary. However, nailing is usually not as secure as it is in fresh holes. High nails may be desirable when there is a long interval between shoeings or the lower hoof border is in poor condition. Toe nails may be driven higher than heel nails since the nail row will then be parallel to the coronary band (hoof wall growth source) and the wall is thicker at the toe than at the bend in the quarters.

2. Place the shoe in position on the hoof and hold it with the edge of your hand on one side while you position the nail between your thumb and forefinger in the center of the opposite heel nail hole.

   The shoe is less likely to slip back from the toe when the heel nails are driven first. The slope of the wall at the bend of the quarter is less than that at the toe and thus the heel nail does not pull the shoe back to the extent a toe nail does.

3. Hold the nail so that the checked pattern or trademark on the beveled head of the nail is facing the center of the foot. The bevel on the point of the nail will then be in a position to force the nail to come out at the point where it is aimed.

   The checked pattern or trademark and slope of the head on the beveled side of the nail makes it possible to shoe a horse by touch or in the dark, if necessary. (However, the Author does not recommend this practice!)

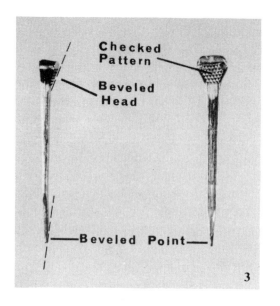

Checked
Pattern

Beveled
Head

——Beveled Point——

3

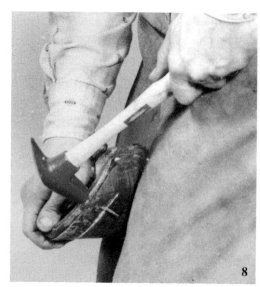

8

4. *Aim* the nail at the chalk line.

Aiming the nail at a line (drawn or imaginary) works much better than haphazardly driving nails, hoping they will come out somewhere on the outside of the foot. With practice, you will place your finger where you want to aim the nail and tell by the sound of the nail where it is going. If the nail should go in deeper than where your finger is resting or sounds like it is going into soft tissue, pull the nail out and redrive it. Move your finger away each time you hit the nail.

5. Start the nail with light taps with the hammer.
6. Once the nail is started, grasp the toe of the foot so that you can safely and securely hold the hoof while driving and wringing off the nail. This allows you some degree of control if the horse suddenly tries to jerk his foot away.
7. Shortly before the nail reaches the chalk line, strike the nail head with harder blows. The bevel on the point of the nail will force it to come out at the desired height.
8. Continue driving the nail until it is seated in the shoe.
9. Turn the nail to a right angle with the wall by hooking the claws of the hammer under it and pulling toward the shoe.

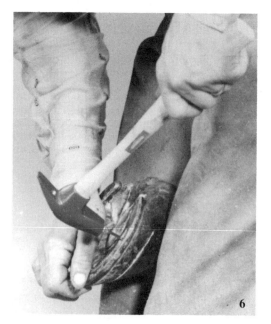

6

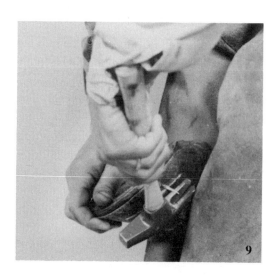

9

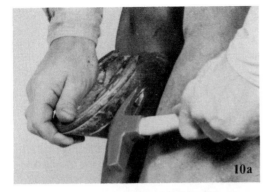

10a

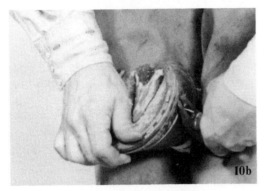

10b

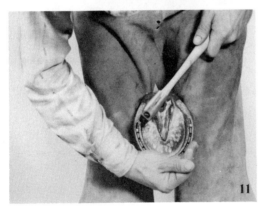

11

The shoe will now be attached solidly so that when the toe nails are driven they will no longer have a tendency to pull the shoe back. However, you can expect the wall to expand about the thickness of the nail at its junction with the shoe after the nails are driven. The shoe should be fit slightly full to allow for this.

The nails should come out on or near the line. If the nails come out consistently too high or too low, something is wrong with the fit of the shoe, the positioning of the nail holes in the shoe, or your nail driving technique. If one nail comes out too high or too low, pull it out with the pull offs and redrive it. A small bend at the point of the nail is sometimes necessary to get the nail

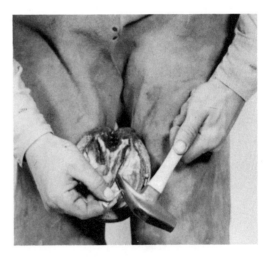

Fig. 20-5.   *Bending the nail in the claw of the hammer.*

10. Wring the nail off. This is done by placing the hammer head against the hoof, sliding the projecting nail point to the bottom of the claws of the hammer, and then shearing the nail off next to the hoof by quickly rotating the hammer head.

    Nails can also be bent over against the wall and cut off later with the nail cutters. The important thing is to make the point of the nail safe immediately after the nail is driven.

11. Line up the shoe by striking it with the hammer and drive the other heel nail.

12. Drive the rest of the nails in alternating succession from heel to toe. The first few nails can be used to further align the shoe.

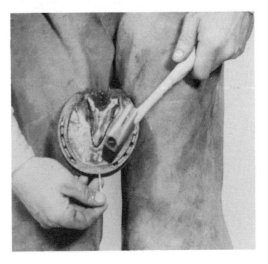

Fig. 20-6.   *Bending the nail on the shoe.*

to come out in the desired place. This bend is made at the top of the bevel on the tip of the nail in the claw of the hammer or on the edge of the shoe.

If you drive a nail down into the crease of a shoe and then decide to remove it, there are several ways of doing so:

1. Wring or cut the nail off, hammer the stub flat against the wall, place the clinching block perpendicular to the nail, and strike the shoe next to the nail with the hammer. This will usually loosen the nail enough so that it can be grasped by the pull offs.
2. Insert the pointed end of the clinch cutter underneath the head of the nail, and strike down on the head of the point. This will usually loosen the nail enough so that it can be grasped by the pull offs.

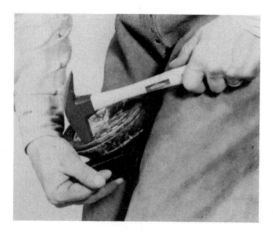

Fig. 20-7. *Removing the nail head from the shoe crease with a clinching block.*

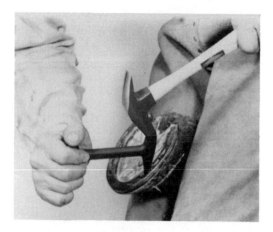

Fig. 20-8. *Removing the nail head from the shoe crease with the point of a clinch cutter.*

3. Pull the nail with a crease nail puller. This method is preferred by the Author because of the ease and speed with which it can be done. However, an extra tool is required.

"Quicking" (also called pricking or nailing), refers to penetration of the sensitive structures of the foot by the nail. Usually the horse will jerk and let you know of your error if you chance to accidentally quick him. However, this may not always be the case. You may note a difference in sound as you drive the nail or you may note blood around where it enters or leaves the foot. Occasionally the nail may be just "close" to the sensitive structures and the resulting pressure causes the horse to be lame later. You can test for a close nail by using your clinchers or hoof testers to create pressure against the wall between the clinch and shoe. It is difficult to isolate a bad nail by tapping with a hammer. A lame horse may flinch no matter where you tap. First aid for quicking is described in Chapter 18.

Clinching the Nails

Steps in clinching the nails:

1. Place the clinching block under a heel nail stub. Hold the block flat against the wall.
2. Strike the nail head once or twice, or just enough to seat the nail and turn the stub. Striking very hard blows causes the wall to be torn away under the stub. This practice may cause pain to the horse and bruising of the sensitive structures if the wall is thin.
3. Alternate back and forth from one side of the shoe to the other in the order that the nails are driven. This is especially important in thin-walled hoofs to prevent lameness

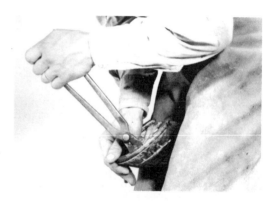

Fig. 20-9. *Removing the nail head from the shoe crease with crease nail pullers.*

caused from unequal tightening of the shoe. Many experienced shoers start on one side of the foot and continue all the way around the foot or start at each heel and move toward the toe. Increased speed can be obtained in this manner and it is not harmful when shoeing sound feet of good substance.

4. Take the foot to the forward position. (Place the foot on a stand, if desired.) Perform all operations on the outside of the foot before proceeding to do the inside on young or nervous horses that may be excited by movement. Do all of each operation with a given tool on gentle horses that are not bothered by your movements.

5. Cut all the turned stubs close against the wall with nail cutters *or* rasp all the stubs until they each project about 1/16 inch from the wall. This will make the clinches square when they are turned. Clinches should be longer than they are wide when shoeing with heavy shoes.

6. File away the burr of the wall which was formed by turning the clinch. This can be done with the edge of the rasp or a fine cut mill file. Hold the fine side of the rasp or the file nearly flat against the foot and remove the burr of hoof down to the nail. By holding the rasp in this position, you will avoid cutting a deep groove in the wall. Be careful not to cut into and weaken the nail.

7. Place the clinchers on the nail stub and roll them over the nail. Dull clinchers usually work best for beginners as they won't grab the nail but will roll off it. Sharp clinchers may turn too much clinch and tear the wall. Note that as the one hand closes the handles on the clinchers and rolls them downward, the other hand holds them in against the wall.

The clinch may be turned with the clinchers or with the hammer and clinching block as a back up. However, young or sensitive-footed horses should be done only with the clinchers. There are several sizes of clinchers for the various sizes and heights of nails. Pull offs can be used as clinchers, if necessary.

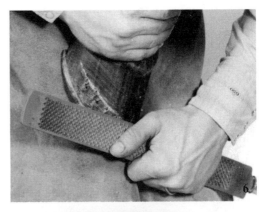

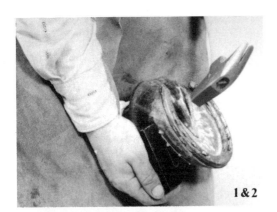

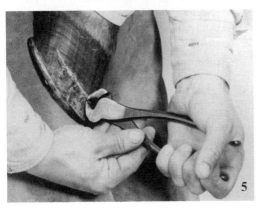

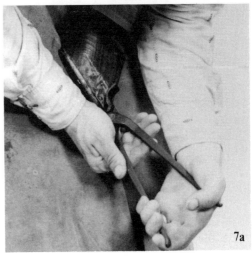

Fig. 20-10. Steps in clinching the nails (1-10).

The clinch may be seated into the wall with the driving hammer and the clinching block. Be careful not to hit too hard on the clinch when seating it into the wall, for the clinch may be weakened, and sensitive tissue underlying the wall may be bruised. Seating the clinches adds to the appearance of the work but is not necessary if the clinchers are used properly.

8. Finish the job with the smooth side of a used rasp (clinching rasp). The clinches should be smooth enough so that when you pass your hand over them, they do not feel rough. Care must be taken so as not to rasp them so much that they are weakened. The lower border of the wall should be rasped until it is flush with the shoe. Again, a finer cut mill file may be used for this work instead of a rasp.

9. Run the edge of the rasp around the hoof between the rim of the shoe and the foot. This is not necessary but it adds to the appearance of the work.
10. Return the foot to the "home position" if the horse is nervous and you are not using a foot stand. The foot of a gentle horse can be passed behind your back.
11. Take the foot forward and finish clinching the nails on the inside of the hoof.
12. Evaluate your work. Make mental notes that will help you improve your next job.

References

Hickman, J. 1977. Farriery. J. A. Allen and Co., Ltd., London.

Simpson, J.S. 1983. The Mechanics of Horseshoeing Simplified. Scott Simpson, Walla Walla, WA.

Springhall, J.A. 1964. Elements of Horseshoeing. Univ. of Queensland Press, Brisbane, AUSTRALIA.

War Department. 1941. The Horseshoer (TM 2-220). U.S. Government Printing Office, Washington, DC.

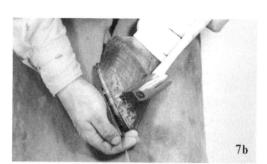

7b

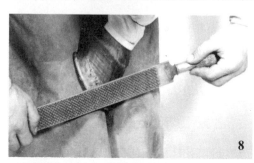

8

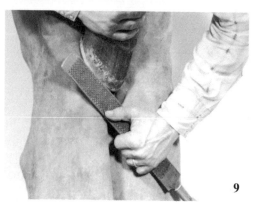

9

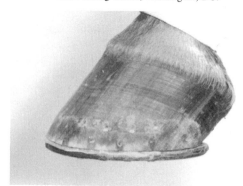

Fig. 20-11. Side view of finished foot.

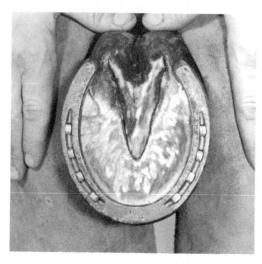

Fig. 20-12. Bottom view of finished foot.

Chapter 21

Shoeing Evaluation

Evaluation of the job is an important part of horseshoeing. Every detail must be considered in shoeing. A small mistake on one part of the job can cause other mistakes to be made as a result of it. When working with a live structure such as the foot, there is little room for error. Learning to evaluate your work and the work of others is an important part of improving the quality of your craftsmanship.

The return of *shoeing competitions* and the awarding of *performance ratings* for participating horseshoers is bringing about a renewed interest in self-evaluation. This will continue to improve the workmanship of those who have the desire to achieve. The winners are setting the standard of excellence for the profession.

The following evaluation or check list was developed by the U.S. Army (War Department, 1941). A "standard to measure to" should include the following questions in the four general areas below:

Hoof Preparation

1. Are corresponding pairs of feet the same size (toe and heel length and angle the same; can be checked with a hoof protractor and dividers)?
2. Is the foot in balance in relation to the leg (not broken in or broken out; broken forward or broken back)?
3. Is the foot in balance in relation to the horse's conformation (weight equally distributed over it; flares removed to shift center of weight distribution)?
4. Is the hoof shaped sufficiently and does the conformation of the foot warrant the amount of rasping done?
5. Has the toe been "dubbed" to cover up poor fitting of the shoe?
6. Is the foot level (not rounded, quarters trimmed too low, or heels unlevel)?
7. Has the frog been trimmed sufficiently to prevent the formation of an environment for thrush and facilitate hoof cleaning?
8. Has only dead sole been removed? Has the sole been trimmed in such a way that it has a natural appearance?

Shoe Fitting

1. Is the shoe the right size for the foot (nail holes in right place, heels correct length)?
2. Does the shoe fit the outer border of the wall and have proper "expansion" at the heels?
3. Are the heels of the shoe of sufficient length and width to cover the buttresses (prevent corns)?
4. Are the heels of the shoe finished smooth (prevent shoe boils)?
5. Is the shoe level (no "sprung" or "eased" heels; prevents cast shoes and lameness)?
6. Has the shoe been concaved or beveled in order to prevent sole pressure?
7. Is the shoe the correct weight for the use of the horse, and will it provide reasonable wear and protection to the foot between shoeings?
8. Are the projections on and/or alterations of the shoe correctly made and fit to the foot (clips, calks, etc.)?

Nailing and Clinching

1. Are the nails driven to the proper height for the size and condition of the foot (at least ¾ in. in average-sized sound hoof, ⅜ in. above old nail holes, or higher if hoof wall chipped or broken)?
2. Are the nails driven to the same height and in a line parallel to the shoe or parallel to the coronary band (for appearance, and so the holes in the wall will grow out evenly for the next shoeing)?

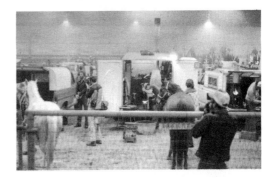

Fig. 21-1. Shoeing competitions have stimulated improvements in farrier craftsmanship. The 1981 American Farrier's Association's North American Challenge Cup Futurity Horseshoeing Contest at Albuquerque, New Mexico. Photo by K. Ball.

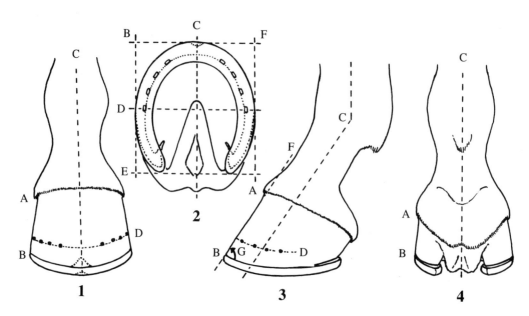

Fig. 21-2. Evaluate the hoof from all directions (1) A should be parallel to B, C perpendicular to B, and D parallel to B or A. (2) C should bisect B, D and E, and D should bisect B and F. (3) F should be parallel to C, D parallel to

B or A. Angle G on the left foot should equal angle G' on the opposite right foot. AB on the left foot should equal A'B' on the opposite right foot. (4) C should bisect A and B, C be perpendicular to B, and A should be parallel to B.

3. Are the nails the proper size for the foot (cause a minimum of wall damage and don't crack or split hoof, yet substantial enough to hold on the shoe)?
4. Do the nail heads seat correctly in the shoe (1/16 in. of the head projecting from the shoe for clinching)?
5. Are the clinches square and strong (not rasped thin)?
6. Are the clinches seated in the wall and smooth?

Overall

1. Does the horse stand square and comfortably?
2. Does the horse move straight and sound?

Score Sheet Format

The American Farriers' Association (1981) has published a booklet which establishes standards by which horseshoeing contests sanctioned by that organization are judged. Following is a way of arranging the categories of concern into a score sheet format that can be adapted to a progressive evaluation of a shoeing job. The foot can be viewed on the ground until the first asterisk (*). The foot can be evaluated off the

ground between one and two asterisks (**). A final study and evaluation can be made with the foot on the ground after the two asterisks. Numerical scores can be totaled and compared.

Speed in Shoeing

Speed in shoeing is essentially achieved by finding the easiest and fastest way to do the job. Accuracy must be developed first, and then cultivated along with speed to achieve real skill and excellence.

The following eight principles will help to make horseshoeing easier and more profitable for you if applied daily in your work:

1. **Leave out any part of the task you can.** Is there any step or part of the job you can leave out and still achieve the same quality results? For example:
   a. Use ready-made cold shoes instead of handmade shoes or hot shoes on normal-footed horses.
   b. Buy horseshoeing supplies ahead in quantity and stock a good assortment of sizes (saves time and money).
   c. Buy shoes with nail holes that fit the nail size you desire to use.

Farriery Competition Score Sheet

Five (5) points possible for each sub-category on each foot.

Competitor Number _____   Judge Number _____

(A) **HOOF PREPARATION**	LF	RF	RH	LH	Subtotal	_____
						100
Lateral Balance	___	___	___	___	_____	
Toe Angle	___	___	___	___	_____	
Toe Length	___	___	___	___	_____	
Dishes/Flares	___	___	___	___	_____	
* Sole/Frog Trim	___	___	___	___	_____	

(B) **SHOE QUALITY**						_____
						100
Shoe Form	___	___	___	___	_____	
Shoe Heels	___	___	___	___	_____	
Nail Holes	___	___	___	___	_____	
Shoe Level	___	___	___	___	_____	
Clip(s)	___	___	___	___	_____	

(C) **SHOE FIT**						_____
						100
Outline Fit	___	___	___	___	_____	
Clip(s) Fit	___	___	___	___	_____	
Heel Length	___	___	___	___	_____	
Sole Pressure	___	___	___	___	_____	
** Heel Expansion	___	___	___	___	_____	

(D) **NAILING AND FINISH**						_____
						100
Nail Height	___	___	___	___	_____	
Nail Alignment	___	___	___	___	_____	
Clinch Shape	___	___	___	___	_____	
Wall Smooth	___	___	___	___	_____	
Clinch Smooth	___	___	___	___	_____	

Fig. 21-3. Suggested score sheet for American Farrier's Association judging standards.

TOTAL   400

   d. Wring nails as they are driven instead of cutting them off later.
   e. Use clinchers instead of hammer to turn and seat the nails.
   f. Arrange truck so you don't have a lot of unnecessary steps for setup and take down.
2. **Make one task out of two or more**. Is there any step or part of the job you can combine with another to eliminate motion and steps and thus save time? For example:
   a. Divide the work into operations and perform all of one type of work while in the same position, i.e., pulling shoes and trimming; nailing and clinching.
   b. Do all of your work at the fire or anvil at the same time by marking shoes and noting changes to be made on them so they can all be worked at the same time.
   c. Trim the frog and bars (if necessary) while the hoof nippers are in your hand instead of changing tools and using the knife.
   d. Educate customers while you are working.
3. **Keep everything within easy reach**. Is everything you need to do the job within easy reach before you start and when you need it? For example:
   a. Make a shoeing box which is the right height for you, in addition to being light, and which puts your tools where you can reach them easily.
   b. When trimming, use a knife pocket on your apron or a trimming box. It saves time and effort by preventing the neces-

sity of picking up each tool individually when you are finished with a foot, and it keeps your tool sharp longer.
   c. Store tools used most frequently together in your truck.
   d. Store tools with supplies they are used with, such as knives and scissors with pads, etc.
   e. Store shoes on a rack that is easy to reach, and which makes it easy to tell what sizes you have and how many of each are in stock.
4. **Make both hands work.** Do you use both hands to make work easier and less tiring? For example:
   a. Use both hands on the knife. Either push it with your thumb or put both hands on the handle. (This also gets your other hand out of the way so it won't get cut!)
   b. Position the foot on your knees or foot stand so that you can use both hands when rasping in all positions.
   c. Practice driving nails and using the rounding hammer with either hand.
5. **Use the best tool.** Keep your tools and equipment in good condition. Do your tools contribute to the ease and speed with which the job may be accomplished? For example:
   a. Buy quality tools. Their design makes the job easier, you don't have to sharpen them as often, they hold up longer, and they aren't as apt to break when you need them most.

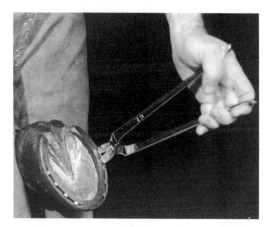
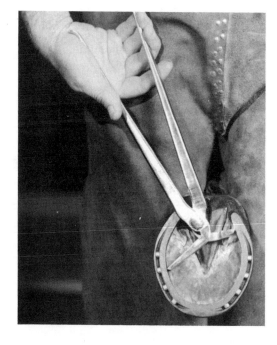

Fig. 21-4. Tools that save time and energy increase efficiency and profit. (Left) crease nail puller, (Right) shoe spreader. Photos by McLain.

b. Use sharp tools; dress them frequently; protect them.

c. Buy or make tools which make the job easier and more accurate. (You can shoe a horse with only a hammer and a rasp; but who wants to!)

6. **Sit to work or rest whenever possible.** Use the best posture when sitting or standing. Do you sit whenever possible to take the strain off your back and legs and allow them to rest? For example:

a. Sit whenever you can. Rest between horses, putting on Borium, waiting for a shoe to heat, sharpening tools, and, if working with another person, when holding a horse.

b. Adjust your anvil, forge, work area, and shoeing box to a height that is comfortable for you.

c. Learn to relax when working. You won't get tired as fast, and the horse will stand better.

7. **Develop smooth, easy, rhythmic motions.** Do you use long, smooth, rhythmic motions to suit your pace instead of short jerky ones? For example:

a. Rasping is much easier and faster when done with long rhythmic strokes.

b. Using the nippers can be easier when a smooth pace is developed.

c. Hammering at the anvil is much less tiring when done with a definite timing and rhythm. Also, a rhythmic sequence in forge work helps make more efficient use of heats.

d. When attention is given to maintaining a rhythm, the last horse of the day can be shod at the same pace as the first.

8. **Improve the order of your work.** If you changed the order of your work or the use of your tools, could you do the job faster and with less effort? For example:

a. Group things in your tool box in the order they are picked up to perform a job. Carry in the box only those tools used on *every* horse. Add and take away tools as needed for special cases.

b. Have a set procedure or way to do a job. It then becomes easy to increase speed.

c. Experiment with the step-by-step order in which you do jobs; time and evaluate various procedures to find the best for you.

d. Arrange tools and equipment so you can set up and take down with minimum lifting and maximum speed.

Implement these principles into your work. They can be applied to most any job. Not only will this evaluation process ease and speed up your work, but you will enjoy doing it more, too.

References

Daniels, B. 1981. Standards for Judging Farriery Competition. American Farriers' Association, Albuquerque, NM.

Evans, J.W. 1981. Horses. Freeman, San Francisco.

War Department. 1941. The Horseshoer (TM 2-220). U.S. Government Printing Office. Washington, DC.

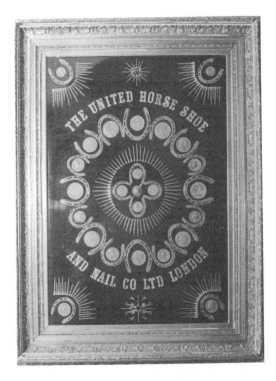

Fig. 21-5. Display boards stimulate craftsmanship as well as gather prizes and awards. Old Globe (Mustad) Nail Company display board. Photo by H. Nilsson.

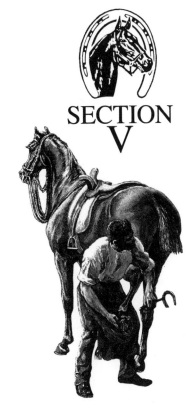

SECTION
V

IRON AND FORGE
WORK

Chapter 22

The Forge Fire and Heats

Fuel Types

Coal, coke and gas are the three popular forging fuels used today.

Charcoal or split hard wood can be used when coal or coke are unavailable. These will produce the heat necessary, but are relatively expensive or labor intensive and produce great quantities of ash. They may even be preferred for heating tool steel.

Forging heat can be obtained from an oxy-acetylene torch or a mixture of oxygen and gas (butane or propane). However, this has limited application due to the expense involved. These heat sources may be used in addition to a con-

ventional forge. An electrical carbon arc torch can also be used to obtain a forging heat, but it is not usually practical due to the special equipment and protection for bystanders necessary. Oil and electricity are used in many commercial furnaces, but are not practical for blacksmithing or horseshoeing.

Coal used for forging should be the best quality bituminous or soft coal available. In many areas it is difficult to obtain and usually must be shipped from long distances in large quantities. The following specifications are useful when ordering coal (Bealer, 1974):

Carbon (high)	55 to 65%
Moisture (low)	2.5 to 3%
Ash (low)	3 to 8%
Sulfur (low)	1 to 2%
Volatility (high)	30 to 40%
BTU (high)	13,500 to 14,500

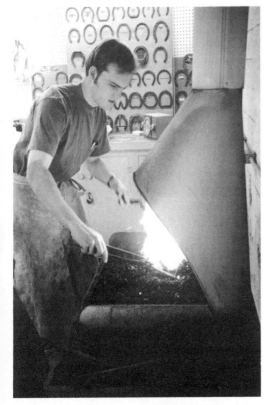

Fig. 22-1. Skill in the use of the forge fire is necessary to produce good craftsmanship. Photo by R. Rankin.

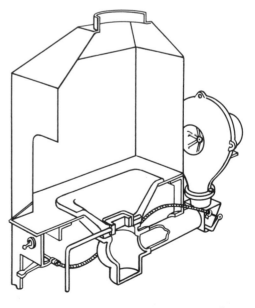

Fig. 22-2. Coal forge design. Drawings by J. Hoffman.

213

If possible, inspect and burn some of the coal before purchasing. Look for the following ideal characteristics:

1. Size—about marble size lumps, referred to as pea coal.
2. Clean—free from dirt, rocks and shale, referred to as washed coal.
3. Texture—crumbles easily rather than layering: uniformly bright and glossy faces without dull streaks.
4. Fines—no more than 25 percent coal dust among the lumps. Some aids in creating a solid fire. Too much may not coke properly and interfere with the blast.
5. Fire—free from green (sulfur) smoke and produces a white flame in the center and a blue flame on the edge of the fire. The coal is self-coking and very little clinker is formed.

Coal is often difficult to obtain except in large quantities (railroad car loads of 50 to 100 tons per car) due to industrial demand. You may have to go together with several smiths in your area to buy the right coal at the right price. Coal can be shipped in bulk or in sacks.[1] Coal should be kept under cover as it is said to lose some of its heating qualities when the sun shines on it continually.

Hard coke may be obtained from steel mills or suppliers to steel mills. In some areas, that is the only fuel that may be conveniently obtained. Hard coke is soft coal after it has been exposed to the intense heat of coke ovens. Coke has the advantage of burning very hot and requiring comparatively less storage space. It has the disadvantage of being hard to start and very dirty. It snaps, crackles, pops and forms large clinkers. Pieces of coke are grey, porous, light in weight and can be broken like chalk.

Gas (propane or butane) has become popular as a forge fuel in recent years. Previously, gas forges were too bulky, too noisy, too cool and too expensive to be seriously considered by most horseshoers. Gas was more expensive and less plentiful than coal.

Times have changed. Modern gas forges permit forge welding as well as limited-temperature safe-heating of several shoes at a time.[2] They have enjoyed a surge in popularity. Bottled gas of uniform quality is available in nearly every part of the country. There are no complaints of air pollution. The relative ease of operation of the gas forge has made it especially popular with beginners. There are even gas forges that require no electric power source to operate. These are called atmospheric gas forges.

However, the relatively high noise level, the fragile inner liner, and increased metal scaling are definite disadvantages of gas forges. The lack of a fast soaking or complete heat necessary for major shoe shaping and welding without excessive fuel consumption is a major concern.

In addition, determining fuel level can be a problem. Tanks must be weighed, consumption must be figured and a time log kept, if accuracy is desired. For example, a 30 pound tank may only have 20 pounds of gas available. The amount of gas that will vaporize and be available for use will vary, especially between cold and warm days.

Forge Design

A hoodless shop **coal forge** which draws the smoke (and fire) to the side may be made from brick or rock with a fire pot made of cast iron or fire clay. An electric reostat-regulated centrifugal blower or a hand-operated bellows supplies a constant regulatable air blast. Ideally, a forge should have both electrical *and* mechanical regulation of the air blast.

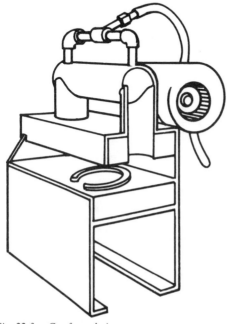

Fig. 22-3. Gas forge design.

[1]*Cumberland Elkhorn Coal and Coke, Inc., Louisville, KY*

[2]*Mankel Blacksmith Shop, Cannonsburg, MI*

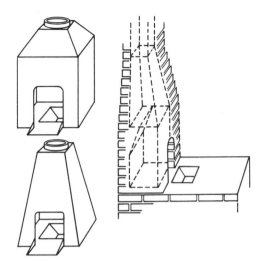

Fig. 22-4. Coal forge hood designs; (Left top) straight-sided, (Left bottom) funnel-shaped, and (Right) side-draft masonry.

Fire pots may be purchased commercially or constructed from scrap. Ash gates may be constructed horizontally or vertically, depending on the clearance available. Tuyeres (twyers) can be simple bar grates or elaborate clinker busters. Fire pots must be constructed of material thick enough to prevent warpage due to heat and premature collapse due to scaling. Fire clay can be used, but it increases the weight of a portable forge.

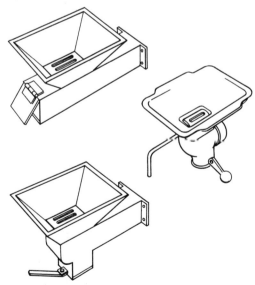

Fig. 22-5. Types of coal forge fire pots; (Left top) horizontal ash trap with removable grate, (Right) vertical ash trap with clinker buster, and (Left bottom) vertical ash trap with removable grate. Drawings by J. Hoffman.

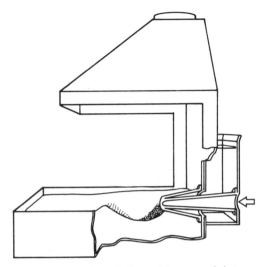

Fig. 22-6. Side-blast coke forge with water-cooled tuyere.

British Alcosa forges (hearths) have no fire pot. The air blast comes from a water cooled tuyere projecting from the side directly into the pile of coke. The size of the fire is regulated by the amount of the blast. Exceptionally fast and long heats on steel can be obtained with this type of forge.

The best type of AC blower is a centrifugal blower. An old Champion No. 50 is ideal, if you can find one. Buffalo[3] and Yant[4] also make this type of blower. They are expensive. A portable squirrel cage blower made from a DC car heater blower is satisfactory if you have no more than one elbow and you have a small fire. (Each elbow decreases the blower blast by 10%). These blowers can be regulated by an on-off switch and reostat. A good hand crank centrifugal blower is better than a weak AC or DC electric powered squirrel cage blower.

Many of the commercial coal and gas forges are unsatisfactory for shoe making. They are designed for intermittent operation for making minor alterations to keg shoes. Proper forge design is critical to the horseshoer desiring to make his own shoes.

The new double-fired (from above or below) **gas forges** with soft super-insulating liners are the hottest and most satisfactory of this type to date. They are comparatively economical to operate and can be adjusted to yield from just

[3]*Buffalo Forge Co., Buffalo, NY.*

[4]*Yant Manufacturing, Ft. Collins, CO.*

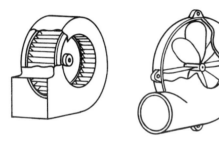

Fig. 22-7. Forge blower types; (Left) squirrel cage, (Right) centrifugal or blade.

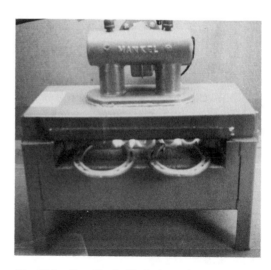

Fig. 22-9. Portable double-fired gas forge. Photo from Mankel.

enough heat for hot fitting all the way up to a welding heat. Welding flux must be used when welding in a gas forge. Follow starting and adjusting instructions supplied by the manufacturer.

Even with modern improvements, gas forges require time and experimentation to obtain maximum efficiency. And, they are especially hard on arm and facial hair. Inaccessibility to the fire with anything other than a plate shoe is a problem. Construction of large shoes for draft horses and swedging long pieces are most difficult if not impossible in many of the portable models.

Well designed gas forges are unexcelled for speed in altering and fitting keg shoes. They are constantly being improved. The addition of hoods, holes allowing proper placement of bar stock, and interchangeable, replaceable parts, make gas forges very attractive to modern horseshoers.

Gas forges must be properly vented like coal forges when used in an enclosed area. They both produce poisonous carbon monoxide.

Building a Coal Forge Fire

Coke is the heating fuel of a coal forge. It must be present or created to obtain the maximum and most efficient forging heats. When building a coal forge fire for the first time, and there is no coke available, you must build a fire of wood or other substantial long-burning material to create enough heat to make coke from coal. It is unwise to try to use the fire until all the coal over the heat source has been consumed or turned to coke. Coke puffs up as it forms. As it is lifted up with the fire rake or poker, more is produced from the coal on the sides of the fire.

Forge coal should be soaked in water before it is used. Wet coal, sometimes called green coal, will form coke much more readily than dry coal. The gases in the coal combine with the water and are released as steam. Also wet coal forms coke that holds together better and thus produces a hotter fire. Wet coal keeps the fire from spreading as it will pack down hard and contain the air blast.

Wet or green coal forms coke as the gases in it are driven off by gradual heating. A good supply of coke is essential for a hot, clean fire. As the coke is consumed, it is replaced by wet coal, thus constantly replenishing the supply of coke. Green coal alone is of little or no use in heating iron or steel because it does not produce

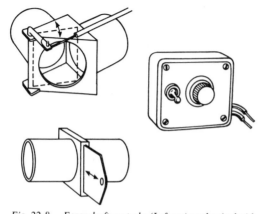

Fig. 22-8. Forge draft controls; (Left top) mechanical with no air flow restriction, (Left bottom) mechanical with air flow restriction, and (Right) electrical speed control with on-off switch and rheostat.

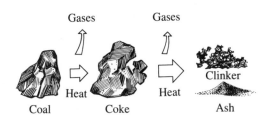

Fig. 22-10. Heating process of a coal fire. Drawing by J. Hoffman.

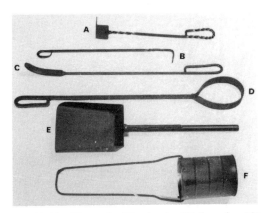

Fig. 22-11. Fire tools. (A) ash rake, (B) fire poker, (C) fire rake, (D) circular fire rake, (E) fire shovel, and (F) water valve or sprinkling can. Photo by G. Poellot.

a high degree of heat, it sticks to the metal, and emits a smoke and smell which interfere with the work. Higher degrees of heat can be obtained only from a coke fire.

As iron or steel is heated, it gives off particles, or scales, which remain in the fire and bind with impurities and particles of consumed coke or coal. These hard, glass-like structures are called clinkers. They gradually become larger if left in the fire, and must be removed as they form. If left in, they will spoil the efficiency of the fire by plugging the blast holes as well as sticking to the metal being heated. Clinkers are so named because of their characteristic clinking sound when struck (after cooling) with the poker.

There are many blacksmiths who are good horseshoers, but there are few shoers who are good blacksmiths. Learn to build and maintain a clean hot fire.

NOTE: Many horseshoers insist on wearing safety glasses when working at the forge. All are advised to do this.

Steps in building a forge fire:

1. Clean the forge pot. Remove all dirt, ashes, clinkers and unconsumed fuel. Pile the coal on the sides and the coke on top of it.
2. Open the slide or ash gate and rock the tuyere vigorously to break up clinkers which may have formed. A straight poker will often be necessary to aid in removing clinkers. In a grate-type forge pot, a curved poker may be useful for this purpose.
3. Remove the ashes. If necessary, turn on the blower momentarily to remove accumulated dust.
4. Place dry newspapers (three or four double sheets wadded up), kerosene-soaked wood shavings, or any other inflammable material in the center of the crater and ignite it. An oxy-acetylene torch may be used to ignite coke placed in the fire box.

5. Place coke on the burning material and turn the blower on at a very slow speed. Care must be taken not to cover the fire so closely that the flames are smothered and have no where to go.
6. As the coke begins to burn, pile wet coal around the edges of the fire (not on top of it).
7. As the coke in the center is consumed and the fire becomes hollow, push the coke which has been forming on the edge of the fire into the center.
8. Replenish the coal at the sides of the fire. Moisten the coal at the sides of the fire periodically with a sprinkler can to prevent the fire from spreading. Fires of various shapes can be made in this way.
9. Repeat Steps 7 and 8 as it becomes necessary. Open the fire with the poker and drag out clinkers as they form.

An alternate fire building method is to place a block of wood or tin can about 4 inches in diameter over the tuyere. Pack wet coal on the sides or around the block or can until the desired height is reached. The block or can is then withdrawn and the fire started in the hole directly over the tuyere with paper and coke.

Characteristics of a Coal Fire

The fire, to a large extent, determines the success or failure of all forging operations. Building and maintaining a good fire are skills which should be acquired by all horseshoers.

The depth of the fire should be 6 to 8 inches for most horseshoeing. The bar stock or shoe should be placed or snuggled into the fire at the point of greatest heat, about 3 to 4 inches above the tuyere or grate. If the metal is too near the

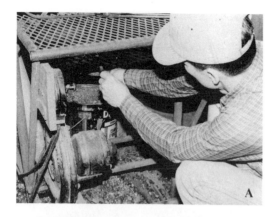
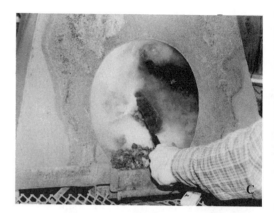
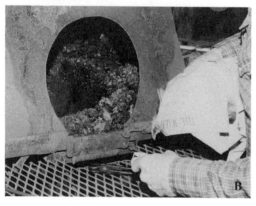
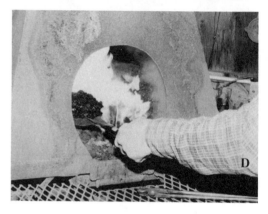

Fig. 22-12. Steps in building a coal forge fire; (A) pile coke on top of coal at sides of fire pot and clean out ashes, (B) ignite several sheets of crumpled newspaper, (C) place coke over and around ignited newspaper in fire pot, and (D) heap coal on the sides of the fire. Photos by J. Graves.

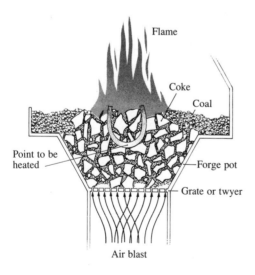

Fig. 22-13. Parts of coal forge fire. Drawing by L. Sadler.

source of air, the cold blast of air will prevent the shoe from getting hot.

Coal fires can be open or hollow. Most horseshoers use an open fire where combustion occurs on top of heaped coke. Many blacksmiths use a hollow fire where combustion occurs in the center with wet coal being packed to form a roofed cave. The hollow fire is hotter but is more difficult to maintain access to with horseshoes.

A good blacksmithing forge fire is known as a reducing fire. This is a fire that has a deep bed of hot coals (coke) and is surrounded on at least three sides with packed wet coal. A reducing fire uses all of the oxygen supplied by the air blast to make the fire hotter. A reducing fire produces less scale and is essential for good forging. As soon as the fire tends toward an oxidizing fire by becoming hollow or oxidizing, it should be built up immediately.

An oxidizing fire is one in which more oxygen is blowing through the fire than is being used for fuel combustion. It is usually characterized by a rim of coke or live coals around the fire pot and a hollow center. An oxidizing fire causes very rapid oxidation or scale formation on the metal. It will not produce a uniform high heat like a reducing fire. A gas forge produces an oxidizing fire.

Procedure for maintaining an efficient reducing fire:

1. Build and maintain the fire at the proper depth by routinely opening the fire with the straight poker and lifting the coke up. Remove clinkers as they form.
2. Contain the fire by keeping the sides of the fire packed with wet coal. Sprinkle the sides of the fire with water.
3. Limit the air blast so that it heats the fire instead of blowing it up the chimney. Shut the blower off when not heating metal. Or run it at a very low speed while keeping the several pieces of metal being worked at once high in the fire.
4. Place the metal high in the fire with a few inches of coke over it but the majority under it.

Banking a Coal Fire

A fire should always be "banked" when it is left for more than a short period of time. To bank or keep a fire, place a stick of hardwood in the center of it and rake the coke into a mound around it. Then cover the coke with wet coal and open the slide or ash gate. This will keep the fire alive for an hour or so and insure plenty of coke for the next fire if it does die out. In the horse and buggy days, the blacksmith used to keep his fire with a broken wagon spoke. Any piece of hardwood will work as well. Upon returning, turn the blast on until the stick and coke catch fire. Rake back the coal and remove the stick. Resume your work.

Breaking Down a Coal Fire

A fire should be broken down at the end of a day or when you move from place to place. If a fire is simply allowed to slowly consume itself and go out, not only will fuel be wasted, but there will also be little if any coke available to start the next fire. Clean the fire by removing

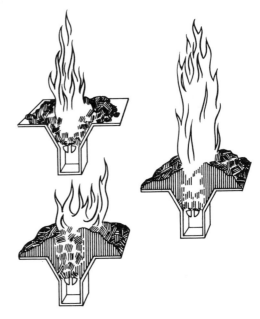

Fig. 22-14. Coal fire types; (Top left) oxidizing, (Bottom left) tight, and (right) reducing. Drawings by J. Hoffman.

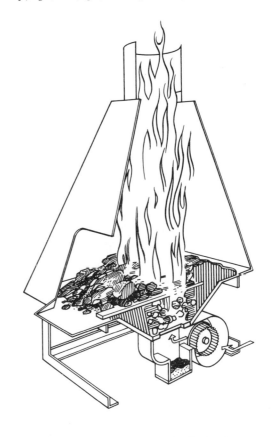

Fig. 22-15. Position of bar stock when heating in a portable coal forge.

the clinkers. Run the coal shovel down the edge of the fire pot and lift the fire up, placing it on the sides of the firepot. If your forge is too small to allow room for this, place the hot coals in a steel bucket. The coke will quickly extinguish itself in the absence of any air blast. Do not open the ash gate.

Characteristics of a Gas Fire

Light the gas forge by placing a match in it and turning on the gas. Then, immediately turn on the fan. A flint striker works well for lighting most gas forges. Many horseshoers wear a glove when lighting a gas forge with a flint striker or lighter.

A gas forge produces an oxidizing fire. Comparatively, a gas fire produces much more scale than a coal fire. However, gas is quick and clean for shaping and altering keg shoes. Alteration of gas forges makes possible heating of straight lengths of bar stock. Shoes should be removed from gas forges as they are brought up to forging temperature to prevent oxidation and subsequent loss of cross sectional area of the steel. Gas forge liners are damaged by excessive scaling. The fire on a gas forge can be turned down to prevent excessive oxidation. A low fire is ideal for hot fitting shoes, but may not be hot enough for major shaping, turning calks or clips.

Forge welding is possible in a modern gas forge designed for horseshoeing. The shoe must be heated until it is hot enough for a welding flux containing iron filings to stick to the metal. The hot shoe should be brushed vigorously to knock off scale and fluxed immediately before scale forms. The flux must stick to the metal and melt (appear wet). The flux should be between as well as around the surface to be welded. Excess flux will damage the gas forge lining. The shoe is placed back in the fire and the gas is turned up and the air shut down until flame is going up as well as out from forge.

Each type of forge may produce different heating characteristics. You must learn them. Periodically glance at the flux. Do not stare at it unless you wear protective dark glasses. When the flux starts to puddle on the top and bottom of the weld, bring the shoe to the anvil. Avoid placing the shoe on the anvil until you are ready to strike it. Strike a sharp blow in the middle at

first and then finish the edges of the weld with lighter blows. Finally, flatten the welded metal to its original or desired thickness. Readjust the fire to be more efficient for heating after welding. Leave the blower on a minute or so after you shut a gas forge off. This will cool the liner and reduce the danger of burning yourself on the forge. The fire should be turned off after each use. It is most efficient to group all of your forging operations together and run the fire for a short time. Many modern gas forges are not designed for constant operation.

Heats

The character (color, temperature, grain size, forgeability, etc.) of metal being forged is referred to as a heat. These are usually identified by color. However, color varies depending on the light source in the work area. Temperatures are general values indicating a range that might be expected for a given color. Exact temperatures are important in heat treating steel and may be detected by special marking crayons (see Chapter 25).

Heat is also the term assigned to any given time a piece of metal is taken from the fire and worked on at the anvil. A blacksmith's efficiency is judged by the number of heats it takes to complete a job.

The **yellow** heat is the highest heat obtainable without melting the shoe. The metal is nearly sparking. Horseshoes and other forgings of mild steel are started at this heat. The metal is approximately 2500 degrees to 2100 degrees F. Major alterations such as turning the toe and branches of a shoe, shaping or cutting heels, creasing, pulling clips, making square toes, etc., are done at this heat. The metal moves easily under the hammer. The bright yellow heat is referred to as the forging heat.

The **lemon-orange** heat is the color the metal becomes after it loses the yellow heat. Lemon may range from 2100 degrees to 1800 degrees F. Orange may range from 1800 degrees to 1600 degrees F. The metal still may be shaped with relative ease in these temperature ranges. Most of the major alterations begun at a yellow heat are finished in these heat ranges. Nail holes should be stamped when the metal is lemon to orange in color.

The **bright red** heat is the color the metal becomes after it loses the orange heat. It ranges from 1600 degrees to 1500 degrees F. The metal may be shaped at this temperature, but it is less yielding to the hammer. Nail holes should be punched out with the pritchel at this heat, especially on thick heavy shoes. It is also the best heat to reform nail holes on machine-made shoes. The bright red heat is as hot as one may heat some types of tool steel without significantly changing their grain structure.

The **cherry red** heat is the color the metal becomes after it loses its bright red color. It ranges from 1500 degrees to 1300 degrees F. In this heat range, major (critical point) changes in the grain structure of the metal occur. Steel becomes nonmagnetic at this point. Some types of tool steels should not be worked above this temperature. The cherry red heat may be referred to as the hardening or annealing heat.

The **dark cherry red** heat is the color the metal becomes after it loses its cherry red color. It ranges from 1300 degrees to 1100 degrees F. This color may be used as an indicator in hardening or annealing of the high carbon steels. It is the coldest color in which pritcheling should be done. The shoe may be leveled and hot fit at this heat.

The **blood red** or **very dark red** heat is the last color to be seen before a shoe turns black. It is an indicator the steel is between 1000 degrees and 1100 degrees F. in daylight (less in darkness). Final leveling and fitting of shoes may be done at this heat. Below this heat filed and brushed shoes will turn blue. This color can be held by stopping the polishing action and quenching the shoe.

The **black** heat is the general term for a shoe which is hot but shows no radiant color. It may be any temperature below 1000 degrees F. in daylight. Minor shaping, opening nail holes and final leveling may be done at this heat. Wiping a shoe or tool with linseed oil at this heat gives it a rustproof mat finish.

The **white** or welding heat is necessary for forge welding two or more pieces of metal together. The metal becomes pasty and melts on the surface. This may occur at 2500 degrees to 2700 degrees F. in mild steel and at 2200 degrees to 2400 degrees F. in high carbon tool steel. Above this heat, steel is burned and destroyed. Only a clean, hot, well-coked fire can produce the even heat necessary to make a good sound weld. The pieces are brought out to weld when they become the same color as each other and the sides of the fire around them. When metal gives off sparks that explode above the fire, it is almost too late. The metal must be positioned quickly and struck immediately after leaving the fire.

A welding flux, consisting of borax, clean sand and metal shavings, is usually used when welding in the forge. This is especially important when welding dissimilar metals (in size or in composition). The flux flows (runs) and carries away iron oxide (scale) which forms during the heating process. It also allows the metal to rise to a higher temperature without oxidizing (burning). Welding in modern gas forges is impossible without flux.

References

Bealer, A.W. 1974. Blacksmith coal specifications and source. The Anvil's Ring. 2(1):9.

Bealer, A.W. 1976. The Art of Blacksmithing (2nd ed.). Funk and Wagnalls, New York.

Coleman, G.J. 1921. Forge Note Book. The Bruce Publishing Co., Milwaukee, WI.

Gerakeris, D. 1979. Starting a fire. The Anvil's Ring. 7(l):16.

Holford, H. 1912. The 20th Century Toolsmith and Steelworker. Frederick J. Drake and Co., Chicago.

Lattin, F.N. 1979. Control of electrically blown forge air. The Anvil's Ring. 7(1):34.

Mankel, K. 1982. Personal Communication. Cannonsburg, MI.

Meilach, D.Z. 1977. Decorative and Sculptural Ironwork. Crown Publ., Inc., New York.

Simpson, J.S. 1978. How to Build Horseshoeing Tools and Equipment. Scott Simpson, Belgrade, MT.

Tempil. 1977. Basic Guide to Ferrous Metallurgy. Tempil Division, Big Three Industries, Inc., South Plainfield, NJ.

Chapter 23

Forging Tools and Skills

Basic forging skill development is a necessary prerequisite to forging tools and horseshoes. Using the forge requires many additional skills not needed when cold shoeing. Each skill or technique requires concentrated study and practice. It is more practical and effective to concentrate on the few specific operations of a forging exercise than it is to begin immediately the complicated process of making horseshoes. By doing simple exercises you can become coordinated in the use of hammer and tongs, learn to maintain the fire and heat the metal in the proper place and to the correct forging temperature. All these operations will be awkward at first.

A blacksmith is always working against the clock. Iron must be worked when it is hot. It cools rapidly in the air and on the anvil. The object in blacksmithing is to get the most work done in the shortest possible time. Thus, the ancient adage, ''Strike while the iron is hot!''

A blacksmith's efficiency is judged by the number of heats needed to complete a job. The fewer heats, the more skilled the blacksmith. Blacksmithing and horseshoeing are piece work. More efficiency and speed mean more income.

Every forging operation should be practiced until you are confident of your ability to perform it. You should mentally plan how much work you expect to do during each heat. Eventually, you can put several operations together and make simple projects. Later, you can make more complex objects like horseshoes.

Forging Tools

The name and uses of tools must be learned by the beginner. Also, the proper method of holding each tool and manipulating the work under it must be learned. Good work requires good tools and technique.

Anvils may be of the shop or portable type. The shop anvil should be heavy. An anvil 200 to 300 pounds in weight causes more hammer rebound and does not move when struck with force. An old anvil with a wrought iron base and a hardened steel face is preferred. The anvil should be mounted on a solid base such as a tree stump. The face of the anvil should be at the level of your knuckles when your hands hang loosely at your sides. The English style or black-

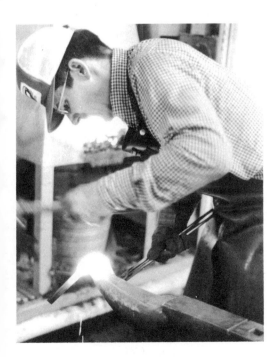

Fig. 23-1. Strike while the iron is hot!

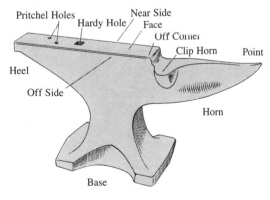

Fig. 23-2. Parts of the farrier's anvil. Drawing by L. Sadler.

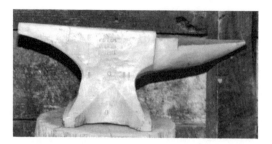

Fig. 23-3. Peter Wright blacksmith's anvil. The numbers on the side tell the weight of the anvil. (Left) The number of hundred weight (112 pounds English), (middle) the number of quarterweights (28 pounds English), and (right) the number of pounds less than a quarterweight. Photo by J. Graves.

smith pattern of anvil is most popular for shop work.

The portable anvil should weigh between 100 and 125 pounds. It should have a narrower face and rounded edges on the heel for cold shaping of shoes. It is desirable to have a swelled horn and a heel hooking hole (if not the hardy hole) as well. These anvils may be mounted on portable stands with foot operated vise clamps. Small anvils are unsuitable for general blacksmith work or shoe making.

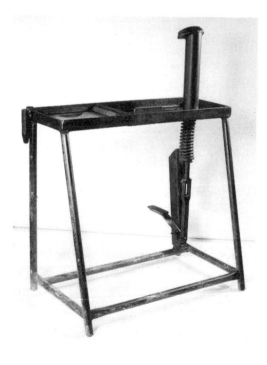

Fig. 23-4. Portable anvil stand with foot-operated spring tension vise. Photos by G. Poellot.

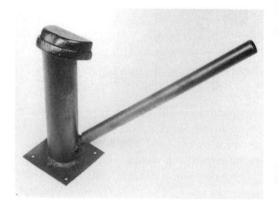

Fig. 23-5. Hand-operated tailgate spring tension vise.

The anvil must be purchased, set up and used with intelligence. It will probably be the most expensive piece of equipment you buy and you will keep it the longest. The edge or horn of the anvil may be chipped or nicked by careless blows. Discourage others from beating on it for the sake of hearing the noise. Chips, dents and deformed edges affect the work and well being of the smith, besides being potentially dangerous to bystanders.

Vises for shop work should be mounted solid on a large post or bench. The heavy box leg type is preferred. It has a spring in it to assist in opening the jaws. The vise should be mounted at elbow level. Portable spring vises operated by the foot or hand should be lower (Miller, 1983). A portable hand-operated vise made from vise-grip pliers can be slipped in and out of the hardy hole of the anvil (Daniels, 1981).

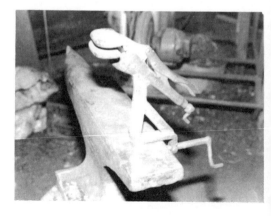

Fig. 23-6. Hand-operated vise-grip anvil vise. Photos by J. Graves.

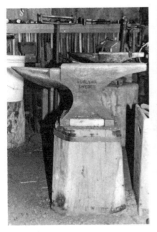
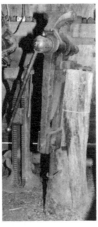

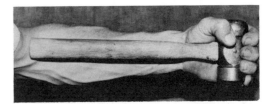

Fig. 23-10.   Proper hand hammer handle length.

Fig. 23-7.   Shop blacksmith's anvil mounted on a wooden block (left).

Fig. 23-8.   Box leg blacksmith's vise.

Hammers are the most important tool of the blacksmith. It requires as much time and dedication to use a hammer with precision as it does to play and master a musical instrument. Blacksmiths have been nicknamed "hammermen." Hammers are made of cast or tool steel. There are many hammer weights and shapes. Hand hammers may range from 1 to 4 pounds. Sledge hammers may range from 6 to 16 pounds. The average horseshoeing hand hammer weighs 2 pounds.

The shapes of hammers vary. Each has a specific use. The rounding hammer is preferred for horseshoeing because it has one round face useful for turning shoes and pulling clips. Other types are the cross-pein, straight-pein, ball-pein, machinists and cats head or turning hammer. The face of a hammer used for blacksmithing must be slightly convex. A flat face, such as that on a machinists hammer, is difficult to control and marks the work.

Most factory-made hammer handles need to be modified. They should be shaped with a rasp to fit your hand comfortably. The proper length for a hand hammer may be determined by holding the head in your hand and laying the handle against your arm. The end of the handle should extend to the elbow joint.

Tongs are used for holding hot metal. There are many types. The handles are called reins. The jaws vary in shape according to the work to be held. Tongs must be properly adjusted to hold the work. The reins should be adjusted so the tongs turn freely in the hand. To avoid frequent adjustment, blacksmiths usually have many pairs of tongs.

Flat-jawed tongs are used for holding horseshoes and flat stock, but may be adapted to hold round or square stock. Hollow bit tongs are used to hold heavy round, square or rectangular stock. They are used, too, for making and repairing pritchels and punches. Pickup tongs usually have long handles and are used to pick up most sizes of stock or move it in the fire. Bill tongs are used for forging tools with eyes, scroll work or wagon tires. Clip tongs are used to hold a long flat piece of steel while forging its end. They are useful for forging calks and for holding steel under a power hammer. Link tongs are used for forging chain links. There are many modifications of each of these basic types of tongs.

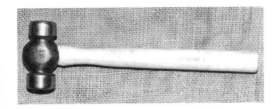

Fig. 23-9.   Two pound rounding hammer.

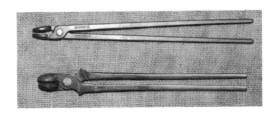

Fig. 23-11.   Horseshoeing tongs.

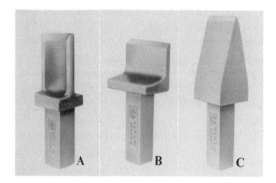

Fig. 23-12. Types of hardies. (A) half-round (curved), (B) straight or cut-off, and (C) chisel. Photos by Diamond.

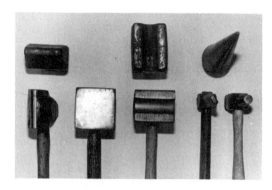

Fig. 23-14. Top and bottom fuller and flatter (left), top and bottom swedge (middle), punches and anvil mandrel (right).

Top anvil tools include top (handled) and bottom (square shank) fullers and swedges. Many of these tools have limited use in horseshoeing except for making tools.

Fullers are for drawing or spreading metal, swedges are for shaping or finishing up drawn metal. The bottom round swedge or swedge block is used to make half-round or swedged horseshoes. However, the handled corresponding top tool is not used. The set hammer is used to draw or finish between two shoulders, the flatter is used to finish flat surfaces. Handled punches are used to punch holes in hot metal. They may be square or round. Heading tools are used for forming the heads on bolts and nails. They may be made (drawn and punched) from axles, springs or other good steel. Hardies or cutting off tools mounted in the anvil are used for cutting off hot or cold stock. A different shape is used for each. The hardy for hot cutting is drawn thin and sharp. The hardy for cold cutting is short, thick and beveled. It is also tempered. Handled top cutters, called chisels, both hot and cold, are used with a sledge hammer. The hot chisel may be used for splitting as well as cutting off.

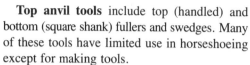

Fig. 23-13. Types of swedges. Photos by J. Graves.

Other hand tools include a center punch, measuring rule, calipers, various punches and drifts. A drift is used to enlarge or shape a hole in hot metal. Nail stamps, called fore punches, and pritchels are among the most important hand tools. They must have the proper shape and be made from tough hot work steel. Tool forging is covered in Chapter 25.

Hammer Position and Control

A blacksmith is a hammerman. You must learn to select and effectively use the right hammer for each job. Hold the handle about two-thirds of the distance between the head and handle end. Control is increased by shortening the handle grip, power is increased by lengthening the handle grip. Use your wrist, elbow and shoulder to swing the hammer.

The velocity of the hammer determines its striking force, not brute strength. Increased velocity is achieved principally by snapping the wrist. It can also be increased by raising the hammer high and rapidly contracting the arm and stomach muscles. Thus, the whole body can be put into the swing. The hammer should be falling of its own weight during the last part of the swing. It is simply guided by you. Look where you intend to hit. Stand balanced on the balls of your feet. Work as close to the anvil as is comfortable.

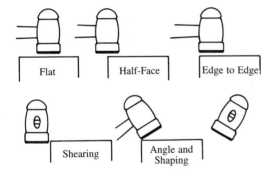

Fig. 23-15. Types of hammer blows.

Control and timing may be developed by striking a board held on the anvil. Practice striking in the same place at various rates and force. Find out what is comfortable for you. Learn to strike rather than push. Be limber rather than tense. Conscientiously try to increase your speed until you achieve a comfortable efficient rhythm. It is a pleasure to watch a hammerman who has achieved such perfection. However, it takes years of practice to be able to use a forging hammer with precision.

The hammer is used to create various effects in the metal. The position of the hammer in relation to the anvil accounts for the variety of results. Many different blows must be delivered rapidly in each heat.

The **flat or upright blow** is made directly over the center of the anvil face. This blow pushes the metal away from the blow in all directions. The thickness of the stock is reduced. This hammer blow can be used to draw, spread and smooth the work. The metal should be worked at right angles to the anvil, in most cases.

The **half-face or overhanging hammer blow** is used to form a shoulder on one side of the stock. The hammer meets the metal halfway over the edge of the anvil. The upper portion of the stock stays flat. The lower portion is indented or shouldered.

An **edge to edge blow** is used to form a tenon or double shoulder. The outside edge of the hammer and anvil line up and thin the metal on the anvil face.

The **shearing blow** is used for cutting iron hot on the hardy or edge of the anvil. The stock is cut into from all sides to prevent distortion of the metal. Then, the last blow is made off to the side, but close to the edge, to shear the stock. The sharp edge of the hardy must not be struck with the hammer. It is possible to shear small diameter stock over the edge of the anvil. However, a set hammer and sledge are usually used for this type of shearing since it is difficult to be accurate enough with a hand hammer. The last blow on a hot cutter or chisel is also made with the tool just off the edge of the anvil.

The **angle blow** is used for drawing out or tapering stock. The point or end of the stock is placed next to the rounded edge on the off side of the anvil. The stock is held up at the same angle that the hammer is swung to create the taper. The anvil face creates the other side of the taper. The stock can be tumbled (moved back and forth in quarter turns) for rapid drawing out and pointing.

The **shaping or leverage blow** is used for bending stock. These blows are struck away from the anvil face or horn. The anvil is used for a fulcrum for these bending operations. A uniform heat over the area to be bent is essential. Iron will bend most where it is hottest. Uneven heating causes uneven bending.

Tong Adjustment and Use

Tongs must be properly adjusted to fit the stock being forged. There are an infinite variety of tongs. Most blacksmith shops have many sizes and styles. Eventually, you will want a pair of tongs adjusted for each size of stock you commonly forge. One pair is sufficient to begin with, if you know how to adjust them. Later, you will make your own tongs.

Heat the jaws of the tongs by rolling them over in the fire until they are red to orange. Place the size stock you want the tongs adjusted for in the jaws flush against the rivet edge. Place the jaws in a vise and close the jaws. The handles must be held apart so they are parallel and close together. An additional piece of stock may be inserted between the handles to keep them apart. The tongs should roll easily in the hand. If the tongs are adjusted properly, very little pressure will be needed to hold the work in them.

Tongs should be held by the upper rein. The forefinger and thumb hold the top rein, the bot-

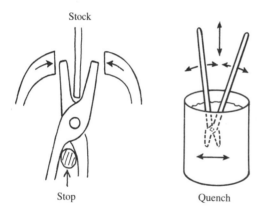

Stock

Stop   Quench

Fig. 23-16. Steps in adjusting tongs.

tom rein works by gravity in the other three fingers. The jaws of the tongs should be cooled frequently in water.

Occasionally, the rivet needs to be tightened or replaced. The rivet should be struck around its outside edge. If the jaws need to be pushed together, a short piece of pipe can be placed over the rivet and struck. Worn rivets can be replaced by grinding off one side and driving the old rivet out with a punch. The holes should be trued by drilling while cold or drifting while hot and a new rivet inserted.

After riveting the tongs will be tight. Heat the jaws and rivet. Work the tongs back and forth vigorously. Plunge the tongs in water while you are still working the handles. Continue to open and close the handles while holding in water until cool. The tongs will now be loose and ready to use.

Forging Operations

There are at least a dozen operations that may be performed on metal stock heated in the forge.

Shearing is cutting the stock hot or cold on a hardy with a handled cutter and sledge or mechanical shear.

Drawing is lengthening and thinning the stock. The metal becomes less compact and its area decreases.

Upsetting is shortening and thickening the stock. The metal becomes more compact and its area increases.

Shouldering is reducing the stock at a given point from one, two or four sides.

Spreading is increasing the width of the stock.

Offsetting is changing the lines of the center of a piece of stock.

Shaping is bending or forming stock over the anvil horn or face.

Punching is shearing from the area of the stock a piece the shape of the punch.

Drifting is enlarging a hole that has already been punched with a tapered drift tool.

Welding is uniting the ends of stock in a cohesive union with hammer blows when they are nearly at their melting temperature. Welding flux is desirable.

Jump Welding is uniting the ends of two dissimilar pieces of stock by hammer blows when they are nearly at their melting temperature. Welding flux is necessary.

Brazing is uniting two ends of stock in a cohesive union by a nonferrous filler material, usually copper or bronze. Borax flux is necessary.

Welding and Brazing Fluxes

A thin film of iron oxide or scale forms when heating iron or steel. This oxide may be mechanically removed or heated to a higher temperature than the parent metal to make it melt and run off before welding is possible. Wrought iron could be heated to a high enough temperature to melt off the scale without being burned. However, steel is oxidized and destroyed if brought to such a high temperature.

A flux is used to lower the melting point of the oxide. It protects the metal from the air. Clean sand is the preferred flux for iron. Borax is the preferred flux for welding steel and also for brazing copper or bronze to steel. Borax and sand mixed with iron filings (commercial welding compound) is preferred for welding in a gas forge. Commercial welding compounds are general purpose products for welding steel of dissimilar sizes and carbon composition.

Fluxes are not cements. Rather, they are antioxidants. Their purpose is to melt and clean the scale from the metal allowing welding at a lower temperature. The flux is applied at an orange or yellow heat just before welding. It forms a coating on the metal that dissolves the oxide present and prevents further oxidation as the metal is brought to a welding heat.

Forging Exercises

Each exercise combines several operations. They are progressive and each should be done several times in succession. It is important to work through the steps several times rather than trying to make the first one perfect.

Metal may be sheared for the exercises hot or cold. Round stock should not be cut in a straight jawed shear. Avoid cutting heated stock with tempered cold cutting tools.

Cold cutting is done by nicking into the stock from both sides and then breaking the stock over the edge of the anvil or vise. Small dimension square or rectangular stock can be twisted off with a vise and large crescent wrench. Hot cutting may be done with a hardy or handled cutter. Stock should be cut into from several sides to prevent distortion of the cut end.

Concentrate on forging the steel at the correct forging heat color. Efficient use of a heat requires planning. Steps must be done in order to get the right things done at the right metal temperature. The hotter metal is when you start to work it, the longer you have to get the work accomplished. Form a habit of working rapidly and efficiently.

Hammer Wedges can be made from ¼ to ½ inch round stock. Forge the wedge while it is still attached to a rod at least 18 inches long. You will perform drawing and shearing operations. Wedges of various sizes can be made.

Steps in forging a hammer wedge:
1. Heat the end of the stock to a bright yellow heat. This project can be made in one heat. However, do not hammer on the stock unless it is an optimum temperature.

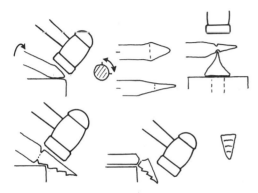

Fig. 23-17. Steps in forging a hammer wedge.

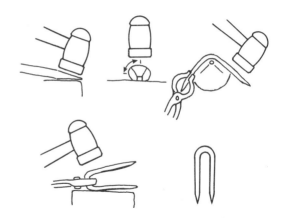

Fig. 23-18. Steps in forging a staple.

2. Hold the stock at an angle so that the anvil and hammer work together to point the stock. Taper and square the end nearly to a point by tumbling (¼ turns back and forth) the stock as you strike. Strike the same number of times each time you turn the stock.
3. Flatten the pointed end to a sharp edge and flatten to the desired thickness and length. Mark the wedge on the edge of the anvil several times on each side.
4. Extend an inch of stock over the hardy. Strike the stock directly over the hardy. Cut one-third of the way through and turn it over. Strike the stock again to nick it one-third of the way through.
5. Cool the wedge end in water. Place the nick line over the edge of the anvil and strike the overhanging wedge until it breaks off.

Staples can be made from ¼ inch or larger round stock. You will perform drawing and shaping operations. This project should be completed in two to three heats.

Steps in forging a large staple:
1. Cut off 4 inches of stock.
2. Heat one end to a bright yellow forging heat and draw and taper it to a point.
3. Heat the other end and point it.
4. Heat the center and bend it over the horn.
5. Cool the points so they won't be deformed and close the staple on the anvil face until its legs are parallel and about ¾ inch apart.

Nails or Rivets can be made from ⅜ inch or larger round or square stock. You will perform shouldering, drawing and upsetting operations. You will need a nail heading tool. These can be made from an axle or machine part and a punch of appropriate diameter.

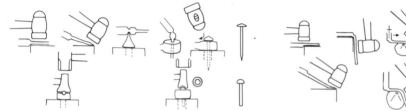

Fig. 23-19. Steps in forging a nail and rivet.

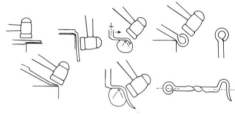

Fig. 23-20. Steps in forging a gate hook.

Steps in making a nail or rivet:

1. Heat about 1 inch of the stock to a bright yellow forging heat.
2. Hold the stock flat on anvil face with less than the desired length of the nail (rivet) over the face.
3. Strike edge to edge blows over the near edge of the anvil while tumbling the stock to shoulder and draw it on four sides.
4. When making nails, point the stock next to the off edge of the anvil by tumbling and striking the stock at an angle. When making rivets or bolts, round the stock with a top and bottom swedge of appropriate size.
5. Hold the shouldered edge over the hardy one-half inch. Strike enough to cut in all around the stock.
6. Push the point into the heading tool and twist the handle piece off.
7. Place the heading tool over the hardy hole and upset the head by smashing straight down until it is about ¼ inch thick.
8. Strike angled blows from four directions to give the head a chamfered (beveled) effect. Rivet heads can be made round with a half-round rivet head set.
9. Cool the heading tool and nail or rivet in water. The nail (rivet) will then shrink and drop out.

Gate Hooks can be made from ⅜ inch square stock. You will perform shouldering, bending, drawing and twisting operations. This project should be completed in five to six heats.

Steps in making a gate hook:

1. Cut off 7 inches of stock.
2. Heat the eye end to a bright yellow forging heat.
3. Shoulder and draw 1¼ inches of stock on three sides. Half-face hammer blows will be necessary to create a flat surface on the back side of the eye. Round this end to ¼ inch diameter by first making it octagonal and then round. The roundness may be made uniform with a ¼ inch top and bottom swedge.
4. Determine how much stock is needed for the eye. This may be determined by the formula: (Inside circle diameter + stock thickness) (22/7) = stock. For a ½ inch inside diameter eye: (½ + ¼) 22/7 = 2.35 inches. If the amount drawn is more than this, cut the excess off with hardy. If less, draw the stock more.
5. Heat the eye end to a forging heat and bend the stock to a right angle over the off edge of the anvil. The flat side of the shouldered area should be down against the anvil. The hammer should hit beyond the bend, not on it.
6. The eye is curved over the horn of the anvil near the pointed end. Start at the extreme end and push the metal over the horn while striking the hammer in the same position to form the circle. The rest of the stock should remain vertical to the anvil face as it is moved across the horn.
7. Close the eye on the off rounded edge of the face or the horn.
8. Round the eye over the point of the horn. Level.
9. Heat the hook end to a forging heat and point it.
10. Put 1⅜ inches on the anvil face and shoulder the stock on three sides with the flat side on the top side. This will be the same side as it was on the eye side. Round this end to ¼ inch diameter by first making it octagonal and then round.
11. Determine the length of stock necessary for the hook. This may be determined by the formula: (Inside semicircle diameter + stock thickness) (11/7) + (length beyond curve) = stock. For a ½ inch inside diameter hook with 1⅜ inches projecting below the curve: (½ + ¼) (11/7) + 1⅜ = 2.55 inches. If the amount drawn and rounded is more than this, cut it off on the hardy. Point the hook.
12. Heat the hook end to a forging heat and bend the stock to a right angle over the off edge of the anvil. The flat side should be down against the anvil. The hook should be bent in the same direction as the eye was.
13. The hook is bent away from the right angle

bend over the horn. The curve should be a semicircle. The sides should be parallel to one another. The point may be bent out slightly.

14. Heat the center and place one side in a vise with about 1 inch of stock from the eye to the edge of the vise. Place a wrench or heavy tongs on the other end equidistant from the hook. Twist the stock one complete turn. The edges should be parallel and the twist uniform. Uneven twisted stock can be heated and straightened on a wooden block with a mallet.

Fire Pokers can be forged with various types of handles. A simple design is described. A piece of ½ inch round stock about 24 inches long makes a good fire poker.

Point one end, then round it. Cool the end. Heat the other end and turn over about 5 inches and form an eye. Other handle shapes can be made. Make one that suits you.

Fire Rakes can be forged from square or round stock. If you choose to use square stock, try twisting it in the center or do other distinctive things to it. About 4 inches of the end of a fire rake is flattened to ⅛ inch thickness and curved. The end to be flattened should be upset first.

Water Valves or sprinklers can be forged from light stock of any dimension. An eye or handle is made on one end. The other end is flattened and drawn out like a fire rake for 2½ times the diameter of the water can. An open eye is formed. This should be slightly smaller than the can and hold it tight. Holes are punched in the side of the can for wetting down and containing the fire.

Fluxing Spoons can be made from any scrap piece of mild steel bar stock several inches long. One end will be upset and peined out to form the spoon. The other will be drawn out and finished to form a handle. The spoon will be used for applying welding flux for forge weld-

ing. A long handled spoon can be used to apply flux to pieces without removing them from the fire. The spoon end may be made by alternately folding a short piece of metal onto itself and welding it. This is called fagot welding.

Heat a short distance of one end of the stock and upset it on the anvil face. Do this several times. Next, flatten the upset end to ⅛ inch thick. Shape and round the corners as you flatten the stock. Pein the center of the spoon with a ball pein starting at the center and moving toward the outside edge. A dish in the spoon is created by the peining and can be increased by peining over the anvil hardy hole or a swedge block.

Chain Links can be made from 7 inches of ⅜ to ½ inch round stock. You will perform bending, scarfing and welding operations. Each link can be completed in four heats. Make a chain of several links in length. A chisel can be used to force the ends of a link open so that others can be placed in it. The weld should always be in the bend for maximum strength. A reducing fire of good depth and quality is required for welding.

1. Bring the center of the stock to a forging heat. Turn the stock over the horn by striking blows beyond the horn and close the stock until the sides are parallel and about 1 inch apart.

2. Heat both ends to a forging heat. Scarf one end using the edge of the anvil or cross-pein hammer. Turn the link over and scarf the second end the same way. Turn the ends in and overlap the scarfs. A left-handed smith will overlap them so that the top one points

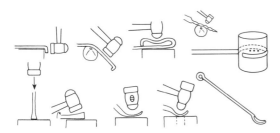

Fig. 23-21. Steps in forging fire tools.

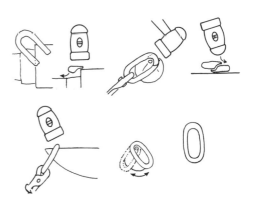

Fig. 23-22. Steps in forging a chain link.

to the left. A right-handed smith will over-lap them so the top scarf will point to the right.

3. Uniformly heat the area to be welded to an orange or yellow color. Wire brush the area to be welded and apply forge welding flux or borax.

4. Heat the area to be welded until the flux begins to melt. Turn the piece over and heat momentarily on the other side. Quickly bring the iron from the fire to the anvil when it is same color as the fire. Strike rapidly, first in the middle of the weld then on the edges. Turn the link over and weld the other side in similar fashion. Hard blows drive the molten welding metal out before it can freeze. Strike softly first and harder as you shape the metal. Do not flatten the weld to more than the original thickness of the metal. Do not try to join the metal after it loses its wet or sparking appearance. Prevent the area to be welded from touching the anvil until you are ready to hit it with the hammer.

5. Quickly move the link to the horn and shape it by moving it back and forth under the hammer at an angle. Flatten and shape the link until the sides are about 1 inch apart. A flattened link is stronger than a round one.

Eye Bolts and Tie Rings can be made from ½ or ¾ inch round stock. These can be installed in your shop or stable to tie up horses.

The eye is bent the same as the gate hook eye. More stock (½ to ¾ in.) is added to the measurement to allow for welding. The eye is welded over the rounded portion of the off edge or horn of the anvil. The first welding blows are struck in the middle, then near the point and finally near the eye. Ideally, the job may be dressed up with a top and bottom round swedge of appropriate size. The other end of the eye bolt should be threaded and fitted with a washer and nut. Or, the pointed end may be clinched over on the back of a post.

The ring should be 3 to 4 inches in diameter. The formula for finding the length of stock to make the ring is 22/7 multiplied by the sum of the inside diameter desired plus the width of the stock. The ends of the ring should be upset and scarfed. The sharp ends should be tapered narrower than the stock for ease in welding. The thickest part of the scarf (where it joins the ring) should line up. The eye is dropped over one end of the open ring before welding. A ring made of heavy stock may require two or more welding heats. Do not thin the weld area to less than the stock's original thickness. The ring may be shaped round on the anvil horn with difficulty or a cone mandrel with ease.

Worn shoes can be forged into projects or stock for making new shoes. Welding and hammer practice can be obtained by folding old shoes in half, inserting them together, and then welding them several times along the length of the fold. The resulting stock can then be forged to size for building horseshoes.

Straightening out used shoes and then turning them into a horseshoe shape is a good exercise preparatory to learning to make horseshoes from bar stock. Old horseshoes can also be made into circles and welded into chains as practice for welding bar shoes. However, building the projects previously demonstrated is an inexpensive and effective way to improve forging skills.

Hoof Picks can be forged from a worn out horseshoe or a pitchfork tine. You will perform shouldering, drawing, pointing or simply bending operations depending on the type of material used.

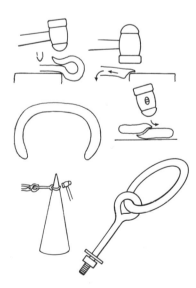

Fig. 23-23.   *Steps in forging eye bolts and tie rings.*

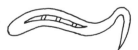

Fig. 23-24.   *A hoof pick can be forged from a worn shoe.*

Steps in forging a hoof pick:
1. Figure the amount of stock necessary to make a hook the size desired (See Gate Latch).
2. Shoulder (if necessary) the stock to approximately ¼ inch round.
3. Point the end of the shouldered stock. This is not necessary when using a pitchfork tine. The end should be pointed but not sharp. Ideally, the end should be broad and flat on the side facing the handle. Such a shape makes removal of foreign material from the hoof easier.
4. Shape the hoof portion of the pick.
5. Shape the handle portion. Make it as personal as possible. You may twist it, bend it back and weld it or create other distinctive variations. Do not try to weld pitchfork tines in the fire. They may be brazed or welded with the oxy-acetylene process.

Tongs can be made with drawn handles or welded on handles. You will perform nearly all of the various forging operations when making tongs and create useful tools. Many styles and sizes of tongs will eventually be needed for blacksmithing and horseshoeing.

Horseshoeing tongs with drawn handles can be made from ⅜ inch x ¾ inch or other horseshoe stock. Drawing out the handles is a good exercise to practice working with a striker. The handle should remain thick where it joins the boss.

The preferred design for tongs may be to forge weld round stock handles to jaws formed from ¾ inch x ¾ inch square stock. Handles can also be drawn out with a striker or power hammer. Make both halves the same.

Steps in making flat-jawed tongs:
1. Heat the end of the stock.
2. Hold the stock flat on the anvil face with about 1 inch projecting on to the face from the near edge.
3. Strike half-face hammer blows with the hammer face tilted away from you. Flatten the stock to one-half its thickness. Shape the stock and maintain a consistent width.
4. Lay the jaw over the off edge of the anvil at a 45 degree angle with the inside of the jaw and boss side facing you. Strike half-faced blows to form the shoulder on the jaw where it meets the boss. The hammer should strike parallel to the anvil face.

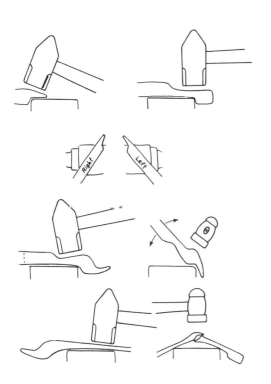

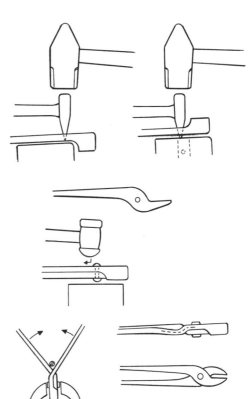

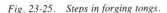

Fig. 23-25. Steps in forging tongs.

5. Heat the stock and place the same amount of metal over the off edge to form the boss as the boss is wide.
6. Strike half-face hammer blows with the hammer face tilted toward you. Flatten and then draw the stock to one-half its thickness. Be sure to leave the reins thick where they join the boss.
7. Round the edges of the boss and make it a uniform width and thickness.
8. Cut the jaw from the stock so that the rein to be welded will be about 2 inches long. Make both reins the same.
9. Upset, scarf and taper the end of the short rein. The scarf should not be more than one and one-half times the stock's width.
10. Upset, scarf and taper the ends on two pieces of ⅜ or ⁷⁄₁₆ inch round stock for handles.
11. Heat, flux and weld the handles to the jaws. Keep the area to be welded off the anvil until you are ready to hit it. Position the sparking pieces by bracing them against the sides of the anvil. The tongs should be in your hammer hand. Drop them and quickly pick up the hammer and lightly strike the scarfed ends until they fuse. Roll the tong jaw handle quickly after it fuses to the jaw and try to weld on both sides. Flatten the welded area so that, like the boss, it is wider than it is thick. Practice jump welding two straightened worn shoes first.
12. Finish the welds by hot rasping.
13. Heat each boss and punch out the rivet hole. Start with the jaw over the edge. Finish with the flat side down against the anvil face and over the pritchel hole. Drilling is more accurate and the preferred method for making rivet holes in tongs.
14. Rivet the jaws together. It works best to get only the small end of the rivet hot. Insert the rivet. Cold rivet it enough to prevent it from falling out. Heat the boss with the end to be riveted down in the fire. Upset the hot end of the rivet. Hit on the rivet center first and then chamfer the edges. Use a rivet set to finish the job.
15. Align the handles one above the other by clamping the tongs behind the rivet in a vise.
16. Adjust the tong jaws to the size stock desired as explained at the beginning of this Chapter.

Forging With a Helper

Forging heavy draft horse shoes, tools or decorative items is much easier and faster when done with a helper. A traditional and effective method of training apprentices has included striking. One who uses a sledge hammer under the direction of a blacksmith is called a striker. Homemade or commercial power hammers of various sizes may be used when working alone. Mechanical, hydraulic or electrical benders may be used. Work done by a horseshoer requiring the use of a human or mechanical helper includes: drawing out weighted shoes, swedging or creasing shoes, turning and punching heavy draft or show horse shoes.

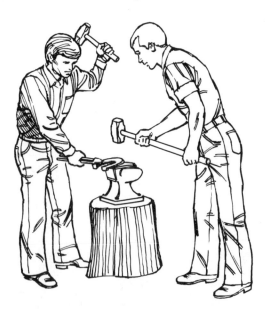
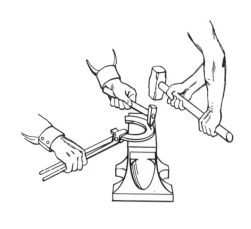

Fig. 23-26. Position when forging with a striker. Drawings by J. Hoffman and K. Burdette.

The **striker** is the person who operates the sledge hammer. He is often called the hammerman. Strikers may use a hammer weighing from 6 to 16 pounds. An 8 pound hammer is most common for horseshoeing work. The anvil being struck against should weigh at least 20 times what the sledge hammer weighs and be mounted solid.

The **blacksmith** (or master) communicates with the striker (or apprentice) by signals made with the hammer. Experience has shown this to be the most effective means of communicating fast and accurately.

Once a blacksmith was said to have told his striker, "When I nod my head you hit it!" Perhaps a tragic incident such as this caused the present system to be developed. These signals may vary slightly from culture to culture. However, the principles are the same.

The call to the anvil is given by several quick taps on the heel of the anvil or by a rocking back and forth and tapping of the place to be hit if the striker is looking on. When the striker is in position, the blacksmith strikes the iron. The striker follows the first hit with a blow from the

sledge matching the position and intensity of the blow by the blacksmith. The iron should be struck in the middle of the anvil except when the work requires another position.

The speed and intensity of the striker's hammer blows are controlled by the blacksmith behind the anvil. Timing is critical. The striker's hammer must be down when the blacksmith's hammer is up and vice versa. The blacksmith's hammer should be drawn back and raised as high as the striker's hammer to avoid collision.

Experienced strikers may hit the forging in a predetermined place at a predetermined force while the blacksmith merely taps the heel of the anvil to keep in time. This is especially common when swedging. A heavy blow struck by the blacksmith upon the work followed by an intermediate light blow on the anvil means heavy sledge blows are required. Double striking with two strikers is advantageous on very heavy forgings. The blacksmith strikes a hand hammer blow between each helper's sledge blow to indicate where the blows are to fall.

The striker's signal to stop is given by the blacksmith by moving the hand hammer off the metal and dropping it on the anvil. Sometimes, the hammer is placed on the end of the heel of the anvil to signal stop if time is being tapped out on the top of the heel. The striker completes the last blow after the signal is given.

Striking a tool is somewhat different than striking iron or swedging. The striker cannot rely on his timing to come from the blacksmith's hammer. He must learn to hit the tool while watching what the tool does. He must never hit the tool when it is not properly aligned. Knowl-

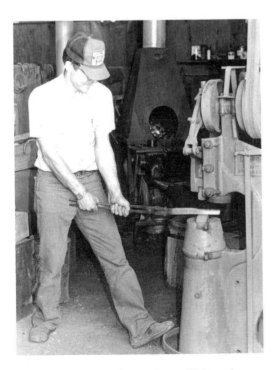

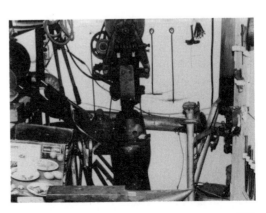

Fig. 23-27. (A) Power hammer in use. (B) Power hammer mounted in Shorty Roberts' truck.

edge of what the tool does and what shape or impression it is to create is essential. The striker should look at what the tool is doing and trust the hammer to hit the top of the tool.

Practice in communicating instructions and swinging accurate hammer blows may be given under mock conditions with a soft board in place of hot steel. This is especially necessary when training beginners. The striker must learn to hit with force exactly where the blacksmith hits. Everything happens (or should happen) very fast and in a predetermined sequence when the iron is hot. As a striker becomes more adept he can learn to run the fire as well as do the striking. This is an efficient way of working and an excellent training experience for the striker.

Power hammers were invented to replace the use of one or more strikers in a shop that did heavy work. There are many types (Fleming, 1979).

The most widely used power hammer is the 25 or 50 pound "Little Giant". These are motor driven, eccentric drive, guided ram power hammers. They are sometimes called trip hammers. However, trip hammers are much larger, permit access from at least two sides and actually are a drop hammer. The guided ram of a Little Giant is connected by means of a spring to toggle arms from a motor driven eccentric. This design reduces a lot of the stress and vibration created by these machines.

A power hammer is most useful to a horseshoer working alone when drawing out heavy weighted shoes, swedging light racing plates, drawing and shaping tong handles and pritchels. They also can be used for punching, shearing and numerous blacksmithing projects. Power hammers should be mounted on a solid base separate from the floor of the shop to absorb vibration.

A few horseshoers have mounted power hammers in their mobile shops. It is best to jack up and block the truck or trailer body when the power hammers are used or when the vehicle stands for any length of time. Suspension springs may lose their elasticity if this is not done.

References

Andrews, J. 1977. Edge of the Anvil. Rodale Press, Emmaus, PA.

Bacon, J.L. 1911. Forge Practice (2nd ed.). John Wiley and Sons, New York.

Coleman, G.J. 1921. Forge Note Book. The Bruce Publ. Co., Milwaukee.

Daniels, B.B. 1981. Shop talk: the American vise for international competition. Amer. Farriers' J. 7(5):255.

Fleming, J. 1979. Powerhammers. . . a survey of the different types. The Anvil's Ring. 7(3):27.

Martin, E. 1982. Profile: Edward Martin remembers apprenticehood. Amer. Farriers' J. 8(3).173.

Miller, B. 1983. Workshop: how to make a hot rasping vise. Amer. Farriers' J. 9(1):38.

Perch, D.G. 1977. Blacksmithing hammer signals. The Chronicle of Early American Industries. 30(1):9.

Roberts, S. 1981. Personal Communication. Lexington, KY.

Schwarzkopf, E. 1916. Plain and Ornamental Forging. John Wiley and Sons, New York.

Selvidge, R.W. and J.M. Allton. Blacksmithing. The Manual Arts Press, Peoria, IL.

Simpson, J.S. 1978. How to Build Horseshoeing Tools and Equipment. J. Scott Simpson, Belgrade, MT.

Staff. 1911. Striking position. Blacksmith and Wheelwright. (Nov.).

Staff. 1911. The blacksmith and the anvil. Blacksmith and Wheelwright. (Jan).

Weygers, A.G. 1978. The Recycling, Use, and Repair of Tools. Van Nostrand Reinhold Co., New York.

NOTES:

Chapter 24

Selecting, Shaping and Fitting Hot Shoes

Review the use of the horseshoe and the terms discussed at the beginning of Chapter 19.

Hot shoes are machine-made shoes made with long heels. They have been called keg shoes because they used to be sold in wooden kegs weighing 100 pounds. Hot shoes can be shaped hot or cold. They are made from the same type of steel as cold shoes. The heels of hot shoes may be cut or trimmed to correspond to the buttresses when a plate shoe is desired. The heels may be turned in and welded to make a bar shoe. A long heel may be turned over to make a blocked heel or calk or it may be turned out to form a trailer.

Hot shoes are available in several sizes, adjacent sizes being 1 inch different in length (½ in. at each heel). The No. 0 size shoe is the smallest and is used on a small horse. It may be cut off and fitted to ponies or foals that need corrective work by using only the first and second toe nail holes on each branch. Modern hot shoes are sized as high as No. 8 for draft horses. However, a No. 2 is the largest commonly used on saddle horses.

Selection of Hot Shoes

Selection of hot shoes is based upon the same factors as those for cold shoes (described in Chapter 19).

After other factors are considered (weight, pattern, etc.), the position of the last or heel nail hole is probably the most important consideration in the selection of a hot shoe. Heel length is most important when selecting a cold shoe. Of course, the lightest-weight shoe that will give satisfactory service is usually the best for the horse.

All hot shoe styles used to be made in front and hind patterns. Several weights of each style were available. Hind shoes were narrower in web and lighter in weight and were preferred by horseshoers when buying shoes by the pound. Also, it is easier to make hind shoes into front shoes than it is to make front shoes into hinds.

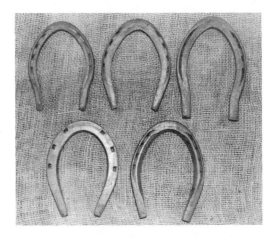

Fig. 24-1. *Types of hot shoes. Top row (left to right) extra light, extra light, and light patterns. Bottom row (left) countersunk, (right) snow pattern. Photo by J. Graves.*

Today, the largest distributor of machine-made horseshoes in America makes hot shoes only in a hind pattern.

Machine-made hot shoes have the same disadvantages as machine-made cold shoes. The principal advantage of long heeled or hot shoes is a savings in time. They are most useful for construction of basic corrective shoes. Also, fewer sizes of shoes need to be stocked than when using ready-made shoes. Most shoers carry an assortment of both types.

Hot shoe sizes most commonly used in America follow the traditional military or cowboy sizing system. Learn to recognize a shoe size at a glance. The most popular sizes in order of popularity are: No. 1, 0, and 2. This order may vary in localized parts of the country.

Inches of Steel	11	11½	12	12½	13	13½	14
Hot Shoes							
(EL and Snow)				0	1		2
Cold or Ready-Made Shoes							
(Bronco)		0	1		2		
(Saddlelite and Rim)	0	1		2			

Fig. 24-2. *Comparison of hot shoe sizes to cold shoe or ready-made sizes (Diamond-U.S.).*

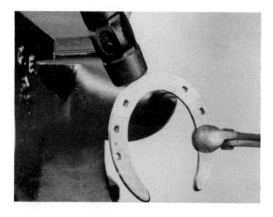

Fig. 24-3. To narrow or point the toe. Photos by G. Poellot.

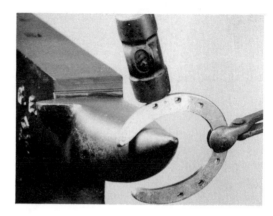

Fig. 24-5. To bring out the quarter.

Shaping Hot Shoes

Shoes should be marked to correspond to the foot they are being shaped for. A system for marking shoes is explained in Chapter 19.

Minor alterations in keg hot shoes may be made cold using the techniques demonstrated in Chapter 19.

Major alterations of light shoes or routine shaping of heavy shoes are best done at a yellow heat. Work toward the goal of being able to roughly shape the shoe in one heat. Practice until you can do this consistently. Try to visualize the shape of the hoof wall as you are working on the shoe at the anvil, and make the shoe conform to that visualized shape.

The following basic principles are applicable to any hot shaping done on heavy or light shoes:

1. **To Narrow or Point the Toe:** Heat the toe. Hold it on the extreme point of the horn. Strike near the toe on the side farthest from you (off side). Reverse the shoe on the horn and strike the opposite side of the toe. This operation can also be done over the heel of the anvil in a manner similar to the cold-shaping method.

2. **To Flatten or Round the Toe:** Heat the toe. Hold it on the horn of the anvil so that the space between the shoe and the horn is proportionate to the amount of change desired in the toe of the shoe. Strike along the toe, not limiting the blows to any one spot. Rotate the shoe with the tongs under the hammer to create a smooth, round shape. To flatten or round the toe on a large shoe when using an anvil with a small horn, hold one side of the toe of the shoe over the horn at a time and strike on the hot toe as you hold the branch solid with the tongs. Keg draft horse shoes have to be worked in this manner on small anvils.

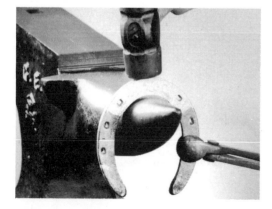

Fig. 24-4. To flatten or round the toe.

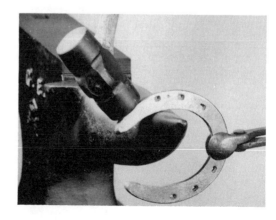

Fig. 24-6. To bring in the quarter.

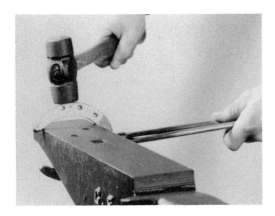

Fig. 24-7. To straighten the quarter.

3. **To Bring Out the Quarter:** Heat the quarter. Hold the heel of the shoe on the horn, while pulling on the opposite branch with the tongs. Strike the point from which it is desired to spread, or throw out, the quarter.

4. **To Bring In the Quarter:** Heat the quarter. Hold it over the point of the horn of the anvil so that the shoe will rest on the inside edge at the point from which the change is to be made. Strike near the heel on the part projecting over the horn.

5. **To Straighten the Quarter:** Heat the quarter. Hold it over the heel or horn of the anvil. Strike directly over the middle of the area to be straightened. (Technique No. 3 may also be used.)

6. **To Round the Quarter:** Heat the quarter. Hold the midpoint of the straight place on the point of the horn and strike alternate blows on each side of, and close to, the point to be rounded.

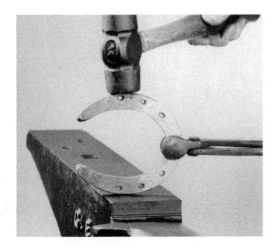

Fig. 24-8. To close the shoe.

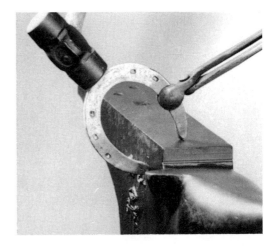

Fig. 24-9. To open the shoe.

7. **To Close the Shoe:** Heat the whole shoe. Hold the shoe on edge on the face of the anvil and strike down on the quarter. This will narrow or close the shoe without changing its general shape. The toe will be narrowed slightly.

8. **To Close One Branch:** Heat the whole shoe. Place the branch you don't want to change in water up to the place in the toe where you want the branch to close from. Then close the shoe. Only the hot side will be affected.

9. **To Open the Shoe:** Heat the whole shoe. Hold one heel on the face of the anvil and one on the side opposite you. Strike the toe. This will open or spread the shoe without changing its general shape.

10. **To Bring Out the Heels:** Heat the heels of the shoe. Hold each shoe heel in turn over the heel of the anvil with the inner rim of the shoe just behind the last nail hole resting on the face of the anvil. Strike the quarter toward the heel of the shoe near the edge of the anvil. (Technique No. 3 may also be used.)

Marking the Heels

The shoe should fit the foot reasonably well before the heels are marked for cutting. Some shaping of the heels can be done while the heat from cutting is still in them. Remember to allow for expansion at the heels when shaping the heels.

Steps in marking the heels:
1. Draw a short chalk line on the hoof extending from the point of each heel or buttress toward the bulbs of the foot.
2. Place the shoe against the foot and hold it flush with the toe.

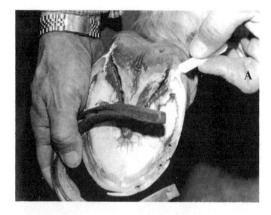

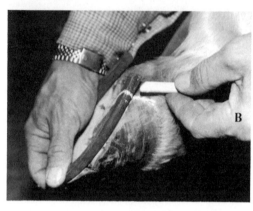

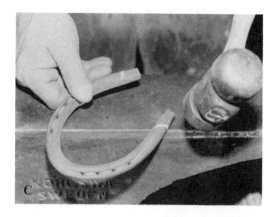

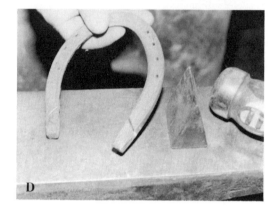

Fig. 24-10. Marking the heels; (A) outline the buttress with chalk and extend the line back up the hoof, (B) hold the shaped shoe in place and mark the outside edge and ground surface with chalk, (C) place the chalk mark over *the edge of the anvil or on a straight hardy and strike the ground surface. (D) A permanent mark that won't come off when heated is transferred to the shoe.*

3. Mark the outer rim of each heel (thickness) of the shoe with a chalk line coinciding to the line on the foot.
4. Extend the previously drawn lines on the outer rim of the shoe across the ground surface of the shoe following the angle of the bars.
5. Hold the shoe on the edge of the anvil with the chalk mark up and line it up with the anvil edge. Strike the chalk mark. The foot surface of the shoe is now marked with a line which will not be destroyed in the fire. The chisel-type straight hardy can be used in a similar manner to the anvil edge to mark the heels.

A center punch may also be used. Only the line drawn in Step 3 needs to be used when using a center punch. The center punch mark should be on the outside edge of the foot surface. The center punch mark works best when using the Sharp style half-round hardy.

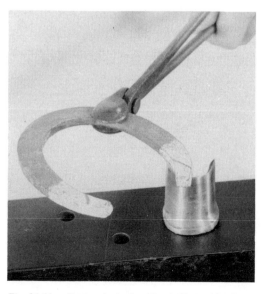

Fig. 24-11. Cutting the heels with a half-round hardy.

Cutting and Finishing the Heels

Steps in Cutting the heels:

1. Heat the heels of the shoe in the fire to a white heat. Most experienced horseshoers cut and finish both heels in one heat. Beginners find it easier to do one heel at a time. The heel must be very hot to make a smooth cut. The open portion of the hardy should face you so that the heels will point away from you when they are cut.

2. Place the shoe on the half-round hardy with the marked or foot surface up. The outside edge of the heel of the shoe at the point to be cut should be perpendicular to the center of the half-round hardy. Only one-half of the hardy is used for each cut. The mark on the shoe should nearly correspond with the sharp edge of the hardy. The end should project over the edge to allow for backward movement of the shoe as it is cut on the beveled hardy.

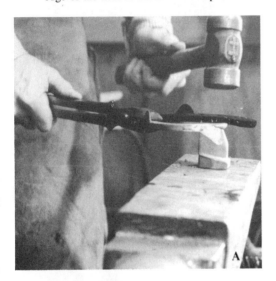

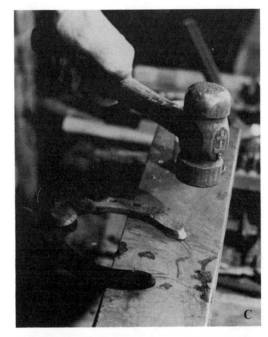

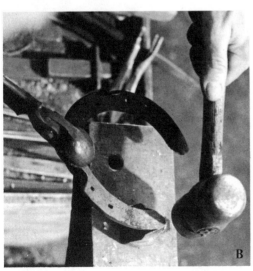

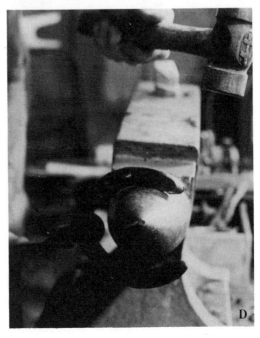

Fig. 24-12. Cutting the heels with a Sharp style hardy; (A) side view, (B) top view, (C) leveling the heel, (D) shaping the heel, (E) hot-filing on the bevel, (F) rounding the sharp edge, (G) removing the burr, (H) the finished heel with the hardy. Photos by J. Graves.

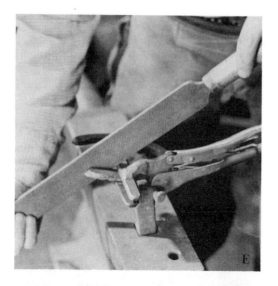

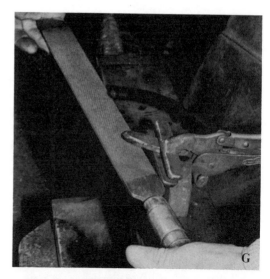

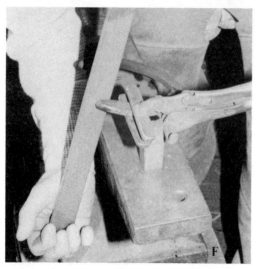

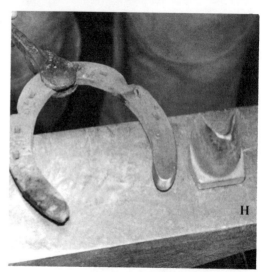

Two-thirds of the hardy is used when using the Sharp style half-round hardy. The center punch mark is placed over the forward edge to allow for the bevel and the outside of the heel is parallel to a line bisecting the V of the hardy.

3. Hold the toe of the shoe level or slightly above the heels to avoid putting a bend in the foot surface at the end of the shoe heel when cutting it off. The bevel of the heel should be approximately the same angle as the sides of the bars of the hoof near the buttresses.

4. Strike the hot metal directly over the hardy cutting edge until just a paper thin piece of metal remains, or until you can see a black line in the hot metal over the cutting edge.

5. Strike on the end of the heel in order to shear it off without dulling the hardy. Many horseshoers use a brass hammer or a soft annealed steel hammer to cut heels, and thus further reduce the possibility of dulling the hardy.

6. Cut the other heel similarly, only place it on the *opposite side* (right or left) of the hardy.

7. Quickly turn the shoe over and place it flat on the anvil face. Strike flat blows on the ground surface of the heel(s). This procedure is necessary to level the foot surface of the heels since it becomes warped in the cutting process.

8. Hold the inside of each heel over the horn of the anvil and strike the outer edge. When

heels are cut on a hardy, the steel widens near the end. By shaping and narrowing the heels in this manner, the amount of hot rasping necessary to produce a finished heel is reduced. Also, some final shaping of the shoe can be done at this time.

9. Place the shoe in the vise with the beveled, or ground, surface of the heel toward you.
10. Rasp the heels with the coarse side of the hot rasp to remove the sharp edges, and then finish them with the fine cut side of the rasp.

There is a sequence of four movements or passes to be made with the rasp. Several strokes are necessary in each pass. The first pass is made with the coarse side against the sharp corners on the end and inside of the heel. The second is made with the fine side on the same angle as the heel. The third is made with the fine side perpendicular to the heel to remove the sharp edge. The fourth pass is made under the shoe against the foot surface side to remove any burrs that have formed. Only pass three and four are necessary with the Sharp style half-round hardy.

It is important to round and finish the heels smoothly so that they won't cause a shoe boil (front shoes) or cut another horse (hind shoes). A shoe boil is a bruise on the point of the elbow of a horse caused by a sharp or protruding shoe heel which hits the horse there when he lies down and folds his front feet under him. A horse can cut another horse badly if he kicks it with sharp heeled hind shoes.

Pritcheling Machine-Made or Keg Shoes

Pritcheling is usually done as the last operation after the heels have been cut and finished and all other major alterations have been made on the shoe.

Steps in pritcheling the nail holes of machine-made or keg shoes:

1. Heat the shoes all over to a dull red or hot black heat. If possible, take advantage of the heat left in the shoe after cutting the heels or shaping.
2. Place the shoe on the anvil face with the foot surface up.
3. Drive the pritchel in the nail holes at an angle which would correspond to the angle of the hoof wall at that point. Hold the pritchel at about a 45 degree angle slanted toward the center of the shoe at the toe. Hold the pritchel nearly vertical but slightly inclined to the center of the shoe at the heel. Drive the pritchel until it is stopped by the anvil face or the holes are the desired size. This is called back punching.

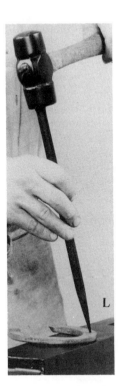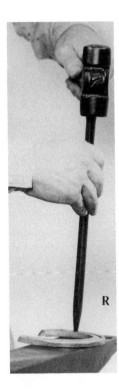

L   R

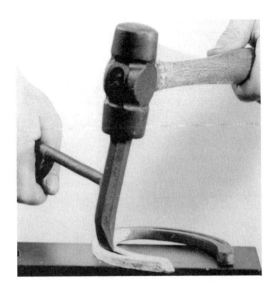

Fig. 24-13. (L) Pritcheling the foot surface of a machine-made shoe. Photos by G. Poellot.

Fig. 24-14. (R) Pritcheling the ground surface of a machine-made shoe.

Fig. 24-15. Opening the crease of a machine-made shoe.

4. Turn the shoe over so that the ground surface is up. Place the nail holes of the shoe over the hardy hole or pritchel hole(s) of the anvil. Drive the pritchel into the nail holes at the corresponding angle of the hoof wall to clean the metal burr formed from the previous operation out of the nail hole. This step may not be necessary if the back punching leaves a clean hole.

5. Drive a pritchel into a heel nail hole (or use fitting tongs), and carry the shoe to the foot to check for a final fit. Many shoers use a different pritchel for each operation, i.e., punching holes, back punching holes and fitting.

The use of the creaser is occasionally necessary to open the crease of shoes which have been severely mangled by beginners during hot or cold shaping. Striking between the nail holes and in more than one place will prevent this. Opening of the crease must be done before the nail holes can be pritcheled out.

Leveling the Shoe

Leveling the shoe is done at a black heat and after all other operations are completed on the shoe. "Concaving" or beveling of the foot surface of the shoe is done at the same time as a part of the leveling process. This is done to prevent pressure on the sole.

In cases of dropped sole or founder (laminitis), the foot surface of the shoe must be beveled excessively. This operation is sometimes called

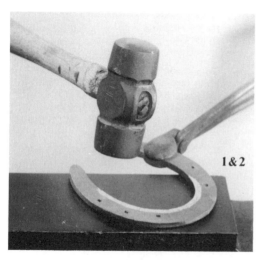

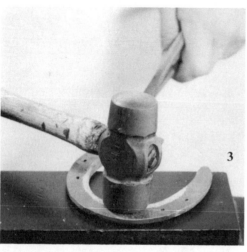

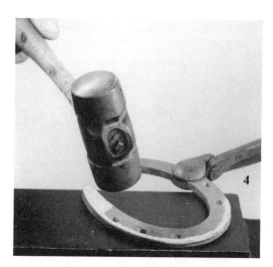

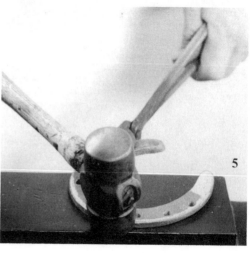

Fig. 24-16. Steps in leveling a shoe. The chalked area shows where to strike flat overlapping hammer blows.

seating out and must be performed at a red heat with the rounded face of the hammer used on the inside half of the foot surface of the shoe. In these cases, the concaving should vary from zero at the nail holes to about one-third the thickness of the shoe at the inner edge of the web.

Steps in leveling the shoe at a black heat:
1. Place the shoe on the anvil with the foot surface up and as much of the shoe on the anvil as possible. This will usually be an arc from one heel to the opposite second or third nail hole.
2. Strike slightly inwardly beveled, overlapping blows on the *inside half* of the web of the shoe starting from one side of the toe and progressing around to the opposite branch to a point about 1½ inches from the heel.
3. Rotate the shoe on the anvil face and strike the foot surface of the other branch similarly.
4. Turn the shoe over and apply slightly outwardly beveled overlapping blows to the *outside half* of the ground surface web from one side of the toe to a point about 1½ inches from the heel. Strike flat blows covering the whole web of the shoe from this point back to the end of the heel.
5. Rotate the shoe on the anvil face and strike the ground surface of the other branch similarly.
6. Sight over the foot surface of the shoe to check to be sure it is level. Hold the shoe by one branch with the tongs and rest the toe on the anvil face. Sight across the foot surface from the heels to the toe, and then from one branch to the other. For a double check, hold the shoe by the toe with the tongs, rest one branch on the anvil, and sight across the branches.
7. If the shoe is not level, lay it on the face of the anvil and strike the highest surface until it is level.

Hot Fitting

Fitting to determine what minor alterations need to be made on the shoe to get a perfect fit can be done with the heat remaining in the shoe from previous alterations. All major alterations on the shoe such as shaping, cutting and finishing heels, punching and pritcheling, concaving and leveling, should be done previous to this time.

Drive a pritchel into a heel nail hole of the shoe, or use fitting tongs, and take the shoe to the foot to check for a final fit. Only hold the shoe on the foot long enough to check the fit and sear the high spots of the hoof. Note any discrepancies which exist, level the foot and/or take the shoe to the anvil to make necessary alterations.

Things to check when fitting:
1. Shoe shaping to fit the foot with allowance for expansion at the heels.
2. Heels of shoe cover the buttresses.
3. Outer half of foot surface of shoe and wall of foot fit tightly against each other. Or, in cases where the wall is broken in the quarters, the shoe does not "rock" from side-to-side.
4. Heels of shoe fit flat against heels of foot.
5. Inner half of foot surface of shoe and sole of foot do not touch each other (i.e., shoe is concaved).
6. Nail holes on shoe are opened sufficiently for the size nail to be used.

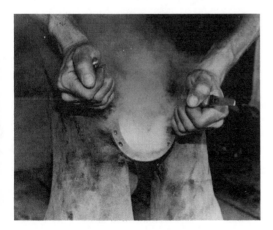
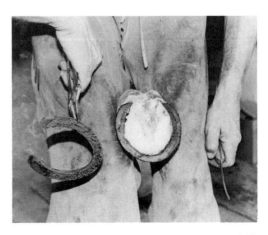

Fig. 24-17. Hot fitting is not harmful as long as enough hoof is present to allow for it. It is helpful in obtaining a perfect fit, especially when clips are needed. Photos by J. Graves.

7. Nail holes are positioned to allow for maximum security and safety when nailing, i.e., so nails will enter the outer border of the white line, and that they are far enough forward to allow for physiological movement (expansion) of the foot.

Hot fitting is necessary when seating clips and rocker-toes and is useful to obtain a perfect union between the hoof and shoe. It has been proven harmless to the hoof and its sensitive structures in numerous experiments by Smith (1971) in Denmark. He showed, using electric thermoprobes, that as long as there was at least 4 millimeters (slightly less than $\frac{3}{16}$ in.) of hoof (sole or wall) between the hot shoe and the sensitive structures, the horse was in no danger. He used a red hot shoe and held it on for much longer than the usual few seconds.

There is no evidence to indicate that hot fitting damages the foot in any way as long as enough hoof is left to allow for it. In fact, there is some evidence that it is beneficial in the shoeing process (Holmes, 1949). And, the sole is easily trimmed after hot fitting.

Hot fitting is done by uniformly heating the shoe to a dull red heat. The shoe will lose its color by the time you get to the foot. Drive a pritchel into a heel nail hole. As the shoe is sitting on the anvil with the toe away from you, a right hander will put the pritchel in the left branch, a left hander in the right branch. Fitting tongs or pliers can also be used. Carry the shoe to the foot and seat the clip.

A rasp or hoof knife is useful to hold the hot shoe level against the foot. Also, the rasp or knife can be used to carve the wall and assist in the fitting process. The matching of the hoof wall and shoe can be checked by quickly brushing your finger against the hoof and shoe. You must bend low to check the coinciding of the hoof and shoe and to avoid inhaling too much smoke. Blowing the smoke away helps also. Some horses don't like a hot fit because of the smoke.

When the shoe and hoof are perfectly matched, set the shoe aside to cool slowly. This will prevent shrinkage and warping that may occur if the shoe is cooled rapidly.

References

Pieh, B. 1981. Horseshoe size comparison chart. Centaur Forge, Ltd. Catalog, Burlington, WI.

Habacher, F. 1928. Der Huf-und Klanenbeschlag. Urban and Schwarzenberg, Berlin.

Holmes, C.M. 1949. The Principles and Practice of Horse Shoeing. The Farrier's Journal Publ. Co., Ltd., Leeds, ENGLAND.

Smith, M. 1971. Temperatursteigerung im Hufe bei der "warmen Anpassung der Hufeisen" (Rise in hoof temperature from fitting hot shoes—translated by L. Gray). Wien. tierarztl. Mschr. 58:155.

War Department. 1941. The Horseshoer (TM 2-220). U.S. Government Printing Office, Washington, DC.

NOTES:

Chapter 25

Tool Forging and Metallurgy

Make Your Own Tools

Every horseshoer should know how to properly make, repair and maintain at least the basic tools used in the business. To successfully do this requires a knowledge of tool steel, proper tool form, forging techniques and use of tools.

Many of the desired tools or designs of tools may be unobtainable, too costly, or of poor quality. In addition, there is a great deal of personal satisfaction and confidence gained from using tools you have created yourself. Scott Simpson's book on the construction of tools is recommended as a basic guide (Simpson, 1978). Books by Richardson (1890) and Weygers (1973) are more advanced and give ideas concerning design. Most engineering books are too technical to be useful.

Used Steel Sources

Wherever you live, you should begin (or continue) to collect pieces of tool steel for your own junk pile. If you have need of a specific material such as springs or axles, you may go to a wrecking yard to obtain it. However, if you collect pieces from discarded implements, machine and tool parts, you will find you can make most anything from used material. Even the city dump may be a good source for some items. Rummage barns and farm sales often sell boxes of old tools containing various types of high carbon steel.

Used Steel Identification

Aids in identifying used steel quality:
1. The former or intended use of the steel. Perhaps specifications are available from the manufacturer.
2. The condition of the head and cutting edge of the steel. A dull, chipped or bent cutting edge may indicate poor quality steel, improper heat treating or abusive use.
3. The appearance (grain structure) of the surface of a break. Fine structure is characteristic of hardenable steel.
4. The forging properties. Soft (low carbon) steel gives more readily under the hammer and will

hold the heat much longer than hard (high carbon) steel.
5. The hardness obtainable by quench from a cherry red heat and tested by a file. If a new file will easily cut the material, it is soft. If the file glances off and will not mark it, the material is very hardenable.
6. The spark test against a grinder.

The spark test must be conducted under as controlled conditions as possible. The light (not daylight or dark), the viewing background, and most important, the pressure applied to the grinding wheel must be the same for each test. An illustrated chart is useful when comparing the various types of iron and steel.

SPARK PATTERNS

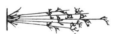

Gray Cast Iron
Length, about 25 in.; spark color red near wheel, straw yellow farther out; volume, small.

Malleable Iron
Length, about 30 in.; spark color same as gray iron; volume, greater than gray iron.

Alloy Steel
Length, variable (depending on alloy) but always shorter than carbon steel stream; color, straw yellow to white.

High-Carbon Steel
Length, about 55 in.; large volume, spark color, white.

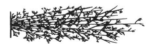

Wrought Iron
Length, about 60 in.; spark color, straw yellow near wheel, white elsewhere. Volume, large, with long straight shafts.

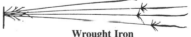

Low-Carbon Steel
Longest of all spark streams, up to 70 in.; spark color, white throughout; moderately large volume (less than medium- to high-carbon steels.) Pattern shown is also typical of most cast steels.

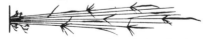

Fig. 25-1. Spark test patterns. Drawing from Union Carbide Co. (1976).

The spark test must be studied and practiced. It is helpful to keep several pieces of material of known composition near the grinder for making these comparisons. Low-carbon steel makes a moderately large volume of relatively long sparks with little branching or sprigs. High-carbon steel makes a large volume of relatively shorter white sparks with numerous sprigs. The higher the carbon, the shorter and whiter the spark. Alloy steels make yellow sparks next to the wheel and white ones away from it. They vary in spark stream length. Alloys tend to suppress carbon bursts. Manganese causes sparks that follow the surface of the wheel. Silicon causes short fuzzy sparks close to the wheel. Chromium causes orange sparks and suppresses the spark stream. Nickel causes small forked tongues or wedges at the end of the spark streams. Cast steel appears much like low carbon steel. Cast iron, which cannot be forged, causes a small volume of red sparks next to the wheel blending to a yellow color away from the wheel with many fine sprigs.

Estimating the Weight of Steel

Steel is usually priced and sold by weight. Charts are figured on the weight per cubic inch (mild steel = 0.283 lb. or 4.528 oz. per cu. in.). However, there is a method that can be used to approximate how much constructed equipment or shoe stock will weigh.

The formula for steel weight in pounds per lineal foot is T x W x 10/3 where T equals steel thickness and W equals steel width (Kugler, 1957).

For example: How much does 1 foot of ½ x 1 inch steel weigh?

½ x 1 x 10/3 = 5/3 = approximately 1.67 pounds.

The formula for steel weight in ounces per lineal inch is T x W x 40/9 where T equals steel thickness and W equals steel width (Manning, 1983).

For example: How much does 11 inches of ¼ x ¾ inch steel weigh?

¼ x ¾ x 40/9 x 11 = 55/6 = approximately 9.17 ounces.

A weight chart is useful when figuring the price of shoeing stock sold by the pound in cut lengths. Some sizes cannot be obtained except by special order of large quantities. Others are not used as shoe sizes, but may be used when constructing equipment or corrective and therapeutic shoes. Plate or sheet steel is used in the construction of horseshoeing equipment and therapeutic shoes.

Steel is heavier than wrought or cast iron. Steel weighs 490 pounds per cubic foot. Wrought iron weighs 480 pounds and cast iron 450 pounds per cubic foot.

Steel Classification

Steel is a mixture of iron and very small amounts of carbon. All modern tool steels, even plain carbon steels, contain other alloying elements in addition to carbon.

Carbon steels contain iron, carbon, manganese, and small amounts of silicon, sulfur and phosphorus. Sulfur and phosphorus, though considered impurities (not more than 0.05% of

WEIGHT OF MILD STEEL BAR STOCK IN POUNDS PER LINEAR FOOT

Thickness in inches	Width (web) in inches										
	¼	⅜	½	⅝	¾	⅞	1	1⅛	1¼	1⅜	1½
⅛	0.11	0.16	0.21	0.27	0.32	0.38	0.43	0.48	0.53	0.59	0.64
3/16	0.16	0.24	0.32	0.40	0.48	0.56	0.64	0.72	0.80	0.88	0.96
¼	0.21	0.32	0.43	0.53	0.64	0.75	0.85	0.96	1.06	1.17	1.28
5/16	0.27	0.40	0.53	0.67	0.80	0.93	1.06	1.20	1.33	1.46	1.59
⅜	0.32	0.48	0.64	0.80	0.96	0.12	1.28	1.44	1.59	1.75	1.92
7/16	0.37	0.56	0.75	0.93	1.12	1.30	1.49	1.68	1.86	2.05	2.23
½	0.43	0.64	0.85	1.06	1.28	1.49	1.70	1.92	2.13	2.34	2.55

Fig. 25-2. Weight of mild steel bar stock in pounds per linear foot.

WEIGHT OF MILD STEEL BAR STOCK IN OUNCES PER LINEAR INCH

Thick-ness in inches	Width (web) in inches										
	¼	⅜	½	⅝	¾	⅞	1	1⅛	1¼	1⅜	1½
⅛	0.14	0.21	0.28	0.35	0.42	0.49	0.57	0.64	0.71	0.78	0.85
3/16	0.21	0.32	0.42	0.53	0.64	0.74	0.85	0.95	1.06	1.17	1.27
¼	0.28	0.42	0.57	0.71	0.85	0.99	1.13	1.27	1.41	1.55	1.70
5/16	0.35	0.53	0.71	0.89	1.06	1.24	1.41	1.60	1.77	1.94	2.12
⅜	0.42	0.64	0.85	1.06	1.27	1.48	1.70	1.91	2.12	2.33	2.54
7/16	0.49	0.76	0.99	1.24	1.48	1.73	1.98	2.23	2.47	2.72	2.97
½	0.57	0.85	1.13	1.41	1.70	1.98	2.26	2.54	2.83	3.11	3.39

Fig. 25-3. Weight of mild steel bar stock in ounces per linear inch.

either is allowed in most steel), can improve the machining qualities of steel. If there is too much sulfur and not enough manganese, cracking after forging known as hot shortness results. If there is too much phosphorus, a brittleness known as cold shortness results. Both manganese and silicon act as deoxidizers during the production of steel and increase its tensile strength.

Carbon steels may be classified as hot-rolled or cold-rolled. Hot-rolled steel still has some scale on it. Cold-rolled or machining steel has the scale removed, has a polished appearance, usually has a higher carbon content and is rolled to closer measurement tolerances than hot-rolled steel. Cold-rolled is more expensive than hot-rolled stock.

Steels are classified primarily by carbon content or by content of alloying elements other than carbon. Carbon is present in every type of steel.

WEIGHT OF MILD STEEL PLATE IN POUNDS PER SQUARE FOOT AND OUNCES PER SQUARE INCH

Thickness in inches	U.S. Std. Gauge	Approx. Wt. in pounds per sq. foot	Approx. Wt. in ounces per sq. inch
1/32	22	1.28	0.14
1/16	16	2.53	0.28
⅛	11	5.10	0.57
3/16	7	7.63	0.85
¼	3	10.20	1.13
5/16	0	12.73	1.41
⅜	000	15.30	1.70

Fig. 25-4. Weight of mild steel plate in pounds per square foot and ounces per square inch.

Carbon steels may be divided into five groups (Kugler, 1957):

1. Low carbon steels: contain 0.05 to 0.15 percent carbon.
2. Mild steels: contain 0.15 to 0.25 percent carbon.
3. Medium carbon steels: contain 0.25 to 0.50 percent carbon.
4. High carbon steels: contain 0.50 to 0.80 percent carbon.
5. Very high carbon steels: contain 0.80 to 1.50 percent carbon.

Low carbon steels are used in baling wire, nails, fencing, rivets and some horseshoe bar stock. They are the most ductile, forgeable, machineable, and weldable of the steels.

Mild steels are used in drop forgings, angle iron, channel iron, strap iron, machinery frames and horseshoe bar stock. They are also very ductile, forgeable, machineable and weldable.

Medium carbon steels, often called forging steels, can be heat treated to extreme toughness. They are used for machine parts, gears, shafts, axles and mower knives.

High carbon steels, commonly referred to as tool steels, are heat treatable to extreme hardness. They are used for most hand tools, springs, chisels, and harrow teeth.

Very high carbon steels are exceptionally hard and brittle. They are used for punches, files, knives, drills and metal cutting tools.

Wrought iron, once the most commonly used material in a blacksmith shop but not manufactured now, has been replaced by mild steel. Wrought iron was very low in carbon (less than 0.03%), and about 3 percent of its weight was noncorroding, glass-like, iron silicate slag. The metal's fibrous structure made it easy to forge weld and very resistant to shock and vibration.

249

Cast iron is very high in carbon (2 to 4 percent) and is unsuitable for forging. It is very hard and brittle. Cast iron may be identified by raised letters, sand mold casting marks or the spark test. It is used for forge-pots and tuyeres due to its high resistance to heat related expansion and contraction.

As the carbon content of a steel increases, its hardness increases. As hardness increases the steel's ductility and melting temperature decrease. Tensile strength increases until the carbon content reaches approximately 0.80 percent, where it begins to decrease.

High carbon content increases a steel's resistance to wear, but reduces strength and toughness. The addition of alloys allows a steel to be hardenable without sacrificing strength and toughness.

Alloy elements alter the steel to (Schroen, 1980):
1. Produce greater strength in large sections.
2. Provide less distortion in the hardening process.
3. Add greater abrasion resistance.
4. Produce greater toughness in small sections.
5. Retain strength at high temperatures.

Alloy steels contain a guaranteed minimum amount of any alloy other than carbon. The most frequently used metals for alloying purposes are manganese, chromium, molybdenum, nickel, vanadium, tungsten and cobalt. Various combinations of these alloys produce remarkably different products.

Manganese improves ductility and toughens steel by producing a fine grain structure and increasing hardness penetration.

Chromium creates hardness without brittleness, refines the grain structure thereby increasing toughness, and increases resistance to wear.

Molybdenum produces the greatest hardening effect of any of the alloys except carbon. It also reduces the enlargement of the steel grain structure.

Nickel increases the strength of steel without decreasing toughness or ductility. Large quantities produce corrosion and shock resistance.

Vanadium inhibits grain growth when steel is heated above the critical point in heat treating. It also adds toughness and strength.

Tungsten increases hardness, especially red hardness, toughness and resistance to wear necessary in metal cutting tools.

Alloy	Melting Pt. Degrees F.	Alloy	Melting Pt. Degrees F.
Tungsten	6150	Copper	2000
Carbon	3500	Gold	1950
Titanium	3300	Silver	1750
Chromium	2925	Brass	1700
Wrought Iron	2800	Bronze	1600
Mild Steel	2750	Aluminum	1200
Cobalt	2700	Magnesium	1200
Stainless		Aluminum	
Steel	2700	Alloys	1050
Nickel	2650	Zinc	800
Silicon	2600	Magnesium	
High Carbon		Alloys	900
Steel	2550	Lead	600
Monel	2400	Babbit	500
Manganese	2300	Tin	450
Cast Iron	2100		

Fig. 25-5. *Approximate melting points of metals (alloys) in degrees Fahrenheit. From Kennedy (1965).*

Cobalt is used in combination with tungsten to develop red hardness in hot work steels. However, it decreases toughness.

The addition of alloys affects the melting point and optimum forging temperature of steel depending upon the combination. Some have a wide melting point range; others may be considered a single point.

Color, surface texture and sound may also be useful aids to the experienced person. Making a tool and using it is a sure test. However, this is usually too time consuming to be practical.

In addition, the specific gravity test is useful in distinguishing between the various types of nonferrous metals found in used castings. Specific gravity is the ratio of the density of the material to the density of water. For example, steel is nearly eight times as heavy as water while aluminum is only three times as heavy. (Steel is three times as heavy as aluminum). Specific gravity may be determined by first subtracting the weight of an object in water from the weight of an object in air. Then divide that difference into the weight in air to determine the specific gravity.

Carbon and alloy steels have number designations assigned by the Society of Automotive Engineers (SAE) or the American Iron and Steel Institute (AISI).

The SAE uses a four digit number to identify the chemical composition of the steel. The first digit represents the general class of steel, based

Metal	Melting Pt. Degrees F.	Tensile Strength Pounds/Sq. In.	Specific Gravity
Mild Steel	2600	65,000	7.82
Tool Steel	2450	50,000	7.81
Wrought Iron	2900	50,000	7.70
Cast Iron	2200	17,000	7.21
Copper	1925	36,000	8.90
Bronze	1692	36,000	8.80
Brass	1692	24,000	8.40
Aluminum	1472	20,000	2.56
Lead	625	3,000	11.35
Tin	445	4,600	7.30
Zinc	775	7,500	6.80

Fig. 25-6. Properties of several metals. From Schwarz-kopf (1916).

on its major alloy ingredient. The second digit gives an approximate percentage of the principal alloy ingredient. The last two digits give the number of carbon points in the steel. A point of carbon equals 0.01 percent or 100 points equals 1 percent carbon content.

For example, a plain carbon steel 1060: 1 means it is plain carbon, 0 means there is no alloy element present, 60 means it contains 60 points or 0.60 percent carbon. Hot rolled bar stock (A-36) is 1008 and cold rolled bar stock is usually 1018. An alloy steel 2511: 2 means it is nickel alloy, 5 means it contains about 5 percent nickel, and 11 means it contains 11 points of carbon.

A leaf spring from a General Motors car is 5160 steel. A coil spring might be a 5160 or 9260 steel. Axles are 1050 steel (Andrews, 1977).

The following are examples of basic SAE number designations of carbon and alloy steels:

Plain Carbon	10____
Manganese	13____
Nickel	20____
Nickel-chromium	31____
Carbon-molybdenum	40____
Chromium-molybdenum	41____
Chromium-nickel-molybdenum	43____
Nickel-molybdenum	46____
Chromium	51____
Chromium-vanadium	61____
Tungsten	7____
Nickel-chromium-molybdenum	86____
Manganese-silicon	92____
Nickel-chromium-molybdenum	93____
Manganese-nickel-chromium-molybdenum	94____

In addition, prefix letters are used to indicate the process used in making steel. They are:

A—Open-hearth alloy steel (90 percent of the steel produced in the U.S.)

B—Acid Bessamer carbon steel

C—Basic open-hearth carbon steel

D—Acid open-hearth carbon steel

E—Electric furnace steel of both carbon and alloy steels

The electric refined tool steels have an AISI numbering system which is based on the quenching method, application, special characteristics, and steels for particular industries. Commonly used tool steels are grouped into six major classifications with 11 subgroups assigned a letter symbol (Clark and Varney, 1962).

1. Water hardening . . . . W
2. Shock resisting . . . . S
3. Cold work: oil hardening . . . . O
     Med. alloy-air hardening . . . . A
     High-carbon, high-chromium . . . . D
4. Hot work: chromium base . . . . H1 to H19
     tungsten base . . . . H20 to H39
     molybdenum base . . . . H40 to H59
5. High-speed: tungsten base . . . . T
     Molybdenum base . . . . M
6. Special-purpose: low-alloy L
     carbon-tungsten . . . . F
     Mold steels: low carbon . . . . P1 to P19
     other types . . . . P20 to P39

Selection of the proper steel for a given tool and use involves consideration of the following factors: hardness, wear resistance, toughness, distortion in hardening, depth of hardening, resistance to deformation at high temperatures, forgeability and cost. Cost is usually closely related to the total alloy content. Performance must merit the cost involved. Plain carbon steels are easy to heat treat. Alloy steels often are difficult to precisely heat treat and erratic results are common. Variation occurs among steels of the same type and grade, due to differences in manufacturing techniques and design purposes.

Tool Steel Properties

Grain structure of tool steel is dependent upon the steel's composition and temperature and mechanical or hammering forces applied to it. As steel is heated or cooled, its crystalline or grain structure changes. Grain size increases or decreases depending upon the heat treatment given

251

Type	Common Name	Common Use	Quench Medium	Degrees F. Hardening Temperature	Degrees F. Tempering Temperature (Rockwell C-55)	C	Analysis %				
							Cr	V	W	Mo	Ni
W1	Carbon tool	General Purpose	Brine/ Water	1432-1514	605	0.60-1.40	—	—	—	—	—
S1	Tungsten Chisel	Punches	Oil	1668-1814	705	0.50	1.35	—	2.50	—	—
H13	Chromium Hot Work	Punches	Air	1841-1896	1014	0.35	5.00	1.00	—	1.25	—
L6	Special Purpose Low Alloy	Hammers	Oil	1450-1550	500	0.70	0.75	—	—	0.25	1.50

Fig. 25-7. Analysis and heat treatment of several tool steels. After Lindberg (1980); Clark and Varney (1962).

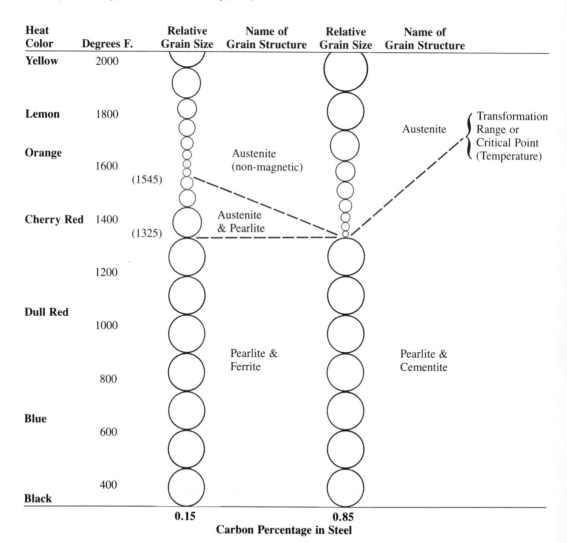

Fig. 25-8. Relationship of temperature (as indicated by color) to grain growth in mild and carbon steel. After Kugler (1957).

252

the steel. Grain size and steel strength are inversely proportional. Fine grain structure is necessary to produce maximum hardness and toughness. Coarse grain structure produces brittleness. Each grain formation has a characteristic pattern and name.

Pure iron crystals or grains are called ferrite. Iron mixed with carbon is called iron carbide or cementite. Ferrite mixed with cementite is called pearlite. Unheated, unhardened steel has a pearlite structure. When steel is heated above the critical (transition) temperature, the ferrite and cementite dissolve to form austenite. Austenite has a small uniform grain structure. This happens at a specific transformation temperature in tool steel but occurs in a transformation range in mild steel.

Slow cooling (normalizing and annealing) from temperatures above and below the transformation range or temperature causes pearlite formation. Normalizing causes pearlite to develop a form known as bainite. Annealing (cooling very slowly) causes the cementite portion of pearlite to become soft and spheroidite (round) in form. Rapid cooling (quenching or hardening) changes austenite directly (avoiding pearlite formation) to martensite, the needle-like type of crystal that makes hard steel. Tempering by slowly heating the steel well below the critical temperature relieves internal stresses and toughens the steel.

Heat treatments are methods used to achieve and hold a fine grain structure. First the steel (tool) is annealed, then hardened and finally tempered. Only steels with sufficient carbon or other alloys will harden sufficiently to hold up as tools, even when the fine grain structure is obtained. The temperature of heat treated steel is estimated by observing the color.

In low carbon steel, grain refinement begins at about 1325 degrees F. or a cherry red heat and progresses over a critical range until the critical temperature is reached (about 1545 degrees F.). At the critical temperature, grain size is its smallest. This point can be detected by:

1. Color change. For mild steel it is a bright red, for high carbon steel it is a cherry red. Alloy steel is usually higher but varies with each type.
2. Interrupted heating. The metal seems to reach a plateau in heating for a few momemts.
3. Magnetic attraction. The temperature at which a magnet will no longer affect the steel is the critical temperature.
4. Grain appearance. Draw out a piece of metal in a thin strip and nick it at ½ inch intervals. Heat it so the color varies along the piece. Quench and successively break off each piece from the hottest end. The color corresponding to the break with the smallest grain size is the critical temperature.

Grain size in high carbon steel changes immediately when reaching the critical temperature (1325 degrees F. for 0.85% carbon steel). Grain size of both mild and tool steel increases slowly as the temperature of the steel continues to increase.

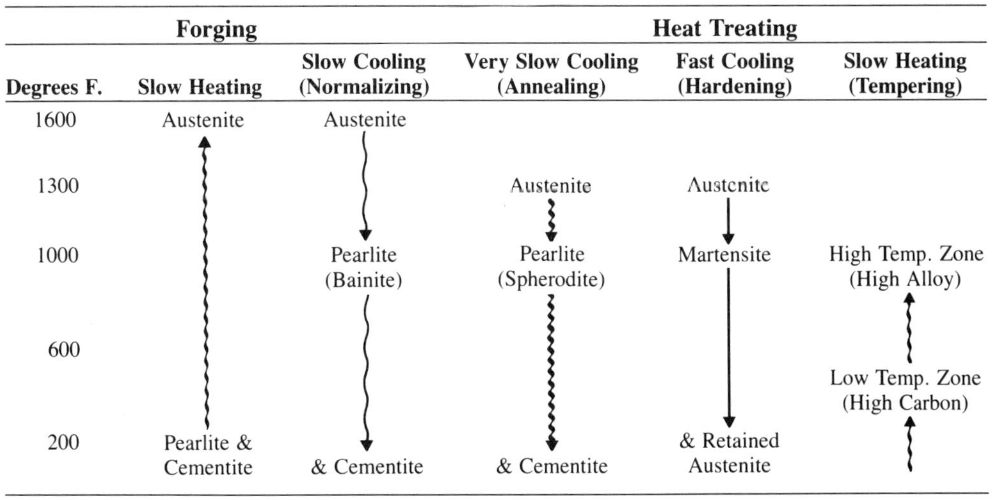

Degrees F.	Forging		Heat Treating			
	Slow Heating	Slow Cooling (Normalizing)	Very Slow Cooling (Annealing)	Fast Cooling (Hardening)	Slow Heating (Tempering)
1600	Austenite	Austenite			
1300			Austenite	Austenite	
1000		Pearlite (Bainite)	Pearlite (Spherodite)	Martensite	High Temp. Zone (High Alloy)
600					Low Temp. Zone (High Carbon)
200	Pearlite & Cementite	& Cementite	& Cementite	& Retained Austenite	

Fig. 25-9. Relationship of forging temperature and heat treating to high carbon steel grain structure. After Schroen (1980).

Packing involves hammering the steel at a dull red color for a long period of time. Hammering the metal above and down to the critical temperature toughens, refines the grain and packs the steel. It is essential for strong, hard tools. Packing is also especially important after forge welding. If properly done, the steel will show a bright black gloss. Either fast or slow cooling will hold a fine grain structure. This is done in several ways.

Hardening is accomplished by immediately quenching in water causing the steel to take on a hard glass-like state. The steel will show a white (mottled gray) appearance when coming out of the water. It is best to harden steel at the lowest heat that will harden it, or in other words at the critical temperature. Without further treatment, many steels are too hard and brittle to be of value for most tools after hardening only.

Tempering should be done immediately after hardening. Tempering reduces the hardness by reheating the steel enough to add toughness but still retain a hard edge. The steel is polished and when heated the colors appear in the following order: yellow, light straw, dark straw, purple, dark blue, light blue, and grey. The steel is quenched when the correct color for the type of steel and tool use is reached. The colors represent the following approximate temperatures (Westbury, 1977):

Bright (polished surface)	below 430 degrees F.
Pale yellow	430
Pale straw	450
Middle straw	475
Dark straw	500
Purple	535
Blue	570
Green gray to black	600 and above

An expanded temperature chart for temper colors may be found in Andrew's (1977) book.

Some tools are hardened and tempered in the same heat. The end of the tool is heated to the critical temperature an inch or so above the cutting edge. The edge is dipped in the water until water will hang on the edge. The portion dipped in the water should be moved up and down slightly to prevent a water line crack. The edge is polished rapidly and quenched when the desired color reaches the cutting edge. When all visible red color is gone from the rest of the tool, it too is quenched.

Tools and springs that need to have elasticity rather than extreme hardness are cooled in oil. Springs are quenched at the hardening temperature and then the oil is burned or flashed off. They are removed from the fire and cooled in the air. Tools are quenched and left in the oil until cold. The tool is polished and the temper drawn.

Casehardening is used to produce a hardened surface or skin on a tough, unhardened steel core. Steel can be surface hardened by carborizing, gas carborizing, nitriding (alloys), and cyaniding. A lower carbon and therefore cheaper steel can be used. However, usually greater skill is required.

Annealing is the opposite of hardening. The steel is cooled very slowly from the critical temperature, instead of very quickly. It is often done to make tool steel softer to facilitate filing or machining. The steel is heated slightly above the critical temperature (cherry red in a room shadow) and buried in slack lime or sifted wood ashes free from dampness. It usually takes several hours for the steel to reach room temperature by this process. Annealing assures uniform grain structure and complete relieving of internal stresses in the steel.

Normalizing is a fast and less complete method of annealing. The steel is cooled in the air after having been heated slightly above the critical temperature in the transformation range (cherry red in room light). It is often more practical since it relieves high stresses, takes less time, and many tools will give satisfactory service with this treatment before hardening. Normalized steel has slightly higher tensile strength and less ductility than annealed steel.

Tool steel may crack during the heat treating process. Possible causes for this are:
1. Overheating (burning) the steel.
2. Uneven heating of the steel.
3. Irregular hammering of the steel.
4. Uneven cooling of the steel.

Critical temperatures are different for each of the alloy steels. It is best to get the metallurgy data from the steel company that made the steel you are forging. The colors described for plain carbon steels do not necessarily apply to the alloy steels.

Uniting the actual temperature with the color can be done using temperature indicator markers (crayons).[1] Marking crayons come in 105 temperature ratings from 100 degrees F. to 2500 degrees F. and have a guaranteed ±1 percent accuracy. Each of the steel companies have specification sheets for their steels. However, the varying amount of light available when viewing the colors makes accurate judgments difficult.

Quenching is the rapid cooling of steel from an elevated temperature. The purpose of quenching is always to harden the steel. The various types of quenching baths cool the steel at different rates. The hardening effect of each may be very different on different steels. Brine (a 10 percent salt solution) is usually thought of as the fastest quench. Water is next, then thin oil, thick oil or animal fat, forced air and finally still air.

When steel is quenched, it must be gently moved while it is vibrating to avoid lines and subsequent cracks in the steel. Moving the steel also prevents the quenching bath from warming up too fast around the steel, and slowing the quenching process. Steel must cool rapidly on the outside in each of the quenching mediums to get the desired edge or surface hardness. The reason for the different mediums is to control the speed the core or interior of the tool cools. The slower the core cools the softer it becomes and thus tougher and more resistant to impact. Since the depth of hardness is also controlled by the quenching medium, thick tools usually need a water bath where thin tools require oil.

In summary, successful heat treating involves a knowledge of the steel (carbon and alloy content), awareness of the proper forging and heat treating temperatures and selection of how fast the steel is cooled (quenched). Maximum hardness *and* toughness are achieved by tempering in the proper temperature range related to the quenching method used.

Hardness of steel is closely related to tensile strength and ductility. Up to a point, the harder the steel, the higher the tensile strength and the lower its ductility.

Hardness of heat treated steel can be measured more readily than ductility or tensile strength. Several methods of hardness testing are used in industry. Three of the most common are:

1. The Rockwell method. A diamond core is pressed into the metal surface with a known force. Hardness is determined by a gauge built into the testing unit which determines the depth of the impression. Designations are given on various scales, depending on the type of point and amount of load. The C scale is most commonly used.
2. The Brinnell method. A steel ball is forced against the metal surface by a known load. Hardness is determined by measuring the diameter of the impression left in the surface. Brinnell values are approximately 10 times Rockwell C values.
3. The Scleroscope method. A diamond-pointed cylinder of steel is dropped onto the surface of the material from a fixed height. Hardness is determined by measuring the height of the rebound. Scleroscope numbers are approximately one-seventh of Brinnell values.

Hardness can be approximated by applying a new fine cut file to the surface of a plain carbon steel. This technique is most useful to the blacksmith when tempering steels of unknown composition. The following filing tests indicate approximate Rockwell C hardness:

File grabs the surface easily. Soft.	10
File removes metal with little pressure. Quite soft.	20
File is resisted by metal. Some hardness.	30
File removes metal with pressure. Quite hard.	40
File barely removes metal with pressure. Very hard.	50
File slides over metal surface and dulled. Extreme hardness.	60

Expansion and contraction must be considered when it affects accuracy. Steel expands when it is heated. Steel contracts when it cools. Expansion and contraction must be considered when it affects accuracy. Steel will expand approximately 1/10 inch per foot when heated from room temperature to a cherry red color. It will expand approximately ⅛ inch per foot when heated from room temperature to a bright red (Selvidge and Allton, 1925).

Forging Tool Steels

Plain carbon, shock resistant and hot work tool steels are used to make creasers, stamps and pritchels.

Plain high carbon tool steels have been used for many years. They may range in carbon content from 0.55 to 0.95 percent. Tools made of plain carbon tool steel are first hardened and then tempered by quenching at the right time in water or oil. Plain carbon tool steel was used in

[1]Tempil, South Plainfield, NJ

most of the old factory-produced punches. It is relatively inexpensive. Its hardness when tempered and its forgeability make it suitable for many tools. However, it's red hardness is not as good as modern alloy tool steels.

An example of plain high carbon tool steel is 1080 steel. The 1 indicates that plain carbon is the major alloy. The 0 indicates the nearest whole percent of the major alloy element other than carbon. The 80 is the hundredths of 1 percent or points of carbon content in the steel.

New bars of tool steel should be cut with a hacksaw. The steel comes annealed, so this is not difficult. A power hacksaw saves time and produces a consistent square end. Hardened steel may need to be annealed or cut with a cutting torch.

Plain carbon tool steels should be forged between 1450 degrees and 1500 degrees F. (cherry red). They should be annealed at this temperature before hardening. They can be quenched in water at 1400 to 1500 degrees F. and tempered at 300 to 650 degrees F. depending on their use.

Shock resistant alloy tool steel makes excellent hot or cold punches, depending on its treatment. S1 steel is an example of this type of steel. The forging and heat treating specifications must be checked for each *manufacturer* as well as *class* of steel you use. Shock resisting steels are comparatively expensive.

S1 is usually forged between 2100 degrees and 1660 degrees F. (yellow to bright cherry red). It should be initially heated very slowly. After the tool is forged it should be brought to about 1475 degrees F. (medium cherry red) and buried in ash to anneal for 4 to 5 hours (overnight is best). This anneals or softens the steel and relieves stresses caused when forging the tool.

The working end of the tool is brought to 1750 degrees F. (between orange and bright red). The whole tool is cooled in oil. This hardens it. The hardened punch is tempered for one hour in a 500 degree F. oven. This steel and treatment will give excellent service for hot or cold work as a creaser, stamp or pritchel. S5 and S7 are also used for punches by some horseshoers.

Hotwork alloy tool steels are popular for making punches for handmade shoes. They retain their shape well when driven into hot shoes. H13 is readily available, cheaper and easier to forge to the desired shape than the others of this class.

H13 is forged between 2000 degrees and 1700 degrees F. (bright orange to bright cherry red). Heating this steel above 2000 degrees F. will destroy its quality. Forging it colder than 1700 degrees F. can cause fractures in it.

The completed tool forged from H13 is brought to 1560 degrees F. (cherry red) and buried in dry, sifted ash to slowly cool for several hours. This relieves the forging stresses and anneals the tool.

Tools should be cleaned of any scale and polished prior to the hardening process. The tool is heated to 1800 degrees F. (orange) and allowed to cool in the air. Cooling in air, until cool enough to handle with bare hands, hardens and tempers the steel. Double tempering (repeating the process) is recommended by some manufacturers. Sudden cooling in water or oil can ruin this type of steel.

Tool Form

The **creaser** is used to groove the ground surface of a shoe for the purpose of increasing traction. The shoe crease fills with dirt, and dirt

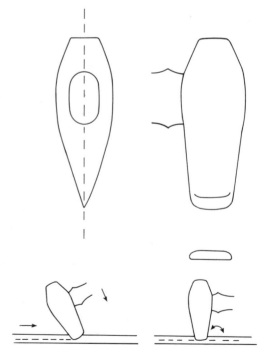

Fig. 25-10. Creaser form. Drawing by D. Manning.

against dirt creates more traction than steel against dirt. Creasing is not routinely done on handmade shoes due to the increased time and skill necessary.

The creaser should be the same width and have the same taper as the specified nail head. It should be slightly rounded on the end to allow it to move through the shoe as the crease is cut. Descriptions of how to make and use a creaser or fuller have been given by Bruce Daniels (1976 and 1981). He suggests making a creaser from a small ball pein hammer head or fence post tamping bar.

The **stamp** or fore-punch is used to form the ground surface of the nail hole that receives the head of the nail.

The stamp can be made from about 2½ to 3 inches of H13 or an old hammer head. The steel is upset in the middle so that there is sufficient thickness to permit punching out an eye for a wood or steel handle. Or a handle can be welded on. The end of the stamp should take the shape of the head of the nail.

The **pritchel** used in making a horseshoe shears the bottom out of the nail hole formed by the stamp or fore-punch. A hot work pritchel needs to be made of a steel least affected by heat since tempering will be drawn out of the tool by the heat of the shoe.

Pritchels are preferably made from flat bar. If round steel is used, it should be flattened on two sides first. This permits use by feel without studying the tip of the pritchel each time a hole is punched.

Ten inches is a good length for a pritchel. A longer pritchel may be desirable to keep your hand cool when punching heavy shoes. A shorter pritchel allows greater control.

The striking surface of the tool may be tapered and rounded. A smaller striking end aids in directing the pritchel and concentrating the power of each blow through the center of the tool. This feature also makes tools easier to tell apart without close examination.

Stubby, square, pointed pritchels cannot form proper nail holes. A pritchel must have a long tapering punching end to avoid distorting the countersunk formed by the stamp.

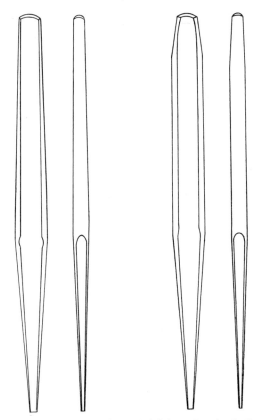

Fig. 25-12. *Shoe making pritchel form. Drawing by D. Manning.*

Fig. 25-11. *Stamp form. Drawing by D. Manning.*

The tip of the pritchel used in forging hand-made shoes is flat and rectangular in shape. The end must conform in size and shape to the neck of the horseshoe nail. The rectangular shape extends throughout the forged portion of the pritchel.

A properly shaped and used pritchel makes back punching (from the foot surface) unnecessary. Back punching of handmade shoes should

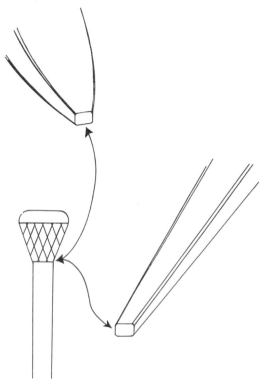

Fig. 25-13. Relationship of stamp end to pritchel end. Drawing by D. Manning.

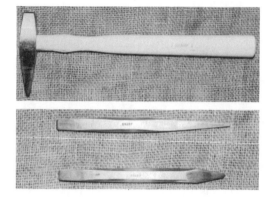

Fig. 25-14. Shoemaking stamps and pritchel made from H13 steel. Photos by J. Graves.

be avoided since it takes extra time and tends to drive a ridge into the nail hole which can pinch the neck of the nail. A flat-tipped, sharp pritchel makes it possible to drive the tool through the nail hole with one or two sharp blows.

A pritchel used in cold shoes for back punching expands holes that were previously punched. Pritchels used in cold shoes need to be tough.

Cold shoes require the use of a pritchel with a point that corresponds to the shank of the nail. This pritchel expands the hole rather than punching it. The smaller tip is also good for removing old nail heads locked in a shoe to be reset. Cold work pritchels should be tempered and thus made harder than hot work pritchels. S1 steel makes a good cold shoe pritchel.

Forging a Center Punch

Center punches can be made from coiled car springs. The springs must be straightened, and 4 inch pieces cut from them. Car springs are usually made of 5160 steel.

Steps in forging a center punch:
1. Heat one end for a short distance no hotter than an orange color. Square up the end by striking upsetting blows as the steel projects over the off edge of the anvil.

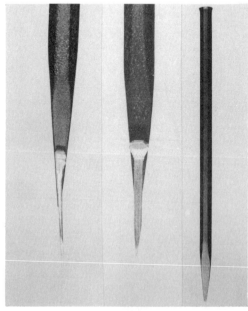

Fig. 25-15. Keg shoe or back punching pritchel form. Photos by G. Poellot.

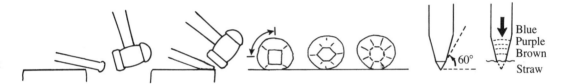

Fig. 25-16. Steps in forging a center punch.

2. Hold the steel at a 45 degree angle next to the off edge of the anvil and bevel the edge of the stock all around. Continue to shape and upset the end.

3. Heat the other end for about 1½ inches to an orange color. Draw and bevel the stock for about 1 inch. First square it, then take it to an octagonal shape and finally round it. Do not hammer the steel after the red color is not visible. Take as many heats as necessary to obtain the shape desired.

4. Heat the entire punch to a bright red color. This helps relieve the internal stresses created by forging the tool. Straighten the punch, if necessary. Let it air cool until there is no color present. Quench in water.

5. Grind the point of the cold punch to approximately a 60 degree angle. Be sure to grind back far enough to remove all cracks that may have formed during the forging process.

6. Heat the pointed end of the punch to a bright red back as far as the start of the bevel. Have a sharp fine cut file handy.

7. Quench about ½ inch of the tip of tool in water until water hangs on the tip. Move the punch up and down and around slightly to prevent a water mark where the tool may later crack.

8. Remove the punch from the water and quickly polish the cooled tip with a fine cut file. Hold the point of the tool near the water and watch the colors run down toward the tip.

9. Quench the tip when it turns a dark straw color. Again move the punch around slightly. Hold only the tempered tip in the water.

10. When all the red heat color is gone from the steel, quench the whole tool.

11. Check the hardness of the tool with a sharp fine cut file. The head and body of the tool should be soft. The file will grab easily. The tempered tip should be hard enough that the file will grab when pressure is applied. If the file slips off, the tool is too hard. Heat it again, following the same process, and let the colors run to the next visible color and try it again. Different steels have different properties, but the file test will allow you to temper most carbon steels accurately.

12. Try center punching a piece of mild steel. If the point dulls easily, retemper it by quenching before the color you used appears. Test again with the file. If the punch is too hard, it will shatter when struck. If it is just right, the point will hold up under normal use.

Forging a Keg Shoe Pritchel for Back Punching

Pritchels for opening nail holes on keg shoes from the ground surface (called back punching) can be made from 6 to 8 inch pieces of coil springs that are unwound and straightened. Round material should be flattened slightly to aid in placement of the tool in nail holes. Other springs or machinery parts of suitable dimension made from spring steel, medium carbon or high carbon steel will make fairly tough pritchels.

Carbon steel must be worked at the correct heat. It should not be heated hotter than an orange color and it should not be hit with the hammer below a dull red heat. If the point gets too hot and burns, cut it off and begin again. It is a good idea to shape the point with a little metal hanging off the edge of the anvil. Tiny fractures that start in the end of the stock during the pointing process can then be ground off with the end blob.

The pritchel is held up on an angle since the anvil shapes the steel from one side while the hammer shapes the other. One side of the pritchel should be wider than the other. The pritchel's dimensions should line up with a No. 5 city head horseshoe nail. The tip should correspond to the cross section of the nail at its midpoint. The taper should correspond to the head of the nail when the mid point of the nail shank is lined up with the end of the pritchel.

Pritchels used only on cold shoes can be tempered like the center punch. Pritchels used for shoe making have a broader and thicker tip corresponding to the base of the nail head and are not tempered. You may anneal the pritchel by heating it to a bright red and burying it in ashes. Leave it until cool to the touch. However, most car spring steel that is cooled in the air after a uniform heating to the critical temperature will hold up as well as that which is annealed.

Forging Round Punches

Round Punches can also be made from coiled car springs. Hot punches should be made 8 to 10 inches in length. The head end is made the same as the center punch. The pointed end is drawn first square, then octagonal and finally round to the size desired. The steel may crack or become distorted if this is not done. The end is then ground off perpendicular and flat or upset and formed with the hammer.

Make a punch that is ¼ to ⅜ inch in diameter on the end. The punch does not need to be tempered since any tempering would be taken out when punching hot steel. This punch may be used for making tongs and could be used for making a rivet header. Headers can be made from car axles or other large diameter medium carbon steel.

Make a second punch that is drawn more than the first. It should be about ⅛ inch in diameter on the end. Rivet holes are often needed in the heels or bars of shoes to secure pads or wedges. Hot fitted shoes may be more conveniently punched than drilled.

Forging a Clinch Cutter

Clinch Cutters or buffers can be made from leaf springs (5160) or old horseshoeing rasps. A used rasp can be cut up with a torch and forged into three clinch cutters.

Heat one end of the rasp piece to a bright orange and fuller it (top and bottom) 1 inch back from the end. This may be done one of several ways. A conventional top and bottom fuller may be used. A spring fuller may be constructed from a piece of round stock. Or, edge to edge blows may be struck on the off edge of the anvil with 1 inch of stock projecting over the edge. The indentations should each be about ½ inch deep. The metal is smoothed up and one end is drawn to a thin edge. The drawing is done with the rounding head of the hammer. The sides of the cutting edge are finished by placing the edge of the tool against the edge of the anvil and striking flat blows. Do not pound the metal when it shows no color. This end will be used to cut clinches.

Heat the other end of stock and fuller it ½ inch back from the end. Draw the end out that is on the same side as the blade. The drawn end should resemble a small pritchel. This end will be used to drive broken nails from the hoof.

The center may be flattened and drawn. This will make the tool longer. Or, you may choose to leave the center handle short and thick.

The blade and point of the clinch cutter need to be tempered. This is best done by doing each end separately. The blade end is heated red all over back to the handle. Remove it from the fire and cool about ½ inch up the tip of the blade. Move the blade up and down and around slightly to prevent a water crack from forming. When water will hang on the tip (or you can touch it), quickly file or polish one side of the blade and watch the colors run. Stop the color on a rasp at brown or purple, a spring at straw by quickly quenching the tip when the desired color is reached. The rest of the end of the tool may be quenched when all the color is gone. Test the

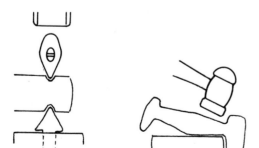 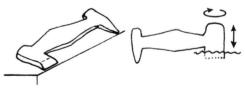

Fig. 25-17. Steps in forging a clinch cutter.

blade with a file. A sharp fine cut file should cut the tempered steel when pressure is applied. Compare the hardness with the striking head. The head should be soft. Lay a horseshoe nail on a board and cut it. If the blade is indented, it is too soft or too sharp. Retemper or resharpen the tool with a steeper bevel.

The pritchel end is tempered in the same way except the blade end is frequently cooled when heating and a wet cloth is wrapped around it while the other end is being tempered. It is also important to avoid grinding either end long enough to draw out the temper. Proper forging technique eliminates the need for excessive grinding. Only a minimum amount of filing should be necessary to sharpen the tool.

Forging a Hot Work Pritchel for Shoe Making

The steel used is ⅝ inch round, H13 air hardening tool steel. Round stock, though not preferred is more easily obtained. Several horseshoeing supply houses sell it in pieces small enough for individual pritchels. Long bars may be cut with a hacksaw or circular metal cut-off saw.

A 7 inch bar will make a 10 inch pritchel if a long taper is forged on the striking end. Use an 8 inch bar if the long tapering striking end is not desired.

The entire length of ⅝ inch round bar is flattened at a bright cherry red to orange heat. A 4 to 6 pound hammer is best for this work. Several heats may be needed to flatten the bar until it is approximately ⅜ inch thick. It will then be ¾ inch wide. This flattened bar makes a pritchel that is easy to direct when punching.

The head end is tapered first to 4½ inches on

the sides. The head will be 5/16 x ½ inch rectangle when viewed from the end. Round the edges formed on the taper with the hammer.

The punching end of the pritchel is drawn out in a long thin blade with a 4 inch taper on each side. Repeatedly upset and compact the steel at the tip. Care must be taken as the steel is heated to prevent the tip from getting too hot. Keep the narrow point out of the direct blast of the forge. Avoid rapid heating of the steel.

The tip of the pritchel is forged to the same size as (or slightly larger than) the neck of the specified nail. The taper must be long enough and thin enough to pass through the nail hole without distorting the countersunk formed by the stamp. Final shaping of the tip should be done with a lighter 2 or 2½ pound hammer. If desired, the edges can be slightly rounded at this time.

Fracture lines can be caused by forging the tool too cold. Take a few extra heats. Don't hit the steel after it cools below a bright cherry red.

The completely forged pritchel is heated to a cherry red and buried in ashes to cool slowly for several hours. This relieves the stress put in the steel during the forging.

All scale is removed after the tool cools. Scale may be kept to a minimum by brushing the tool with a wire brush each time it is brought from the fire. Some final shaping may be done with a grinder. However, it is best to do the shaping with a hammer while the steel is at the proper heat since all marks in tool steel are potential cracks.

The cleaned pritchel is heated to an orange and allowed to cool in the air. This will harden and temper it. Double tempering (doing this twice) is recommended.

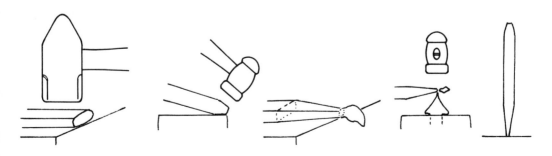

Fig. 25-18. Steps in forging a pritchel.

Punching a Nail Hole

A nail hole is made in a horseshoe using a stamp and a pritchel. Use scrap horseshoes or leftover short pieces of shoeing stock for testing your punches. Keg shoes can be altered by punching nail holes between the existing ones.

The stamp forms the hole to receive the nail head by being driven into the hot shoe (yellow-orange) until you can feel it stop or until the top (ground surface) of the nail hole is the correct size for the specified nail. If the steel is very thick and regular or city head nails are used, a second punch between the stamp and pritchel may be needed to drift the holes to the bottom. The stamp should be quickly removed from the shoe after striking it to prevent deformation of the tip.

The pritchel's purpose is to punch out the bottom of the nail hole. Set the pritchel into the stamp hole and quickly move the pritchel and shoe over a corner of the hardy hole in the anvil. One or two sharp blows on the pritchel will shear the small metal plug from the bottom of the nail hole. Immediately place the tip of the pritchel on the anvil face and strike down on the hot

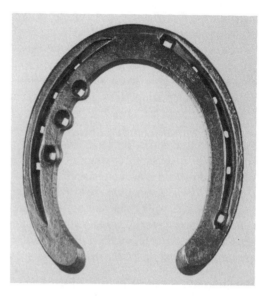

Fig. 25-20. Keg shoe with altered nail holes. Photo by G. Poellot.

shoe. This releases the pritchel from the shoe.

Pritcheling over a corner of the hardy hole is easier than aligning the shoe over one of the small pritchel holes of the anvil. Very light shoes may need to be pritcheled over a small hole to

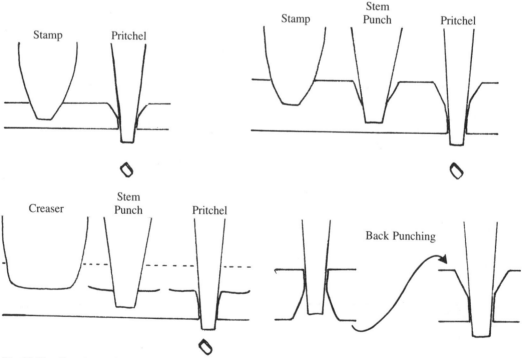

Fig. 25-19. Steps in punching a nail hole.

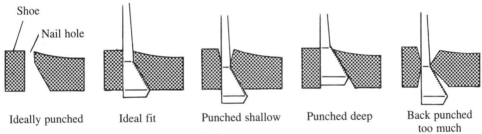

Shoe
Nail hole

Ideally punched   Ideal fit   Punched shallow   Punched deep   Back punched
too much

Fig. 25-21. Nail hole evaluation. Drawing by L. Sadler.

prevent distortion. Some shoers prefer pritch-eling thin shoes over a groove or slot cut across the anvil face.

Pritcheling is done as the color is leaving the shoe from fore-punching with the stamp. The thicker the shoe, the hotter it must be for pritch-eling. Thin shoes may be pritcheled at a black heat. Thick shoes must be at least dull red for pritcheling. The pritchel should be allowed to remain in the hot shoe only a few seconds at a time. A shoe with any color showing is at least 1000 degrees F. The tip of an H13 pritchel may soften if it reaches temperatures above 600 degrees F. Minor distortion of the pritchel tip can be corrected while it still has heat in it. Major rebuilding requires reheating of the tool.

Strike flat overlapping blows on the foot surface of the shoe to remove any bulges caused by the punching process. Try a nail in the hole. A push tight fit with no wobble is most desirable. The checking or trademark on the nail head should be buried in the hole and the nail should be immovable when driven into the shoe with a driving hammer.

References

Althouse, A.D., C.H. Turnquist and W.A. Bowditch. 1976. Modern Welding. The Goodheart-Willcox Co., Inc., South Holland, IL.

Andrews, J. 1977. Edge of the Anvil. Rodale Press, Emmaus, PA.

Boye, D. 1977. Step-by-Step Knifemaking. Rodale Press, Emmaus, PA.

Brewer, P. 1982. How to make a plating hammer. Amer. Farriers' J. 8(6):360.

Canfield, D.M. 1968. Elements of Farrier Science. Enderes Tool Co., Inc., Albert Lea, MN.

Clark, D.S. and W.R. Varney. 1962. Physical Metallurgy for Engineers (2nd Ed.). American Book-Van Nostrand-Reinhold, New York.

Daniels, B.B. 1976. Fullering. Amer. Farriers' J. 2(3):40.

Daniels, B. 1977. Shop talk. Amer. Farriers' J. 3(3):45.

Daniels, B. 1981. Making hand-held stampers and creasers. Amer. Farriers' J. 7(3):129.

Dollar, J.A.W. and A. Wheatley. 1898. A Handbook of Horseshoeing. David Douglas, Edinburgh.

Hickman, J. 1977. Farriery. J.A. Allen and Co., Ltd., London.

Holford, H. 1912. The 20th Century Toolsmith and Steelworker. Frederick J. Drake & Co., Chicago.

Holmes, C.M. 1928. The Principles and Practice of Horseshoeing. Frederick Duffield & Sons, Leeds, ENGLAND.

Johnson, H.V. 1979. General Industrial Machine Shop (3rd Ed.). Chas. A. Bennet Co., Inc., Peoria, IL.

Kennedy, G.A. 1975. Complete Book of Welding. J.W. Sams, Inc., Indianapolis.

Kugler, H.L. 1957. Arc Welding Lessons (2nd Ed.). James F. Lincoln Arc Welding Foundation, Cleveland, OH.

Lindberg. 1980. Tempering Chart for Tool Steels. Chicago.

Lungwitz, A. and J.W. Adams. 1913 (1966 Reprint). A Textbook of Horseshoeing (11th ed.). Oregon State University Press. Corvallis, OR.

Manning, D.C. 1981. The pritchel. Unpublished paper. Sul Ross State Univ., Alpine, TX.

Manning, D.C. 1983. Personal Communication. Roosevelt, UT.

McQueen, H.J. and W.J.M. Tegart. 1975. The deformation of metals at high temperatures. Sci. Amer. 232(4):116.

Rice, B. 1977. Treatment of steel for hot work. Farriers' Assn. of Washington State Newsletter.

Richardson, M.T. 1890. The Practical Horseshoer. M.T. Richardson, New York.

Schroen, K. 1980. The hand forged knife. The Anvil's Ring. 8(4):46.

Schwarzkopf, F. 1916. Plain and Ornamental Forging. John Wiley & Sons, Inc., New York.

Selvidge, R.W. and J.M. Allton. 1925. Blacksmithing. The Manual Arts Press, Peoria, IL.

Simpson, J.S. 1978. How to Build Horseshoeing Tools and Equipment. Scott Simpson, Belgrade, MT.

Turley, F. 1977. Introduction to toolsmithing. Amer. Farriers' J. 3(2):33.

Union Carbide Co., 1976. The Oxy-Acetylene Handbook. Union Carbide Co.-Linde Div., New York.

Westbury, E.T. 1977. Gentry's Hardening and Tempering Engineers' Tools. Argus Books, Ltd., Watford, ENGLAND.

IRON AND FORGE WORK

Chapter 26

Forging Handmade Shoes

Why use handmade shoes? Today's machine-made or keg shoes are superior to those first produced over a century ago. They come in a variety of sizes, can be shaped without heating, have the heels rounded and smooth, and have the nail holes slightly graduated from the outside edge from toe to heel (to correspond to the varying thickness of hoof wall on an average horse). Keg shoes applied by a skilled craftsman may do an adequate job of protecting the wall of an average sound horse's foot. Many horses have given years of useful service wearing only keg shoes. Why learn to make and use handmade shoes?

Advantages of Handmade Shoes

Handmade shoes are specific and exact. They can be made specifically for each foot. They can be made to exactly meet an individual horse's needs. More secure nailing and less interference with natural hoof function are possible with handmades. The making and applying of handmade horseshoes requires a dedication to craftsmanship and skill perfection not found in farriers using machine-made shoes.

Hand forged shoes can be made with the nail holes punched in a variety of positions and for various sized nails. Differences in hoof wall thickness, shape, size and condition may be allowed for when making a handmade shoe. It is desirable to have all nail holes fit directly over the outside border of the white line. Since there is so much variation in feet, it is impossible to retain maximum bearing surface on the wall and exactly follow the outline of the hoof wall on every horse without using a hand turned and punched horseshoe.

Hand forged shoes can be punched to correspond to the angle of the hoof wall. Nails are best driven at an angle slightly greater than that of the wall so they will exit about one-third of the way up its height and parallel to the coronary band. All nail holes in keg shoes are punched perpendicular to the shoe. This makes driving a high toe nail especially difficult.

Hand forged shoes can be made to allow for the natural expansion of the hoof at the heels. The last or heel nail hole can be punched to correspond to the bend in the quarters (the widest point of the shoe). Nails placed behind this point retard the natural expansion of the foot. If all

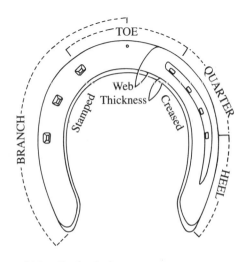

Fig. 26-1. Front and hind handmade pleasure horse shoes made from 12 inches of ⁵⁄₁₆ x ¾ inch stock. Photos by J. Graves.

Fig. 26-2. Handmade shoe terms.

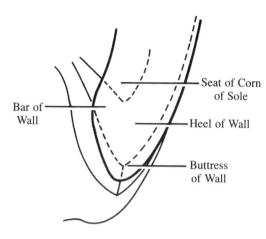

Fig. 26-3. Handmade shoe heel fit.

nails are placed far in front of it, insecure nailing may result. Also, exact heel fit including maximum cover or protection is possible with the hand forged shoe. Exact heel fit means easier hoof cleaning, and less chance of corns or lost shoes.

Handmade shoes can be made in a variety of widths, thicknesses and styles of bar stock. The lightest shoe that will properly protect the hoof and wear for the interval between shoeing periods is usually preferred. However, heavier shoes may be desirable to enhance action, protect the foot or prolong wear. Factors considered when selecting size and type of bar stock to make handmade shoes for each individual horse are: intended use of the horse, stage of training, terrain to be worked on, size of the horse and interval between shoeings. Conformational and/or pathological problems are also considered and

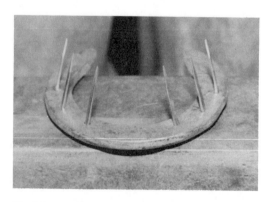

Fig. 26-4. Pitch and position of nail holes in a handmade shoe allow more secure nailing.

266

when needed, therapeutic shoes can usually be most appropriately handmade from bar stock.

The craftsmanship required to accurately make handmade shoes is infinitely more than is necessary to do an acceptable job of cold shoeing with keg shoes. Repeated practice over a long period of time is necessary. Frequent evaluation by yourself and especially a qualified teacher is an absolute necessity. Apprenticeship has its merits. There is no substitute for guided experience. Hand-eye coordination is slowly developed. Until one can accurately make a handmade shoe, it is probably best for the horse that the farrier use machine-made shoes. However, machine-made shoes are at best a compromise and should be only a step in professional development. Rather, precision and craftsmanship should be sought each day by rote practice, critical evaluation and applied learning until you can efficiently produce an attractive and functional horseshoe.

Selecting Material

Horseshoes can be made from many types of metal. In days past, almost all shoes were made from wrought iron. It was much softer and easier to forge than today's steel due to its lack of carbon content and unique fibrous structure. Keg shoes are now made from low carbon or mild, hot-rolled steel. Some companies make their shoes from a higher carbon steel. Shoes made from higher carbon and alloy steels wear longer than conventional shoes but are more expensive, may be difficult to shape, and fracture if not cooled slowly.

Handmade shoes can be made from almost any size or shape of stock depending on the use of the horse and the material available. Round, square, or flat stock can be shaped to form horseshoes. U.S. Army horseshoers were once taught to improvise under field conditions by learning to make a horseshoe from strands of baling wire twisted together and then fused in the forge.

New shoes can be made from old ones by folding the worn shoes at the toe, inserting one inside the other and forge welding them together. The pieces are then welded several times and drawn out. Straightening and then re-turning worn keg shoes is also a good exercise for beginners.

The weight of the finished shoe is often a

factor for consideration when selecting material. A light horse doing fast work (racing) requires a shoe made from light stock. A heavy horse doing slow work (pulling) requires a shoe with substance, and thus increased weight. A show horse, which needs to be shod in order to enhance his action, often requires a heavy shoe. As a rule, pleasure horses are shod with the lightest shoe which will provide adequate protection to the horse's feet for the interval between shoeings.

Pleasure horse shoes are usually made from ¼ to ⅜ inch thick hot-rolled bar stock. Traditionally, front shoes have been made with a wider web (¾ to ⅞ in.) than hind shoes (½ to ⅝ in.) because the front foot bears more weight and the sole is flatter and may require more protection than the hind foot. Thickness and width usually graduate from smaller to larger along with shoe size. Today, most front and hind pleasure and performance horse shoes are made from the same size bar stock.

Width of stock (web) may be selected for the average pleasure horse by making it about twice the width of the wall at the toe. Thus, for a horse with a ⅜ inch wide wall, ¾ inch wide bar stock would be selected. Thickness may be chosen by considering the size of the horse, the strength of the foot, and the probable wear the shoe will get between shoeings.

Determining Bar Stock Length

Bruce Daniels of Mullica Hill, New Jersey, has developed a formula for determining the length of bar stock necessary to make a horseshoe (Daniels, 1980). Reduced to its simplest form it may be stated: $3D - 2W - H =$ Bar Stock. D equals the average diameter of the ground surface of the foot. W equals the width of the bar stock. Thickness is not considered. H equals the width between the buttresses or the place where you want the shoe to end.

Rather than multiply these numbers out each time you figure steel, try the following simplified procedure. Use a ruler or a tape. A hook on the zero end of a ruler is handy.

1. Measure the foot across its *longest* diameter. Usually this is from one side of the toe to the opposite buttress. Read at the buttress. Grasp the ruler with your right thumb nail pointing to this measurement. Average the two different distances on odd feet.

2. Measure the foot across its *shortest* diameter. Usually this is across the quarters from quarter bend to quarter bend. Read on the right side. Grasp the ruler with the left thumb nail pointing to this measurement. Halfway between your thumbnails is the average. Round up to the nearest ⅛ inch, if necessary. Place your left thumbnail on the mark.

3. Multiply the whole number by three. Put your right thumbnail on the answer. Multiply the fraction by three. Move your right thumbnail to the new mark.

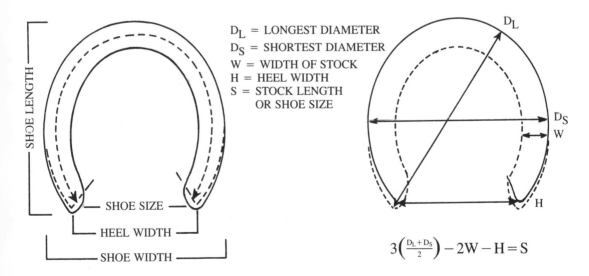

D_L = LONGEST DIAMETER
D_S = SHORTEST DIAMETER
W = WIDTH OF STOCK
H = HEEL WIDTH
S = STOCK LENGTH
    OR SHOE SIZE

SHOE LENGTH

SHOE SIZE

HEEL WIDTH

SHOE WIDTH

$$3\left(\frac{D_L + D_S}{2}\right) - 2W - H = S$$

Fig. 26-5. Bruce Daniel's formula for correct bar stock length for handmade shoes.

4. Now subtract off (moving to the left and mark with your left thumbnail) the two widths of bar stock. If you are going to make a bar shoe you can stop at this point and read your steel length. If not, place your right thumbnail on the mark.
5. Place the rule with the measuring edge between the heels and your right thumbnail at the right buttress or where you want the shoe to stop on the right side.
6. Read the rule on the left buttress or where you want the shoe to stop.
7. Cut your bar stock this length.

The addition of heel calks or extensions are extra and must be figured accordingly. Clips require no extra stock, but must be set into the wall so that the hoof and shoe circumference coincide.

An alternate way of measuring feet around 5 inches wide on a short ruler is to use the five as a 15 after multiplying the whole number by three. Then add or subtract two more of the fraction to or from the product of the whole numbers, subtract two times the bar stock width, place the ruler on the heel opening and read your bar stock length.

Jack Kohler of St. Louis, Missouri, noticed that, according to Daniel's formula, for each ⅛ inch the width of stock increases, the length of stock decreases by ¼ inch. And, vice versa, for each ⅛ inch the width of stock decreases, the length of stock increases by ¼ inch. Kohler fig-

ured that a flexible tape could be used for figuring the amount of stock to use for a handmade shoe by subtracting 2⅛ inches (for ¾ in. stock) from the heel to heel circumference. He then made a tape with ¼ inch marks on it for each ⅛ inch change in the stock width. To date, this is the most rapid and accurate way of determining bar stock length of handmade shoes.

Cutting Bar Stock

Bar stock can be cut with an anvil devil, tempered hardy, cold cutter or chisel, twisted off with a wrench, sheared with a shear or heavy bolt cutters or burned off with a cutting torch.

An anvil devil is a tempered piece of three-cornered file or other high carbon steel that is sharpened and placed on the top of the anvil. Cold steel is placed on it and struck with a hammer. When the steel is bent it will break at the indentation. A tempered hardy may also be used for this purpose.

The cold cutter or cold chisel is used with a helper swinging a sledge. This is the best method of cutting heavy steel cold if a heavy stationary shear or cutting torch is not available. Again, the steel is not cut all the way through, but only until it may be broken by hand over the edge of the anvil.

Shoeing stock may be sheared by twisting it

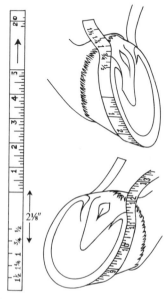

Fig. 26-6. Jack Kohler's foot measuring tape.

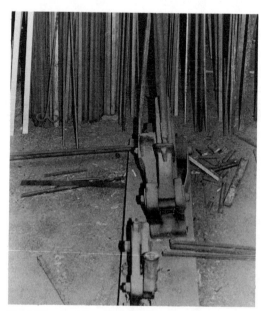

Fig. 26-7. An Edward's No. 5 shear is useful for cutting bar stock.

off using a heavy vice or slot shear and a large adjustable wrench. Heavy bolt cutters will also shear stock sizes up to 5/16 inch in thickness.

A heavy stationary shear, such as an Edwards No. 5, is necessary for fast cutting of stock over ⅜ inch thick. Power shears are used in large metal fabrication shops. Portable electric circular metal cut-off saws have become popular in recent years.

Nail Hole Layout

The beginner will find it useful to lay out the toe nail holes in a flat or plate shoe. This is a most useful aid in aligning the nail holes and centering the toe bend of the shoe.

Dennis Manning of Roosevelt, Utah, has developed a formula for determining the distance the toe nail holes should be from the center of the bar on shoes made from 10 inches or more of bar stock. Round the length of bar off to the nearest inch. The first digit equals the number of whole inches. The second digit equals the number of eighths of an inch. Thus, the toe nail holes on a 10 inch bar would be chalk marked 1 inch from center and those on a 16 inch bar would be marked 1¾ inches from the center. Generally, the toe nail holes of a hind shoe should be slightly less than those of the front since the more pointed toe of the hind shoe places the toe nails farther back in the turned shoe. The chalk mark is stamped with a center punch the thickness of the wall in from the outside of the shoe.

Even though many experienced horseshoers do not mark their toe nail holes, they usually will mark the center of the bar to aid them in placing the toe nails in the first branch that is turned (usually the outside branch). Such a mark also serves as a guide for positioning toe clips. The center of a bar can be found by balancing it on the hardy and striking the edge of the bar to make a mark or by measurement and a center punch. Another method is to lay the two bars of a pair side by side, draw a line across them near the center and turn one bar end for end. The center is halfway between the two lines.

Nail holes are usually placed in the front half of a shoe so that they won't interfere with the physiological movements of the foot. Heel nail holes are positioned at or slightly forward of the bend in the quarters. They are positioned in from the outside of the shoe the thickness of the shaped wall at that point. One or two (may be more on draft horses) nail holes are punched equidistant between the toe and heel nail holes in each branch.

The position of the heel nail hole of the second branch (usually the inside branch), may be determined by positioning the shoe so that the edge of the anvil can be seen through the toe nail holes. Sight across from the heel nail hole to the unpunched branch and place the stamp on the projected line of sight. The intermediate nail holes are lined up by placing the stamp on a line of sight through the center of the toe and heel nail holes. The distance is divided in half when punching three nail holes per branch and divided in thirds when punching four nail holes per branch.

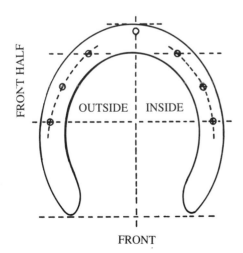
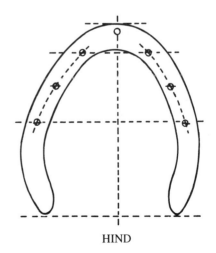

Fig. 26-8. Nail hole layout in the shoe.

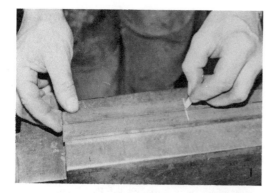

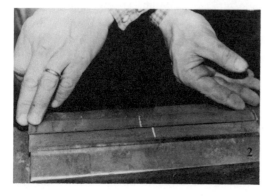

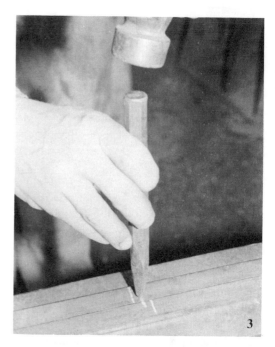

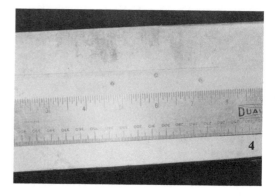

Fig. 26-9. Finding the center and marking the toe nail holes in bar stock.

Shoe Shape

The shoe should be shaped to fit the outer rim of the trimmed and shaped hoof. The shoe should follow the outline of the hoof exactly from one bend in the quarter around to the other. From the bend in the quarter to the end or buttress of the heel the shoe should be fit slightly full to provide a place for the rear of the hoof to expand upon as the foot bears weight. This fullness is called expansion. Usually more expansion is provided on the outside heel than on the inside heel, especially on performance horses. The full or extended portion of the shoe may be boxed (foot surface beveled) to prevent any possibility of the horse catching and casting the shoes.

Handmade shoes are made to fit each foot. However, most horse's feet have a distinctive front and hind pattern. Note the comparative differences. These differences govern how the shoe is made. Shoes are made and fit from toe to heel. A balanced shoe is formed in five equal sections.

The front foot has a round toe compared to the more pointed toe of the hind foot. The front foot has a slightly rounded and straighter quarter than the hind foot. The widest part of the front foot is usually in the middle of the foot. The widest part of the hind foot is usually in the rear third of the foot. The heels of the front foot are more rounded or turned in than those of the hind foot. Usually there is less distance between the heels (buttresses) of the front foot than those of the hind foot. The hind foot is usually smaller and therefore it takes less stock to cover it than a front foot on the same horse.

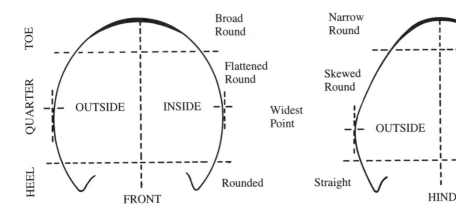

Fig. 26-10.   Front and hind hoof shape govern the form of the shoe.

Shoe Turning

A flat plate shoe can be turned (forged) in two or three heats. It is possible to completely forge a shoe in one heat. Work toward the goal of completely forging a shoe in three to four heats.

Shoes are turned in pairs. One shoe of the pair should always be heating while the other is being worked on the anvil. Experience in the use of the forge will teach you timing and the best placement of the steel in the fire to achieve maximum efficiency.

Speed must be combined with accuracy when making handmade shoes or even their advantages will not be sufficient to encourage their use in place of machine-made shoes. Visualize and review in your mind the progression of the operations to be performed at each heat before the steel is taken from the fire. It is best to do the necessary operations at the correct heat, even if it takes more heats to do them. A beginner will take many more heats than an experienced blacksmith.

Shoes should be heated from toe to heel. They should be rolled in the fire so that the toe is heated first and the heel is heated last. This will create an even heat that will greatly facilitate the turning of a smooth and properly proportioned shoe. Some shoers punch the toe nail holes in the same heat as the toe is turned to make maximum use of each heat and to reduce the length of the heat necessary to turn and stamp the branch.

Steps for turning a flat, stamped **front** shoe in four heats:

Heat (1) the center half or two-thirds of the bar to a white heat (nearly sparking).

1. Position the bar sloping toward you and at a 45 degree angle to the anvil face or horn. The end of the bar touching the anvil should ex-

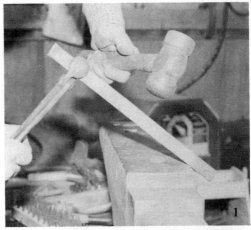

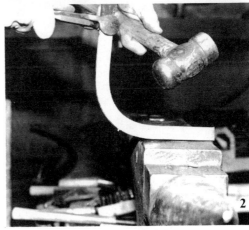

Fig. 26-11.   Steps in turning the toe of a front shoe.

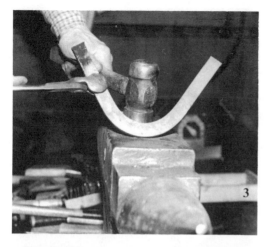

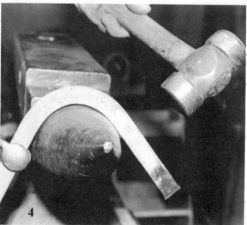

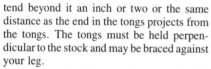

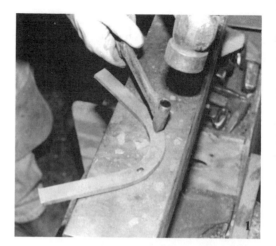

tend beyond it an inch or two or the same distance as the end in the tongs projects from the tongs. The tongs must be held perpendicular to the stock and may be braced against your leg.

2. Strike alternating blows on the upper (inside) edge of the bar with the round head of the turning hammer on the inside of the toe nail hole center punch marks until a smooth, round bend is created and the branches are at a 90 degree angle to each other. The toe bend of the shoe should match the curvature of the toe of the dressed (previously trimmed and shaped) foot.

3. Level the toe to straighten any twisting that may have occurred in the turning process.

4. Check to be sure the toe bend is centered and symmetrically turned. If necessary, change the position of the toe bend while heat is still in the toe. This may be done by placing the toe bend over the horn with the long branch toward you. Strike the high point of the toe, driving more metal into the shorter branch. Open and smooth the toe bend over the horn.

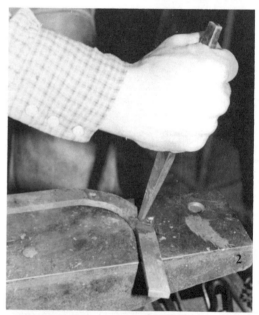

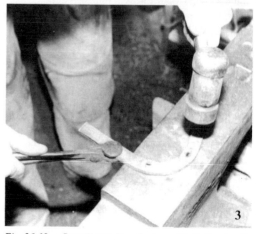

Fig. 26-12.   *Steps in punching the toe nail holes (optional).*

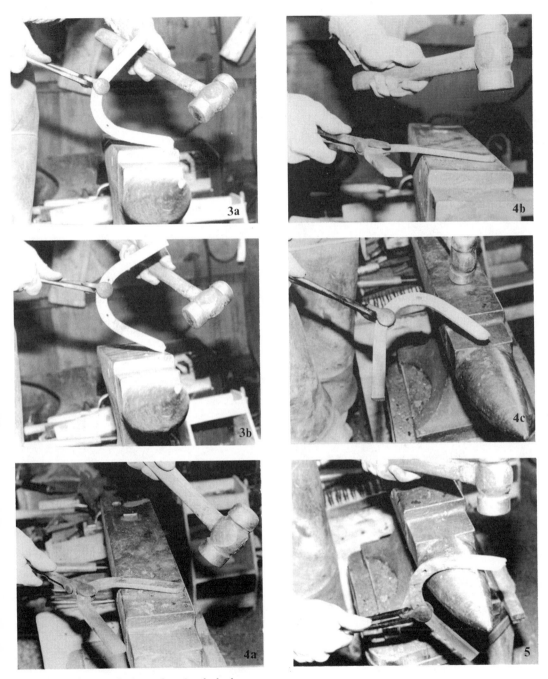

Fig. 26-13. Steps in shaping and turning the heel.

Heat (2) the outside branch from toe to heel. Remove from the fire when the heel is white or nearly sparking.

1. Grip the shoe with the tongs on the side of the toe opposite the branch to be turned. Position the handles of the tongs in line with where the edge of the frog would be if the toe of the shoe were fit to the hoof.

2. Lay the end of the branch (inside edge up) near a rounded portion of the off edge of the anvil.

3. Strike a couple of blows on the inside corner of the heel at a 45 degree angle. Then raise the tongs as you strike a couple more blows. This shapes the heel to conform to the shape of the ground surface of the hoof.

273

4. Strike the ground surface and level the shaped heel on the anvil face to the same thickness as the bar stock. Quickly hammer dress the heel again. You may desire to bevel the heel by striking it at an angle. This reduces the amount of rasping necessary to finish the heel.

5. Place the heel of the shoe (outside edge up) on the heel or horn of the anvil. The entire heel portion of the shoe from the position of the last nail hole back should be extending over the anvil face or horn. Strike the end of the heel as the tong hand drops. This turns the heel of the shoe.

Heat the branch of the shoe again. Eventually you will be able to finish the entire branch (heel and nail holes) in one heat. However, beginners should take an extra heat when needed.

1. Place the toe of the shoe over the horn with the hot branch extending over and perpendicular to the horn and with the tong handles up. The position across the horn (toward the base or point) is determined by the size of the shoe. Large shoes are turned near the base, small shoes nearer the point.

2. Bend the hot metal over the round fulcrum point formed by the top of the horn as the tong handles are moved down beneath the horn. The tong jaws may remain in contact with the anvil horn as the hand is dropped. The hammer hand applies the force as the tong hand forms the shoe.

3. Stamp the toe nail hole at the appropriate distance from the center of the toe. Line the toe nail hole up with the inside web of the shoe at mid-toe. Stamp the heel nail hole at the widest point in the turned branch. It will be approximately halfway between the toe and heel borders of the shoe. Equally space (and stamp) the other one or two nail holes between the toe and heel nail holes. All nail holes should be in from the outer edges the width of the wall and pitched at the angle of the wall at that point. Mark the branch by turning the stamp crossways between the second and third nail holes and striking it once.

4. Punch out the bottom of all the stamped holes with the pritchel. Start with the coldest hole. The branch should still show a dull red heat for this operation. On light shoes it can be done when the shoe is black. Heavy shoes

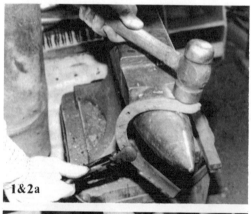

1 & 2 a

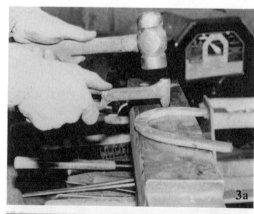

3a

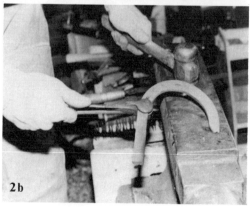

2 b

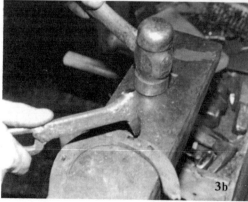

3 b

Fig. 26-14. *Steps in turning the outside branch and punching the nail holes.*

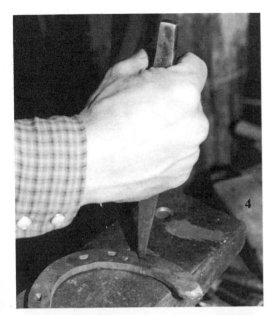

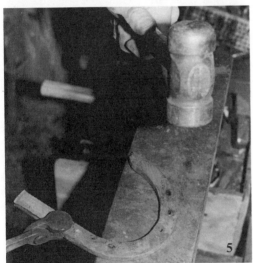

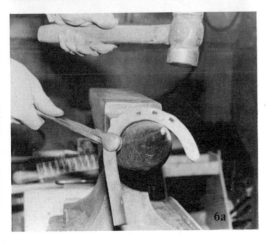

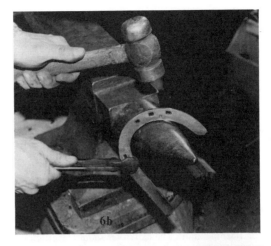

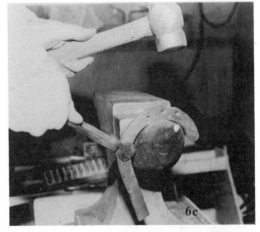

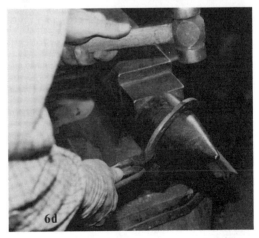

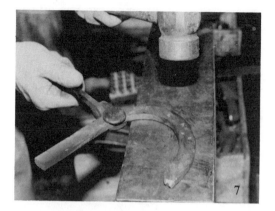

are best done when the shoe is at a higher temperature. The nail holes should be pritcheled at an angle corresponding to the angle of the wall at that point. Stamping and pritcheling are covered in Chapter 25.

5. Turn the shoe over and flatten the bulges on the foot surface formed by punching the nail holes. Hammer overlapping blows on the inside half of the foot surface from mid-toe to the heel nail hole. Turn the shoe over and hammer overlapping blows on the outside half of the ground surface from the toe to heel. These operations concave the inner foot surface of the shoe to prevent sole pressure and speed up the final leveling process.

6. Lightly hammer the edge of the branch of the shoe as you move it over the high point of the anvil horn from toe to heel on first the ground surface edge and then the foot surface edge. This flattens bulges created by stamping and puts smoothness on a shoe without excessive filing. It is a sign of good craftsmanship.

7. Level the outside border of the shoe by striking overlapping blows on the ground surface.

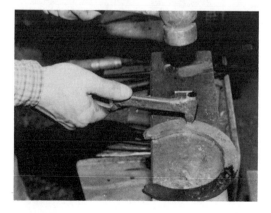

Fig. 26-15. *Line up the inside heel nail hole by sighting from the heel nail hole in the outside branch. Lining the shoe up with the edge of the anvil face helps the alignment process.*

Heat (3) the inside branch. Follow the same steps as on the outside branch. Do not mark.

Heat (4) both heels by placing them down in the fire and bringing them both to a yellow heat. The shoe should not show color any farther forward than the heel nail holes.

1. Place the shoe in the vise with only the last 1½ inches of the heel projecting from it.
2. Bevel around the heels at a 45 to 60 degree angle with the coarse side of the rasp. The angle of the bevel is determined by the angle of the hoof between the buttress and heel bulb.
3. Finish the heels by holding the fine side of the rasp perpendicular (90 degree angle) to the shoe and removing all sharp edges.
4. Remove the burr or feather formed under the heel by running the rasp fine side up under and across the heel.
5. The shoe may be turned around and the outer ground surface edge rounded with the smooth side of the rasp.

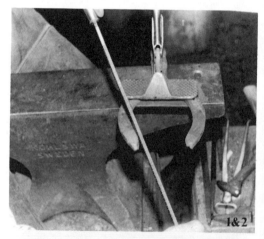

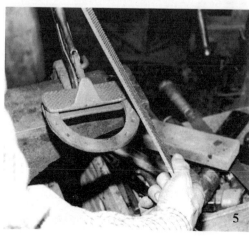

Fig. 26-16. *Steps in finishing the heels and shoe.*

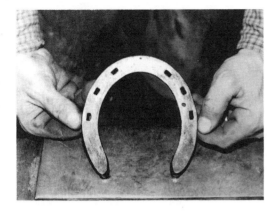

Fig. 26-17. The finished left front shoe.

6. Finish leveling the shoe on the anvil face.
7. Try (fit) the shoe to the hoof.
8. Make minor adjustments and check for levelness.

The shoe is now ready for hot fitting (See Chapter 24).

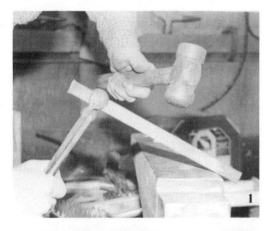

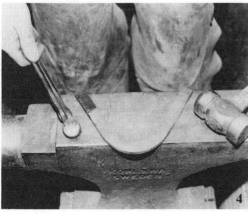

Fig. 26-18. Steps in turning the toe of a hind shoe.

Steps for turning a flat, stamped **hind** shoe in four heats:

Heat (1) the center third of the bar to a white (nearly sparking) heat.

1. Position the bar sloping toward you at a 45 degree angle to the anvil face or horn. The end of the bar touching the anvil should extend beyond it an inch or two or the same distance as the end in the tongs projects from the tongs. The tongs must be held perpendicular to the stock and may be braced against your leg.
2. Strike alternating blows on the upper (inside) edge of the bar with the round head of the turning hammer on either side of the center of the toe. Shoes for small pointed-toed feet may need to be struck only in the center. The branches of the completed toe bend should form slightly less than a 90 degree angle. The toe bend should coincide with the curvature of the toe of the dressed hind foot.
3. Level the toe to straighten any twisting that may have occurred in the turning process.
4. Check to be sure the toe bend is centered and symmetrically turned. Change its position, if necessary, as described for front shoes.

Heat (2) the outside branch from toe to heel. Remove from the fire when the heel is almost sparking.

1. Grip the shoe with the tongs on the side of the toe opposite the branch to be turned. Position the handles of the tongs in line with where the edge of the frog would be if the toe of the shoe were fit to the hoof.
2. Lay the end of the branch inside edge up near a rounded portion of the off edge of the anvil.
3. Strike a couple of blows on the inside corner of the heel at a 45 degree angle. The outside

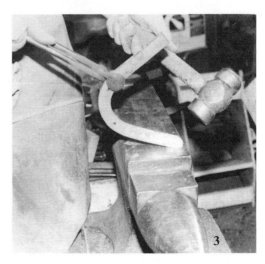

Fig. 26-19. Steps in shaping and turning the outside heel.

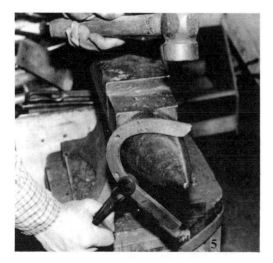

heel may be left with a little more cover (width) than the inside heel as it may be fit with more expansion than the inside heel. Or, it may be shaped as the front heels.

4. Strike the ground surface and level the shaped heel on the anvil face to the same thickness as the bar stock. Quickly hammer dress the heel again. You may bevel the heel slightly with the hammer to reduce the amount of rasping necessary.

5. Place the heel of the shoe (outside edge up) on the heel or horn of the anvil. The entire heel portion of the shoe from the position of

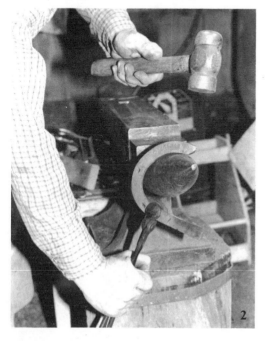

Fig. 26-20. Steps in turning the outside branch and punching the nail holes.

the last nail hole back should be extending over the anvil face or horn. Strike the end of the heel as the tong hand drops. This turns the heel of the shoe.

Heat the branch of the shoe again, if necessary.

1. Place the toe of the shoe over the horn with the hot branch extending over and at a 45 degree angle to the axis of the horn with the tong handles up. The position of the metal across the horn (toward the base or point) is determined by the size of the shoe. Large shoes are turned near the base, small shoes nearer the point.

2. Bend the hot metal over the elongated fulcrum point formed by the top of the horn as the tong handles are moved downward. A tong jaw remains in contact with the anvil horn as the hand is dropped. Hammering on the edge of the branch between the anvil horn and tongs may be necessary to straighten the quarters or further point the toe on some hind shoes.

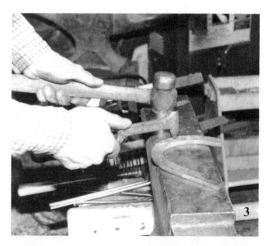

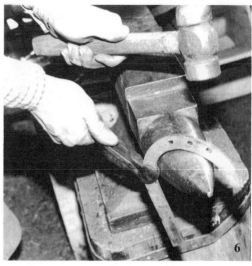

3. Stamp the toe nail hole at the appropriate distance from the center of the toe. Line the toe nail hole up with the inside web of the shoe at mid-toe. Stamp the heel nail hole slightly forward of the widest part in the turned branch. It will be approximately halfway between the toe and heel borders of the shoe. Equally space and stamp the other one or two nail holes between the toe and heel nail holes. Leave a larger space between the first and second nail holes if side clips are to be drawn. All nail holes should be in from the outer edge the width of the wall and pitched at the angle of the wall at that point. Mark the branch by turning the stamp crossways behind the last nail hole and striking it once.

4. Punch out the bottom of all the stamped holes with the pritchel. Start with the coldest hole. The branch should still show a dull red heat for this operation. On light shoes it can be done when the shoe is black. Heavy shoes are best done when the shoe is at a higher temperature. The nail holes should be pritcheled at an angle corresponding to the angle of the wall at that point.

5. Turn the shoe over and flatten the bulges on the foot surface formed by punching the nail holes. Hammer overlapping blows on the inside half of the foot surface from mid-toe to the heel nail hole. Turn the shoe over and hammer overlapping blows on the outside half of the ground surface from toe to heel.

6. Lightly hammer the edge of the branch of the shoe as you move it over the high point of the anvil horn from toe to heel on first the ground surface edge and then the foot surface edge.

7. Level the outside border of the shoe by striking overlapping blows on the ground surface.

Heat (3) the inside branch. Follow the same steps as on the outside branch. Shape the inside heel as the front heels. Do not mark.

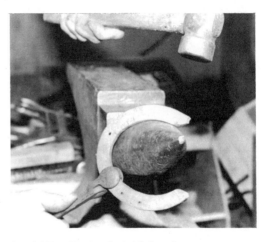

Fig. 26-22. *Turning the inside branch.*

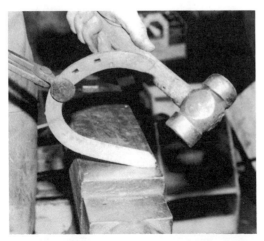

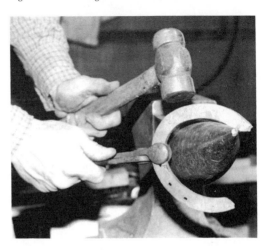

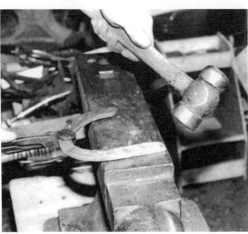

Fig. 26-21. *Steps in shaping the inside heel.*

Fig. 26-23. *Lift up on the tongs to flatten a quarter that is accidentally turned too much.*

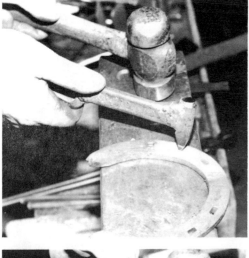

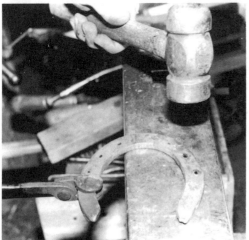

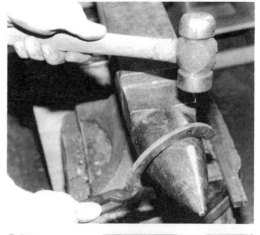

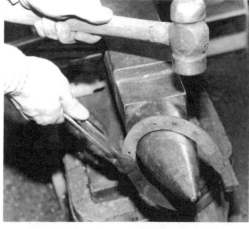

Fig. 26-24. *Steps in punching the nail holes in the inside branch.*

Heat (4) both heels by placing them down in the fire and bringing them both to a yellow heat. The shoe should not show color any farther forward than the heel nail holes.

1. Place the shoe in the vice with only the last 1½ inches of the heels projecting from it.
2. Remove the sharp corners and slightly bevel the heels with the coarse side of the rasp. Both heels may be finished the same. Or, the outside heel may be rasped with less of a bevel than the inside heel. The inside heel may be rasped like those on the front shoes.
3. Finish the heels by holding the fine side of the rasp perpendicular to the shoe and removing all sharp edges.
4. Remove the burr or feather formed under the heel by running the rasp fine side up under and across the heel.

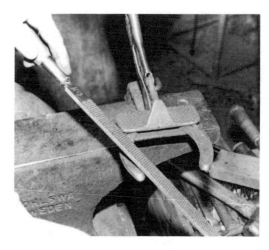

Fig. 26-25. *Rasping the heels smooth.*

5. The shoe may be turned around and the outer ground surface edge rounded with the smooth side of the rasp.
6. Finish leveling the shoe on the anvil face.
7. Try (fit) the shoe to the hoof.
8. Make minor adjustments and check for levelness.

The shoe is now ready for hot fitting and evaluation.

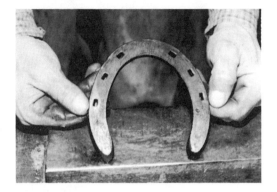

Fig. 26-26. The finished left hind shoe.

Shoe Evaluation

The completed shoe(s) should be smooth when handled and level. Nails should drop in the nail holes and seat tight. Only the portion of the nail head above the bevel or checked pattern should be exposed. All nail holes should be the same depth and size. The pitch of the nails when pushed into place should be the same as the hoof wall. Nail holes and shapes of shoe pairs should coincide when placed foot surface to foot surface. Front and hind shoes should form an egg shape when lined up at their widest point with a toe at each end.

Turn as many shoes as possible. Practice mak-

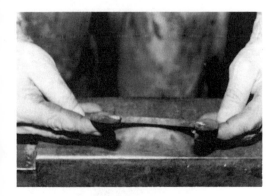

Fig. 26-27. The completed shoe should be smooth and level.

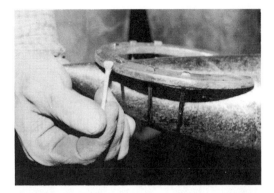

Fig. 26-28. Nails should drop to the same level in all the holes and seat tight.

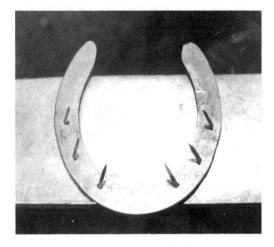

Fig. 26-29. The pitch of the nails should be the same as the hoof wall.

ing shoes in pairs. Challenge yourself. Trace your progress by identifying your best shoe from each day and comparing it to previous work.

Shoes can be completed in three heats by combining the heel finishing into the same heat as the branch is turned in. Shoes can be completed in two heats by combining the toe bend with the turning of the outside branch and finishing the heels when the branches are turned. A shoe can be completed in one heat, but this is rarely done in routine shoeing. Strive to get as much work done as possible in each heat. Turn each shoe more efficiently and make it better than the previous one. Hopefully, the advantages of handmade shoes will soon cause you to desire to put them on every horse you shoe. At least, you will be able to make them when their use would enhance the horse's performance.

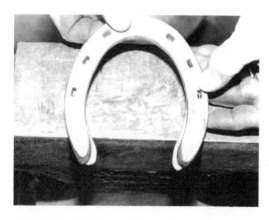

Fig. 26-30. Nail holes and shapes of pairs should coincide when placed foot surface to foot surface. The heels of a front shoe are closer together than those of a hind shoe of the same size.

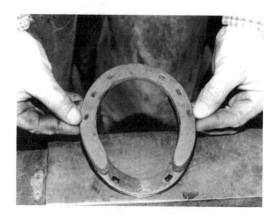

Fig. 26-31. Front and hind shoes should form an egg shape when lined up at their widest point with a toe at each end.

References

Butler, D. and D. Manning. 1981. Why handmade horseshoes? Amer. Farriers' J. 7(5):262.

Daniels, B.B. 1979. Shoptalk. Amer. Farriers' J. 5(3):81.

Daniels, B.B. 1980. Shoptalk—measuring stock for shoes. Amer. Farrier's J. 6(2):50.

Dollar, J.A.W. and A. Wheatley. 1898. A Handbook of Horseshoeing. David Douglas, Edinburgh.

Duckett, D. 1984. Shoemaking Clinic. Olympia, WA.

Hickman, J. 1977. Farriery. J.A. Allen & Co., Ltd., London.

Hoffman, J. 1982. Measuring tape. Gateway Farrier's Association Newsletter. (June):3.

Hoffman, J. 1984. Jack Kohler's hoof measuring tape. Anvil. (Jan/Feb):9.

Holmes, C.M. 1949. The Principles and Practice of HorseShoeing. The Farrier's Journal Publ. Co., Ltd., Leeds, ENGLAND.

Manning, D.C. 1980. Personal communication. Alpine, TX.

NOTES:

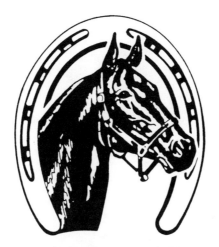

PART
II
CORRECTIVE, THERAPEUTIC
AND
SPECIALIZED SHOEING

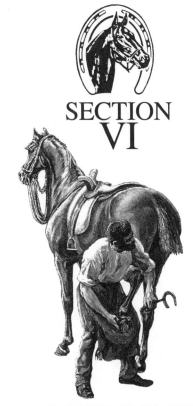

SECTION VI

SHOEING THE CROOKED HORSE

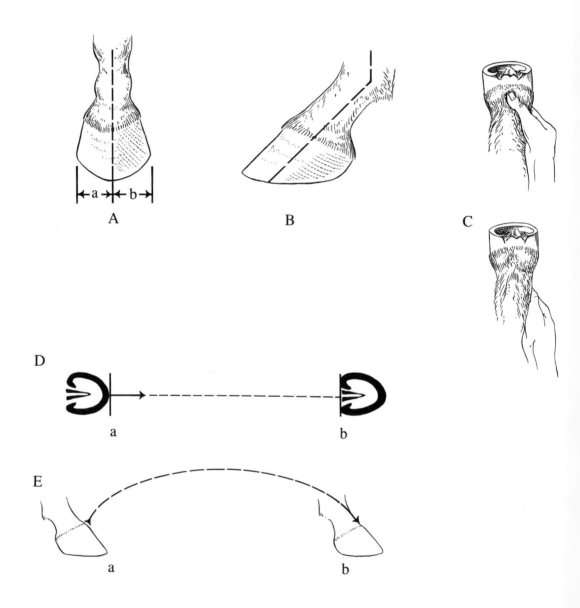

Fig. 27-1. Balanced stance and gait. (A) balanced lower leg and foot viewed from in front; a should equal b. (B) balanced lower leg viewed from the side; axis of the foot should be parallel to the hoof wall at the toe. (C) balanced lower leg and foot viewed from the rear when sighting a foot. Two methods of holding the leg are shown; the bottom one is preferred. (D) balanced breakover and landing; (a) breakover in the center of the toe, (b) landing with equal force on both heels of the hoof, foot moves in alignment with the body without lateral swing. (E) ideal foot flight pattern when viewed from the side. Drawing by L. Sadler.

Chapter 27

Principles of Corrective Shoeing

Next to religion and politics, there is perhaps nothing more controversial than corrective horseshoeing. The reason for this difference of opinion can often be attributed to a lack of understanding of the principles involved. The purpose of this chapter is to explore these principles and gain an understanding. We will begin by defining terms.

Correction means change. It may or may not mean change to an ideal. We must first distinguish between correction (or change) of stance and gait. Stance refers to the position of the foot on the ground. Gait refers to the flight pattern, sequence and timing of the hoofs in motion.

Frequently, corrections (or changes) of stance or gait may adversely affect one another. They often *do not* work together. This is because diverse combinations of limb deviation may cause similar deviations in gait where deviation is defined as departure from the ideal. And, similar hoof flight patterns may not respond to the same correction procedures. Generally, the higher up the leg that the deviation from the ideal occurs, the more severe the procedure needed to affect a change or correction.

Ideally, the weight placed on each leg of the horse is distributed equally over the foot. A horse has a balanced stance when such is the case. When viewed from the side, a balanced stance is defined as one having the angle of the

pastern equal to the angle of the hoof wall at the toe. When viewed from the front, a balanced foot is usually defined as one that can be divided into equal halves by a plumb line passing through the axis of the limb bones. The latter definition may be modified in unusual combinations of upper limb deviation.

Crooked limbs cause unequal weight distribution on the epiphyseal or bone growth plates. Unequal weight disturbs the circulation of the plate and causes uneven growth of the bones. A defect that might be minor at birth may become serious by neglect. The feet of a horse must be kept balanced from an early age to help prevent environmentally caused conformation problems. Inherited deviations from the balanced stance rarely can be corrected. However, there is a possibility of positive change when feet are regularly balanced at an early age before the epiphyseal plate closes in the maturing horse. Some horses will grow out of limb deformities if they are kept balanced.

The time for epiphyseal plate closure varies between limb joints and among breeds of horses. The average time for closure of the bones of the digit (fetlock and below) is less than a year in Thoroughbreds and Quarter Horses. It takes slightly longer in slower maturing breeds like the Arabian. The knee end of the radius closes at about 2 years of age. Since it is one of the

Front Limb Location	Plate Closure Time in Months	Hind Limb Location	Plate Closure Time in Months
1st phalanx (proximal)	6 to 9	1st phalanx (proximal)	6 to 9
2nd phalanx (proximal)	6 to 9	2nd phalanx (proximal)	6 to 9
3rd metacarpal (distal)	8 to 12	3rd metatarsal (distal)	9 to 12
Radius (distal)	24 to 30	Fibular tarsal (proximal)	4 to 7
Radius (proximal)	15 to 31	Tibia (distal)	18 to 24
Ulna (distal)	6 to 9	Tibia (proximal)	24 to 30
Ulna (proximal)	24 to 36	Fibula (distal)	24 to 30
Humerus (distal)	6 to 9	Femur (distal)	24 to 30
Humerus (proximal)	18 to 30		

Fig. 27-2. Radiographic evidence of epiphyseal plate closure time varies between limb joints and among breeds of horses. From Adams (1974).

287

last plates of the limb to close, the radiographic appearance of the distal radial epiphyseal plate may be used as an indicator of fitness for strenuous work such as racing. After closure, change in the stance is difficult if not impossible to achieve without surgery.

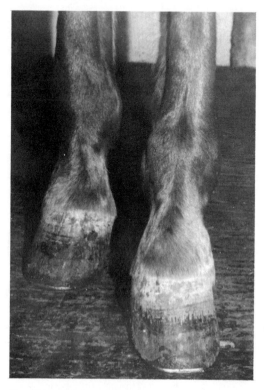

Fig. 27-3. Result of corrective shoeing after the epiphyseal plates close. Note the difference between the medial and lateral hoof growth on the hind feet of this crooked-legged weanling colt.

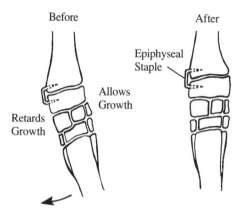

Fig. 27-4. Epiphyseal stapling limits the growth and expansion of the epiphyseal plate on the stapled side. The plate continues to grow and expand on the unstapled side.

Two types of surgery that have received some publicity are epiphyseal stapling and prescribed fracture. Epiphyseal stapling is accomplished by placing a stainless steel staple over the growth plate with the greater angle (usually the medial side). This limits the growth and expansion of the epiphyseal plate on the stapled side and allows it to grow and expand on the unstapled (usually lateral) side. This is not effective unless done at least several months before the epiphyseal plate closes. It takes several months for the limb to straighten using this method. The results are sometimes disappointing. Prescribed fracture is a designed breaking of the bone, usually by drilling holes in it, and then rotating or bending it to the desired position. Of course, the difficulty of keeping the patient inactive until healing takes place makes this technique impractical in most equine cases.

Limitations

Economic reality must be considered when prescribing a correction in cases of severe limb deviations. For humans, we say save life and limb at any cost. But for horses, even though all of us tend to be somewhat anthropomorphic, we must always say, "Save life (or straighten limb) at what cost?" For as Dr. J.R. Rooney points out in his book *The Sick Horse*, consideration must be given to "...cost in terms of money, time, effort, future usefulness, etc....the prognosis is (often) a function of what the horseman is able and willing to do....(Besides,) the owner who says to save the animal no matter what the cost...doesn't care what the cost is, since he has no intention of paying anyway!!" Another consideration must be the limitations imposed by Nature upon us to affect a change. Occasionally, limitations are self imposed by our own lack of knowledge.

Certainly education of horsemen as to the limitations of any corrective measure on horses of more than a year of age is most important to the solution of this problem. Convincing breeders of the importance of mating only horses that possess straight sound legs is another significant challenge. Bone and limb deformities are highly heritable. Predisposition to unsoundness is something that can be better controlled by the breeder than by the farrier. This fact has been

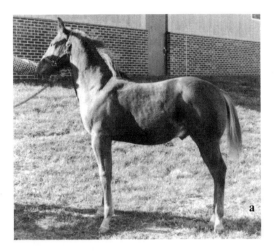

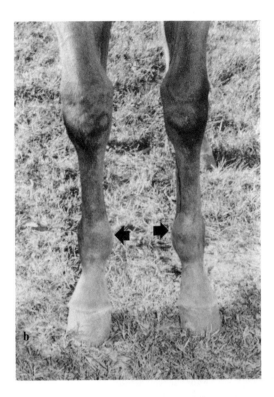

Fig. 27-5. An overfed weanling colt with epiphysitis: (a) side view—note contracted tendons—especially in the hind legs, (b) close-up of front legs—note swelling above fetlock joint.

classically demonstrated to us in recent years by the high incidence of navicular disease in small-footed horses.

The responsibility often falls upon the farrier or veterinarian to educate and inform his clients of the above facts. This presupposes that the farrier and veterinarian know the facts themselves and are prepared to communicate them tactfully to the horseowner. They must appreciate the limitations of the horse as well as their own and then explain these to the owner. Most important, they must get across the idea that a farrier or veterinarian is not a magician that can simply "say the word" and the horse will be arrow straight possessing ideal conformation. Most people are reasonable and will understand that the best a competent horseshoer can do is to help the horse do its best with what Nature has provided.

There are basically only two things a horseshoer can do to help or "correct" cases where limb bone deformities are present resulting in an impaired gait. One is to alter the balance of the hoof by trimming. The other is to alter the stance or gait by shoeing.

Stance Correction

Changing the balance of the hoof by so-called corrective trimming causes a strain at the joints of the limb. The pastern and coffin joints are arthrodial joints (with gliding surfaces) and will give to the limit of the elasticity of their collateral ligaments. The pastern joint is stiffer and has less side to side give than the coffin joint. The fetlock joint has a medial condyle (ridge) on the end of the cannon bone and a matching groove on the long pastern bone and thus will not give laterally or twist.

In the very young horse, the growth plate may be affected by changing or neglecting hoof balance, but after the first year of life bone changes are negligible. Thus, any change made by corrective hoof trimming is of a temporary nature and places excessive strain on the ligaments of the pastern and coffin joints and the articular surface of the fetlock joint. The hoof is often deformed and sheared heels and epiphysitis may result due to the strain of imbalance.

A general rule that applies in all but a few special cases of lateral balance (side-to-side) is to lower the hoof on the side it points. In other words, a hoof that points out, whether it be toed-out or broken-in, would be lowered on the outside. The amount it is lowered is determined by the change desired or thought wise at one trimming.

Always keep in mind you are trying to shift the axis of weight distribution to the center of the limb. Most feet which are out of balance laterally have flares (outward deviations of the wall) which must be removed to bring the foot into balance. Usually flares are on the same side as the foot points, i.e., on the same side which must be lowered. Upper limb deviations may make it necessary to move the shoe laterally or medially to place the weight in the center of the limb.

Flares should be removed to help straighten the foot. When removing flares, it is usually best

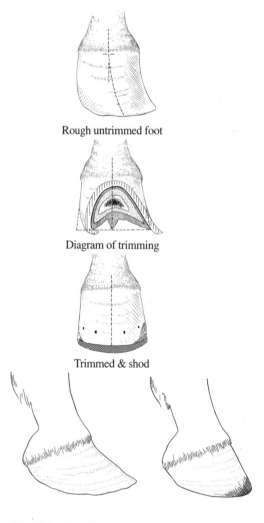

Rough untrimmed foot

Diagram of trimming

Trimmed & shod

Fig. 27-6. The object of shoeing to correct stance is to shift the axis of weight distribution to the center of the limb. A flared toe should also be reduced to correct the axis of weight distribution and relieve tendon stress.

to remove no more than one-half the thickness of the wall at each trimming. This allows the bearing strength of the wall to be retained and thus prevents further spreading or flaring. It also allows a shoe to be safely nailed on the foot. However, flares can be rasped as far down as the white line on severely distorted feet. Horses that are worked must have their feet protected by shoeing after such radical sculpturing. The direction of new hoof growth will follow the consistently-shaped and balanced hoof wall.

Ideal limb conformation and possible deviations from it must be studied and understood to appreciate the merit of various corrective procedures. Generally, the higher up the limb or the farther away from the foot the deviation from the ideal occurs, the more difficult it is to correct (change or compensate for). A deviation at the coffin joint is easiest to correct, those at the knee or hock and higher are more difficult. The principles of correcting front or hind limbs are slightly different because of the difference in action of the knee and hock joints and the function of the stay (reciprocal) apparatus of the hind limb.

Gait Correction

The second general way in which a horseshoer can affect limb stance and gait is by shoeing. Shoes may: (1) prevent wear and thus maintain balance or designed imbalance, (2) have a shape or projection(s) which affects the placement and movement of the foot at the moment of landing or breaking over, and/or (3) increase the flight arc of the foot by the addition of weight. The effect of corrective shoes is temporary. The moment they are removed the horse will usually return to its former gait defect.

Corrective trimming and shoeing may help a horse look and do his best. This is the reasonable expectation of a horse owner. However, the use of shoes of an obvious corrective nature is discriminated against by most horse show judges. Shoes will not create a permanent change in a mature horse. The owner's decision to use them on show horses should be based upon an interpretation of the following questions: (1) Will corrective shoes attract attention to a defect that could be compensated for (and thus go unnoticed) by clever showmanship?, or (2) Will the judge view the use of corrective shoes as an honest effort to improve the horse's performance?

Limb interference poses a different problem. The horseshoer must make a decision to use a corrective measure based not so much on how it looks as how it works. Anything that will prevent the problem from impairing the horse's utility is considered valuable. Several seemingly opposite methods may work on a particular problem. Here again, shoes are a temporary measure and when removed the horse usually returns to his original vice(s).

When shoeing horses for the purpose of correcting conformation stance and confirming or altering gaits, it must be remembered that there are as many variations in conformation, hoofs, and gaits as there are horses. Several horses may have the same fault of conformation or gait, but each may require a different method of shoeing. Methods suitable in one case may be unsatisfactory in another. Even when skillfully done, corrective shoeing should not be represented as a creator of perfection. Its purpose should be to help the horse do its best.

Changes should be made gradually in most cases. Do not try to change the horse's gait too radically in one shoeing, as the added strain on the ligaments, tendons, and joints and other structures of the foot may cause the horse to go lame.

Horses suspected of needing correction should first be observed at rest to determine if any conformational predispositions to faults of gait exist. Then the path of the feet in motion should be studied. The horse should be observed at the gait which will best show the fault of gait (usually the trot) from three positions: (1) going straight away from you, (2) coming toward you, and (3) from the side as the horse goes by you. You may have to observe the horse several times to determine exactly what the feet are doing and how a corrective measure would affect them. A smooth impressionable surface to move the horse over is useful. A video tape camera and recorder is very helpful when available. Slow motion pictures may be necessary to detect the more subtle faults of gait.

The point of breakover on a hoof can usually be determined by examining wear on the ground surface of the wall or the shoe. The point where the center of breakover takes place is worn the

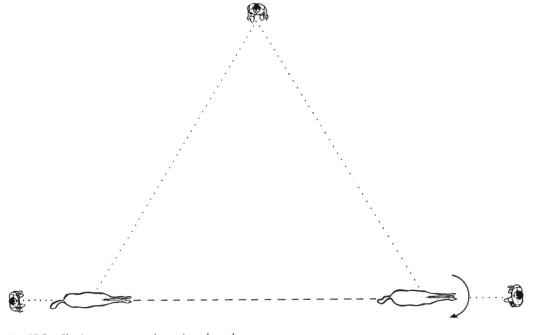

Fig. 27-7. *Shoeing to correct gait requires close observation of the moving horse from three directions while it is moving at the gait(s) in question.*

most. The point of a lateral extension or square-toe should be placed just behind (to the side of) this point for maximum effectiveness in giving lateral support to the toe.

The point of interference may not be observable at the faster gaits or at the moment it happens. However, it can easily be detected by coating the inside of the hoof walls and edge of the shoe with livestock marking crayon, chalk, or lipstick. The crayon will rub off at the point of interference. It will show where the horse is hitting the opposite leg. Such a procedure is useful when determining where to cut away the hoof or shoe or to place a protective pad or boot.

Changes in the angle of a hoof affect its vertical flight pattern. Lowering the heels or lengthening the toe (decrease the hoof angle) decreases the speed of breakover, shifts the center of weight distribution back toward the heels, increases the stride height at the beginning of the arc of foot flight when viewed from the side. Lowering the toe or increasing the height of the heels (increase the hoof angle) increases the speed and ease of breakover, shifts the center of weight distribution forward toward the toe, increases the stride height at the end of the arc of foot flight when viewed from the side.

Most gait problems where the hind feet interfere with the front feet, such as forging, can be corrected by the application of some variation of the principle of "speeding up the front feet and slowing down the hinds." However, each situation must be considered individually and limits recognized (before the horse comes apart!).

Some faults of gait in young horses, especially forging, are simply the result of lack of coordination or lack of maturity. The horse is not "set in his gait." The awkwardness of youth displayed by "green" horses will cure itself in time. Corrective shoes on such horses may be of value to help stabilize the animal until it becomes confirmed in its gaits.

Occasionally there are faults of gait, and even habits of standing, that are caused by an unskilled rider or handler and/or improperly adjusted equipment. Even though the horseshoer has no control over these factors, he must be aware that such problems can exist. When a problem is not obvious, ask to see the horse ridden or worked before shoeing it.

Start at an Early Age

It is much easier to keep legs and feet straight from birth than it is to try to straighten them when they become crooked from neglect or other causes. Good care and management of the foal are a must.

The recommended age to start to trim the foals varies between two weeks to three months, averaging about one month, and then about once a month thereafter. Only severely crooked animals should be trimmed sooner than one month of age. The newborn foal's hoof is still quite soft up until a month or so due to the presence of neonatal horn, and the joints are very weak. Some large horse farms and ranches wait until the animal is at least two months old and has been halter broken and handled a few times. Ideally, foals should be handled enough that they will not be frightened by the horseshoer and will stand for trimming.

Light rasping and rounding of the hoof wall is usually all that is necessary the first time or two that a straight-legged foal is trimmed.

Alterations on the feet of foals which are crooked from the fetlock down should be gradual and consistently maintained. In many cases this will mean rasping the foot every two weeks to keep one side shorter or out of balance over the period of time it takes to make the desired correction.

Foals with conformation defects above the fetlock should be maintained in a balanced condition. Trying to correct upper limb deviation is more likely to create a crooked (wry) hoof and other problems without correcting the original defect. Time is the best treatment for these kinds of problems.

After the epiphyseal plates close, only slight and temporary changes can be made by trimming or shoeing without risk of causing more severe problems. Older horses which have conformational defects above the fetlock should not be trimmed out of balance. Generally, changes that must be made on horses that interfere are incorporated into the shoe design. Corrective shoes are then nailed onto a balanced foot.

Don't Overdo It!

There are many opinions on the degree of correction which should be applied when changing lateral balance. Some (especially Standardbred horsemen) say that a "horse goes the best the way he is naturally made." They maintain that leveling and balancing the foot is all that is required on a young horse, and that he will learn to live with any faults he may have. They are interested in making the horse's foot hit the ground flat at speed to prevent lameness, and do most of their correction with shoe design.

Others (particularly show horse fanciers) consider everything but a pipe wrench to twist the leg to correct horses that aren't perfectly straight, and often carry trimming and shoeing of the foot out of lateral balance to the extreme, especially on young horses.

People who raise Thoroughbreds and Quarter Horses for racing sometimes overdo lowering a horse's heel in an effort to get more length of stride. Bowed tendons often result from such a practice.

Guidelines

Guidelines for applying corrective trimming and shoeing:

1. Start corrections at a very young age, at least several months before the epiphyseal plate is to close at the joint where the deviation occurs.
2. The farther from the foot or higher up the leg a conformational deviation is, the more difficult it is to correct (change) by corrective trimming or shoeing.
3. Avoid changing the lateral balance of the foot more than ¼ inch each trimming or shoeing. It takes time for the ligaments to adjust to a change in lateral balance even when making a slight correction. A horse should not be worked hard for several days after changes in lateral balance or hoof angle.
4. Avoid changing the hoof angle more than 2 degrees each trimming. Exceptions include neglected or chronically foundered hoofs and cases of interference between the front and hind hoofs. Generally, its best to keep the hoof angle parallel to the pastern angle.
5. Avoid removing more than one-half the thickness of the hoof wall when shaping a flared hoof. Exceptions include severely distorted or foundered hoofs where it may be necessary and desirable to reduce the wall to the horny laminae to bring the foot into balance. However, this procedure requires much judgment and knowledge of the internal foot structures.
6. Use the least severe corrective trimming or shoeing method necessary to prevent limb interference. Do not change the balance of the foot or the type of shoe unless the horse is interfering.
7. Keep records of the changes made at each trimming or shoeing. Record the method(s) used, the results and the rate of change. This information is valuable in determining the usefulness of a corrective method.
8. There are few invariable rules in corrective horseshoeing. Even basic principles may sometimes have special conditions or need to be modified by common sense according to a given situation.

Corrective trimming and shoeing are extremely controversial, mainly because they are not well understood. Many of the problems confronting the shoer involving the position of the foot at rest or in motion can be solved by skillful trimming and shaping of the hoof. However, the basic principles of balance and the limitations of both the horseshoer and the horse's body must be appreciated before achieving a solution of maximum benefit to both the horse and rider (owner). There are no shortcuts for obtaining this understanding. It comes only by study and experience.

References

Adams, O.R. 1974. Lameness in Horses (3rd ed.). Lea and Febiger, Philadelphia.

Catcott, E.J. and J.F. Smithcors. 1972. Equine Medicine and Surgery (2nd ed.). American Veterinary Publications, Inc., Wheaton, IL.

Rooney, J.R. 1974. The Lame Horse. A.S. Barnes and Co., Inc., Cranbury, NJ.

Rooney, J.R. 1977. The Sick Horse. A.S. Barnes and Co., Inc., Cranbury, NJ.

Siegmund, O.H. (Ed.). 1979. The Merck Veterinary Manual (5th ed.). Merck and Co., Inc., Rahway, NJ.

Sisson, S. and J.D. Grossman. 1953. The Anatomy of Domestic Animals (4th ed.). W. B. Sanders Co., Philadelphia.

Skewes, A.R. 1966. Stapling to straighten legs. The Blood Horse. 91:776.

Swenson, M.J. (Ed.). 1977. Duke's Physiology of Domestic Animals (9th ed.). Cornell University Press, Ithaca, NY.

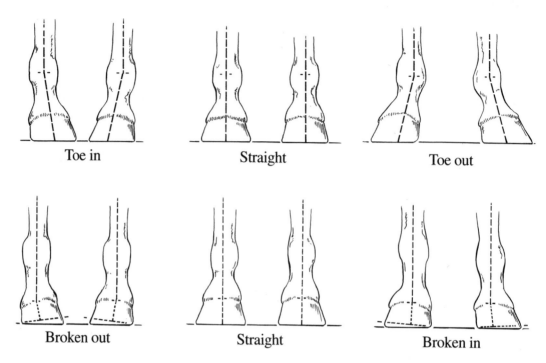

Fig. 28-1. Digit conformation and axis viewed from in front (dotted lines show where to trim).

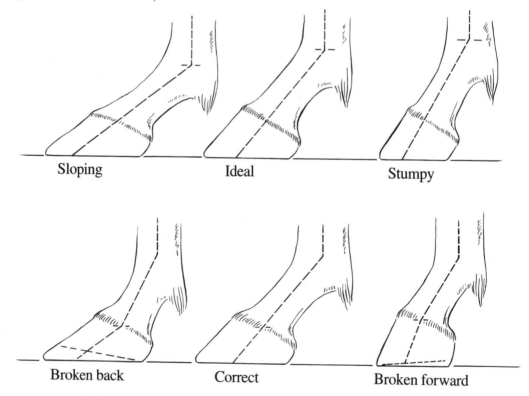

Fig. 28-2. Digit conformation and axis viewed from the side (dotted lines show where to trim).

Chapter 28

Foot Conformation Types

Foot conformation is the result of genetic or environmental effects. Genetic hoof or limb defects may be passed from one or both parents to the foal. In either case, they are highly heritable and are usually passed on to the next generation. Foot conformation defects may predispose a horse to lameness.

Environmental effects may have several causes. The environment of the uterus (congenital) may be responsible for creating some limb defects before a foal is born. Or, the environment after birth (developmental) may be a problem. Nutrition, exercise, hoof care and management all are important to ideal hoof formation.

The horseshoer must learn to define the problem. You must become a critical observer and make decisions about hoof problems. You must learn to judge how far you can go toward bringing a deformed hoof to an ideal condition. A horseshoer changes the conformation of the foot to some extent every time he trims or shoes the horse. You must learn to make that a positive change.

Suggested corrections must be applied with judgment. They vary in degree on each individual horse. The hoof is not a static organ. It is constantly changing due to differences in weight bearing, age, diet, moisture content and injuries. When in doubt about the merits of a particular procedure, it is best to balance the foot and let the horse take care of itself.

Horses have preferences for their right or left limbs. The hoof that is used most will be the larger of a pair. For example, many horses have a slightly larger right front foot than left. A lame horse will often show a difference in size between the lame and sound hoofs. The lame hoof will be smaller.

Digit Conformation Viewed From in Front

Foot conformation may be influenced by a deviation of the axis of the digit. When the digit axis is plumb, straight or ideal, the foot is in balance. When the pastern is toed-in, the foot is pushed out of shape by uneven weight bearing. The outside half of the hoof grows slower and the inside half grows faster. A flare is created on the inside. When the pastern is toed-out, the most weight is borne by the inside of the foot and the hoof is pushed to the outside. Pastern conformation deviations from the ideal are fixed by heredity. They may also be due to improper nutrition or disease. The deviations occur at the fetlock joint. Slight changes can be made only before the epiphyseal plates close in the very young horse. The fetlock joint is not laterally flexible due to its hinge-like structure.

Digit Axis Viewed From in Front

Foot conformation may be influenced by a deviation of the axis of the digit. When the digit axis is plumb, straight or ideal, the foot is in balance. When the axis is broken out, the hoof appears toed-in. The foot is pushed out of shape by the uneven weight bearing. A flare develops on the medial side. When the axis is broken in, the hoof appears toed-out. The hoof is pushed to the outside. Digit axis deviations from the ideal are caused by uneven wear or growth resulting from unequal weight distribution due to upper limb deviations, disease, trauma or neglect. Faulty hoof preparation may also cause axis deviations. The flexibility of the coffin joint permits immediate and sometimes drastic changes to be made by hoof trimming. However, the possibility of ligament and tendon strain should be considered when making changes.

Digit Conformation Viewed from the Side

Foot conformation is influenced by digit conformation or pastern slope. When the pastern is at an ideal or average slope of about 50 degrees in front and about 52 degrees hind, the foot is usually normal and symmetrical in shape. When the pastern is very acutely angled or sloping (for example, 45 degrees or less), the hoof may flare at the toe and have sloping, underslung or weak heels. A large frog is characteristic of sound feet of this type. When the pastern is very stumpy or upright (for example, 55 to 60 degrees or more), the hoof may be short and narrow. The frog may be small and the heels vertical. The conformation of the pastern and hoof is inherited. The foot is said to be in balance when viewed from the side if the toe of the hoof is parallel with the axis of the digit. Hoofs should be trimmed to correspond to their various pastern conformations.

Digit Axis Viewed from the Side

Foot conformation may be influenced by a deviation of the axis of the digit. When the axis of the digit is parallel to the toe of the hoof, the foot is correct or in balance. When the axis is broken back, the hoof appears sloping. The toe elongates and the heels are often bent under the foot. When the axis is broken forward, the hoof appears stumpy. The toe may be rounded or broken off and the heels vertical. Digit axis deviations are caused by uneven wear or growth resulting from unequal weight distribution on or circulation to the coronary band. This may be the result of upper limb deviation, disease, trauma or neglect. Faulty hoof preparation may also cause axis deviations. The flexibility of the coffin joint permits immediate change by hoof trimming. However, the possibility of ligament and tendon strain should be considered when making drastic changes in axis angles.

Ideal Foot Conformation

The ideal foot is one that is functional and symmetrical. The outer surface of the wall is smooth and straight from the coronary band to the ground. The wall is angled about 50 degrees at the toe. The quarters are symmetrical and the heels from the buttress to the bulbs form an angle similar to that at the toe. The sole is concaved, the frog is large, free from disease and in contact with the ground. The heels are open and strong. The front feet are characteristically larger and rounder than the hind feet. An ideal foot is created by an ideal combination of genetics, nutrition, cleanliness, moisture and health. It can be maintained by routine balancing and attention to detail.

Flared Foot

A flared foot has an outward distortion of the hoof wall. It may be lateral or medial or at the toe. Flares are caused by unequal weight bearing on the wall due to neglect or upper limb deviation. Flares should be removed and compensated for at each shoeing. Severely flared hoofs may require removal of the wall down to the white line. Usually, no more than one-half the thickness of the wall should be removed per shoeing. A foot that is flared at the toe is called a dished foot. Club feet may be dished.

Hoof Rings

Rings which circle the hoof wall and are parallel to the coronary band are called fever, growth or grass rings. These rings are normal and associated with nutritional, seasonal, climatic or systemic changes. They are sometimes rasped away on show horses. Wavy lines, especially near the heels, may be the result of founder. However, thrush, yeast infection, low ringbone, side bone, hoof abscesses or uneven weight distribution can cause uneven hoof rings. The rings will be widest apart at the point where growth is greatest. Founder rings are widest apart at the heel.

Club Foot

Club feet vary in severity. They may have an angle of more than 60 degrees with the heels high in relation to the toe. The foot may be knuckled over with the horse walking on the front of the hoof wall. Or, there may be only slight contracture of the tendons causing a concave deformation of the hoof wall at the toe. The horse may be born with the condition or it may be caused by injury or overnutrition. The combination of overnutrition and lack of exercise in young growing horses is a common cause of club feet. Occasionally, surgery involving the desmotomy of a check ligament of the affected tendon is necessary. Usually, reducing the feed intake and frequent shoeing with an extended toe will return most affected animals to normal. Severe congenital birth defects may be helped by some type of "beaked" shoe. The beak is an extended toe which prevents the horse from walking on the front of its foot or fetlock joint.

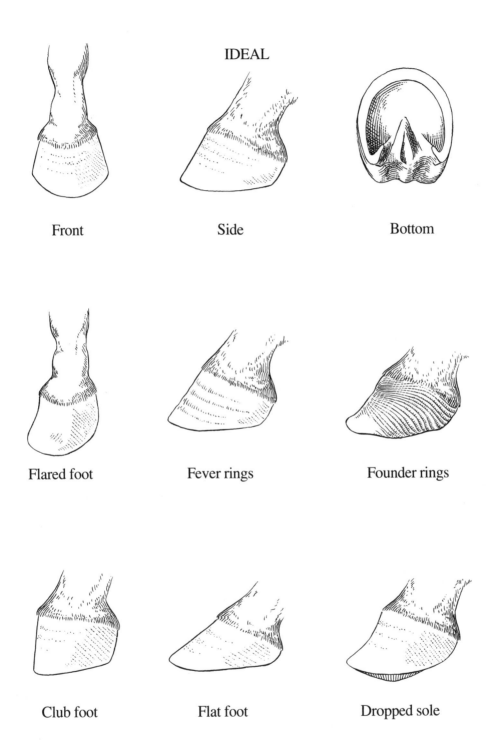

IDEAL

Front   Side   Bottom

Flared foot   Fever rings   Founder rings

Club foot   Flat foot   Dropped sole

Fig. 28-3.   Foot conformations (a).

Beaked shoes usually need heels and may need clips and a band to hold them on, since the hoof wall of a horse with an inherited club foot often is of poor quality. A major consideration with club feet is to make the ground surface of opposite feet in a pair cover the same area. This may require applying acrylic hoof repair material to the club foot at the toe. •

Flat Foot

The sole of a flat foot lacks normal concavity. It usually is very acutely angled and flaring with a long toe and low heels. Horses are sometimes born with this condition. However, many cases are caused by poor environmental conditions. When the ground is wet and the feet are not regularly trimmed, they have a tendency to become flat. The condition is more commonly seen in the front feet of heavy horses and may be related to mild cases of founder. Horses with flat feet should be regularly shod with a wide-webbed shoe. The foot surface of the shoe should be beveled or concaved on the inside so that there will be no sole pressure. Horses to be used in rough terrain should be padded. The wall of flared flat hoofs should be shaped at each shoeing.

Dropped Sole

A sole that has dropped protrudes below the ground surface of the wall. This condition is associated with chronic founder and the downward rotation of the coffin bone. The sole's thickness may be checked by exerting thumb pressure. A thin sole will give readily. It must be trimmed very carefully. The sole should be padded with a full pad of hard plastic or metal. A rim pad may be added between the hoof and pad for extra protection. A wide-webbed shoe concaved away from the sole is also desirable.

Retained Sole

Retained or false sole does not flake away. It grows down with the wall and at the same rate. It is most prevalent in horses with well arched soles. A retained sole may be a desirable trait for a horse that is used in rocky terrain. The extra thickness of sole protects the coffin bone. A retained sole is an undesirable trait for a stalled horse. Anaerobic bacteria create subsolar abscesses that can make the horse lame. Proper

shoeing interval is more difficult to estimate. Toe length records should be kept. Retained sole should be removed from the foot of a stalled horse with the sole knife and hoof knife. After each pass of sole shaving with the knife, press the sole with your thumb near the toe. When the sole gives to firm thumb pressure, you have gone far enough.

Thin Wall and Sole

This condition is inherited and is usually associated with a light or fine hair coat. The sole may need to be padded. Some horses will respond to several applications of turpentine to the sole. This toughens a thin flexible sole. Horses with thin walls will do better with handmade shoes with the nail holes punched fine or close to the outside edge. Shoes should be fit so no outside wall is removed in the shoeing process. Shoes should be punched for the smallest size nail that will hold the shoe in place. Clips are helpful.

Thick Wall and Sole

This condition is usually associated with a heavy or coarse hair coat. It is very desirable.

False Quarter

False quarter is the name given to a vertical indentation in the wall parallel to the horn fibers. These are not true cracks but are the result of a defect in the coronary band. Injuries from barbed wire or other sharp objects heal and produce this type of wall. As long as the wall is closed and does not move, there is no need for special shoeing. However, most feet with this type of problem should be kept moist, balanced and shod.

Cleft

A hoof cleft is a horizontal separation or hole in the hoof wall. Clefts are caused by injuries to the coronary band. The most common are tread wounds from the opposite foot, especially when wearing sharp calks. Abscesses will produce clefts when they break out at the coronary band. Overreaching by the hind feet onto the heels of the front feet will also cause them. Clefts grow down and out of the foot as the hoof grows. When they reach a point where they interfere with nail-

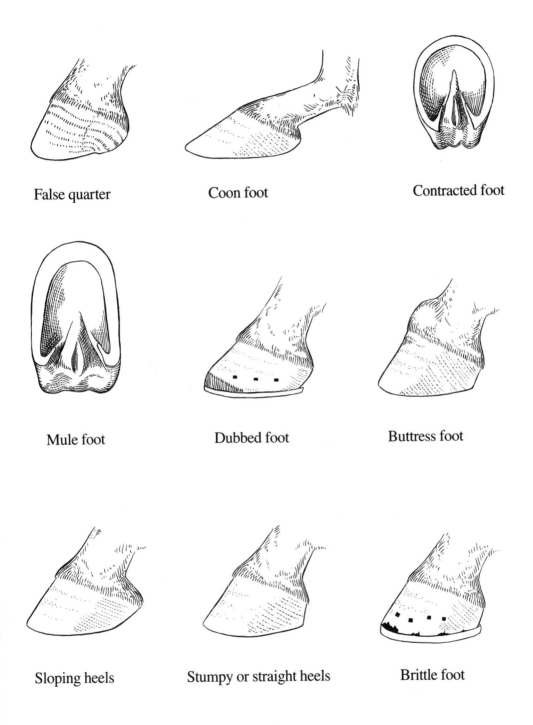

False quarter

Coon foot

Contracted foot

Mule foot

Dubbed foot

Buttress foot

Sloping heels

Stumpy or straight heels

Brittle foot

Fig. 28-4. Foot conformations (b).

ing, handmade shoes with appropriately spaced nail holes may be necessary.

Coon Foot

Coon footedness usually appears in the hind feet. The pastern angle is lower than the hoof angle. It is usually the result of "run down" (a spraining or tearing of the suspensory ligament). A horse with congenitally weak pasterns may have it in all four feet. The condition may also be associated with chronic founder where the horse rocks back on its heels to relieve pressure at the toe. These horses may be helped with run down bandages which support the fetlock joint. They can be shod with an egg bar shoe on front feet and extended heels on the hind feet. Race horses are occasionally shod with a hind shoe called a run down shoe. It has extended heels that are twisted 90 degrees and welded together like an extended egg bar.

Contracted Foot

A contracted foot has buttresses closer together than normal and a frog that is atrophied or smaller than normal. The U.S. Army had a rule which said that a foot was contracted if the buttresses came inside of parallel lines projected back from the first (toe) nail holes on issue shoes. Contraction may be caused by lack of moisture or weight on the foot. Normal weight distribution may be disturbed by foot or limb disease and lack of exercise. Contraction may be in one foot or both feet. It may be on one side or both sides of a foot.

Occasionally, contracted feet are inherited. These small feet predispose the horse to a host of limb unsoundness. Contraction is treated by restoring moisture to the foot and restoring weight bearing to the atrophied hoof structures. Moist clay packs in the bottom of the foot will moisten the hoof in a few days. Anything which improves the circulation of the foot will probably help contraction. A bar shoe that places one-eighth to one-quarter of an inch pressure on the frog is sometimes recommended. Hoof springs and expanding shoes have been recommended, but are usually not practical. The beveled-edge shoe, having the foot surface gradually sloped from the last nail hole back to the buttress, helps the hoof expand as weight is borne by the hoof.

Mule Foot

A mule-shaped foot is narrow and straight in the quarters. The frog is usually large. The horse is born with this conformation. It may be altered slightly by consistent shoeing and adequate hoof moisture.

Dubbed Foot

A dubbed foot, sometimes called a bull-nosed or dumped foot, is a foot with the toe rasped or worn at an abrupt angle. The horseshoer may produce this condition, rasping the foot to fit a shoe smaller than the regular size for the foot. The horse may cause the condition by dragging and wearing off the toe. Lameness of the upper limb, especially the hock, may produce this condition. Properly sized and fit shoes will prevent the man-made condition. Treatment of the lameness may reduce the wear on the toe. The bull-nosed foot with a convex wall surface may be inherited or the result of excessive hoof length. Horses with a concave club foot on one side and a convex bull-nosed foot on the opposite side are very difficult to balance.

Sloping Heels

Sloping heels are very weak and gradually sink causing deformation of the foot. They may predispose the horse to quarter cracks, bowed tendons or navicular disease. Sloping heels can be congenital or caused by neglect of long feet, very sloping pasterns and overlowering of the heel for an extended period of time. The toe must be frequently trimmed leaving all the heel possible. Shoes with extended heels and heel elevation supplied by wedge pads may be helpful. An egg bar shoe is especially useful when the bulbs are near the ground and need protection.

Stumpy or Straight Heels

Stumpy heels are usually congenital and may accompany a club foot. Wire cuts in the heel area and some leg lamenesses may cause them. Feet with stumpy heels should be treated like club feet. The heels of the shoe should end exactly at the point of the buttress and slope underneath the foot. A horse with stumpy heels in front is more likely to pull a shoe if it is not shod short.

Brittle Foot

Brittle, "shelly", or "seedy" hoofs are defective and readily split when nails are driven into them. The hoof wall chips off in layers and separates from the sole near the bearing surface. The condition is associated with seedy toe. The worst cases apparently are inherited. Brittle foot is especially prevalent in some types of Pinto horses. White feet seem to be more commonly affected than black feet. Nutritional deficiencies, filthy stabling conditions and lack of moisture have also been incriminated. The best treatment is frequent shoeing with small nails and clips to prevent strain on the nails. Large broken out areas can be filled in by acrylic hoof repair materials. Horses with hoofs that are susceptible to chronic cracking should be kept shod all the time.

White, Black and Striped Feet

There are sound and unsound feet of any color. There is no evidence to indicate that one color is more preferred to another. Traditionally, black feet have been considered superior to white feet. Striped feet have been said to be superior to both. There are too many exceptions to these rules. Consider each hoof individually. Beware of optical illusions regarding the size of opposite black and white feet. When in doubt, measure them.

Sheared Heels

Sheared heels are a result of uneven weight bearing on the hoof. One side of the hoof is shoved up due to an increase in weight bearing. This displaces the coronary band and causes a distortion of the frog. Severe twisting may cause tearing of the sensitive structures in the heel region and lameness. Weight bearing must be

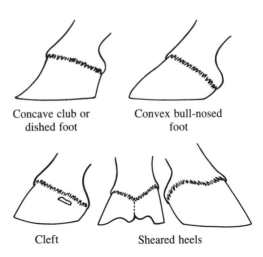

Concave club or dished foot   Convex bull-nosed foot

Cleft   Sheared heels

Fig. 28-5. Foot conformations (c).

equalized on the hoof. Lower the high side of the hoof when the distance is measured between the coronary band and the ground surface. The hoof will twist as weight is placed upon it and eventually the heel will "settle" to its natural position.

References

Adams, O. R. 1974. Lameness in Horses (3rd ed.). Lea and Febiger, Philadelphia.

Butler, D. 1978. Foot notes-shoeing club feet. Amer. Farriers' J. 4(3):68.

Lungwitz, A. and J.W. Adams. 1913. A Textbook of Horseshoeing (11th ed.). Oregon State University, Corvallis, OR.

Moyer, W. and J.P. Anderson. 1975. Sheared heels: diagnosis and treatment. J.A.V.M.A. 166(1):53.

Rich, G.E. 1890. Artistic Horseshoeing. M.T. Richardson, New York.

Ruthe, H. 1969. Der Huf (2nd ed.). VEB Gustav Fischer, Jena, W. GERMANY.

U.S. War Dept. 1941. The Horseshoer (TM 2-220). U.S. Government Printing Office, Washington, DC.

NOTES:

SHOEING THE CROOKED HORSE

Chapter 29

Limb Conformation Types

Bone and limb conformation are some of the most highly heritable traits. Very little if any change can be made in limb conformation by so called corrective shoeing. However, horseshoers must learn to see the source of problems that ultimately affect the feet. Limb problems affect the growth, wear and flight of feet. Conversely, the condition of the feet affects the development and soundness of the limbs.

The epiphyseal growth plates of long bones close at varying times. The plates closest to the ground close first, when the horse is about 3 months of age. All the growth plates are closed in the lower limb before the animal reaches 1 year of age (see Chapter 10). If any change can be made in limb conformation, it must be done before the animal becomes a yearling. Severe

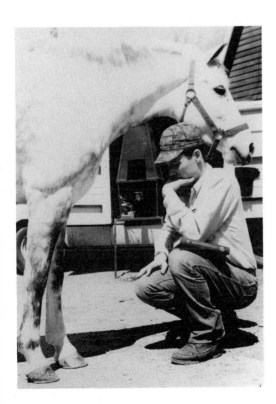

Fig. 29-1. Horses should be observed by viewing the feet first and then evaluating up the limb. Photo by L. Butler.

twisting created by unbalanced hoofs may cause epiphysitis, joint soreness and/or ligament damage.

As a rule, the closer to the hoof the problem is, the more likely corrective trimming or shoeing will be of some value. Limb deviations are best viewed and analyzed from the ground up. High limb deviations are rarely affected by foot alteration.

Accurate and frequent balancing of the hoofs encourages the legs to grow as straight as possible and minimizes the effects of unequal weight bearing on immature bones.

Front Limb Conformation Viewed From In Front

Ideal front limbs are perfectly straight and allow the weight of the horse to be equally distributed over the feet. There is no excessive strain on any structure of the limbs. A plumb line from the point of the shoulders bisects the leg bones, knees, fetlocks and hoofs. Such a horse does not exist. The ideal is used as a standard to discuss and measure conformation deviations.

Toed-out or splay-footed conformation is an outward twisting of the pastern and hoof away from the plumb line. The deviation originates at the fetlock joint. The majority of the weight is placed on the inner half of the foot causing it to wear more than the outside, which flares out. Toed-out horses tend to wing-in when moving, and in severe cases, interfere. The condition is sometimes called toe-wide. However, toe-wide is a general term that means a hoof points out or deviates outward from the plumb line for any reason.

Toed-out can be congenital or it can develop from excessive stress on the epiphysis while the animal is growing. A short-necked, narrow-chested foal that must eat off the ground may make the condition worse. Frequent balancing of the foot to account for differences in wear or growth is necessary. As a general rule, the hoof must be trimmed on the outside to shift weight distribution to the center of the limb. The flare on the outside is removed.

Radical trimming of the outside which places the foot out of balance in an effort to "correct" the conformation defect is unwise. Joint soreness, sheared heels and collateral ligament damage may result. In addition, epiphysitis may also result on young growing horses. Only in rare cases where the owner recognizes the possible consequences and still insists should one trim a horse so that it is purposely out of balance. Usually, it is not worth the risk.

Toed-in or pigeon-toed conformation is an inward twisting of the pastern and hoof away from the plumb line. Greater weight is placed on the outside of the foot causing it to wear more than the inside, which flares in. Toed-in horses tend to wing-out or paddle when moving. Paddling is much less serious than winging-in, since an animal will not interfere. Toed-in conformation is inherited and is usually associated with a wide chest and base-narrow conformation. Frequent balancing of the foot to account for differences in wear and growth is necessary. As a general rule, the hoof must be trimmed on the inside to shift weight distribution to the center of the limb. The flare on the inside is removed. Radical trimming of the inside in an effort to "correct" the conformation defect is unwise.

Knock-kneed or knee-narrow conformation is a deviation of the knees toward each other. The condition may be congenital or develop due to nutritional deficiencies. The feet should be balanced. The feet usually wing-in and may cause high limb interference. If the horse hits or interferes (called knee-knocking) then jar calks can be attached to the shoe. The calks tend to hold the foot and prevent it from twisting at the moment of breaking over. Occasionally, severely deformed foals are corrected by surgery, epiphyseal stapling and/or an externally applied limb cast.

Bowlegged or knee-wide conformation is an outward deviation of the knees from each other. It is often associated with base-narrow conformation. The feet may wing-in or wing-out. The condition is usually congenital, but may be caused by nutritional deficiencies. Rickets are often blamed for this deformity. However, it is very

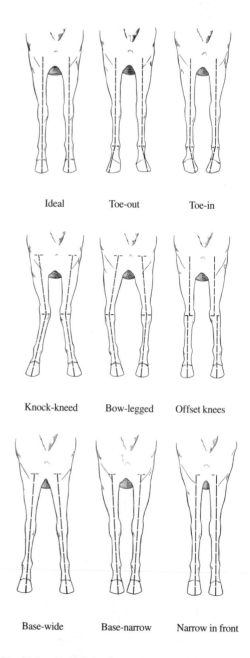

Ideal   Toe-out   Toe-in

Knock-kneed   Bow-legged   Offset knees

Base-wide   Base-narrow   Narrow in front

Fig. 29-2. *Front limb conformation types viewed from in front. Drawings by L. Sadler.*

difficult to produce rickets in the horse. Casting or bracing the limbs may be helpful in some cases. Proper feeding of the mare during gestation and the mare and foal after birth will prevent all but inherited conformation defects. Frequent balancing of the hoof will prevent uneven weight bearing and stress on the limbs.

Offset knees or bench-kneed conformation is highly heritable. The cannon bone comes down from the lateral side of the radius instead of directly under it. Such an animal is likely to develop knee or splint problems. Frequently balance the hoofs to prevent uneven weight bearing on the knee bones.

Base-wide, also called toe-wide, is a deviation of the entire limb outward from the plumb line created from the point of the shoulder to the ground. The feet are farther apart than the points of the shoulders. The feet tend to wing-in slightly at speed. Base-wide conformation is usually associated with a narrow chest and long legs. Feeding and exercising a horse to develop the chest may help the condition. A larger chest reduces the deviation from the plumb line. This conformation may result in limb interference at the faster gaits, especially if it is combined with a toed-out condition. Frequently balance the feet. Usually, more hoof will be trimmed from the outside wall.

Base-narrow, also called toe-narrow, is a deviation of the entire limb inward from the plumb line created from the point of the shoulder to the ground. The feet are closer together than the points of the shoulder. The feet tend to wing-out or paddle slightly at speed. Base-narrow conformation is usually associated with a wide chest and short legs. Frequently balance the feet. Usually, more hoof will be trimmed from the inside wall.

Narrow in front is characteristic of weak, underdeveloped horses. The horse has a narrow chest and legs that are nearly parallel. Such horses are usually limber and may interfere at speed. Their weak condition may be congenital or it may have been caused by poor development due to inadequate nutrition or disease. The feet must be frequently balanced and rounded on the inside to prevent interference.

Base-narrow combined with **toed-out** conformation is a symmetrical multiple limb deviation. The legs deviate inward from the plumb line down to the fetlocks and then they twist outward. It is most common in some families of Quarter Horses. These horses must be properly conditioned before hard work in order to stay sound. The feet should be balanced in relation to the plumb line of the leg. Flares are usually

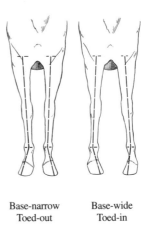

Base-narrow   Base-wide
Toed-out   Toed-in

Fig. 29-3. Front limb symmetrical multiple deviations.

present on the inside of the feet. They should be removed. Shoes should be flat and fit full to the outside. A handmade shoe punched fine on the inside and coarse on the outside works well for this condition. Every effort should be made to get the horse balanced over the plumb line. Only a horse that is interfering should be placed out of balance by trimming or shoeing. The object should be to allow the horse to perform the best it can and stay sound in spite of its conformation. Many horses that have this conformation are excellent performance horses.

Base-wide combined with **toed-in** is a less common symmetrical multiple limb deviation. The legs deviate outward from the plumb line down to the fetlocks and then they twist inward. The feet should be balanced in relation to the plumb line of the leg. Flares may be present on the outside of the feet. The feet should be balanced by trimming and shoeing in an effort to get the weight of the horse over the plumb line. Rarely will a horse with this conformation interfere at speed. However, there is a great possibility of joint damage when a horse with this conformation is worked.

Asymmetrical limb deformities will occasionally be seen. These horses are difficult to keep sound. The weight placed on the limb should be kept balanced over a plumb line drawn through the limb. Shoes with nail holes punched appropriately are a necessity. An evenly worn shoe indicates the foot is bearing weight uniformly across its surface. Shoe position and design may

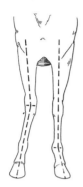

Fig. 29-4. *Front limb asymmetrical limb deviation.*

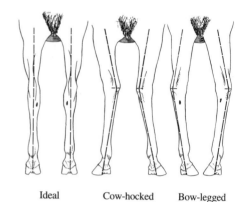

Ideal   Cow-hocked   Bow-legged

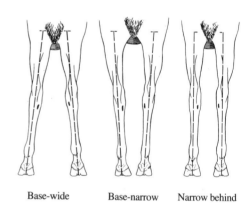

Base-wide   Base-narrow   Narrow behind

Fig. 29-5. *Hind limb conformation viewed from behind.*

need to be changed at each shoeing, especially on young horses, to achieve this uniform wear. Hoof size may change with these types of deformities. The crookedest leg will usually have the smallest foot. Rarely, a horse will be born with one leg shorter than the other. The short leg must be built up (use rim pads) to make it equal in length to its opposite.

Hind Limb Conformation Viewed From Behind

Ideal hind limb conformation shows parallel plumb lines bisecting the pin bones (tuber ischii), the hocks, cannon bones, fetlocks and hoofs. It is said that the weight of the horse on the hind leg is equally distributed over the foot and there is no excessive strain on any structure of the limb. However, the practical ideal that is desired by many horsemen has the cannon bones inside the plumb lines but parallel to one another. Such a horse can move straighter and more efficiently. The hocks are said to be stronger than those of the traditional ideal. When this ideal horse moves, the hocks have a tendency to go out. This is especially true on a young unconditioned horse. Horses with the cannon bones closer than plumb tend to move straighter and maintain sound hocks. The feet should be frequently trimmed and balanced. Often, the inside wall will require more trimming than the outside.

Cow-hocked, or close at the hocks, is an inward deviation of the hocks from the plumb line toward each other. Cow-hocked horses may also be toed-out. These horses tend to wing-in and may interfere. Cow-hocked conformation predisposes a horse to ligament sprain and spa-

vin in the hock region. The condition is congenital and very common, even selected for, in some breeds. Frequently balance the feet. More wall is usually trimmed off the outside. Most wear and wall distortion may be on the inside. Cow-hocked horses are traditionally shod with a square-toe or lateral extension placed on the inside toe. A short trailer is often used on the outside heel to give lateral support to the heel at the moment the hoof contacts the ground.

Bowlegged, out at the hocks or bandy-legged, is an outward deviation of the hocks from the plumb line away from each other. Bowlegged is usually accompanied by a base-narrow conformation. The horse tends to wing-out or "rope walk." The hocks are limber and rotate as the horse moves. Frequently balance the feet. More wall is usually trimmed from the inside. The inside is usually flared. A square-toe or lateral extension on the outside toe may be used. An outside heel calk or blocked heel on a trailer is most helpful.

Base-wide conformation is characteristic of horses with narrow hips and lightly muscled, long legs. The entire limb deviates outward from the plumb line. The base is wider than the origin of the limbs. The feet tend to wing-in as the horse moves. Young horses with this conformation will improve as they fill out and put on weight. Frequent balancing of the feet is usually all that is necessary. Occasionally, fitting the shoe full on the inside will help. However, this should be done only if there is no evidence of limb interference.

Base-narrow conformation is characteristic of horses with heavy hind quarter muscling. It is common in draft and Quarter Horses. The entire limb deviates inward from the plumb line. The horse tends to wing-out or rope walk, sometimes called plaiting. The feet should be frequently balanced. The shoes should be fit full on the outside. Calks are sometimes used on an extended outside branch. A toe calk extended to the outside is often used on draft horses that are severely affected.

Narrow behind is characteristic of weak, underdeveloped horses. The horse has narrow hips and the legs are nearly parallel. These horses usually suffer from a lack of coordination and may interfere at speed. Frequently balance the feet and round the inside wall or shoe. Special attention must be given to feeding and parasite control. Gradual conditioning for work is essential.

Front Limb Conformation Viewed From The Side

Ideal front limb conformation when viewed from the side is said to exist when a plumb line bisects the leg and falls slightly behind the bulbs of the heel. The weight of the horse is equally distributed over the foot, and there is no excessive strain on any structure of the limb. This is the ideal or standard that all other conformations are compared to. The ideal pastern angle in front is about 50 degrees.

Sloping or weak pasterns are usually related to excessively long pasterns. These horses may also have a sloping shoulder and are very smooth

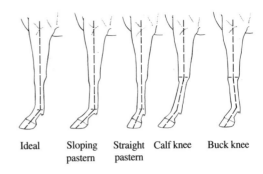

Ideal   Sloping pastern   Straight pastern   Calf knee   Buck knee

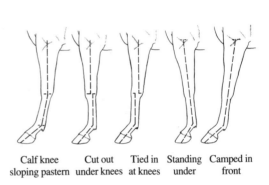

Calf knee   Cut out sloping pastern   Tied in under knees   Standing at knees   Camped in under   front

Fig. 29-6. Front limb conformation viewed from the side.

gaited and comfortable to ride. However, they may be subject to tendon and muscle strain. Frequently balance the feet. As a rule, more toe must be trimmed off than heel. These horses may need to be shod with extended heels to support the leg and prevent excessive tendon strain.

Straight, steep, upright or stumpy pasterns are usually related to short pasterns. These horses may also have a straight shoulder. They are very rough gaited and uncomfortable to ride. This conformation predisposes horses to bone and joint unsoundnesses. Frequently balance the feet. As a rule, more heel must be trimmed off than toe. Rocker-toed shoes and pads may be helpful.

Occasionally, one will see a horse with one front limb sloping pasterned and one straight pasterned. This usually indicates that one leg is shorter than the other. It can also indicate injury in the straight limb. Check closer when you see this type of conformation.

Calf-kneed, also called back at the knees, is a most serious congenital defect. The knees deviate back from the plumb line. Horses with this deformity rarely stay sound when worked. The knee joint is damaged and/or the flexors are strained. Calf-kneed horses should be shod with short toes and a steep angle. Rocker-toed shoes can also be used. Calf-kneed horses are not valuable for breeding or work. The defect is highly heritable. These horses will break down when worked.

Buck-kneed, knee sprung, over at the knees or goat knees, are the opposite of and more desirable than calf-knees. The knees deviate forward from the plumb line. Buck-knees are often selected for in an effort to get away from calf-knees. The feet should be balanced frequently and the heel may need to be lowered due to uneven growth caused by excess weight on the toe.

Calf-kneed and **sloping pasterned** is a multiple deviation that accentuates the seriousness of calf-knees. This is a very undesirable conformation and should be considered an unsoundness.

Cut out under the knees is an undesirable inherited condition. The weight of the horse is not evenly distributed over the bones of the knee. The cannon bone is offset to the rear of the radius and makes a "cut out" appearance just below and in front of the knee.

Tied in at the knees is also a serious inherited fault. The flexor tendons may be constricted and unsoundness may result. The cannon bone is offset to the front of the radius. The leg appears to be "tied in" just below and in back of the knee.

Standing under may be associated with buck-kneed conformation. The entire limb deviates behind the plumb line. This conformation may predispose a horse to forging or overreaching, especially when combined with sickle-hocked conformation.

Camped in front may be associated with calf-kneed conformation. The entire limb deviates forward of the plumb line. Standing under and camped in front conformations are affected by the length and angle of the humerus bone. Camped in front may cause low underslung heels due to the unequal weight distribution on the front feet. The heels of the shoe may need to extend slightly behind the buttress. A rocker-toe may help the action of a horse with this conformation.

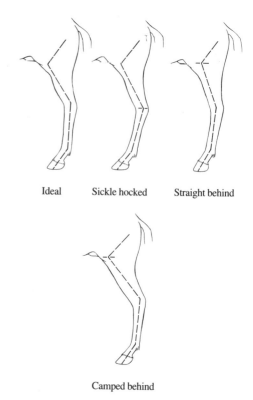

| Ideal | Sickle hocked | Straight behind |

Camped behind

Fig. 29-7.   Hind limb conformation viewed from the side.

Hind Limb Conformation Viewed From The Side

Ideal hind limb conformation when viewed from the side is said to exist when a plumb line dropped from the pin bones (tuber ischii) touches the back of the hock and fetlock and falls slightly behind the bulbs of the heel. Actually, most well conformed horses have the leg (from hock to ground) positioned slightly forward of this plumb line. The hock must be slightly bent in order to function properly. Ideally, the weight of the horse is equally distributed over the foot and there is no excessive strain on any structure of the limb.

Sickle-hocked or saber-legged is a congenital deformity that in its severest form predisposes a horse to curb and spavin problems. However, if it is minor and the hocks are strong and sound, this conformation is considered desirable by trainers of Western performance horses. The leg is deviated forward from the plumb line below the hock. The horse is standing under from the hock down.

Standing under is considered desirable by stock horse trainers. The leg is properly conformed but under the body more than the ideal described. The horse appears collected. Collection refers to a shifting of the horse's weight to the hind limbs when working.

Straight behind or post-legged is a very undesirable conformation defect. The hock receives such jar and concussion that rarely will these horses stay sound when worked. The stifle joint may also be injured on these horses. The excessively straight rear limbs are usually associated with short upright pasterns. Frequently balance the foot and shoe the horse to prevent excessive wear on the toe. Be alert for signs of hock and stifle lameness.

Camped behind is an inherited condition that is considered desirable in some breeds of show horses. Breeders often "stretch" their horses when showing them creating a camped behind conformation. The entire leg deviates back behind the plumb line.

References

Adams, O.R. 1974. Lameness in Horses (3rd ed.). Lea and Febiger, Philadelphia.

Edwards, G.B. 1973. Anatomy and Conformation of the Horse. Dreenan Press Ltd., Croton-On-Hudson, NY.

Goody, P.C. 1976. Horse Anatomy. J.A. Allen and Co., Ltd., London.

Goubaux, A. and G. Barrier. 1892. The Exterior of the Horse (translation by S.J.J. Harger). J.B. Lippincott, Philadelphia.

Lungwitz, A. and J.W. Adams. 1913. A Textbook of Horseshoeing (11th ed.). Oregon State University, Corvallis, OR.

U.S. War Dept. 1941. The Horseshoer (TM 2-220). U.S. Government Printing Office, Washington, DC.

NOTES:

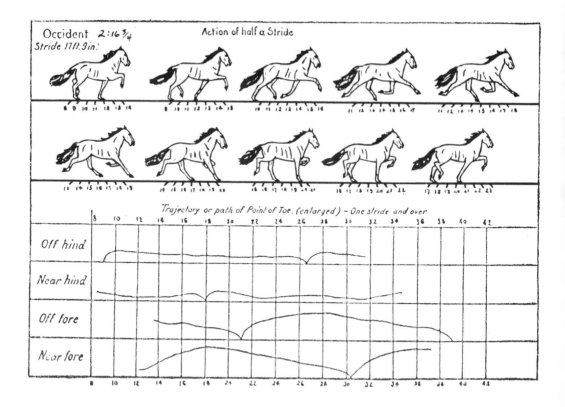

Fig. 30-1. Early gait research by E. J. Muybridge from Jordon (1910).

Chapter 30

The Gaits of Horses

A gait is a pattern of movement or way of going. Gaits may be natural and simply improved and maintained by conditioning. Or, they may be artificial and man-made by training and shoeing.

The gaits of horses can be changed by shoeing. However, improvements are often of a minor or subtle nature. A poor horse cannot be made into a great horse by a horseshoer or anyone else. But a good horse can be allowed to give his best performance. Several exaggerated and cruel practices have resulted from attempts at producing champions from mediocre animals.

Recent research suggests that the natural gaits of the horse are controlled by a "program" present at birth in the motor nerve "wiring" of the spinal cord. Conditioning may improve an individual horse's ability to perform but the program apparently cannot be changed significantly. Effective training and shoeing consists of allowing a good horse to do his best.

A horse's usefulness to man is determined by his ability to move efficiently at the gait desired. Gaits range from the slow and powerful walk of the heavy draft horse to the swift and fluid gallop of the light runner. The horse's body is balanced around its center of gravity at each gait. The center of gravity is located about 6 inches behind and above the elbow in a standing horse. The horse distributes about 60 percent of its weight onto the front limbs and about 40 percent onto the hind limbs. The center of gravity moves forward as the horse increases speed. It moves backward as the horse acquires collection.

Advocates of each breed or specialized type of horse have a preferred ideal form of gait. Recognized judges for each of the types are looking for an animal that matches their ideal. Breeding, Selection, Feeding, Management, Training, Conditioning and Shoeing all must work together to create this ideal. Horse show judges and the clock (in timed events) probably most influence the current form (conformation) and function (gait) of our horses.

Characteristics of Gait

Gaits are characterized by variations in the stride. Stride is the term given to the action of the leg between successive footprints or tracks made by the same foot. A step is the distance between front or hind pairs of footprints. Flexion is the decreasing of a joint angle. Extension is the increasing of a joint angle as the horse moves. Hyperflexion refers to over bending of the joint, especially the fetlock joint.

A stride may be characterized by its: 1) length, 2) height, 3) trueness, 4) speed, 5) sequence of hoofs striking the ground and 6) hoof beat sounds (number and timing) made during a stride. Each of the legs has its own stride pattern. A stride's length is usually measured from the toe of one track to the toe of the next track of the same foot.

A stride's height may be observed from the side as an animal passes by the observer.

Trueness of gait refers to a lack of lateral or medial deviation from the horse's line of travel. A gait that has no deviation is said to be perfectly true. Trueness of gait may also refer to the equal forward and backward swing of the leg and the smoothness of the arc made by the foot when viewed from the side.

Each stride of a horse (pattern of movement of one foot) may be divided into a swing phase and a stance phase. Swing is when the foot is off the ground and moving. Stance is when the foot is on the ground and bearing weight. The time of the swing phase is constant for most animals at similar gaits. The stance phase varies at the various gaits and affects the efficiency of movement.

A lateral gait is one in which the front and hind foot on the same side of the horse move or work together. A diagonal gait is one in which the opposite front and hind foot move together.

Gaits are spoken of as animated, collected, extended, and irregular, or off. An animated gait is one that shows a lot of snappy, rapid, exaggerated up and down movement. A collected gait is one where the horse is compact and working off his hind quarters with precision and control. An extended gait is one where the horse is strung out and covering ground at a higher speed and a longer stride than in a collected form of the same gait. A horse that is irregular or off in his gait is probably lame or very uncoordinated.

The Gaits of the Riding Horse

The **walk** is a slow, lateral four-beat gait. Each foot strikes the ground separately. The average length of stride at a walk is usually less than 6 feet. The horse is moving at about 6 fps (feet per second) or 4 mph (miles per hour). The

track of the hind foot is made just in front of or on the track made by the front foot. Other maneuvers that are precisely executed may be taught to the horse for Western reining and English dressage classes. However, the horse is incapable of delicate muscle adjustments or manipulations.

The **back** is a slow, diagonal two-beat gait.

The **trot** is a faster diagonal two-beat gait. It is very balanced and lameness is often most detectable at this gait. The average length of stride is about 9 feet. The horse is moving at about 12 fps or 8 mph. The horse can maintain this gait for long periods.

The rider may post to a trot. This is required in most English riding classes. Posting is the

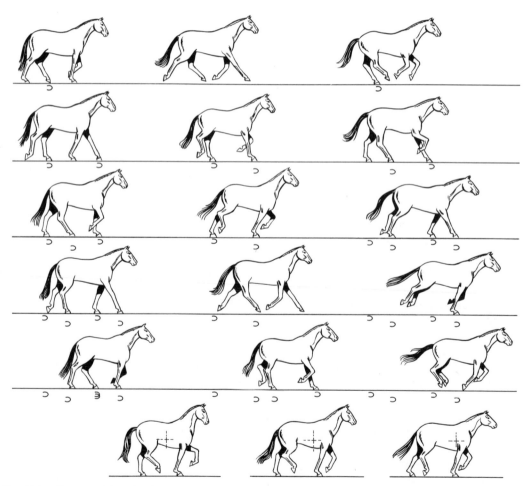

Fig. 30-2. The gaits of the riding horse; (Left) the 4-beat walk, (Middle) 2-beat trot and (Right) 3-beat gallop. (Bottom) Center of gravity shifts forward as the speed increases. Drawings by J. Hoffman and K. Burdette.

synchronization of the rider's up and down movement with the diagonal movement of the horse's legs. The rider may check which diagonal he is moving with by glancing down at the slope of the shoulder. For example, when the right shoulder goes forward, the rider is thrust up by the left hind leg and is on the right diagonal. It is so named because the left hind and right fore make a diagonal line pointing to the right of the direction of the horse. The rider may sit one bounce to change diagonals. Changing diagonals is something the rider does, not the horse.

The rider usually sits to a slow collected trot called a jog. The horse moves at about 9 fps or 6 mph. This form of the trot is required in Western riding classes.

The various breeds of horses have distinctive variations to the trot. For example, the Thoroughbred, characteristically, has a trot in which it carries the feet very close to the ground. They are sometimes referred to as "daisy cutters". Whereas, the Arabian has a very free moving trot with a pronounced dwell when the front feet are completely extended.

The **gallop** is a fast diagonal three-beat gait. It may be collected or it may be extended. The average length of stride is 10 to 15 feet for a slow gallop or canter. (A collected gallop is called a canter in English riding and a lope in Western riding.) The cantering horse travels at about 18 fps or 12 mph. A riding horse going at an extended gallop is moving at the rate of about 24 fps or 16 mph. Its length of stride may be 15 to 20 feet.

The lead leg determines the sequence of hoof beats at the gallop. A horse is said to gallop on the right lead when the right fore track is placed ahead of the left fore track and the right hind track is ahead of the left hind. Usually, a horse that is on the right lead will be traveling an arc in a clockwise direction so that the lead leg is on the inside of the circle. This is referred to as a true gallop. The lead leg supports and propells the horse as the last leg to leave the ground before the moment of free flight when all four feet are in the air. The sequence of beats for a horse in the right lead from free flight is: left hind, right hind and left fore, right fore, free flight.

Leads may be changed by slowing or stopping

a horse and giving various cues as the transition is made back to the gallop. A flying change is made when the horse changes leads in mid-air. This can be effortless and smooth in a well-trained horse.

Horses may gallop on the opposite lead in a straight line or in large circles and still be balanced. This is often done when training horses. It is referred to as a false gallop or counter canter.

A horse is disunited or crossed up when he gallops on one lead with his fore feet and the opposite with his hind feet. This gait is very rough to ride and is hard on the horse. The horse is out of balance and may stumble when turning. When a horse does this during the training process, it should be reined back to a trot and the cues firmly applied as it is pushed into the gallop. Most untrained horses will go disunited during training. Even well-trained horses will occasionally do it with unskilled riders. It may be mistaken for lameness.

The Gaits of Race Horses

Running horses are raced with jockeys and harness horses are raced with drivers. They are conditioned, paced and steadied by their trainers and drivers or riders. They move as fast and efficiently as their individual gait program will allow them.

Race horses place tremendous stress on their feet and legs. The foot of a running horse moving at 55 fps accelerates and stops very abruptly. The stress on the limbs is most influenced by track condition and shoe style. Much stress is due to the unevenness of the surfaces horses race on. Some stress is created by the use of stickers and toe grabs on horseshoes.

The extended gallop or **run** is the principal gait of the running horse. It is a diagonal four-beat gait in its most efficient form. The run is differentiated from the gallop only by an increase in speed. The gallop is a conditioning gait of running horses, not the performance gait. Horses frequently change leads in a race to reduce fatigue and strain. The world record running mile of 1:32⅕ (one minute, thirty-two and one-fifth seconds) was set by *Dr. Fager* in 1968.

Running horses may be divided into Thoroughbred flat track and steeple chase runners and Quarter Horse sprinters.

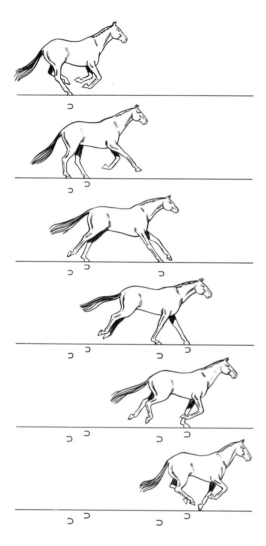

Fig. 30-3. The 4-beat gallop or run.

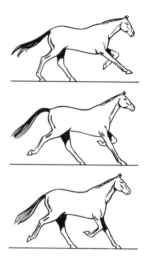

Fig. 30-4. The gaits of race horses; (Top) the run, (Middle) the racing trot and (Bottom) the racing pace.

The average stride length for a Thoroughbred is about 22 feet. Recent studies indicate that a stride of 23 to 23½ feet is ideal and one of 25 feet is rarely any good. Thoroughbred running horses move at about 55 fps or 38 mph, running a quarter mile in 24 seconds or one-eighth mile (furlong) in 12 seconds. This is spoken of as "going at a 12 clip."

Steeplechase horses (running and jumping) move at about 52 fps or 35 mph.

Quarter Horses very quickly reach a velocity of 60 fps and may move at 80 fps (54 mph) when running a quarter mile in 19 seconds.

Harness race horses, usually of Standardbred breeding, may be divided into trotters and pacers.

The extended or **racing trot** is a fast diagonal two-beat gait with the diagonal front and hind feet working together. The racing trot is characterized by extreme extension and length of stride. There is a time when the animal is air borne between diagonal movements. The hind foot hits slightly before the fore foot as it also does in the pace. The feet must slide when they hit the ground to avoid joint strain. The stride length of the racing trot is about 20 feet. The speed of the horse may approach 44 fps or 29 mph. The world record mile of 1:54⅗ was set by *Nevele Pride* in 1969.

The **racing pace** is a fast lateral two-beat gait with the lateral front and hind feet working together. The stride length is about 16 feet. Hobbles which tie the lateral legs together are necessary on most pacers. However, there are some natural or free-legged pacers. Exaggerated side and back motion is required to do the symmetrical pace. Pacers are sometimes called sidewheelers. They are very uncomfortable to ride. Good footing and a light load encourage the pace. Many trotters can be trained to pace. Pacers are usually a little faster than trotters and have less foot balancing and limb interference problems. They may travel at 30 or more mph. The world record mile of 1:49 was set by *Niatross* in 1980.

The Gaits of Show Horses

Many of the gaits of show horses are enhanced by training, artificial appliances and shoeing. In most cases gaits are a characteristic of a breed or type.

The gaits of show horses are characterized by animation. Animation consists of 1) a high elevation of the feet (especially the forefeet), 2) a reduction in relative duration of contact of the forefeet with the ground, and 3) high carriage of the head, neck and tail. Other specific matters of style may apply to each breed or type. Animation is the result of a combination of breeding, training, health, grooming and shoeing.

Three-Gaited Horses are mostly of American Saddlebred breeding. However, Morgan horses are also trained to perform these gaits. Morgans may be shod with less weight than Saddlebreds, since they have rules limiting shoe weight and toe length in some classes. Saddlebred three-gaited horses are shown with roached manes and tails. They are often called walk-trot horses or plain gaited. Three-gaited pleasure horses (a separate horse show division) should have an easy ground covering action without laboring action. They are shown with full manes and tails.

The **walk** is an animated four-beat gait.

The **trot** is a highly collected, animated and square two-beat gait.

The **canter** is a slow, smooth and straight three-beat gait.

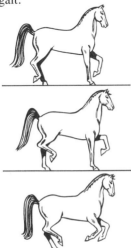

Fig. 30-5. *The gaits of three-gaited show horses; (Top) the animated walk, (Middle) the square trot and (Bottom) the rolling canter.*

Five-Gaited Horses are exclusively American Saddlebreds. They are often called gaited saddlers or society horses. They are shown with full manes and tails and quarter boots to protect them from crossfiring at the rack. Their characteristically brilliant performance has earned them the title of "Peacock of the Showring."

The **walk** is an animated four-beat gait.

The **trot** is a highly collected, animated and square two-beat gait.

The **slow-gait** is a slow, high stepping lateral four-beat gait where the front foot is raised very high, hesitates (dwells) and then lands after the hind foot on the same side. It is performed with great animation and is also called the stepping pace or amble.

The **rack** is a fast and flashy lateral four-beat gait. The foot sequence is the same as the slow gait but much faster and with rounder, ground covering strokes and no hesitation at the peak of flexion. The gait has a beautiful form and is smooth and pleasant for the rider, but very tiring to the horse. Few horses can hold it for more than a few minutes. The rack is sometimes called the single-foot. It is so named because while one front foot is in contact with the ground, the other three are in action off the ground.

The **canter** is a slow, smooth and straight three-beat gait.

Fine Harness Horses may be American Saddlebreds, Morgans, or Arabians. Each breed has its own competitions. The Morgan and Arabian division have Park Horse Driving classes. These breeds have weight and other shoeing limitations. Horses are shown with full manes and an undocked tail. They wear a fine harness with a

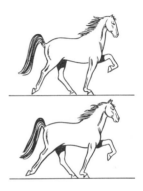

Fig. 30-6. *The additional gaits of five-gaited show horses; (Top) the slow gait and (Bottom) rack.*

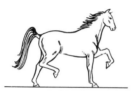

Fig. 30-7.   The animated trot (parade gait) of a parade horse.

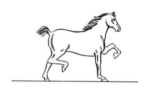

Fig. 30-8.   The very animated trot of the Hackney.

breast strap instead of a neck collar and they pull a light vehicle called a viceroy.

The **animated walk** is animated and graceful.

The **park trot** is an animated gait that is airy and bright. Extreme speed is undesirable.

Parade Horses are mostly of American Saddlebred breeding although any breed may be shown. The palomino or pinto colors are preferred. These horses are shown with silver appointments on fancy stock saddles and colorful cowboy style costumes.

The **animated walk** is a brisk and graceful four-beat gait. It is slow but is not to be a jog or two-beat gait.

The **parade gait** is a high prancing trot. It is a square and collected diagonal two-beat gait. The maximum speed of the parade gait is 5 mph.

Roadster Horses are mostly of Standardbred breeding and Standardbred/Saddlebred crosses are popular. Roadsters are shown in light harness pulling a light two-wheeled bike or sulky. Sometimes they are shown with a road wagon or buggy. Speed at the trot is emphasized. Only occasionally will roadsters be asked to walk and then only to rest.

The **slow jog** trot is a balanced, slow, diagonal two-beat gait.

The **road gait** is a more animated and brilliant but balanced and square trot.

The **full speed** trot done in form and at the command "drive on" is very fast.

Hackney Ponies and Horses exhibit extreme flexion of the hocks and extreme snap and fold in the knees, elbows and fetlocks of the front limbs. Hackneys excel in height, precision and symmetry of action. Hackney ponies are divided from Hackney horses by the 14.2 hand (58 in.) measurement. Under 14.2 are registered as ponies, 14.2 and over are registered as horses. They are almost exclusively shown to a vehicle and

usually have docked (short) tails. They are shown in light or heavy harness. Light harness refers to a breast strap and corresponding harness for light vehicles. Heavy harness refers to a padded neck collar and corresponding harness used to pull heavier vehicles.

The **park pace** is an animated and snappy two-beat trot producing a smooth draft.

The **smart trot** is a faster trot with extreme flexion and fold in the legs. It is done at the command "show your pony." Speed is not as important as form and manners.

Fox Trotters are most popular for trail riding, but are also shown under Western tack. Saddlebreds used to do the fox trot as an optional gait. Saddlebreds, Fox Trotters, Racking Horses and Walking Horses have similar ancestry. Fox Trotters were developed in Missouri.

The **fox trot** is a medium speed diagonal four-beat gait. The hind foot is slightly behind the movement of the diagonal fore foot. The hind foot stays on the ground longer than the fore and it strikes the ground after the fore foot. It is said that the horse is walking in front and trotting behind. Formerly, it was desirable for the hind foot to cap or cover the track of the front foot. Now, overstepping is thought desirable. A good fox trot is easy on both horse and rider. The slow form of this gait is done at 5 mph, the faster speed walk may be done at 6 to 8 mph or more.

Paso Finos are horses developed in the Caribbean and South America from Spanish stock.

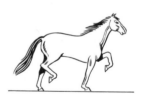

Fig. 30-9.   The trot of the Fox Trotter.

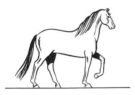

Fig. 30-10. The paso fino gait showing termino (swimming motion with the front legs).

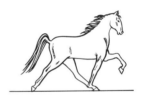

Fig. 30-12. The running walk of the Walking Horse.

They are increasing in popularity as show horses and are shown in traditional tack and costumes. They are to be shown barefoot (hoof length 4 in. or less) or shod with very light shoes weighing under 10 ounces (hoof length 4½ in. or less). Paso Finos are shown at three gaits but may also trot and canter.

The **paso** is a highly collected and smooth broken pace. The front feet wing-out (called termino) and the hind feet wing-in as a result of the characteristic cow-hocked conformation. The paso gait is very smooth and easy on the horse and rider. It is performed at three speeds.

The **paso fino** (fine walk), is a highly collected show gait.

The **paso corto** (short walk), is a less collected, more relaxed and slightly faster gait.

The **paso largo** (long walk), is a long, extended, highstepping speed gait.

Arabians are shown with short hoofs (under 4½ in. overall) and light shoes (under 12 oz.). Most gaits of the Arabian are similar to those done by many of the other light horse breeds. However, the extended trot of the English pleasure and park horse is unique.

The **extended trot** is very balanced; the front legs reach as far forward as the shoulder allows and then hold the extended position momentarily before coming to the ground. This is called dwelling and is characteristic of the Arabian trot.

Walking Horses are bred and trained to perform a very fast and very smooth gait. Walking horses were developed in Tennessee and are

sometimes called plantation horses. Generally, walking horses are shod with excessive weight and length of foot. However, plantation or trail horses are shod with a natural foot and no pads are allowed.

The **flat-foot walk** is the natural walk (faster than normal) of the Tennessee Walking Horse. The horse exhibits a cadenced head motion in both the flat-footed walk and the running walk.

The **running walk** is a fast, lateral four-beat gait characteristic of Tennessee Walking Horses. It is a very smooth, gliding, long striding walk (stride may be 15 to 17 ft.) with the hind feet landing several feet forward of the tracks of the lateral front feet. The front feet may have a step of 6 feet and the hinds of 7 feet or more. The gait is like a pace, but the horse is shod to trot by adding weight and increasing hoof length to break it up into a four-beat gait. The horse may approach 8 mph when the gait is done at speed and will average 6 or 7 mph. A horse that performs this gait well is said to be doing "the big lick." The horse characteristically reaches up under itself with its hind legs and nods its head as it walks.

The **canter** is a smooth rolling motion diagonal three-beat gait.

The flat-foot walk, paso, slow gait, rack and running walk are all lateral four-beat broken pace gaits. They vary in form and speed. Generally, the slower the gait the more up and down motion, and the faster the gait the more stretching of the step and the greater the overstep. Truly great horses can incorporate both features into their stride. There are other more subtle differences. For example, the slow gait and rack differ from the running walk in the way the feet break in cadence. In the slow gait, the break is between lateral fore and hind feet. In the running walk, the break is between diagonal fore and hind feet.

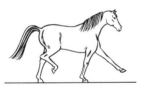

Fig. 30-11. The Arabian extended trot.

317

SHOEING THE CROOKED HORSE

The Gaits of Draft Horses

Draft horses are used at slow steady gaits for pulling a load. Cart horses and coach horses (called hitch horses) may be used at the trot. Halter horses may also be shown at the trot.

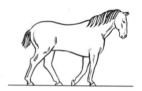

Fig. 30-13. The pulling walk of the draft horse.

The **walk** is a slow diagonal four-beat gait. The step is short in heavy pulling. A front foot usually moves first but most of the pulling is done with the hind quarters.

The **trot** is a slow prancing two-beat gait used in the show ring by cart horses or coach teams on the highway.

References

Bradley, M. 1981. Horses: A Practical and Scientific Approach. McGraw-Hill, Inc., New York.

Chief of Field Artillery. 1933. Elementary Mounted Instruction. The Field Artillery School. Fort Sill, OK.

Dalin, G., S. Drevemo, I. Fredricson, K. Jansson. 1973. Ergonomic aspects of locomotor asymmetry in Standardbred horses trotting through turns. ACTA Vet. Scand. Suppl. 44.

Ensminger, M.E. 1977. Horses and Horsemanship (5th ed.). Interstate, Danville, IL.

Evans, J.W. 1981. Horses. Freeman and Co., San Francisco.

Fredricson, I., G. Dalin, S. Drevemo, G. Hjerten, G. Nilsson and L.O. Alm. 1975. Ergonomic aspects of poor racetrack design. Equine Vet. J. 7(2):63.

Goubaux, A. and G. Barrier. 1892. The Exterior of the Horse (translation by S.J.J. Harger). J.B. Lippincott, Philadelphia.

Hildebrand, M. 1965. Symmetrical gaits of horses. Science 150(3697):701.

Horse and Mule Association of America. 1949. Horse Gaits. Film.

Jordan, R. 1910. The Gait of the American Trotter and Pacer. William R. Jenkins, New York.

Leach, D. 1981. Factors influencing horse locomotion. Amer. Farriers' J. 7(1):22.

Leach, D. 1981. Locomotion in the front and hind limbs. Amer. Farriers' J. 7(2):76.

Muybridge, E. 1957. Animals in Motion. Dover Publ. Inc., New York.

Nilsson, G., I. Fredricson, S. Drevemo. 1973. Some procedures and tools in the diagnostics of distal equine lameness. ACTA Vet. Scand. Suppl. 44.

Plumb, C.S. 1917. Judging Farm Animals. Orange Judd Co., New York.

Pratt, G.W. 1982. Analyzing the movement of the horse. Proceedings of Florida Horsemen's Seminar. 1:52.

Rooney, J.R. 1969. The Biomechanics of Lameness in Horses. Williams and Wilkins, Baltimore.

NOTES:

Chapter 31

Correcting Faults of Gait

Altering foot flight patterns or the timing of gaits generally involves some change in the position, length or angle of the foot. Changes in riding or training technique accentuate any gait changes that can be made. Undesirable gaits can often be improved using a combination of training and shoeing. However, rarely can a severe deviation be corrected to a straight ideal. We must use judgment to achieve a balance between the undesirable effects of the problem and the possible undesirable effects of the solution. Overzealous corrective shoeing (commonly referred to as "jacking horses around") can cause strained joints, ligaments or tendons and muscles.

Limb interference can occur at the various gaits of the horse. Corrective hoof trimming or shoeing are often useful tools to stop limb interference. A slight change in foot flight or gait is usually all that is necessary to allow a horse to clear himself. The old adage, "an inch is as good as a mile" applies when speaking of limb clearance. The goal of corrective shoeing should always be to achieve the functional gait desired with the least degree of deviation from a balanced condition. In many cases, it may only be necessary to bring the horse to a balanced condition to correct the fault of gait or stance caused by uneven growth or wear of the hoof. In other instances the condition of the feet may not be the cause of the problem.

Most of the solutions suggested for correcting faults of gait are either one or the other. They are not to be applied all together. You must judge wisely when choosing a correction procedure.

Your opinion will be most valued as you discover what will work and what won't work for you on the horses you shoe. Keep in mind that the following information is presented as the Author's opinion based on his experience to date.

John Dollar (1898) said:

The necessary knowledge cannot be learnt from books....without much practice and steady observation of living horses, both at rest and in motion, printed instructions are of little value. The best means of all is study under the direction of a competent teacher, who will amplify his lectures by demonstrations on the living animal.

The horse should be observed walking and trotting directly away from and toward you and from the side. The horse handler should be instructed to first walk and then trot the horse straight away from you and back to you. It often helps if you point to some distant object and ask him or her to go toward it and then come back to you. The lead rope should be held about 18 inches from the halter with sufficient slack to allow the head freedom to move. The handler should stand to the side of the horse's head and in line with its ears. When turning, the horse should be pushed away from the handler for safety's sake.

Foot Flight Patterns Viewed from in Front or Behind

Ideal or straight foot flight patterns are the result of perfectly straight leg and foot confor-

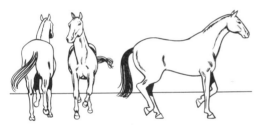

Fig. 31-1. The horse should be observed moving away from you, toward you and from the side.

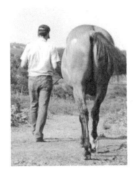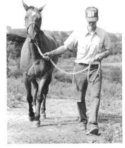

Fig. 31-2. Viewing the horse moving on the line.

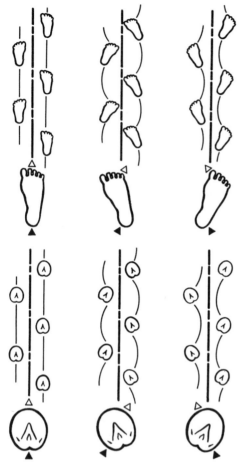

Fig. 31-3. Foot flight patterns result from conformation and breakover point in humans (top) as well as horses (bottom).

mation allowing the hoof to breakover in the center of the toe. However, perfect does not exist. So, we use the ideal to measure and discuss existing conditions. An animal possessing near ideal conformation and gait would be the result of perfect genetic and environmental conditions. Regular hoof care and balancing are a vital part of an ideal environment.

Winging-In is usually associated with a toed-out conformation. The feet usually breakover the inside of the toe and move in an inward arc. In severe cases, interfering results. Mild cases are usually caused by a base-wide conformation in the front or hind feet. Severe cases may be due to a toed-out condition in front or a cow-hocked condition behind.

Front feet may be helped by lowering the outside of the hoofs to bring them into balance, the use of rocker-toed or square-toed shoes, or lateral extension-toed shoes. Use the least severe measure that gets the results desired.

Hind feet may be helped by lowering the outside of the hoofs and applying square-toed shoes with lateral (outside) trailers (projections). A trailer on the outside heel of a shoe provides lateral support and braking action to the hind foot. A lateral extension-toe may be used on the inside toe in place of a square-toe on a winging-in horse.

Winging-Out is usually associated with a toed-in conformation. Winging-out is often called

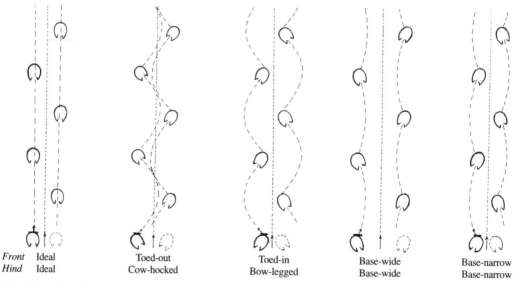

| Front | Ideal | Toed-out | Toed-in | Base-wide | Base-narrow |
| Hind | Ideal | Cow-hocked | Bow-legged | Base-wide | Base-narrow |

Fig. 31-4. Foot flight patterns viewed from in front or behind.

paddling. It is not considered as serious as wing-ing-in. However, it is more easily seen by the horseowner and therefore causes undue alarm. A horse paddling in front rarely interferes. The feet usually breakover the outside of the toe and move in an outward arc. Mild cases are caused by a base-narrow conformation. Severe cases may be due to a toed-in condition in front or a base-narrow condition behind. Some cases of winging-out in front, especially when unilateral, are the result of habits formed due to lunging, ponying (leading from a horse), or hot walking in one direction. Heavy shoes and unbalanced riding can also cause winging-out. Base-narrow behind horses may actually "rope walk". This condition is usually accompanied by weak hocks and may produce hind limb interference at the trot or crossfiring at the pace.

The front feet of a horse that wings-out may be helped by lowering the inside of the hoof to bring it into balance. The use of more severe measures including corrective shoes should be done only at the request of the owner.

The hind feet of a horse that wings-out may be helped by lowering the inside of the hoofs, lateral extension-toed shoes (extension on out-side toe) or square-toed shoes. Calks are turned on the outside shoe branches. They are trailered (turned) outward to provide lateral support to the heels and delay the twisting of the foot.

Foot Flight Patterns Viewed from the Side

Ideal elevation of a hoof during flight creates efficient movement. The foot breaks over easily, is carried in a rounded arc (stroke) at a moderate height between the elbow and the ground, and lands easily. Ideal elevation is a product of an ideal hoof axis (for example, 50 degrees) and an ideal pastern and shoulder angle. The action (elevation) of the front feet is normally higher and more exaggerated than that of the hind feet. However, the action of one foot affects the action of the others.

Vertical Breakover, Horizontal Landing is characteristic of a very acute-angled or sloping hoof and pastern axis (for example, 45 degrees or less). The shoulder will also be sloping and may equal the pastern angle. The foot stays on the ground longer and breaks over in a snappy

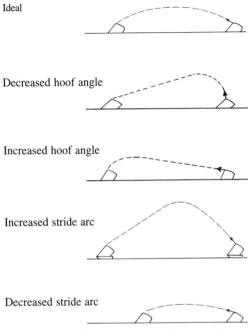

Fig. 31-5. *Foot flight patterns viewed from the side.*

manner. This results in higher action or fold than the ideal. More leverage is necessary to break-over. This results in increased strain and a higher initial stride arc. The foot lands easily producing little concussion. The toe may grow faster than the heel and must be trimmed to prevent strain on the deep flexor tendon and navicular bone. The heels may be raised by wedges or calks. The heels may be prevented from sinking with a bar shoe.

Horizontal Breakover, Vertical Landing is characteristic of an upright or stumpy hoof and pastern axis (for example, 55 degrees or more). The shoulder is usually steep as well. This con-formation produces concussion. The foot breaks over fast resulting in less action or fold than the ideal and increased elevation near the end of the stride arc. The decreased leverage required re-sults in decreased strain and a lower initial stride arc. The foot reaches high and lands hard, in-creasing concussion. The heels can be trimmed in an effort to transfer some of the concussion to the flexor tendons. Pads may be used to lessen concussion.

Increased Stride Arc is characteristic of show horses shod with extra toe length and added weight. The foot stays on the ground due to weight, length and angle and then breaks over relatively fast due to a rolled-toe and training. This results in a snappy action and high initial elevation. The snappiness of the breakover and resulting action is referred to as animation or motion. The increased leverage required to move the foot and/or the unsteadiness created by long feet and roller-motion shoes results in increased tendon strain. Momentum developed by the increased mass and weight of the foot increases the elevation and may lengthen the stride at speed. This effect is produced through a combination of breeding, training, conditioning and shoeing.

Decreased Stride Arc is characteristic of a lame horse. The foot breaks over and is raised with difficulty, has a decreased elevation and decreased length of stride.

Foot Flight or Stride Alteration

The stride (foot flight) of a horse may be shortened by fatigue or lameness. Ideally, a horse will bear its entire weight on each supporting foot when performing each gait. If a horse becomes fatigued or sore, it may take shorter strides in anticipation of pain upon hoof impact. Forward speed and ground surface also affect stride length.

If a horse with an average stride of 24 feet steps short just 1 inch on each stride in a 12 furlong (1½ mi.) or 330 stride race, there will be a loss of 330 inches. This amounts to more than a 9 yard or three length loss. If a horse went 4 inches short in each stride, at the same distance it would lose 13 lengths. The above figures are based on experiments reported by Miles (1846).

Shoe weight should be proportioned to the weight and work of the animal. Race horses are shod with the lightest shoes possible in an effort to prevent fatigue. It has been said that 1 ounce at the toe equals 1 pound at the withers. Recent research shows that 1 ounce on the foot may be more like 30 ounces on the withers (Pratt, 1982).

Show horses are shod with heavy shoes to produce animation. The acceleration and momentum resulting from the weight increases the stride arc, not necessarily the stride length. Even with careful conditioning, these horses fatigue quickly.

A horse shod with shoes weighing 32 ounces each and traveling at a jog has been shown to lift its feet (all round) once each second or 60 times in a minute. If the horse lifts each foot 60 times per minute and each foot weighs 2 pounds, then the horse lifts 480 pounds per minute. In one hour the horse will lift over 14 tons, in five hours it will lift 72 tons. The possibility of injury due to the fatigue caused by excessive weight on the feet is directly related to the rate of speed. The above figures are based on work reported by Russell (1899).

In general, the lightest shoe that will give reasonable wear and support to the foot for the use desired is the most practical. Show horses and race horses are exceptions on each end of the spectrum.

Most cases of limb interference can be improved by corrective shoeing. For occasional interference, protective boots are often more desirable than changing hoof angles or shoe designs. Many limb interference problems can be improved by skilled riding or driving. Some horses cannot be corrected, others will improve only temporarily. A few will require assistance from the veterinarian. Good judgment must be developed in order to tell what should be done about a problem.

Limb Interference at the Walk and Its Correction

Stumbling is interference with the ground. The horse may have a clumsy gait and trip or stumble. The hoof may be long and need trimming. Various methods of increasing the breakover speed may be used including rounding a shortened toe on a barefoot horse, or applying extra light rocker-toed shoes to a short hoof trimmed to an angle steeper than the natural pastern angle. Young horses that are unconfirmed in their gaits may stumble, especially when they get fatigued. Collected horses take time to train. Spurs may help a lazy horse that drags its feet. A balanced rider with common sense can stop most stumblers.

Stumbling

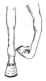

Brushing

Brushing is a mild form of interfering or overreaching. At a faster gait, the horse would probably interfere. Mild forms of correction procedures used for interference and overreaching are usually effective. Interfering or overreaching are rare at the walk.

Limb Interference at the Trot and Its Correction

Interfering is interference between opposite limbs. The shoe or foot strikes the inside of the opposite leg anywhere from the foot to the knee or hock. Interfering most commonly occurs in the fetlock area. Brushing is a mild form of interfering.

There are several approaches to preventing interfering. Horses that interfere may breakover the side of their front or hind hoofs. This can be detected by examining the wear on the hoof or shoes. Lateral support of the toe at the moment of breakover can be achieved by a square-toed or lateral extension-toed shoe. Horses that interfere behind may land on the outside heel of their hind hoofs. Lateral support of the heel at the moment of landing can be achieved by fitting the shoe full on the outside and turning a trailer at the outside heel.

The flight pattern of the feet will need to be widened in some cases of interfering. The foot flight pattern of toed-out front feet may be widened by lowering the outside wall and rasping off flares, especially those on the inside of the hoof. Corrective shims or wedges may be used in extreme cases to increase the distance between the limbs during movement. Jar calks or grabs may be attached to the shoe to prevent twisting

of the hoofs at the moment of breakover. To widen an interfering horse with cow-hocked conformation behind, similar techniques can be used in conjunction with square-toed shoes. To widen an interfering horse that has bowlegged or base-narrow conformation behind, a calk on a trailer fit full on the outside branch is effective. A lateral extension-toe on the outside toes may also be needed. In addition, flares on the inside of the hoof should be reduced. The inside half of the hoof may be trimmed slightly lower than the plane of balance.

Horses that interfere only occasionally in hard going or on turns should not be trimmed or shod out of balance. Rather, they should be protected from injury by interfering boots or making a shoe safe by rounding and hot rasping the edge that may cause damage. The shoe can also be set under the wall or cut out in the area where it is likely to hit. Fatigued horses commonly interfere. Extra light or aluminum shoes may help. However, the rider or driver must learn each individual horse's limit and avoid exceeding it. Traces of unequal length or uneven pulling on the reins may cause a driving horse to interfere.

Forging is interference between the bottom of the front shoe and the toe of the hind shoe on the same side. Forging may be identified by a clicking sound. It can be seen when a horse is viewed from the side at a fast trot.

Conformation is a common cause of forging. Horses that have short backs and long legs, or that stand under, or that have long hind legs and short front legs, should be suspected as forgers. Horses that are shod infrequently will often forge when their hoofs become too long.

The principle behind many of the techniques used to stop a horse from forging may be summed up in the phrase "speed up the front feet and slow down the hind feet." The breakover of the front feet can be speeded up by increasing the angle of the toe and/or using an extra-light rocker-toed shoe. The breakover of the hind shoe can

Interfering

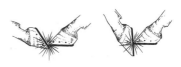

Forging

be slowed down by decreasing the angle of the toe and by using a shoe with extended heels. Leaving the toe of the hind foot ¼ inch longer than the toe of the front foot will help create this effect.

Removing the noise may be enough to stop some horses who have the forging vice. This can be done by squaring the toe of the hind shoe and fitting it back under the toe. The edge of the overhanging wall is rounded. The shoes can also be removed to temporarily stop the noise.

The principle of speeding up the front and slowing down the hind feet doesn't always work. An alternative procedure is to increase the elevation and decrease the forward extension of the hind feet. This may be done by applying heel calks and a rocker-toe to the hind feet. A Memphis bar placed between the first and second nail holes is sometimes used on gaited horses for this purpose. Another possibility is to increase the elevation and forward extension of the front feet. A heavier shoe with a rolled or rocker-toe will cause this effect. The momentum created by the additional weight increases the stride arc.

Many horses forge due to poor horsemanship. The saddle may be positioned incorrectly on the back or the forward speed of the horse may be incorrect for the degree of collection. The horse may be overworked and fatigued or the rider may be out of balance and only a passenger instead of a rider. These things can be corrected without changing the shoeing.

Overreaching is interference between the toe of the hind shoe and the bulb or heels of the front shoe on the same side. In severe cases, the bulbs of the front heels may be damaged and/or the shoes may be wrenched off the front hoofs.

The principles of correcting overreaching are the same as for forging. In addition, the heels or the front shoes should end at the buttresses and be beveled to the slope of the heel of the hoof. Spooned heels or spurs extending toward the bulbs may be drawn from or welded to the

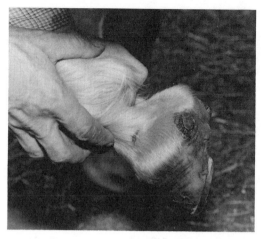

Fig. 31-6. An overreach wound on the bulb of the left front foot.

heels of heavier shoes to prevent shoe pulling.

Overreach boots or bell boots should be worn by horses that have a tendency to damage themselves. Horses that overreach only occasionally when they get out of balance due to a sudden change in terrain or position (such as may happen when roping or jumping), should be protected by overreach boots.

Scalping is interference between the toe of the front foot and the coronary region of the hind foot on the same side. The top of the hoof is known as the hoof head. Damaging this area is therefore called scalping. High scalping (in the pastern area) is often called speedy-cutting. Interference of front and hind legs on the same side may be progressively visualized by noting that overreaching occurs when the front foot is on the ground, forging immediately after breakover, and scalping when the front foot is flexed. Scalping correction by shoeing follows the same principles as forging.

Scalping damage, which mostly occurs in trotting harness race horses, can be prevented by using scalping boots. These are elastic and held in place by the hind hoof. They protect the hoof head or coronary region. Speedy-cut boots protect the pastern and cannon regions and may be used to prevent damage from high scalping.

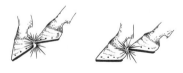

Overreaching

Scalping

Knee-hitting

Knee-hitting, also called knee-knocking, is interference between the inside of a front foot and the knee region of the opposite leg.

In most cases, a foot must twist at the moment of breakover in order to come in enough to strike the knees. Grabs or jar calks welded or brazed on in the direction of movement will delay the twisting of the foot in firm ground. Borium spots can also be used. They are especially good on very hard ground. Borium can be put on small rivets and attached to aluminum shoes. Studs (round screw-in or drive-in jar calks) can also be used on any style shoe. Jar calks or borium spots hold the foot on the ground for an instant at the moment of breakover and reduce the amount of twisting. Square-toed or lateral extension-toed shoes may also be used to make it easier for the foot to breakover in the center of the toe. If it is necessary to widen the foot flight pattern of the front feet, they may be trimmed or shimmed out of balance. Usually, the inside is lowered and/or the outside is shimmed. However, no set rule can be given. Experimentation on each horse is necessary. Sometimes, four short jar calks or grabs are used (two on each branch) on harness horses. Usually, one long grab is placed on the outside toe and one short one on the inside heel on gaited horses.

Damage to the knees of horses that occasionally hit their knees at speed and in turns can be prevented by the use of knee boots. Suspenders which pass over the withers are used to hold knee boots in the proper position on the inside of the knees.

Elbow-hitting is interference between the shoe and the elbow of the leg it is on. This condition may cause a horse to develop a capped elbow or shoe boil.

The height of foot flight or fold can be decreased by reducing the weight of the shoe and increasing the hoof angle or raising the heels. A faster breakover with less momentum helps many elbow hitters. Extending the stride by slacking the reins and changing speed may also help.

Elbow hitting

Damage to the elbows may be prevented at speed by elbow boots held up by suspenders. Shoes may be removed, but this is usually not possible on a performance horse. Horses that damage their elbows in the stall when they fold their legs under themselves may be protected by a sausage-shaped shoe boil boot that fastens around the pastern.

Limb Interference at the Pace and Its Correction

Crossfiring is interference between opposite (diagonal) front and hind feet. This fault of gait may occur at the true two-beat racing or road pace or at any of the broken four-beat gaited horse paces at speed. Principles of correction vary depending on the performance speed and type of horse.

Crossfiring frequently occurs on horses that toe-out or are base-wide in front and toe-in or are base-narrow behind. The front moves inward on the first part of its stride and the opposite hind foot moves inward during the last part of its stride. Crossfiring occurs when the feet meet as both feet are off the ground. The twisting of a pacer's back and the pendulum effect of the feet hanging from the suspended horse accentuate this fault of gait.

The foot flight pattern or outward arc of the hind feet may be widened enough to miss the front feet by applying a side weight on the outside of the hind shoes. The momentum created by the weight and the resulting increased stride arc is enough to cause the hoofs to miss each other. The side weight can be combined with an outside lateral extension-toe. Such a shoe was a common means of correction for crossfiring car-

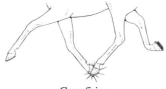

Crossfiring

riage horses early in this century. A more common means of correcting crossfiring pacing harness race horses of today is to use a half-round half-swedge shoe on the hind feet. This widens the foot flight pattern of the hind feet. The outside swedge with a sharp outer rim tends to hold the foot on the ground and slightly delays breakover. The inside half-round portion of the shoe encourages the horse to break toward the inside and prevents damage.

Other alternatives include speeding up the breakover of the front foot with a half-round shoe or a rocker-toed shoe, widening the foot flight pattern of the front feet by lowering the outside wall and/or applying a low calk to the inside branch. Shoes may be set under the inside wall where it is hitting and the inside shoe branch can be hot rasped smooth.

Prevention of damage to the front shoes of a crossfiring gaited horse may require spoons or spurs extended up from the heels against the bulbs of the foot. Padded overreach or quarter boots are also worn.

A severe form of crossfiring which could be called scalping, is rare. If conventional methods of treating crossfiring and speeding up the front and slowing down the rear fail, irritation between the hind legs with a special harness or irritant may be necessary to train a horse to travel wider.

Limb Interference at the Gallop and Its Correction

Speedy-cutting is high limb interference at speed. Usually the inside of the hind leg is "cut" by the front leg on the same side. However, the inside of the front leg is sometimes injured by the hind leg on the same side. High scalping in the pastern area at the trot is also called speedy-cutting by harness horsemen.

Horses that speedy-cut only rarely when they are accidentally bumped or in a turn, on unbanked turns, or in loose and/or slippery footing should be protected by speedy-cut boots. Boots may need to be individually tailored to each horse to protect the specific site where it hits.

Each horse folds its feet at the gallop in a slightly different way. The placement of the limbs when running must be determined for each horse. Some horses fold their front limbs between their

Fig. 31-7. Corrective shoes for various faults of gait and foot conditions.

1. *RF Aluminum Racing Plate with Toe Grab*
2. *LF Aluminum Racing Plate with Toe Grab*
3. *RH Aluminum Racing Plate with Toe Grab and Heel Sticker*
4. *LH Aluminum Racing Plate with Toe Grab and Heel Sticker*
5. *"Level Grip" Front Aluminum Racing Plate*
6. *Aluminum Racing Plate with Toe Grab and Blocked Heels*
7. *Hand-Swedged Steel Racing Plate*
8. *Hand-Swedged Steel Racing Plate with Forge-Brazed on Toe Grab and Hand-Turned Block and Sticker*
9. *Full-Swedged Bar Shoe (high outer rim)*
10. *Half-Swedge, Half-Round Hind Shoe with Trailer*
11. *Half-Round Front Bar Shoe*
12. *Half-Round Hind Shoe with Trailer*
13. *Flat Hind Shoe*
14. *Knee-Knocker Shoe*
15. *Full-Swedge Egg Bar Shoe*
16. *Front Steel Training Plate Rim Shoe*
17. *Flat Shoe with Creased Square-Toe*
18. *Half-Round Front Shoe*
19. *RH 15 oz. Side-Weight with Trailer*
20. *Ice or Sharp Shoe*
21. *Half-Shoe with Heel Pad*
22. *Pony Shoe*
23. *Draft Shoe*
24. *Plate with Roadster Pad*
25. *Plate with Borium Spots*
26. *Front Saddle Horse Plate*
27. *Hind Shoe with Calks and Clips*
28. *Keg Hind Sliding Plate*
29. *Handmade Hind Sliding Plate with Rocker-Toe and Spooned Heels*
30. *Front Saddle Horse Rim Shoe*
31. *Polo Plate (high inside rim)*
32. *Steel Training Plate*
33. *Square-Toe with Trailer and Inside Blocked Heel*
34. *Rocker-Toe with Swelled Heels (Roller Motion Shoe)*
35. *Lateral Extension with Swelled Heel*
36. *Heart-Bar Shoe with Rocker-Toe*
37. *Keg Bar Shoe with Rolled-Toe*
38. *Handmade Bar Shoe with Rocker-Toe and Jar Calks*
39. *Bar Shoe with No Nail Holes in Quarter*
40. *20 oz. Toe-Weight with Rolled-Toe*
41. *20 oz. Hind Toe-Weight with Memphis Bar and Calk*
42. *18 oz. Heel-Weight with Welded-Toe*
43. *Shoe for Stifled Horse to Prevent Weight Bearing*
44. *30 oz. Toe-Weight with Rolled-Toe*
45. *EEL 8 oz. Hind Shoe*
46. *14 oz. Creased Pony Toe-Weight with Rolled-Toe*

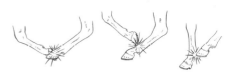

Speedy-cutting

hind limbs. Others fold their hind limbs between their front limbs. Many fold one front leg between the hind legs.

The hind foot flight of a running race horse can be widened by lowering the inside of the hoof and placing a calk (sticker) on the outside

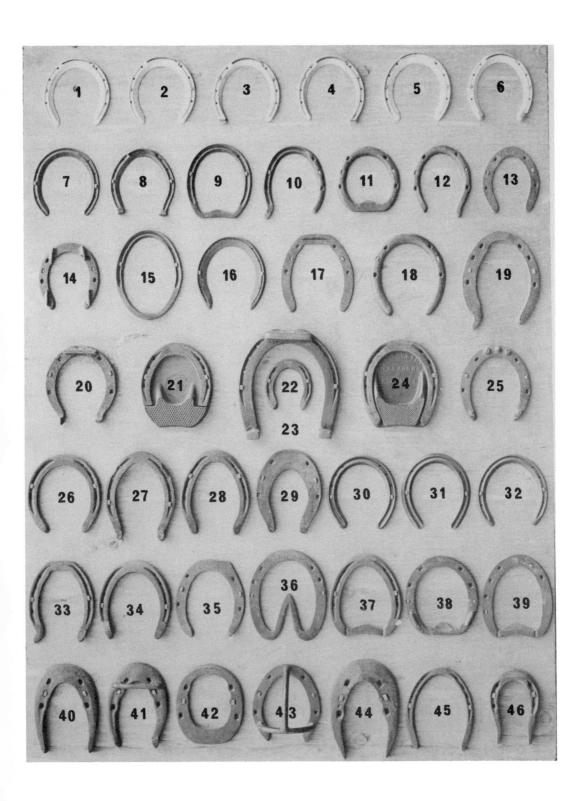

heel. The hind foot flight pattern can be narrowed by lowering the outside of the hoof and placing a calk or sticker on the inside heel. This can be achieved by reversing rear aluminum racing plates with a sticker. The toe grabs of front or hind racing plates can be ground at an angle to create a widening or narrowing effect.

The front foot breakover may be speeded up by increasing the angle of the foot with shims and/or shortening the toe. The front toe grabs of a racing plate can be ground off. Racing plates with calks or level grip plates can be put on the front feet. The hind foot breakover can be slowed by leaving a long toe and toe grab. The heel calks or sticker on a racing plate can be ground off.

When a horse is scrambling in the gate at the start of a race, in a turn, or when it is accidentally bumped, severe but rare limb interference can occur. Overreaching, scalping and crossfiring have all been reported under these conditions.

References

Dollar, J.A.W. 1898. A Handbook of Horseshoeing. W.R. Jenkins, New York.

Harrison, J.C. 1968. Care and Training of the Trotter and Pacer. The United States Trotting Association, Columbus, OH.

Hickman, J. 1977. Farriery. J.A. Allen, London.

Holmes, C.M. 1949. The Principles and Practice of Horse Shoeing. The Farrier's Journal Publ. Co., Leeds, England.

Miles, W. 1846. The Horse's Foot and How to Keep it Sound (4th ed.). Longman, Brown, Green and Longman, London.

Pratt, G.W. 1982. Analyzing the movement of the horse. Proc. of Florida Horsemen's Seminar. 1:52.

Russell, W. 1899. Scientific Horseshoeing (4th ed.). The Robert Clark Co., Cincinnati.

War Department. 1941. The Horseshoer. United States Government Printing Office, Washington, DC.

NOTES:

Chapter 32

Forging and Applying Corrective Shoes

Corrective shoes compensate for a defect in the stance (conformation) or gait (movement) of a horse. Corrective Shoes may have one projection or alteration or a combination of them, depending on the problem(s). Ideally, a corrective shoe should be applied to a balanced foot. In most cases, corrective shoes are effective only while they are on the feet. The horse usually reverts back to the original fault(s) when the shoe(s) are removed. Only in special cases when a horse is very young does the direction of bone growth change enough to "straighten" the leg(s).

Always use the least severe corrective measure to create the desired effect.

Shoes to help diseased conditions of the foot or leg are sometimes called corrective shoes. We will refer to these as therapeutic shoes. Forging and application of therapeutic shoes is covered in Chapter 37.

Corrective shoes are best made from bar stock appropriate to the size and use of the horse. Handmades are especially useful when nail holes need to be placed differently than those found in a machine-made or keg shoe. However, because of the time involved in making handmade shoes, most saddle horse shoers fashion corrective shoes from keg shoes. For this reason, all corrective shoes that are regularly encountered by a saddle horse shoer are described on the keg

shoe. In cases where handmade shoes have some particular advantage, steps for making them are also presented.

There are several sequential steps to making each projection or alteration on the shoe. These must be reviewed and practiced often if a shoer is to become proficient in making and fitting them. Practice in basic iron and forge work, such as the making of handmade shoes, is a necessary prerequisite to the making of corrective shoes. Practice in making corrective shoes fit the foot in the desired manner is as important as learning to make the shoes.

Clip(s)

Clips take the strain off the nails and thus prevent slippage (or twisting) of the shoe on the foot. They should be used whenever there is a projection or feature on a shoe that puts excessive strain on the nails when a foot is weak or broken, or when a horse does not easily keep shoes on because of his way of going or use. Toe clips are usually used on front shoes and side clips on hind shoes.

Horses that twist and turn on their hind feet and/or have projections on their shoes should have a clip on each side of the toe between the first and second nail holes. Included are cutting and reining horses, as well as hunters and jumpers.

When traction producing devices are only on one branch of a shoe, such as an outside calk or half-swedge, the clip is placed on the same side as the traction device between the first and second nail holes.

Clips will vary in height and size according to the size of the shoe and foot, and their use. Clips on a saddle horse shoe may be from one to two times the thickness of the shoe in height and a little wider than they are high. They should taper from about 3/32 inch at the base to 1/32 inch at the tip. They should not be sharp at the tip. As a general rule, clips drawn on heavy stock (3/8 to½ in. thick) with a ¾ to 1 inch web should be as high and wide as the web is wide.

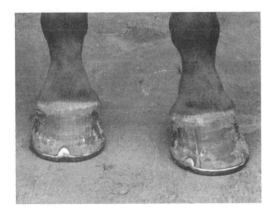

Fig. 32-1. Toe clip and side clips.

Clips are welded on instead of being pulled from the shoe metal when an extra long clip is desired. Clips can be forge welded onto the shoe by a process known as "jump welding," or they can be welded on with an oxy-acetylene or electric welding outfit. This is routinely done on gaited horse shoes (See Chapter 41).

Long clips are fit against the hoof. Standard clips should be set into the hoof and fit at the same angle as the hoof wall. Clips are fit easiest when they are hot. However, they can be fit cold by notching the hoof with nippers, knife or rasp.

Clipped shoes are more difficult to fit but are easier to nail on than flat shoes. However, be careful when nailing on shoes with clips. If the horse should take his foot while the first nail is being driven and the shoe accidentally turns so that the clip is under the foot, the sole may be punctured when the horse puts weight on the clip. Shoes with clips should not be allowed to remain on a horse until they become loose and fall off. Be careful when fitting shoes or resetting. Some horseshoers will not shoe a horse with clips which is difficult to shoe or may be neglected.

Steps in drawing a clip on an anvil with a clip horn:

1. Heat that part of the shoe to be clipped to a white heat and place it on the edge of the clip horn. Place tongs across the shoe and grip the branch opposite from your hand for greater stability. Allow ¼ inch of the shoe to project over the edge of the anvil facing you. Hold the shoe at a 45 degree angle to the anvil face.
2. Stand facing the anvil so that when you hold the hammer at your side the handle is perpendicular to the anvil edge. This position allows you to strike steady, evenly applied blows in the same place, and to draw the clip at a right angle from the shoe toward your body.

3. Strike the first blow with the flat face of the hammer to seat the shoe on the clip horn of the anvil, and thus prevent it from moving while the clip is being drawn out.
4. Use the rounded face of the hammer to draw the clip. A good clip is tapered from the base to the tip. Be careful not to thin the base out too much by hitting only in one place. This will weaken the clip and reduce its effectiveness.
5. As the last few drawing blows are made, turn the shoe down slightly with each one until it is parallel with the side of the anvil when finished.
6. Place the clip down in the hardy hole and level the shoe. Turn the shoe over and level it by striking behind the clip, if necessary.
7. Place the clip over the horn in such a way that the inner edge of the shoe is flush with the horn and pound down the ridges which have formed on each side of the clip until they are even with the curvature of the shoe. Hammer around the toe and shape the clip toward the foot surface until it is sloping at the angle of the wall.
8. The nail holes may need to be reformed by pritcheling after drawing side clips. Pritchel with the clip in the hardy hole or hanging off the side of the anvil. A slot in the face of an anvil is especially handy for pritcheling holes next to side clips. If the clip must be heated a second time to complete or fit it, heat the shoe with the clip up in the fire in order to avoid burning it.

Steps in drawing a clip on the edge of the anvil with a cross pein or ball pein hammer:

1. Heat the area of the shoe to be clipped white hot and place the ground surface up over the off-edge or heel of the anvil. About ¼ inch of the shoe should project over the edge at the point where the clip is to be drawn.
2. Hold the shoe down flat on the anvil and strike the cross or ball pein down repeatedly in one place. As the metal begins to bend, turn the hammer and strike at a 45 degree angle. Stop when the edge of the anvil can be felt at the base of the clip. Continue pulling the metal down below the edge of the anvil for a few hammer blows with the ball pein.
3. Turn the shoe over and grip the branch opposite from your hand. Place the turned down ear of metal on the anvil face with the shoe

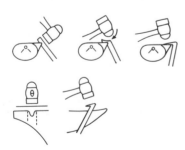

Fig. 32-2. Steps in drawing a clip using a clip horn.

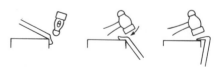

Fig. 32-3. Steps in drawing a clip with a ball pein hammer.

hanging down at a 30 degree or less angle. Draw the clip by flattening the ear or bubble of metal with the flat face of the hammer.

4. Place the inner rim of the clipped branch of the shoe against the horn of the anvil and shape the clip to the angle of the hoof wall.

Steps in drawing a clip with a bob punch:

1. Heat the area of the shoe to be clipped to a white heat. Place the shoe with its ground surface up on the anvil face near the hardy hole.

2. Sight over the bob punch and hold it on the shoe with about 1/16 inch of the edge of shoe visible on a ¾ inch web shoe and about ⅛ inch of the edge visible on wider webbed shoes. Drive the punch down with one or two blows to seat it.

3. Move the shoe over the corner of the hardy hole with the punch. The exact position over the hardy hole is determined by the width of the clip desired. Wider clips must be formed over the edge of the anvil. Tilt the punch and drive it toward the corner of the hardy hole. Several blows are sufficient to push a bubble of metal down. Do not drive the punch all the way through.

4. Turn the shoe over and cut the edges of the bubble on the foot surface with a hammer blow on each side. This controls the width of the clip.

5. Turn the shoe over. Grip the branch opposite from your hand and place the bubble above the anvil face at the opposite edge or heel. Smash and draw the clip with the heel of the flat face of the hammer. Move the shoe away from the anvil after the desired base width is obtained.

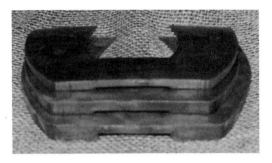

Fig. 32-5. Heel wedges.

6. Place the shoe over the horn and shape the clip to the angle of the hoof wall.

Steps in fitting a clip:

1. Make a seat for the clip(s) with the hoof knife, nippers, or rasp.

2. For a perfect fit, heat only the clip to a dull red heat and pull it back into position against the wall. Be sure to hold the hot shoe on the hoof only momentarily. Check the depth of the seat and then complete the seating process.

Lifts or Wedges

Lifts or wedges are placed between the shoe and hoof to change the lateral balance or toe to heel angle. Wedges for a single heel[1] or bar wedges for both heels[2] are available. Full wedge pads are less desirable for this purpose.

Occasionally, a horse may have one leg shorter than its opposite. This may occur in the front or hind limbs. It is common for diagonal limbs to be affected. The difference in height can be recognized by comparing landmarks on opposite bones such as knee prominences and chestnuts. Mismatched feet may indicate a difference in leg length. Heel wedges may correct some cases. Others will require rim pads or lifts. Full pads

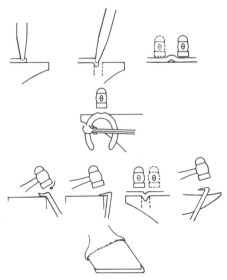

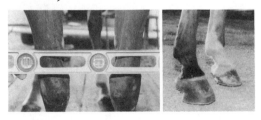

Fig. 32-6. (Left) Horse with front legs of unequal length. Note height of chestnuts compared to the level. (Right) Another horse with front legs of unequal length shod with lifts.

Fig. 32-4. Steps in drawing and fitting a clip with a bob punch.

[1]Multi-Chem, Studio City, CA
[2]Curtis Hamilton, Easley, SC

suitable for lifts are made in ¼, ⅜ and ½ inch thicknesses. The rim pad lifts can be cut out with nippers or a saber saw. The center can be cut out by drilling a hole through them large enough to insert a saber saw blade through. Several thicknesses of pads are fit like they would be on gaited horses (See Chapter 41).

Rocker-Toe

The rocker-toed shoe is used whenever it is desirable to speed up the breakover of the foot and/or relieve the stress of breaking over the toe. It may be used on a plate shoe or in conjunction with swelled or wedged heels to help correct forging or stumbling. A rocker-toed shoe is sometimes used on the front feet of young horses in training to aid them in developing the habit of picking their feet up and breaking over in the center of their toe. The rocker-toe is also a mild reminder for older horses to breakover and travel straight and true.

Steps in making a rocker-toed shoe:
1. Note the thickness of the wall of the horse's foot at the toe. This is usually about half to three-quarters the thickness of the web of the shoe. The toe should be "rocked" this amount. It can be turned from 10 degrees to 45 degrees, depending on the effect desired. Some shoers use a piece of string run from the fetlock to the toe to scribe an arc as an aid in determining the proper angle for an individual horse.

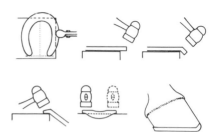

Fig. 32-8.   Steps in making and fitting a rocker-toed shoe.

2. Heat the toe of the shoe white hot and place it over the off-side of the anvil, allowing the web of the shoe to project over the edge of the anvil the thickness of the hoof wall at the toe.
3. Holding the hammer at the angle desired to rock the toe, strike alternate blows on the outside edge of the shoe projecting over edge of the anvil.
4. Work the blows toward the center of the toe until the desired angle is obtained.
5. Level the rest of the shoe surface where it may have warped in the rocking process.
6. Place the shoe in the vise and hot rasp the toe smooth. This adds to the appearance of the work and makes a smoother breakover possible.
7. Check to be sure both shoes of a pair are rocked the same amount and in the center of the toe.

Steps in fitting a rocker-toed shoe:
1. Heat the toe of the shoe dull red and carry it to the foot.
2. Hold the hoof rasp at the same angle to the bottom of the foot as the rocked portion of the shoe is to the ground surface of the hoof.
3. Carefully rasp the wall at this angle until you reach the white line.
4. Press the hot shoe to the foot momentarily. The edge of the toe of the shoe should be flush with the wall.
5. Rasp the scorched areas until the toe seats properly and the shoe rests flat on the foot.

Blocked Heel(s)

The blocked heel is perhaps the most popular style of handmade heel on horseshoes. Its biggest advantage is that it is easy to make. Blocked heels provide some traction but are most useful when height is needed at the heel as in cases where the axis of the foot is broken back. A blocked heel may be turned on one branch of the shoe as a corrective measure in cases where the foot is broken-in or out or toed-in or out.

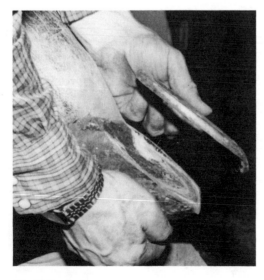

Fig. 32-7.   Rocker-toe.

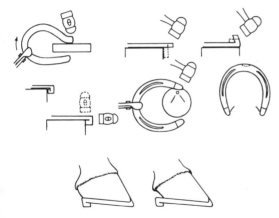

Fig. 32-9. Steps in turning and fitting a blocked heel.

Blocked heels may be created on thin extra light pattern shoes by folding the metal over twice instead of once as described.

Steps in turning a blocked heel:
1. Fit a size larger keg or hot (long heeled) shoe to the foot. At least ½ inch of metal should project beyond each buttress of the foot.
2. Heat the heel of the shoe to a white heat.
3. Extend the hot heel of the shoe over the off-edge or heel of the anvil about an inch with the foot surface up.
4. Bend the heel over until it is against the side of the anvil.
5. Turn the shoe over and hammer the turned heel down against the ground surface of the shoe. On extra light shoes, fold the heel again. Then, upset (smash) and square until the desired height is obtained.
6. Turn the shoe over so that the foot surface is up. Place the part of the heel now nearest to the toe against the off-side of the anvil and hold the shoe flat against the anvil face. Strike squarely on the end of the branch and the turned heel. This will have the effect of squaring and thickening the heel.
7. Place the inner edge of the blocked heel on the heel or horn of the anvil and draw and shape the heel. Next, shape it to fit the curvature of the outer edge of the hoof wall.
8. Hot rasp the heel of the shoe to make it round and smooth.

Blocked heels should extend beyond each buttress no more than ⅛ to ¼ inch when applied to the front feet, and no more than ¼ to ⅜ inch on the hind feet. Excessively low, sloping heels may require more length to reach back to a perpendicular line dropped from the base of the bulbs.

Swelled Heel(s)

A swelled heel is similar in shape to a blocked heel, except that the end of the turned heel is beveled so that less traction is provided by the heel. This is very useful in cases when height of heel is necessary but no traction is desired. The swelled effect can also be created by up-setting or swelling the heel before a handmade shoe is turned. Often a rocker-toe is used in conjunction with swelled heels. Such a shoe is sometimes referred to as a roller-motion shoe.

Swelled heels are useful in compensating for conformational defects and correcting faults of gait, such as forging and interfering. They are also used (especially in conjunction with a rocker-toe) to relieve various pathological conditions. However, bar wedges are preferred to swelled heels by most horseshoers.

Steps in making a swelled heel:
1. Fit a size larger keg or hot (long heeled) shoe to the foot. At least ½ inch of heel should project beyond each buttress.
2. Heat the heel of the shoe to a white heat.
3. Hold the hammer on about a 45 degree angle and taper or scarf the end of the heel next to the off-edge of the anvil.
4. Place about an inch of the heel over the off-edge of the anvil. The ground surface of the shoe should be up.
5. Hammer the heel over flat against the side of the anvil.
6. Turn the shoe over and pound the projecting end down against the foot surface. When striking the heel to get it flat against the shoe, hit on the beveled edge. Much of the height of the heel will be destroyed if you hit on the bent part of the heel.
7. Place the edge of the heel over the horn or heel of the anvil and swell or thicken the heel. If the scarfed end springs away from

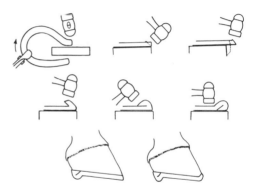

Fig. 32-10. Steps in making and fitting a swelled heel.

the shoe, strike on the bevel to bring it back in position.

8. Place the foot surface of the shoe on the anvil face and level it by striking forward of the base of the heel. The scarfed edge is now against the foot surface. An extra heat may be required to do this.

9. Hot rasp the heel smooth.

Swelled heels should extend beyond each buttress no more than ⅛ inch on normal hoofs. If the hoof heel is sloping, the shoe heels may be extended ¼ inch or more.

Welding of swelled heels is unnecessary when made in the above manner.

Trailer(s)

Trailers, sometimes called donkey or mule heels, give lateral support to the foot as it lands. They are used most frequently on the outside heel of the hind feet of horses with a cow-hocked conformation. They may vary in length from ⅜ to ¾ inch. Most trailers are turned to a 45 degree angle from the medial line of the foot. This varies, of course, according to the conformation of the foot and the correction to be made. Trailers are often applied in conjunction with a square-toe. Calks are often applied to an outside trailer on the hind feet of base-narrow horses. Calks should be turned first and then trailered the length of the calk.

If a horse has a tendency to kick other horses, it should be stabled away from other horses when it wears this type of shoe. Heels of this type can cut another horse very easily. Horses that are fence kickers, stall kickers, or pawers are a poor risk for this type of shoeing. Horses should not be turned loose in a stall or a pasture with a halter on. They may catch the heel of a

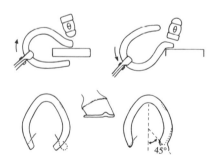

Fig. 32-11. Steps in making and fitting a trailer.

hind shoe in the halter when scratching their head. **Always alert horse owners to the dangers involved with this type of shoe.**

Steps in making a trailer:

1. Fit the shoe and allow for a small amount of metal to project beyond the buttress (doesn't have to be as long as the trailer is to be).

2. Mark the shoe with chalk as though you were going to cut the heel.

3. Take the shoe to the anvil and center punch the outer rim of the shoe one-half the width of the shoe at that point toward the toe from the outside point of the chalk mark.

4. Heat the heel of the shoe to be trailered white hot.

5. Place the outside edge and heel of the shoe on the face of the anvil. Line up center punch mark with the edge of the anvil.

6. Strike the end of heel on the face at angle to miss the upper shoe branch. Drop your tong hand as you strike until the heel turns out or is trailered the desired amount.

7. Cut the trailer to the desired length on the half-round hardy. With the foot surface of the shoe up, make the cut in the middle of the hardy so that the trailer is round on the end and the bevel is on the ground surface.

8. Taper the cut end of the trailer slightly. This is not necessary but it is good craftsmanship. The Sharp pattern halfround hardy does this as the heel is cut.

9. Hot rasp the trailer smooth.

Extended Heel(s)

Extended heels are used on the hind feet of horses that forge or overreach. As the horse moves, the heel of the foot usually comes in contact with the ground a split second before the toe. Extensions of the heels act as a "brake" and thus shorten the stride.

Extended heels may also be used on front or hind feet of horses which have very sloping heels. In cases of this type, the extension should come back to where a perpendicular line dropped from the bottom of the bulb will touch the end of the shoe heel. This is routinely done on gaited show horses. There is a possibility of causing shoe boils when applying extended heels to the front feet. The sausage shaped shoe boil boot will prevent this.

Extended heels differ from trailers in the angle to which the heel is turned. Extended heels are

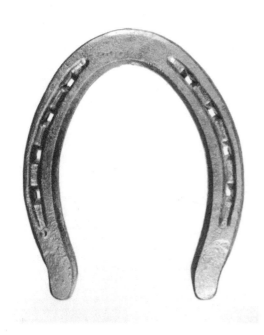

Fig. 32-12. Extended heels.

turned until they are parallel with the center or mid-line of the shoe. **Remember to alert owners to the dangers involved with this type of shoe on the hind feet (see dangers under "Trailers").**

Steps in making an extended heel:
1. Fit the shoe and allow for the desired amount to project beyond the buttresses.
2. Mark the shoe with chalk as though you were going to cut the heels.
3. Center punch the outer rim of the shoe one-half the width of the web of the shoe toward the toe from the chalk mark on each heel.
4. Heat the heels of the shoe to be shaped white hot.
5. Place the inside edge of the heel of the shoe on the heel of the anvil and locate the center punch mark.
6. Strike the heel of the shoe just back of the center punch mark and lift up on the shoe with the tongs until the heel is turned to a position parallel to the mid-line of the shoe. Trailers can also be turned this way.
7. Cut the heels to the desired length and/or hot rasp them smooth.

Spooned Heel(s)

Spooned heels may be used on the front shoes of a chronic overreaching horse to prevent them from being pulled off by the hind feet. They may be used on both front and hind feet to prevent bruising of the bulbs when riding in rocky terrain. Front shoes for gaited horses are sometimes made with long drawn-out spoons ("spurs"), to prevent them from being pulled due to crossfiring at the rack. Spooned heels are often used on the hind feet of reining or stock horses in conjunction with a rolled-toe to encourage collection and sliding stops. It is important to allow for the backward movement or sinking of the back of the foot under load when fitting spooned heels.

Steps in making a spooned heel:
1. Fit a shoe to the foot and allow ½ to ¾ inch to project beyond the buttresses. Taller spoons may be welded to or drawn from a longer heel.
2. Heat one heel of the shoe to a white heat and trailer the projected portion of the heel until it is parallel to the mid-line of the shoe (i.e., in the position that an extended heel would be).
3. Draw and bevel the ground surface of the heel on the face of the anvil so that it graduates from half the thickness of the shoe, at its extremity, to the full thickness of the shoe at the buttresses of the foot.
4. Place the shoe on the face of the anvil with the ground surface up and the heel to be "spooned" projecting over the off-side. The mid-line of the shoe should be perpendicular to the anvil's edge. The end of the bevel or taper (i.e., the part of the shoe coinciding with the buttress of the foot) should be directly over the anvil edge.
5. Strike the shoe so as to bend the heel of the shoe at the same angle as the slope of the heel of the foot. Strike heaviest on the outside of the heel of the shoe. This is necessary to make it fit flat against the heel of the foot.
6. Place the shoe in the vise and hot rasp the heel smooth.

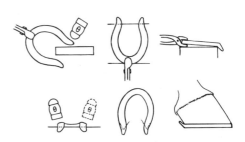

Fig. 32-13. Steps in making and fitting spooned heels.

335

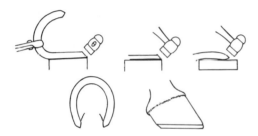

Fig. 32-14. Steps in making and fitting penciled heels.

Penciled Heels

Penciled, sometimes called beveled, under-slung, racing or jumping heels, are used when the shoe needs to end exactly at the end of the buttress. Horses that forge, overreach, paw the fence or step on themselves should be shod in this manner. The heel is shaped to coincide to the angle of the buttress as viewed from the bottom and from the side. The heels must fit flat against the foot. When making handmade shoes, most of the work in making these heels can be done with a hammer. When using keg shoes, most of the work must be done with a rasp or grinder. Racing plates come with sharply pointed underslung heels.

Steps in making a penciled heel on handmade shoes:

1. Heat the end of the heel white hot.
2. Place the end of the heel even with the rounded off edge of the anvil. Bevel the inside of the heel at a 45 degree angle with several hammer blows.
3. Turn the shoe over and bevel the outside of the heel at a 45 degree angle.
4. Hold the heel close to the edge of the anvil with the foot surface against the anvil and bevel it at the angle of the hoof from the buttress to the bulbs.
5. Repeat Step 2 and 3.
6. Hot rasp the heel smooth.

Jar Calk(s)

Jar calks or grabs are used to create traction and delay the twisting action of the foot at the moment of breakover. Jar calks may be attached to the shoe by forge brazing with copper or bronze, by brazing or welding with an oxy-acet-ylene torch, or by arc welding. The shoe should be level before brazing on the jar calks.

Jar calks can be made from flattened ¼ or ⅜ inch round stock. Coiled springs from old farm

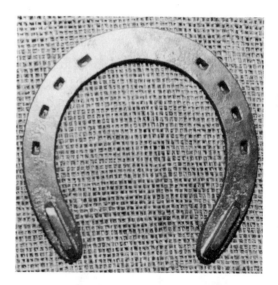

Fig. 32-15. Jar (jumping) calks brazed on with copper by D. Manning.

equipment make excellent calks. Grab steel can be purchased from the racing plate companies. Jar calks can also be formed by depositing bor-ium spots on toe, heel(s) or branch of the shoe.

Steps in brazing on jar calks with copper wire:

1. Form the calk(s) from a high carbon steel. Make a nib on one edge of the calk.
2. Heat the branch of the shoe to a yellow heat and drive the nib of the calk into the shoe. Place a piece of old copper wire ⅛ inch in diameter and the same length as the calk on the inside edge of the calk.
3. Place the shoe in the fire at a slight angle with the copper up. Heat until the shoe and calk are red.
4. Take the shoe from the fire and pour borax powder over the calk, shoe heel and wire. The flux will begin to melt and stick to the shoe.
5. Continue heating the heel until the flux all melts off and the copper begins to get glossy. The copper will melt all at once. When it gets glossy it is going to melt immediately.

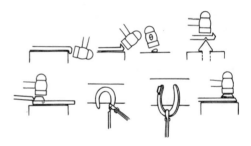

Fig. 32-16. Steps in brazing on jar calks with copper wire.

Grasp the shoe with the tongs and remove it from the fire as soon as the copper begins to flow.

6. Place the shoe on the anvil and press down on the calk with the hammer. This encourages capillary attraction to pull the copper under and around the calk before it sets up and cools.

7. Dip the shoe in water. This loosens the scale. Wire brush the scale and remaining flux off the grab and shoe.

8. File smooth as necessary.

Heel Calk(s)

Heel calks, also called corks, are used whenever height and/or traction is desired. Calks of any kind are not recommended as part of a standard shoeing job because of the extra strain they place on the foot and leg. However, they are often necessary on hunters, trail horses and other types of horses needing traction traveling across country. Most calks should be low and thick. Clips are usually put on shoes that have calks because of the extra strain placed on the nails by a traction creating device.

Keg shoes come in heeled, and toe and heeled patterns. Occasionally, you may need to turn calks. It takes a lot of practice before you can consistently make a perfect calk or clip. You can practice making them on a long piece of bar stock. Cut off each heel after you make it. Strive to increase your speed and efficiency in making calks.

Steps in making a heel calk:
1. Fit the shoe (preferably a hot pattern with tapered and thickened heels). Allow about ¼ to ⅜ inch on each heel of the shoe to project beyond the buttresses for front calks and about ½ to ⅝ inch for hind calks. If there is too much metal, you can cut the excess off with a straight hardy or select a

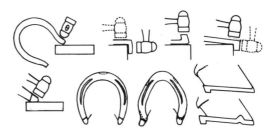

Fig. 32-18. Steps in making and fitting heel calks.

smaller shoe. The reason for the difference in front and hind lengths is the position the calk occupies under the foot. A full-creased (rim) shoe or flat borium application is preferred to calks for the front feet due to the danger of corns resulting from concussion.

2. Heat the heel of the shoe white hot. If the heel is not tapered and thickened so that it is about square on the end, make it so by working it over the horn of the anvil before turning the heel.

3. Trailer about 1 inch to the position of an extended heel.

4. Place the shoe with the foot surface up in such a way that the center or mid-line of the shoe is perpendicular to the anvil edge, and the heel to be calked projects over the off-edge or heel 1 inch.

5. Bend the projecting heel down against the off-side or heel of the anvil so that it forms a right angle to the shoe.

6. Turn the shoe over so that the ground surface and turned heel are up.

7. Strike squarely on the end of the turned heel to upset (swell and thicken) it. It may be necessary to place the shoe in the same position as Step 5 after this operation to straighten the turned heel.

8. Turn the shoe so that the calk is on its edge over the heel of the anvil and smash it so that it is slightly longer than it is wide. This shape gives the calk more length and further stabilizes the lateral movement of the foot.

9. Trailer the calks on hind shoes to the position of extended heels. This gives the horse more lateral support at the heels. The outside calk should be trailered out more than the inside calk. Calks on front shoes should follow the outline of the wall.

10. Again, hammer on the end of the calk until it is the height you desire. As a rule, calks should be no more than about one and a half times the thickness of the shoe.

11. Hot rasp the calk smooth.

12. Draw a toe clip on front shoes and side clips on hind shoes with calks.

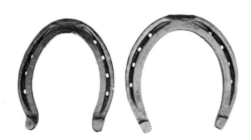

Fig. 32-17. Heel calks.

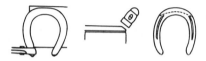

Fig. 32-19.   Steps in making and fitting a rolled-toe.

Rolled-Toe

A rolled-toe, or some form if it, is widely used on show horses to increase the breakover speed of a weighted shoe. It is also used in conjunction with spooned heels on a sliding plate for stock horses to decrease the friction between the shoe and the ground. A rolled-toe may be used on harness racing shoes where one does not want to change the ground surface of the foot.

Steps in making a rolled-toe:
1. Fit the shoe fuller and rounder than the hoof shape at the toe. This allows for the pointing of the shoe that occurs as the rolled-toe is formed.
2. Heat the toe to a white heat.
3. Place the toe of the shoe on the anvil face and near to the off-edge of the anvil.
4. Starting at the outside of the toe, strike overlapping blows at an angle all around the toe of the shoe.
5. Continue beveling the toe in the above manner until the shoe is about ⅛ inch thick at the toe.
6. Hot rasp the shoe in order to further round the edge of the shoe and give it a uniform curvature.

Square-Toe

The square-toe gives lateral support to the toe at the moment of breaking over. The square-toe is used as an aid in making the horse breakover in the center of its foot. It is usually used on the hind feet. The points on the edge of the toe act like little levers. They have a tendency to twist or turn the foot, and thus cause it to breakover in the flattened portion of the toe. Its most common use is on the hind feet of saddle horses as an aid in correcting the cow-hocked condition. It is often used in conjunction with a trailer.

Square-toed shoes may be used on the front feet when they are narrow and pointed in shape instead of lateral extension-toed shoes. Square-toed shoes are fit under the toe of the hind feet in some cases of overreaching to prevent damage

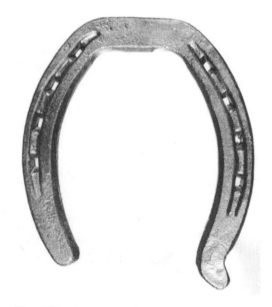

Fig. 32-20.   Square-toe and trailer.

to the front foot. They may be fit under the toe of the front foot to increase breakover speed.

Steps in making a square-toe:
1. Heat the toe of the shoe white hot.
2. Place the toe of the shoe near the point of the anvil, with the heels hanging down perpendicular to the floor.
3. Line up the point of the crease (on most keg shoes) so that it is directly over the point of the anvil.
4. Pull the shoe toward you against the anvil horn while the shoe is in the above position to steady it. Strike flat blows on the toe of the shoe.
5. When half of the toe is flat, strike diagonally against the side of the toe over the horn. This makes the corner square instead of rounded.

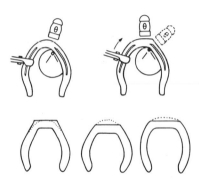

Fig. 32-21.   Steps in making and fitting a square-toe.

6. Turn the shoe around and repeat the process on the other side of the toe. The other side can also be done by moving the shoe away from you into position. However, many beginners find this position awkward and less accurate than turning the shoe around.

Frequently the toe nail holes of a keg shoe cannot be used as they are closed during the shaping process or they are too close to the outer edge of the wall. Only the rear three nails are used on each side of these cases. The square-toe should be fit flush with the center of the toe in order that the pointed projections may give the toe lateral balance.

In some cases of forging and overreaching and other faults of gait, it may be desirable to place the corners flush with the wall and let some of the toe wall project over the square-toe of the shoe. The overhanging wall may be rounded to prevent chipping. Handmade shoes work best for this type of fit. Side clips prevent the shoe from sliding back farther off the toe.

Diamond-Toe

A diamond-toe is beveled on both sides of the toe about half the width of the web. It could be said to be a divided rolled-toe. The heels of the shoe are thinned to break the axis of the foot back and slow the breakover time. It should only be used on a forging horse that is hitting its hind toe on the outside branch of its front shoe.

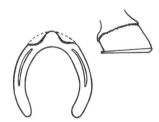

Fig. 32-22. Diamond-toe.

Lateral Extension-Toe

The lateral extension-toe is actually one-half of a square-toe. Its action is more severe than a square-toe, and it is used mostly on round-toed (front or hind) feet that are severely toed-in or out. The point on the extension acts as a lever to turn the toe so that it will breakover in the center. Sometimes a severe measure such as this

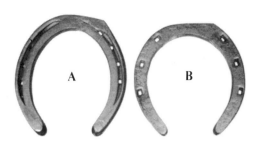

Fig. 32-23. Lateral extension-toe shoes. (A) Keg, (B) handmade.

is the only thing which will stop a chronic interfering horse from hitting itself.

Steps in making a lateral extension-toe on a keg shoe:

1. Heat the toe of the shoe to a white heat and place it on the off-corner of the anvil with the ground surface up.
2. Strike down on that portion of the shoe on the corner of the anvil and draw the extension to a point slightly toward the heel from the place where the foot is breaking over. This location can be determined by noting the wear on the old shoe or the foot, and observing the horse travel.
3. Continue striking until you have flattened the projection to one-half the thickness of the shoe.
4. Hot rasp the toe square. This provides a flat surface for the horse to breakover. If the horse is interfering, hot rasp the inside branch of the shoe as well.

Some shoers fill in the space formed on the foot surface of the shoe with weld metal. This isn't necessary, but it does make the shoe last longer. Others draw the extension with the foot surface up and fill in the recessed area on the ground surface with Borium.

Often, it is wise to build the shoe as described in the above steps and then put it on the foot to see if it will be effective. If it is, you can build another pair when the trial shoes become worn sufficiently to warrant it, and coat the lateral extension on them with Borium.

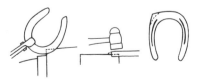

Fig. 32-24. Steps in making a lateral extension-toe on a keg shoe.

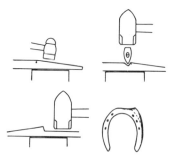

Fig. 32-25.   Steps in making a handmade lateral extension-toed shoe.

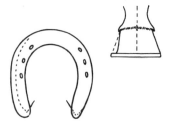

Fig. 32-26.   Lateral balance shoe punching and fit.

Some shoers prefer handmade lateral extension-toed shoes. They have the advantage of allowing individualized placement of nail holes, and a full thickness of metal at the point of breakover.

Steps in making a handmade lateral extension-toed shoe:

1. Cut a piece of ¼ inch x 1 inch stock about 2 inches shorter than the measurement calculated as necessary to cover the hoof with the 1 inch stock.
2. Make a center punch mark on the straight piece of bar iron about where you think the extension should go.
3. Heat the half of the bar which has the center punch mark closest to the end to a white heat.
4. Taper this branch from the center punch mark to the end, drawing the metal out as you go and thus keeping the stock the same thickness. Continue this process until the end of the stock is about ½ inch wide.
5. Heat the other end of the bar white hot up to and slightly past the center punch mark.
6. Fuller down about ⅜ inch on the untapered side of the mark. Another method is to place the untapered portion of the shoe on the anvil face perpendicular to the anvil edge with the center punch mark directly over the anvil edge. Then strike edge to edge flat blows on the edge of the stock on the anvil face. This will put a shoulder in the metal.
7. Draw the stock out until it tapers from ⅝ inch at the shoulder to ½ inch wide at the end and has its original ¼ inch thickness.
8. Heat the stock white hot in the center, making sure that the wider-webbed portion gets the hottest. Dip the narrow branch in water before bending.
9. Turn a toe bend in the stock just as you would a regular horseshoe.
10. Complete the shoe punching the nail holes to allow the extension to project beyond the wall an appropriate amount.
11. Fit the shoe and cut the heels.
12. Hot rasp the heels smooth and hot rasp the toe square. If the horse is interfering, also hot rasp the inside ground surface edge of the shoe smooth.

Lateral extension-toe shoes can also be made by welding a projection on the edge of the shoe just back of the point of breakover and grinding it to conform to the shape of half a square toe. Another way, used mostly on the hind feet of draft horses, is to weld a toe calk on the shoe extending to the outside. Keg shoes can be heated and bent sharply at the point the extension is desired and fit to allow the point to extend over the edge of the hoof.

Always remember that a lateral extension-toe is a most severe corrective measure, and judgment should be exercised when using it.

Lateral Balance Shoe

The lateral balance shoe is a handmade plate shoe punched coarse on one side and fine on the other side. A wide-webbed keg shoe can be adapted by punching extra nail holes inside or outside of the machine-punched nail line. This shoe is applied to a level and balanced foot. The object is to shift the center of weight bearing on the leg. This is usually a better alternative than stressing the limbs by trimming the hoofs out of balance or applying projections to shoes.

Interfering Shoe

The interfering, speedy-cutting, feather-edged, dropped crease or knocked down shoe has its inner branch straight from toe to quarter away from the point of interference. It could be said to be a square-quartered shoe. The edge of the shoe is beveled to a featheredge and rounded off by hot rasping. This style of shoe may be used

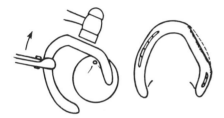

Fig. 32-27. Steps in making and fitting the interfering shoe.

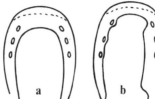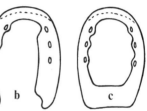

Fig. 32-28. Weighted shoes. a) toe, b) side, and c) heel weighted.

on a horse that occasionally hits itself after other measures have failed. The shoe prevents the horse from being seriously damaged. The wall is rounded off at the point of interference. Usually nail holes must be punched near the end of the heel due to the fit of the inside branch. If no nails can be safely placed in the heel, a bar shoe can be constructed. All the nails are then placed in one side and toe of the hoof.

Steps in making the interfering shoe:

1. Heat the area of the shoe where the horse interferes.
2. Hold the heated portion of the shoe over the heel of the anvil. Flatten the branch from the toe to the bend in the quarter as you would when making a square-toe.
3. Bevel the straightened section of the shoe next to the off-edge of the anvil. Hot rasp this edge smooth.
4. Heat the inside heel.
5. Shape the heel to conform to the foot and stamp one or two nail holes in it. The holes should be pritcheled with the punch corresponding to the angle of the wall in this region of the hoof.

Weighted Shoe

A weighted shoe increases the stride arc of a horse. Weight may be added in an effort to:

1. Increase the animation of a horse.
2. Balance and true the gait of a horse.

Usually, weight must be accompanied by special training and an extended hoof length to produce animation. Animation is exaggerated, graceful movement. Weight, no matter how added, increases muscle strain and produces fatigue.

Weight can be added in ways other than in the shoe. Weights fastened to the toe of the hoof with screws are available and are used quite extensively by harness horsemen. Weight can be added between leather pads on a long-footed

show horse or secured with screws between the shoe and the pad on a horse in training.

There are several types of weighted shoes. Weight may be placed in the toe, on the side, or in the heel of the shoe. There are factory-made patterns available, but most horse owners and horseshoers prefer custom handmade shoes. Weighted shoes are drawn out of heavy stock and custom made when they are called for. Drawing and turning weighted shoes is covered in Chapter 41.

A keg shoe can be easily converted to a weighted shoe for use in cases requiring only a small amount of weight. A widewebbed shoe of heavy stock can be cut with an oxy-acetylene torch or forge heated and cut with a handled chisel on the anvil. The area of the shoe where the weight is wanted is not touched, and the rest of the shoe is cut to one-half the width of the web. Oblique cuts must be made when graduating from the full thickness of the web to one-half thickness to prevent fracture at this point when shaping the shoe. Side weight shoes can be made from keg shoes by welding one-half of a light hind shoe to one-half of a heavy front shoe. A toe or heel weight can be made by welding the toe or heels of a heavy front shoe to the light toe or heels of a light hind shoe. These shoes look very crude and the nail holes are usually in the wrong place. Few horseshoers use them.

References

Gonzales, A. 1983. Proper balance movement. Amer. Farriers' J. 9(5):397.

Hickman, J. 1977. Farriery. J.A. Allen and Co., London.

Holmes, C.M. 1949. The Principles and Practice of Horse Shoeing. The Farrier's Journal Publ. Co., Ltd., Leeds, ENGLAND.

Manning, D. 1984. The art of punching clips. Amer. Farriers' J. 9(6):490.

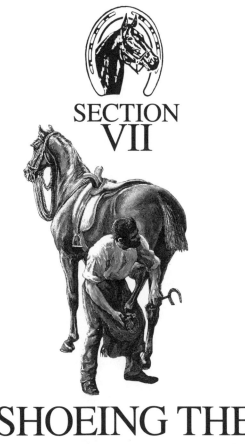

SECTION VII

SHOEING THE LAME HORSE

SHOEING THE LAME HORSE

Chapter 33

Principles of Therapeutic Shoeing

Therapeutic Shoeing, often called pathological or surgical shoeing, involves treating the diseases of the horse's feet or limbs by trimming or shoeing the feet. The need for it is usually manifested by an impairment in the stance or gait of the horse. This condition is called lameness. Often the problem causing the lameness is an unsoundness. Horses with unsoundnesses may be made serviceably sound by the treatment of a horseshoer or a veterinarian. Treatments, as administered by the horseshoer, generally are of a protecting, supporting, or weight-shifting nature applied to the feet or limbs. One or a combination of these three methods may be used on any given horse.

Relationship Between the Horseshoer and Veterinarian

Often there is a fine line in the determination of the realms of the horseshoer and veterinarian. The horseshoer's realm in terms of surgery is usually limited to the horny hoof. Horseshoeing requires great skill and a surgical operation is performed each time the living hoof is trimmed or shod.

The veterinarian's role is usually one of prescribing what is necessary for treatment of the pathological condition, and the horseshoer's role is to carry out the instructions and apply them

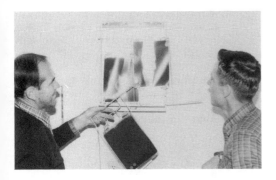

Fig. 33-1. The horseshoer and veterinarian are each in a position to help each other achieve the goal of a sound horse and a satisfied owner.

to the hoof in the form of special trimming or shoeing. The veterinarian writes the prescription, the horseshoer fills it.

One of the horseshoer's closest business associates and friends should be the veterinarian. They are each in a position to be of great help to each other. The horseshoer and veterinarian frequently must work together to effectively treat the more complicated and systemic disease conditions affecting the horse's legs and feet.

The goal should be a sound horse and a satisfied owner.

Historically, horseshoers and veterinarians have exhibited various degrees of jealousy and rivalry. At one time their professions were one in the same. They were called farriers. After they split into two distinct groups, they viewed each other with contempt. There was no division of realms until early in this century (See Chapter 3).

Today, the horseshoer's realm has been properly described as being limited to the horse's foot. The degree to which the horseshoer practices in this realm is largely dependent upon the relationship the individual horseshoer has with a horse's veterinarian. Veterinarians have the welfare of the entire animal as their responsibility. Specialized knowledge concerning the foot and its diseases may not be readily available except from a competent horseshoer.

The horseshoer and the veterinarian can be assets to each other and benefit the horse and its owner, providing each recognizes the other's abilities and realms. Honest mistakes are made in every field of endeavor. Horseshoers are guilty of mistakes from carelessness, lack of knowledge or skills, and circumstance. So are veterinarians. There is a need for both to own up to their ignorance and assist each other in order to maximize the benefit to the horse.

Some veterinarians quickly convict the horseshoer whenever any lameness occurs. Statements frequently quoted, and originally given as someone's opinion, claim that 75 percent of all lameness can be attributed to improper shoeing procedure. So few hours are devoted to horseshoeing and diseases of the feet in modern veterinary college curricula, few recent graduates can tell the difference between a good and a poor shoeing job, to say nothing of distinguishing between a lame and a sound horse. Those veterinarians who are very competent in diagnosing and treating foot lamenesses are, for the most part, self-taught.

It is possible for a trained and experienced individual horseshoer to be more competent than an individual veterinarian in diagnosing and caring for the problem in a given horse's foot. Veterinarians should realize this and regard competent horseshoers as professionals. The horseshoer should in turn acknowledge his dependence upon the veterinarian.

Whenever competent horseshoers and veterinarians that respect each other have the good fortune to work together, each in his own realm, the outcome will always be beneficial to the horse and its owner.

The information in this section is presented in an effort to aid both horseshoers and veterinarians (and horseowners and trainers) so that they may each appreciate what the other can do for the benefit of the horse.

Horseshoeing an Art and a Science

There are often many different ways or variations of ways to accomplish the same end in therapeutic shoeing. Several methods are listed for each problem. Not all are of equal value in the experience of the Author, but sometimes valuable in individual cases. There are few subjects that are more individual, varied and controversial than therapeutic shoeing. There are often several ways to get the same observable result. Results are what count.

Russell (1887) has said:

It is impossible in any art—and shoeing is no exception to this rule—to acquire a veritable

Horseshoeing is not only an art; it is also a science. It has for its object the surgical treatment, if you please, of the foot as well as the mechanical work of shoeing. Three-fourths of the successful work of the farrier depends upon his knowledge of the anatomy of the foot, and practical acquaintanceship with its diseases, their causes and cures.

Fleming (1870) stated:

It is impossible in any art—and shoeing is no exception to this rule—to acquire a veritable

superiority, if its theory as well as its practice be not combined and exercised together. Practice without theory is simply routine without improvement, and theory alone is often impotent to confer advantages without the crucial test of experience.

Hayden (1910a) maintained:

A proper mode of shoeing the horse's foot is certainly of far more importance than the treatment of any disease, or, perhaps, of all the diseases incident to horses...if this art of shoeing be judiciously employed, the foot will not be more liable to disease than any other organ of the horse....To be a successful farrier, theory and practice must work in harmony with one another. With a thorough knowledge of practical skills and theory we, as farriers, could defy the world to produce a craft equal in skill, pride, practice, or knowledge.

The horse's only real value is the work he can perform, whether it be showing, racing or pleasure riding. His ability to perform is limited by our ability to properly understand and care for him. We must unite art and science, as well as work together, to achieve the goal of a sound horse.

Definitions

The following terms are frequently encountered when discussing therapeutic shoeing and should be well understood.

1. **Blemish:** an observable abnormality which does not interfere with the intended use of the horse. May be an inherited characteristic or the result of a past injury. May diminish value, but not function.
2. **Soundness:** a state of excellent health, usually refers to the locomotor system. May refer to the visual, respiratory, nervous, reproductive or other body systems.
3. **Serviceable Soundness:** a state of health where no abnormality is obvious at the time of examination which will predispose to or immediately interfere with the intended use of the horse.
4. **Unsoundness:** a deviation from the ideal (soundness). May or may not render the animal unfit for intended use. May predispose to (cause or result in) or may actually be a pathological condition. Not serviceably sound at the time of examination. May be hereditary, usually a persistent or chronic condition.
5. **Lameness:** an observable change from sound motion or stance due to pain or mechanical dysfunction. A sign (symptom) of a pathological condition. Not sound. May be tem-

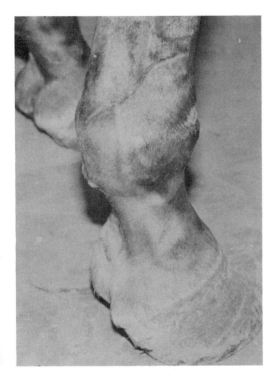

Fig. 33-2. Learn to distinguish between blemishes, lamenesses and unsoundnesses.

porary. May be graded as to severity from 1 to 5. (A.A.E.P., 1982)

6. **Lesion:** specific damage or pathology causing pain or discomfort. Lameness results from a lesion. Lesions may or may not be due to an unsoundness.

7. **Acute Lesion:** relatively short duration. Severe course characterized by pain, heat and swelling.

8. **Chronic Lesion:** relatively long duration. Less severe than and may follow acute course. Often recurring and less obvious than acute.

9. **Congenital Condition:** acquired by foal during development in the mare's uterus.

10. **Hereditary Condition:** acquired by foal at conception by uniting of the genetic material of both parents.

General Location and Incidence (Frequency) of Lameness

A lameness examination should consider the whole horse first, then the apparent affected part of the horse. The following should be considered as background information.

We can usually expect the frequency of lesions or unsoundnesses to be three times as great in the front limbs (about 75 percent) as the hind limbs (about 25 percent). The front limbs carry 60 to 65 percent of the horse's weight and at least 60 percent of the rider's weight. The front limbs also are subject to greater concussion due to their position on impact and their supporting function. Standardbreds are an exception to this rule, due to their balanced trotting or pacing gait. They may have a lameness lesion frequency of 60 percent in the front and 40 percent in the hind limbs.

A very high percentage (many say 90, some say 99 percent) of the lamenesses in the front leg are in the knee or below. A high percentage (about 75 percent) of lamenesses below and not including the knee are in the foot. *The foot should always be inspected and checked out first as the possible site of lameness.* Much embarrassment and disappointment can be avoided if this is routinely done.

Most lamenesses of the hind leg are in and above the hock, including the stifle, hip or back. This is due to the propelling function of the hind legs as opposed to the supporting function of the front legs. It has been stated that 80 percent of hind limb lameness will be seen in the hock or stifle. *However, always check the foot first as a possible site of lameness.*

Lameness producing lesions in one site on a limb may cause the horse to injure a second area in the same limb, or to stress and injure the opposite limb in an effort to avoid the pain caused by the original lesion. This condition is often referred to as a compensatory or complementary lameness. For example, a horse with navicular disease that has pain in the heel may produce a concussion induced pedal osteitis at the toe of the foot. Or, a horse with a broken leg may produce a founder in the opposite foot due to the compensating increase in weight bearing by the sound leg.

There were two distinct peaks of age incidence in 1000 lameness cases reported by Yeates(1968) in England. One was at 8 to 10 years and the other at 16 to 18 years. In America, we see more lameness in animals that are raced or otherwise stressed at too early an age. Racing of immature 2 year olds, especially those that are overfed and underconditioned, is most detrimental to the limbs. Under 20 percent of these animals will be lame in the foot (Milne, 1967).

Common Causes of Lameness

Type of work or use often determines the site of the lameness producing lesion. Fatigue is usually a predisposing factor to work related injuries. Over stressing young horses may create fatigue and limb injury.

The various breeds are subject to injury as a result of their specialized uses. Thoroughbreds that principally run or jump may develop popped knees or carpitis, osselets, popped sesamoids or sesamoiditis, flexor tendon or suspensory ligament injury, shin splints, pedal osteitis or navicular disease. Quarter Horses that run, turn and stop hard may develop bone spavin, navicular disease, ringbone, side bone or fractures of the phalanges. Standardbreds that trot or pace at speed and pull a sulky may develop back trouble, whorl bone or hip lameness, stifle conditions, bone spavin, osselets, suspensory ligament sprain or popped sesamoids, inflamed tendon sheaths or navicular disease.

Today's show horses are more heavily campaigned than they used to be. Exhaustive showing or racing schedules, coupled with a lack of slow and lengthy conditioning, have been responsible for an increase in use related lamenesses.

Hereditary predisposition refers to the susceptibility a horse has to a lameness causing lesion as a result of its inherited characteristics. We most commonly think of conformation faults, since they are so highly heritable (about 0.6 or a 60 percent chance of passing from generation to generation). Crooked (medial, lateral deviation) limbs and feet cause unequal weight distribution and increased stresses on joint surfaces, ligaments and foot structures. Upright, short and stumpy pasterns increase concussion to the same areas. Small feet in relation to body size concentrate concussion upon the constricted structures of the foot. Individuals with poor limb conformation are especially susceptible to bone diseases. Systemic imbalances or weaknesses may make animals more susceptible to some lameness causing diseases.

Breeding horses for a particular goal, such as speed, color, muscling or a beautiful head, without emphasizing well conformed limbs and feet, brings on lamenesses of epidemic proportion.

Diet deficiencies and sometimes toxicities may cause lameness. Adequate calcium and phosphorus consumption, especially in fast growing foals, is of greatest concern. The amount of these minerals, their ratio to each other and the presence of vitamin D should be considered. The amount of feed including adequate protein, energy, vitamin and mineral level is often critical.

A well-balanced ration is necessary for proper bone formation and maintenance. Nutritional requirements vary considerably according to the age, use and condition of the horse. Toxic minerals and fat soluble vitamins may be a problem in some areas, and especially when commercial supplements are fed indiscriminately. Hypersensitivity to feed additives or elements may produce lameness. Selenium toxicity is a serious problem in some areas. Various poisonous plants or chemicals such as urea may be a problem.

However, the most common problem by far is overfeeding. Laminitis or founder and sometimes protein, vitamin or mineral toxicity in addition to obesity may result from this practice.

Environmental conditions that affect the condition of the horse and its feet may be directly or indirectly responsible for foot health and lameness. Climate affects ground moisture, temperature and outside stabling conditions. Soil surface type and moisture content affect hoof condition. Horses that are stabled in stalls are affected by the type of bedding provided, the frequency of stall cleaning and especially the frequency of hoof cleaning. Pampered horses lose much of their ability to cope with the environment. Of course, frequency and quality of hoof trimming and shoeing are very important.

Injury due to trauma inflicted while working, in the stable, on pasture or being shod may be a cause of lameness. Be aware of possible ways this could occur. For example, equipment may rub or irritate, other horses may kick, barbed wire may cut and mutilate, trash may trap, unsafe surfaces and unskilled riding may cause slipping and falling which may result in lesions of varying severity. Incompetent or careless shoeing may temporarily and sometimes permanently injure a foot.

Infection may cause lameness due to filling of the limb (edema) that results from the reaction of the horse's body to bacterial invasion of tissues. Some infections are the result of neglect (e.g., thrush). Others may be contagious and

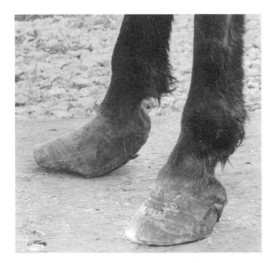

Fig. 33-3. Neglect is a common cause of lameness.

need special attention by a veterinarian (e.g., fistula withers).

Neglect of regular hoof care and trimming or shoeing is detrimental to a horse's health and a leading cause of lameness.

Health Indicators or Vital Signs

Built into each horse are indicators of his state of health and soundness. The horseshoer must observe and understand these indicators to be able to detect the various lesions of lameness. Everyone working with horses should know the difference between conditions requiring veterinary attention, those requiring a professional horseshoer and those that can be adequately treated by a lay horseman.

General appearance includes posture of the upper body and resting position of the limbs, hair coat and skin condition, alertness of the eyes, and color of the mucous membranes.

Normally, the horse stands squarely on his front legs and is alert with his head and ears up. He often rests his hind legs alternately. However, when this is done in front it is called pointing and is a sign of lameness. Shifting the weight from both front limbs to both hind limbs may indicate bilateral front limb lameness.

The horse may sleep standing due to the presence of a unique stay apparatus, but a deep sleep requires the horse to lie down. The horse normally lies on its side with its legs and head extended. Horses also lie on the side of their chest with their legs folded and their head resting on the chin. When the horse rises, the head is thrown up and back, the front legs thrust forward and the body pushes up from the front legs.

A horse that has a listless attitude and stands stiff may be showing signs of a systemic disease. Horses that paw or roll frequently may be expressing pain. Alternating depression and hyperexcitation and altered sensory perception may indicate poisoning by toxic plants.

The hair coat should be fine, glossy and smooth during warm weather and heavier during cold weather. A coarse coat lacking oil indicates a poor nutritional state and often internal parasite infestation. Hair loss or scaliness may be due to external parasite infestation. Excessive hair growth may be due to pituitary or adrenal gland tumors. The skin should be pliable and elastic. When picked up in a fold, a slow return of the skin to its original position indicates dehydration or nutritional deficiency. Sweating after exercise is normal. Cold sweating, especially in patches, may be due to nervousness or great pain. Excessive sweating (may accompany growth of long hair) may be due to pituitary or adrenal gland tumors.

The eyes should be bright, clear and alert. Runny eyes may be a result of respiratory infections, reaction to irritations, or nutritional deficiency. If only one eye is runny, the nasolacrimal duct, from the eye to nose, may be clogged. The normal wetness in the nostrils of a horse is due to drainage from these ducts. The horse has a third eyelid that becomes visible in cases of tetanus.

The mucous membranes are normally moist and have a pink color. Those regularly observed include the nasal, eyelid and lip membranes. Pale color may indicate anemia or poor health. Red indicates irritation or infection. Blue indicates a lack of oxygen to the tissues caused by toxicity or sickness. Yellow indicates jaundice caused by liver damage and increased bilirubin (bile pigment) in the blood.

Pulse Rate can be taken anywhere on the body where an artery is close enough to the surface that it may be lightly compressed against a bone or by listening to the heart. Under the jaw, above the knees, and behind the fetlock are commonly used sites. Pulses are counted for 15

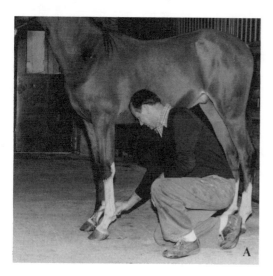

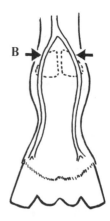

Fig. 33-4. The pulse rate may be taken (A & B) behind the fetlock, or (C) under the mandible.

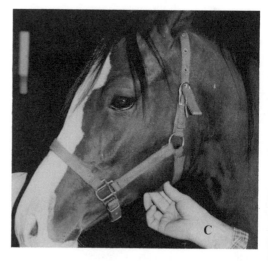

seconds and then multiplied by four to determine the pulse rate. The pulse throb results from the increased pressure in the arteries resulting from each heart beat. Irregular heart beat, detected by stethoscope or electrocardiogram, is an indicator of heart disease.

Age, sex, condition, excitement, exercise, weather, digestion, fever and pain all influence the pulse rate. Age has a marked effect. Newborn foals have a normal rate of 80 to 120 beats per minute. Two-month old foals, 60 to 80 beats is average; yearlings, 50 to 70; 2 year olds, 45 to 65; 3 years, 40 to 60; 4 years, 35 to 55, and 5 year olds, 30 to 50. Adult horses may be normal and have pulse rates of 28 to 48 beats per minute (average 44).

Mares tend to have a slightly faster pulse than stallions or geldings. A horse in very good condition has a pulse rate slightly lower than others of the same age and temperament. Factors that cause the pulse rate to decrease are sleep, cold weather, old age, dehydration and exhaustion. Factors that cause the pulse rate to increase are excitement, fright, exercise, hot weather, fever and pain. During exercise the pulse rate may be as high as 120 to 150 beats per minute. Rates of 80 to 100 at rest may be associated with fever. Some say the pulse rate increases at the rate of eight beats per minute for each Fahrenheit degree of fever.

Comparison of the strength of the pulse in opposite legs may be helpful in diagnosing some insidious lamenesses.

Respiration Rate can be determined by counting the rise or fall of the rear flank or ribs. The breaths are easily counted in cold weather. A relaxed horse will take 8 to 12 breaths per minute. Younger horses (yearling and twos) may breathe faster at 10 to 15 breaths per minute. Respiration rate increases after exercise, in hot weather, with poor condition or with great pain. Persistent coughing, runny nose and watery eyes are signs of respiratory disease.

Labored breathing, especially that associated with heaves, creates a "heave line" on the under side of the rib cage in the flank. Heaves may be due to an allergy or emphysema or both. It can usually be greatly improved by feeding a specially formulated feed containing sugar beet pulp (such as New Hope) instead of hay, pelleted feeds, drugs and/or turning the horse out in a green pasture.

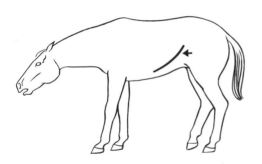

Fig. 33-5. A "heave line" (arrow) can be observed in the flank of horses with heaves.

Body Temperature is determined by placing a heavy duty animal thermometer in the rectum. A piece of string should be tied on the end of the thermometer to a clamp such as a clothes pin for attaching to the tail. The thermometer should be shaken down below 95 degrees F. and lubricated with petroleum jelly. The thermometer can be inserted before the other vital signs are taken to save time. It should be left in the rectum for at least 3 min. The normal temperature for an adult horse should be 99 to 101 degrees F. (average 100.4 degrees F. or 38 degrees C.). Temperature rises during the day and falls during the night. Body temperature may be higher than normal in younger animals and during exercise and hot weather. It may be 99 degrees in very cold weather. Lower temperatures indicate shock. Temperatures over 101 degrees F. indicate the presence of fever, usually due to infection. A fever is considered mild at 102 degrees F., moderate at 104 degrees F., and high at 106 degrees F. Higher fever due to heatstroke, tetanus or influenza usually means impending death.

Urine volume for a normal horse is 3 to 9 quarts daily, average 5.5 quarts. When expressed as ml/kg (milliliters per kilogram) of body weight, it is given as 3 to 18 ml per kg body weight. The horse usually urinates or voids five to seven times daily. A mare in heat will void more often and display a characteristic "winking" posture. Amount of urine excreted may be influenced by diet, exercise and climatic conditions. The pH of urine is often influenced by the level of conditioning. Horses in training may have more acidic urine than horses out of training.

Urine is normally yellow and cloudy. It may be deep yellow or brown. It is very viscous and cloudy due to the presence of calcium carbonate crystals, mucus and epithelial debris. Change in color to blood red may indicate a urinary tract infection. Azoturia creates a port wine (dark red) colored urine due to the presence of myoglobin, a result of muscle breakdown. Hind limb lameness is also present.

Straining in urination may be due to muscle, nervous, or (rarely) kidney disease. The presence of a bean (smegmolith) in the glands penis of a stallion, or (more commonly) a gelding, may cause straining.

Feces volume varies from 30 to 50 pounds per day for the average horse. A horse will usually defecate 8 to 10 times a day. The normal texture of feces is a soft ball form that will flatten when dropped. The feces are normally dark yellow to green in color depending on the diet composition.

Constipation may be due to parasite infestation or toxicity and may lead to impaction or gaseous colic. Diarrhea may be due to malabsorption or other disease and may cause dehydration. Runny droppings (loose feces or diarrhea) can also be caused by nervousness, overwork and fatigue. Laxative feeds (such as bran, alfalfa and green pasture), and especially finely ground pelleted feeds, result in feces with a more watery consistency.

A change in odor may indicate sickness. Blood in the feces may indicate parasite infestation or other gut injury. Dry, mucus-covered droppings may indicate dehydration due to lack of water, dry indigestible feed, or lack of exercise.

Whole grain visible in the feces may indicate the horse's teeth need floating, the horse is bolting its feed, the feed needs processing, or the animal has a digestive disorder.

Listening to gut sounds (on the right side near the flank) may be useful in determining the activity of the gut. These sounds are at first hard to distinguish. It may be necessary to compare the normal horse to the sick horse. Excessive intestinal noises are not as serious as a lack of sound. It is a serious condition when the gut slows down and stops its waves of muscular contractions (peristaltic movements).

Loss of appetite, either partially or completely, is a prime indicator of disease.

Diagnosis of Lameness

The concept of examination should be to view the problem as a lame horse. Next determine the specific lame area(s). Finally, combine your findings into a diagnosis you can feel confident in expressing. If you don't feel confident, it is best to suggest a differential diagnosis (other possibilities) until each can be followed up. The primary objective should be to assist the horse. If you can't do that, you should be wise enough to express your feelings and refer the case to someone who can.

It is most important to follow a step by step system or routine when conducting an examination. Essential information may be overlooked and you may fail to correctly diagnose the problem and effectively treat the horse if you don't follow a system. A complete physical examination may take 45 to 60 minutes.

Request a history. Gather as much information as possible and evaluate it according to what you see and feel. Information that is most useful (after Vaughan, 1980):

1. The horse's breeding, use, diet, age, sex, temperament, physical condition-training schedule, performance record, and value-intrinsic/aesthetic; real/imagined.
2. The complaint or clinical signs as perceived by the owner, rider or trainer.
3. The onset (sudden or gradual), course (acute or chronic), stage (degree of severity and new or recurrent) and duration.
4. Response to previous and present treatment (if any), to rest, to work.
5. Number of horses in same or similar environment affected.
6. Possible explanation of cause (whereabouts and activity of horse before clinical signs first observed).

Observe the horse at rest. Don't overlook the obvious! Walk around the horse and squat to observe the legs closely. Feel the legs with your eyes. Observe from the ground up to the back. Note conformation traits and mentally relate them to possible predisposed lamenesses. Note the balance and condition of the feet. Note the general condition of the horse, especially its attitude or posture.

Pointing of either fore foot, placing weight on the toe, may indicate pain in that foot, usually in the heel area. Pushing back with the front feet, placing weight on the heels, indicates pain in the toe area. Cramping the hind limbs under

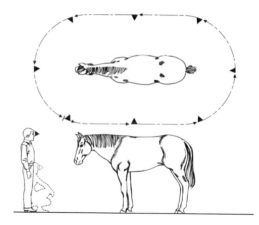

Fig. 33-6. *Observe the horse at rest from several directions. Feel the legs with your eyes.*

the body indicates both front feet or limbs are in pain. Holding the front leg back, especially with the head leaning toward it, suggests shoulder lameness.

Shifting weight from one front leg to another may indicate lameness. Shifting weight or resting first one hind leg and then the other is natural.

Feel the back. Note sensitivity over the withers, loin and spinal area.

Observe the horse from the rear sighting over the sacroiliac area. Check for knock down hip or bump.

Observe the horse in motion. Bone and joint lameness may be more evident when the horse first moves out from a resting position. Observing subtle differences requires practice and skill development. Video tape recorders with slow motion capability may be helpful, if available.

The horse handler should be instructed to first walk and then trot the horse straight away from you and back to you. It often helps if you point to some distant object and ask the person to go toward it and then come back to you. The lead rope should be held about 18 inches from the halter with sufficient slack to allow the head freedom to move. The handler should stand to the side of the horse's head and in line with its ears. When turning, the horse should be pushed away from the handler for safety's sake.

The horse should be observed walking and trotting directly away from and toward you and from the side.

The first priority should be determination of the lame limb.

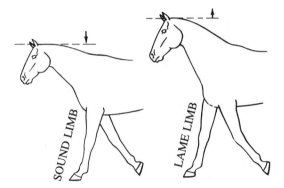

Fig. 33-7. The head of an unrestrained lame horse will nod or sink as the sound leg bears weight and bob up as lame leg hits the ground.

Lameness in one front leg causes the horse's head to nod or sink as the sound leg bears weight and causes it to bob up as the lame leg hits the ground. The flexion of the neck and the position of the ears may change as weight is carried on the lame leg. These changes are usually most recognizable at the trot. You might think of the bobbing action as a form of flinching. It can be more easily detected when viewed from in front or behind.

Lameness in one hind leg is more difficult to detect, since the head will show a similar action for diagonal front and hind legs at the trot. If the hind leg is suspected, it is better to watch the top of the croup than the head. The hip topline will sink as the sound leg bears weight. The hip will bob up sharply (though perhaps subtly) when the lame leg bears weight. To further distinguish between the hind limbs, the spavin test may be used to stress the limb.

Lameness in both front legs may be detected by the presence of a stiff, stilted action known as a choppy or pottery gait, a short stride and lack of desire to step out. The horse will appear stiff in the shoulders and the head is often carried high but does not bob. The hind feet may be lifted higher than the front and carried farther forward and more under the body than normal.

Lameness in both hind limbs results in an awkward gait producing a shortened stride. The head is usually lowered with a jerky motion in an effort to transfer weight to the front limbs. The front feet may be raised higher than the hind feet and the horse will often be difficult or impossible to back.

The relative movement (flexion-fold and extension-reach) of the front and hind limbs can be compared to the pendulum on a clock.

Additional observation tests that are sometimes helpful in determining the lame limb, type and specific site of lameness are:

1. Lunge or lead the horse both directions in tight circles. The limb on the inside of the circles will receive the most stress. This comparison can also be made by turning the horse sharply in opposite directions.
2. Trot the horse over several surfaces. Hard surfaces such as concrete or asphalt emphasize concussion type lamenesses, especially those in the foot. Uneven surfaces such as gravel or a transverse incline will often emphasize ligament or joint lameness. Larger stones may emphasize foot soreness. Wedges under one side or at the toe or heel may be used as stress tests by raising the opposite for a time and then noting any change in gait. An incline may emphasize shoulder lameness when going up and foot and knee lameness when going down. The soft ground of deep arenas, race track cushions and especially moist turf courses make foot lamenesses more difficult to detect.
3. Determine if the horse has a swinging leg (when limb does not bear weight) lameness or supporting leg (when limb bears weight) lameness. Swinging leg usually indicates high lameness above the knee or hock, supporting leg usually indicates low lameness below the knee or hock.
4. Observe progression of the lameness. If the horse warms out of the lameness (gets progressively sounder) you may suspect arthritis, bursitis or navicular disease. If the horse gets progressively lamer with use you may suspect muscle, tendon, or ligament damage, pedal osteitis or bone fractures.
5. Observe the horse while being ridden under tack or driven in harness by its *regular* rider, driver or trainer. Then if necessary, ride or drive the horse yourself.
6. Listen to the rhythm and intensity of hoof placement.
7. Observe the horse step over obstacles to determine shoulder or carpal flexion and corresponding height of foot flight arcs.
8. Observe the horse back up. Stringhalt is often more noticeable.
9. Observe the horse move side to side. Ringbone may be accentuated this way.

Examine the foot. The detailed examination to determine the specific site(s) of lameness begins with the foot. There is a greater chance of finding lameness in the foot. (See Incidence of

Lameness). The rest of the exam will proceed up the leg once the foot is checked out.

Clean out the foot with the hoof pick and check the obvious. Look for nails or evidence of sole puncture or irritation. Note the condition and firmness of the sole, frog and bulbs. If shod, note the condition and position of the shoe. Note the position and extent of the wear on the shoe.

Hoof testers allow one to compress a specific site of the foot without measurably affecting the other parts. They should always be applied to the sound hoof first to gain a "feel" of the pressure than can be applied without causing the horse to flinch or withdraw the foot. Then the same degree of pressure should be applied over the suspected area of the unsound or lame foot. Some practice is required in order to get the "feel" of the instrument. Several types are available.

Note the presence or absence of tenseness in the horse or his flinch from the pain produced by varying degrees of compression. Apply pressure slowly and firmly. Wait a few seconds between tests. Subtle muscle tension may be detected best by having an assistant hold the leg in the pastern area.

Try not to squeeze on or directly adjacent to the coronary band since the horse will give a false impression of pain in the hoof. Test the coronary band by thumb or finger pressure. Remember, two areas are being tested by the hoof tester. If possible always have one jaw on a sound area of the foot. Compression must be especially light if the sole gives to thumb pressure. A subtle problem can often be made obvious by applying continuous pressure to a suspected area of the foot for 30 seconds or more and then immediately jogging the horse.

The hoof testers should be applied in a routine sequence. If the horse is shod, the nails should be examined first. Use the same sequence on each foot to avoid leaving any step out.

Steps in using a hoof tester:

1. Place one jaw of the hoof tester against the inner edge of the shoe, the other just below the clinch of each nail. Compression of the wall under the nail will detect a nail driven in error (may be close to or in the quick), and/or an abscess or bruise at the white line or under the wall. If an abscess is suspected, nails in the area should be pulled individually and checked for wetness or discoloration.

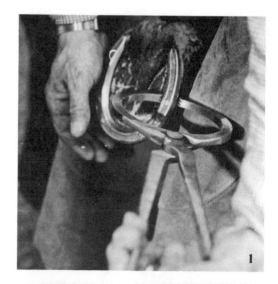

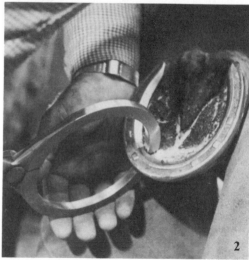

Fig. 33-8. Steps in using a hoof tester.

2. Place one jaw on the sole, the other on the middle of the hoof wall at the toe. Move around the foot from one angle of the sole to the other. Compression of the sole will detect tender soles, sole bruises, pedal osteitis or abscesses.

3. Place one jaw on the right bar, the other on the middle of the hoof wall at the heel. Compression of the bar will detect corns or heel abscesses. However, pain here may indicate internal shearing of the lamina at the heels. Further differentiation may be necessary.

4. Same as Step 3 except on the left bar.

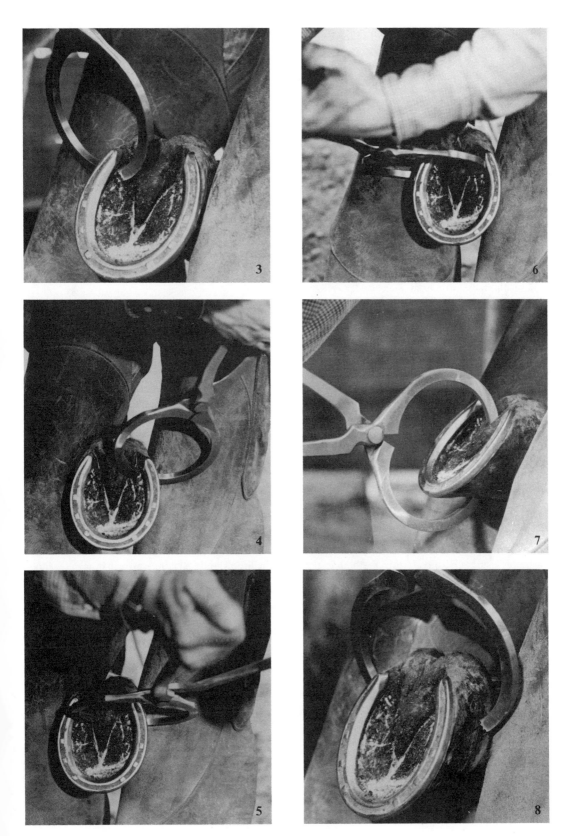

5. Place one jaw on the left side and in about the center of the frog, the other on middle of the hoof wall at the quarter. Compression of the frog will detect navicular lameness due to bursitis, bone remodeling, or pain in the distal navicular ligament, and deep flexor tendon.
6. Same as Step 5 except on the right side of the frog.
7. Place one jaw in the center of the frog, the other on the middle of the hoof wall at the toe. Compression of the frog will detect the same type of navicular lameness as Step 5, but rules out the possible differential diagnosis of sheared heels. Other areas of the frog can be tested to rule out a bruised sensitive frog.
8. Place the jaws on the ends of the navicular bone. Compression of the wings of the navicular bone will detect navicular lameness due to bone remodeling or pain in the suspensory ligament of the navicular bone. This step can also be performed manually if the hoof testers cannot be properly positioned.

Compressing the bulbs of the heel and the coronary band can be done with the thumbs while holding the foot. Thrush, cracked heels or bruises resulting from over reaching or other limb interference may be detected in this manner. Heat in the foot can be detected at this time. Press on the tops of the lateral cartilages and compare their resiliency. Stiffness indicates possible sidebones. Wire scars should be palpated, especially those that include the coronary band.

Tapping the hoof (percussion) with a ball pein or special hoof hammer may be more specific for some hoof conditions such as seedy toe than the hoof testers. However, this method is not always suitable because some horses will flinch no matter where you tap. In addition, this technique requires a great deal of practice and skill to apply and interpret. It relies on interpretation of subtle changes in sound and response to impact pressure.

Measuring the hoofs and comparing them is a means of detecting foot pathology. Calipers, rules or tapes, protractors and close observation may be used. Differences not due to previous unskilled trimming suggest pathological change. An abscessed or inflamed foot will usually grow faster. One that bears more weight will spread out and become larger at its base. A foot or portion of a foot that is not bearing its share of the weight will atrophy (shrink) as in cases of navicular disease, contracted heel(s) and sidebone. Hock or stifle lameness may produce a short or dragged off toe. Unusual parallel rings on the hoof are evidence of environmental or systemic disturbances. Marks or clefts may indicate limb interference.

All of the above observations may and probably should be made before the shoe is removed.

Paring of the sole should be done after removal of the shoe. The frog should be lightly pared, especially in the sulci, to check for evidence of thrush, puncture wounds, or foreign objects. The junction of the wall and sole at the white line should be pared when an abscess or nail puncture is suspected. Cavities in the sole should be inspected with a hoof knife or searcher when suspected as seats of lameness. Avoid cutting large holes in the sole when digging for abscesses. Any hole made should be packed with an antiseptic or poultice and the sole padded to prevent further injury. The larger the holes are, the longer the period required until the sole cover is sufficient for adequate protection of the sensitive sole and coffin bone.

Examine the limb. After examining the foot, the limb should be palpated and manipulated. Start at the foot and progress upward. Manipulate each joint and palpate the surfaces of the leg. Feel each superficial ligament, tendon and corresponding tendon sheath.

Experience will teach you to differentiate between the feel of a sound and an unsound leg. Texture and temperature of the various areas of the limb should be noted on each horse you shoe. Every horse should be your teacher.

Palpate and differentiate between the superficial flexor, deep flexor, suspensory ligament and check ligament on the back of the cannon bone. Press on and note the resistance of the synovial sac of the fetlock joint and the flexor tendons. Run your hand down the front of the cannon bone to check for evidence of shin splint(s). Check the sides of the cannon bone for high and low splints. These are considered blemishes. Feel the distal ends of the splint bones. Occasionally, one of these will be broken and must be removed by the veterinarian.

The hoof can be twisted to test the range and limit of its motion. Every joint should be manually stressed to the limit of its motion in all

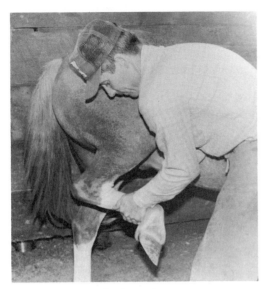

Fig. 33-9. Position for the spavin test.

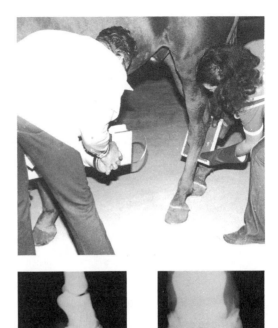

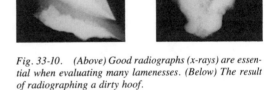

Fig. 33-10. (Above) Good radiographs (x-rays) are essential when evaluating many lamenesses. (Below) The result of radiographing a dirty hoof.

directions. Crepitation (crackling or grating sound) may be heard in dry joints or fractures. After manipulating or stressing a suspect joint, jog the horse and observe if lameness becomes more noticeable. Always compare the suspected joint or area with a corresponding test on the sound leg. Note any increase in the strength of the pulse, pain, heat or swelling.

Flexion tests may be performed on the ankle (fetlock), knee (carpus), elbow and shoulder of the forelimb. The ankle, hock, stifle and hip tests are recommended for the hind limb. The tests which have the best percentage of success are the ankle, knee and hock tests. The interior of the knee joints can be palpated by facing the head of the horse and holding the hoof between your knees.

Flexion tests are made by holding the flexed joint under constant heavy pressure for 30 seconds or more and then releasing it and immediately jogging the horse. Lameness will be more noticeable if present in the stressed joint(s). The hock flexion test, often called the spavin test, may not be specific. Upper limb flexion tests should be done for comparison. The hock should be flexed for 60 or more seconds for the spavin test.

Adjunct diagnostic procedures. Additional diagnostic procedures which may be used by a

veterinarian to confirm a clinical diagnosis include:

1. **Radiography (x-ray)** is usually necessary to confirm most physical diagnosis of the lower limb. Limiting the lameness to a specific site with the physical exam will save time and money when doing an x-ray exam. Good radiographs are especially important in order to distinguish between fractures and periosteal new bone growth. Proper treatment cannot be given without this distinction.

There are a series of standard views to be taken for each suspect area. At least two views must be taken of each area. Loss of quality due to poor technique or positioning decreases the diagnostic usefulness of radiographs.

The digit is the most frequently radiographed area of the horse and requires special positioning. Specially notched wooden blocks are frequently used to position the digit. The object is to take sharp, interpretable radiographs from a consistent position for each view. The opposite foot is usually held up to keep the radiographed leg in place.

Routine radiation safety precautions should always be observed.

Cleanliness of the leg and foot is essential. They should be thoroughly brushed and washed to remove all soil, manure and iodine. It is best to pack the sulci of the frog and the sole of the foot with children's Play Doh (modeling clay) to eliminate contrasting shadows. A similar effect can be achieved by use of a water bath when taking radiographs of the foot.

Horseshoers should learn how to properly evaluate radiographs. They need to examine them to properly perform the shoeing procedure for many pathological cases.

A radiograph is a picture of the number of x-rays passing through the animal's body. The parts that are the densest (bone, teeth) absorb the most x-rays. Less dense parts (muscle, fluids, fat, etc.) absorb a lesser amount, and air the least amount. The variation in absorption records images of body parts on radiographs.

First, view the radiograph from a distance, glancing back and forth over it comparing anatomical differences to normal views you have studied of the same area. Next, study suspected areas closely. A magnifying glass may be beneficial. Shading the light from the illuminator around the radiograph is also helpful. A spot light is especially useful when examining over-exposed areas such as soft tissue structures around bones. Periosteal new bone growth can be made more visible by this technique.

2. **Local and regional anesthesia** including bursa, joint and nerve blocks may be necessary to separate the differential diagnosis of an obscure lameness case into a definitive diagnosis. Most blocks are made with procaine or one of its pharmaceutical relatives since it is mildly toxic and it has an affinity for sensory nervous tissue. Toxic action is further reduced by slowly injecting the anesthetic solution. The anesthetic is injected through a fine 24 gauge needle around and in direct contact with the nerve. Blocks should be started low and proceed up the leg until the horse goes sound.

Regional anesthesia is often used in the horse to determine if a neurectomy of the nerve supplying the area will be successful in relieving pain. If the lameness is not completely relieved by blocking, neurectomy will be of no benefit. After nerves are blocked, the degree of anesthesia of the area and its extent may be determined by use of a sharp needle, hemostat, ball point pen or nail.

Effective use of nerve blocks in the diagnosis of lameness is only possible by a thorough study of nerve distribution and variations.

3. **Rectal examination** is necessary to diagnose obscure lameness due to pelvic fracture(s).

4. **Thermography (heat sensing)** is a means of detecting and recording the infrared radiation emitted from an object directly related to its temperature. It has been used for several years for diagnosing breast cancer in women. Its principal use in veterinary medicine has been detection of soring in show horses and tendinitis in race horses. Thermovision machines are sensitive enough to detect temperature differences up to one-tenth of one degree. The passage of the original Horse Protection Act in 1970 brought the device into the horse industry by the USDA's Animal and Plant Health Inspection Service (APHIS) to enforce the law. The machines are presently too expensive to be routinely used by individual veterinarians.

5. **Video tape recordings** of lame horses in motion are a valuable diagnostic and teaching aid. Slow and stop motion features on portable equipment make this medium all the more valuable. High speed movies (slow motion film) may also be useful but are mostly confined to experimentation since they are more expensive than video tape and require film development time.

6. **Force or pressure plates** which use sensitive strain gauges to detect variations in pressure applied to the ground by lame limbs have been recently developed. Changes in pressure on the various parts of the bottom of the hoof can be detected. Strain gauges can also be applied to the hoof in special shoes for testing track surfaces and on the sides of the hoof for evaluating hoof wall movements. An accelerometer has also been used to study hoof movements through the weight bearing and nonweight bearing phases of a stride. However, these techniques are still experimental.

7. **Electrical activity of leg muscles** can be measured to determine strain on stressed legs. This requires special instrumentation.

8. **Ultrasound** can be used to measure bone density and strength. This may be especially valuable in young horses and horses in training.

9. **Arthroscope** measurements of the interior of a joint are feasible at some veterinary hospitals. An arthroscope allows the veterinarian to look into the joint of the horse to find pathology radiographs fail to show or to evaluate joints before surgery is per-

formed. It utilizes the principles of fiber optics. It has the disadvantage of requiring general anesthesia for the horse and sterile technique. Arthroscopy has been used on the carpal, fetlock, stifle, and tarsal joints to find pathology that could not be seen on radiographs.

10. **Blood, urine, feces, tissue or synovial fluid analysis** are also available to veterinarians to produce a definitive diagnosis for any given problem.

Any one or combination of these procedures may be effectively used as an adjunct (aid) to substantiate the physical examination. But, they should not, indeed they can not, be substituted for a careful clinical examination. Clinical (observed) signs of lameness are always the most significant. The horse's marketable product is work energy. The ability to produce this product is dependent upon physical soundness.

In summary, first determine *where* the horse is lame, second determine *what* caused the lameness, and finally *select* and *apply* an effective treatment.

Treatments Available for Lameness

Treatments for lameness may be categorized by their administrators: the owner or trainer, the veterinarian or the horseshoer. Each should understand what treatments are available and possible for the benefit of the horse.

By the Owner or Trainer. Rest is probably the most important factor in helping a horse recover from a lameness causing lesion. Most lamenesses would not occur if the animal was not stressed beyond the limits of its conditioning and structural makeup. Good judgment prevents many lamenesses. Stall rest or lay-up and pasture turn out are usually the responsibility of the owner or trainer. Some treatments require the animal to rest and thus bring about recovery, often in spite of the treatment.

Physical therapy may be prescribed by the veterinarian but carried out by the owner or trainer. Forms of this may include swimming and controlled exercise.

Swimming is especially helpful in maintaining condition of the cardiopulmonary and muscular systems without stressing bones and joints. However, it is not a complete exercise. Horses must be brought back slowly by controlled exercise to be able to withstand concussion induced

pressures on the limbs. Also, since different muscles are used for swimming than for running, a certain amount of retraining must take place. Horses suffering from lameness associated with weight-bearing, and who must maintain fitness during convalescence, benefit most by swimming. Some trainers use a combination of swimming, track work and hot walking.

Treadmills have become popular for controlled exercise. They are less expensive and provide a more complete exercise than swimming pools. However, they have the same drawback as lunging and hot walkers in that they tend to over develop some muscles at the expense of others.

Feed supplements and so called blood builders have never been shown to have any measurable effect on the hoof or body health of horses receiving a balanced diet. If a deficient diet is fed, they may have a beneficial effect. However, it is usually much cheaper to feed a balanced diet than to supplement a poor one. Reliable recommendations for preparing balanced diets may be found in the current National Research Council publication on horse nutrition.

Chemical refrigerants such as alcohol, ether and menthol may be used instead of cold water for cooling out sore legs. Commercial cooling out boots are an improvement over cold water to cool out hot or inflamed legs. These boots contain cold pack inserts which can be frozen in the freezer and then allowed to thaw slowly on the leg. Ice packs are also used.

Poultices create a drawing effect and are especially useful on abscesses of the foot. They may be applied hot or cold by owners, trainers, horseshoers or veterinarians. They work best when replaced frequently and when applied hot. Poultices are also known as cataplasms.

Counterirritants are agents which cause irritation, hyperemia and some tissue destruction with the objective of relieving an inflammatory process by vasodilation. They may be divided into chemical and mechanical.

Chemical counterirritants include rubefacients and blisters. Rubefacients produce hyperemia and heat by increasing circulation to the area of application. A liniment is a rubefacient and implies a rubbing application. A wash is very mild and used after work outs. A brace is usually twice as strong as a wash. A tightener is stronger than a brace. A sweat causes moisture accumulation on the skin and is often applied under plastic. A paint is stronger than the above, but weaker than a blister. These are all mild rubefacients that can be applied repeatedly. They create warmth and dry the skin but have no blistering effect.

Blisters or vesicants produce hyperemia and increased capillary permeability with leakage of fluid into surrounding connective tissue. This eventually collects and coalesces under the epidermis in the form of vesicles. Blisters may be in liquid, paste or injectable form. Great care must be used with these preparations since they are caustic and may destroy tissue.

Mechanical counterirritants may be administered by the owner, trainer or veterinarian, depending on who owns the mechanical equipment required.

Ultrasound therapy uses high frequency sound to cause deep mechanical irradiation of tissues resulting in increased blood flow to the part. It creates a deep heat. Ultrasound can be overdone causing pain and reduced bone strength. Ultrasound is most useful in reducing periosteal new bone formation. It should not be used over bony prominences such as the sesamoids or near the epiphysis of growing bones.

Diathermy is a process using high frequency short wave electrical current to create deep heat. The internal warmth relieves pain. It is used in the treatment of muscle, tendon and ligament strain.

Muscle or nerve stimulators are used in treating strained or damaged muscles. Portable units are available which can be strapped to the horse and used while it is being exercised.

Hydrotherapy may be applied hot or cold, usually in the form of a whirlpool bath on the affected leg or part. There are boots available for the leg(s) or tubs for the whole horse. Hand or mechanical (vibrator) massage may also be used to relieve muscle soreness.

Radiotherapy and thermocautery should usually be done only by a veterinarian. Radiotherapy is a method of producing deep inflammation which can last over a month. Cobalt 60 needles, radon needles or seeds, or therapeutic x-rays may be used. Chronic arthritis and periosteal new bone formation may respond to this therapy. Radiotherapy is potentially damaging to growing bone.

Laser therapy has been successfully used in recent years. It is said to promote new cell growth to repair a damaged area. Besides being more effective than old methods, there is no pain or disfigurement.

Thermocautery or firing is the severest form of counterirritation. It has been used by trainers and veterinarians when other measures have failed. Its purpose is to transform a chronic inflammation into an acute form to promote circulation. However, the scar tissue produced has a decreased blood supply. Other reasons for firing include local desensitization and production of a supporting layer of connective (scar) tissue around an affected part. The major benefit of firing usually turns out to be the enforced rest. A minimum of 4 months rest is usually required for all major firings. The pattern for firing may be a series of points, lines or combination of points and lines. Firing is a severe procedure and frequently has complications such as exuberant granulation (proud flesh).

By the Veterinarian. In addition to most of the above treatments, the veterinarian may use prescribed drugs, acupuncture and surgery.

Osteum is an injectable inflammatory drug that acts as an internal blister. It has been useful in treating splints and other exostoses where ankylosis (joint fusion) is desired.

Bute (phenylbutazone) is one of the most popular anti-inflammatory drugs. It can be injected or fed orally. It has a systemic effect and may be used to treat more than one problem. It is illegal to administer it to race or show horses in some states because of its stimulating effect. Since bute's detection in the urine can be masked by the simultaneous administration of the diuretic furosemide (Lasix), at least one state (Louisiana) has allowed trainers to orally administer bute or arquel on the day of a race.

DMSO (dimethyl sulfoxide) is an anti-inflammatory superpenetrant. It is an extract of lignin and a by-product of the paper industry. DMSO has been most effective in treating burns and various types of bursitis and arthritis. It is also useful for transporting injectable drugs to hard-to-reach areas. It will carry small molecular compounds through the skin into the blood stream and tissues. However, DMSO will also carry dirt or even soap residue deep into the dermis and cause allergic skin reactions. It has been banned from human use because of lens damage and cataracts occurring in laboratory animals that received large dosages. One should clip the application area, wash and rinse it thoroughly and wear rubber gloves when using this drug. DMSO has the advantage of not suppressing the body's immune response as steroids do. DMSO is often mixed with counterirritants. This is dangerous since it can be explosive if not mixed in proper proportions.

Cocaine and synthetic analgesic drugs injected locally completely desensitize an area, but the effect wears off within hours. Their use is principally diagnostic. Crushing or freezing a nerve or perineural (around the nerve) injection of alcohol or phenol may cause short term (days, weeks or months) loss of pain sensation. However, in most cases these techniques are of unsatisfactory reliability.

Corticosteroids have increased in popularity in equine practice for the past 20 years. They can be administered systemically (orally or by injection) or intra-articularly (inside the joint capsule). Previously, the veterinarian had no alternative but counterirritants and rest to offer the client. Today, treatments which extend over a long period of time are not economically feasible. Injection into a joint is routinely done even though there is a great danger of introducing infection. Chemicals released by infecting bacteria gradually erode the articular cartilage.

Corticosteroids suppress the usual inflammatory response of edema and pain in a lesion and allow the horse to keep going. However, they also suppress healing and may make the treated area more susceptible to degenerative joint disease and infection. They do not cure a lesion, but only retard its progress and prolong a horse's useful working life. A typical repeatedly injected joint radiographically displays a diminished joint space and cloudy synovial fluid. Counterirritants should not be used for at least 30 days in the area of joint injection. Orthopedic surgery should not be done on horses kept going a season by intra-articular use of corticosteroids. One study concluded that when sterile joint in-

jection technique for corticosteroids is coupled with proper aftercare the disease process is stabilized in a majority of cases. Corticosteroids are injected into a joint after an equal volume of synovial fluid has been drawn out by tapping.

Acupuncture has only recently become an acceptable adjunct to conventional medicine and surgery in the Western hemisphere. Many equine practitioners consider it a valuable clinical tool. Most don't look upon it as being curative, but they note a great improvement in the animal's ability to move in a normal gait. Researchers agree that acupuncture points involve both the somatic and autonomic nervous system. These points have been correlated with motor points. Motor points are sites where a muscle is most accessible to percutaneous electrical excitation at the lowest intensity of current. Acupuncture points may also correspond to trigger points. Trigger points are cutaneous tender spots which reflect pathologic changes elsewhere in the body. Trigger points and motor points may be the same for many musculoskeletal structures. Electrical stimulation at the acupuncture points, either manually or by machine, is believed to cause the release of endorphins in the central nervous system. Endorphins (neurohormones) are natural opiates that exert a pain relieving action. Injections of various solutions into acupuncture points have been successful in treating some lamenesses.

Cryosurgery is the destruction of tissue by the application of extreme cold. It may be done with cryospray or cryoprobe instruments. The principle use of cryosurgery in equine medicine is for removal of skin tumors, especially those created by proud flesh or sarcoids. The advantages of cryosurgery, when it is applicable, are: it is relatively bloodless, no local anesthetic is required in a sedated horse, there is rapid healing, there is little scar tissue and rate of recurrence is low.

Surgery for musculoskeletal lameness problems has become very sophisticated in recent years. Cases that were considered hopeless and caused horses to be destroyed a few years ago are now being cured and brought back into useful service by successful surgical technique.

Neurectomy is the severance or removal of a section of nerve resulting in the structures sup-

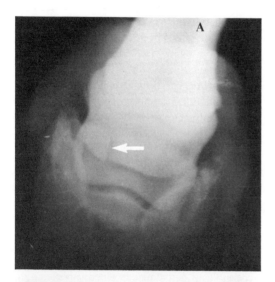

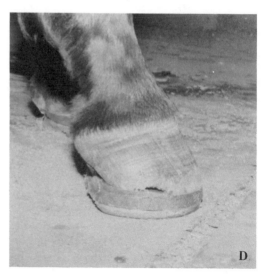

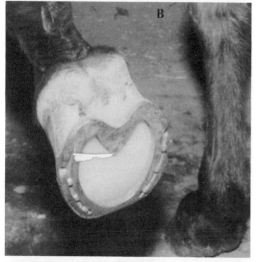

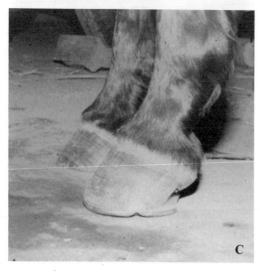

Fig. 33-11. A horseshoer must be an imaginative and skillful mechanic. An unusual case where a Standardbred mare had fractured her navicular bone because of unequal leg length. (A) Radiograph, (B) foot with broken bone shod with protective bar shoe with side clips and pad with silicone under it, (C) side view showing support given by bar shoe, and (D) wedge and lift applied to opposite leg.

plied by its distal portion being deprived of sensations. It has been considered the last resort in many cases of lower limb lameness. Low volar (palmar) or posterior digital neurectomy is most common. It is often of limited duration and may be dangerous to horse and rider. Recently the Federation Equestrian International (FEI) reported that according to survey up to 5 percent of 3-day event horses, 10 percent of dressage and driving horses and 20 percent of show jumpers have been nerved at least once.

Nerving may be performed as high as the elbow in the front limb and the gaskin of the hind limb. Horses nerved this high up are dangerous to ride. In addition, there are other complications arising from neurectomy such as neuromas (a painful tumor on the cut end of the nerve), further injury of the insensitive area, return of sensation, and sloughed hoofs. The area desensitized may be outlined by pinching, prodding or pricking the skin with a pointed instrument such as a horseshoe nail.

Orthopedic surgery involving compression bone screws and plates to set fractures or the removal of chips or joint defects is now common in valuable horses. Tendon transplants and carbon fiber implants have been recently introduced. An equine veterinarian can only keep up with current techniques by regular study, attending meetings and taking courses to learn new techniques.

The veterinarian must always keep in mind the present and future value of an animal when proposing surgery. The physician may say: save life or limb at any cost. But the veterinarian must always say: save life or limb at what cost? Investment of time, effort, money in the perspective of the future usefulness of the horse must be evaluated. Surgery may be a good idea for an expensive race horse, but a not so good idea for a ranch horse. Alternate techniques or euthanasia may be more practical. In addition, the prognosis for recovery and possible complications should always be considered when contemplating surgery. Proper padding is essential for horses when under general anesthesia.

By the Horseshoer. There are three principal ways the horseshoer may treat pathological conditions:

1. Protect the foot with a pad or shoe or both. Foot soreness caused by concussion, bruising, sole penetration or internal disease can be helped by the use of pads. Pads may be of leather, rubber, steel, aluminum or plastic (neoprene, neolite, nylon, or polyurethane). Pads are usually applied between the shoe and hoof. Wide webbed shoes are also used to protect the sole.

2. Support the limb, foot or foot parts. Support may be incorporated into the shoe as with clips or bar shoes. It can be given in the form of a brace or splints of various types. If only one leg is injured, it may be necessary to give support by wrapping the cannon region of the opposite leg to prevent a tendon bow or ligament strain.

3. Shift the weight distribution of the horse over the limb and foot structures. This may be necessary due to increased stress brought about by foot imbalance or conformation defect. Hoof angles, lateral balance or shape of the hoof may be changed to shift stresses (temporarily or permanently) from one area of the limb or foot to another. This technique must be applied with experienced judgment.

One or a combination of these three principles may be used on any given individual horse. There are many variations of each. One must be an imaginative and skillful mechanic to excel as a therapeutic horseshoer. The next four chapters describe the application of these principles to specific lamenesses.

References

Adams, O.R. 1974. Lameness in Horses (3rd ed.). Lea and Febiger, Philadelphia.

Adams, O.R. 1980. Equine lameness and surgery videotapes. Colorado State University, College of Veterinary Medicine, Fort Collins, CO.

Alexander, J.E. 1968. Effects of X-irradiation on growing bone. Modern Veterinary Practice. (Feb.):41.

American Association of Equine Practitioners (AAEP). 1982. Definition and classification of lameness. Newsletter (March) 1:38.

Bobylev, I., H. Gerber, J. Hickman, J.A. Wosowski and R. Zeller. 1980a. FEI veterinary committee report on neurectomy (Part 1). Horse Show. May:13.

Bobylev, I., H. Gerber, J. Hickman, J.A. Wosowski and R. Zeller. 1980b. FEI veterinary committee report on neurectomy (Part II.) Horse Show. June:14.

Burns, S.J. and W.C. McMullan. 1977. Junior Clinics-Equine Section. Texas A & M College of Veterinary Medicine, College Station, TX.

Cannon, R. 1968. What became of the rub-on wonder drug DMSO? Sci. Dig. (Sept.):7.

Carson, D. 1910. A plea for reciprocity. The Farriers' Annual. 1:35.

Cunha, T.J. 1974. Calcium and phosphorus for sounder feet and legs. Horse and Rider 8(12):49.

Delahanty, D.D. 1969. Diagnostic aids in lameness. American Veterinary Conference. Cornell University. 61:35.

Delahanty, D.D. 1975. Counterirritation. Cornell Veterinary College. Ithaca, NY.

Downer, A.H. 1976. Ultrasound therapy for animals. Modern Vet. Practice. 57(7):523.

Fleming, G. 1870. Observations on the anatomy and physiology of the horse's foot. The Vet. 43:13.

Frank, E.R. 1964. Veterinary Surgery (7th ed.). Burgess Publ. Co., Minneapolis.

Gideon, L. 1977. Acupuncture: clinical trials in the horse. J.A.V.M.A. 170(2):220.

Gillette, E.L., D.E. Thrall, and J.L. Lebel. 1977. Carlson's Veterinary Radiology (3rd ed.). Lea and Febiger, Philadelphia.

Hayden, W.F. 1910a. Wilts county council. The Farrier's Annual. 1:40.

Hayden, W.F. 1910b. The lateral cartilages in health and disease. The Farriers' Annual 1:42.

Hill, R.R. 1980. Letters-Back to drawing board. Equus. 38:7.

Holscher, M.A., R.L. Linnabary, M.G. Netsky, and H.D. Owen. 1978. Adenoma of the pars intermedia and hirsutism in a pony. Vet. Med./S.A.C. (Sept.):1197.

Jones, D. 1971. Ethics and honesty. Proc. Amer. Assoc. of Equine Practitioners. 17:234.

Joyce, J.R. 1976. Cryosurgical treatment of tumors of horses and cattle. J.A.V.M.A. 168(3):226.

Kirkpatrick, A. 1980. Veterinary advances-detecting invisible soreness. Horse Show. (Nov.):7.

Knowles, J.H. 1976. The struggle to stay healthy. Time. (Aug. 9):60.

Kraus, S.E. and K.D. Butler. 1977. The realm of the horseshoer. Amer. Farriers' J. 3(1):4.

Lakin, R. 1980. Custom-made hoof testers. Equus. 30:42.

Leitch, M. 1977. Lameness of the horse. National Horseman's Seminar Proc. 2:116.

Lieberman, B. 1980. DMSO: horses yes, humans maybe. Equus. 35:56.

Lorscheider, L. 1980. Color-coded hot spots-thermography offers vibrant view of body heat. Equus. 42:33.

Mackay-Smith, M. 1977. Locating lameness. Equus. 2:47.

Maetz, H.M. 1968. What about licensing procedures? Modern Vet. Practice. (Jan.):23.

McGuire, B. 1977. Horse Health Primer. Instructional Materials Service, Cornell University, Ithaca, NY.

McIlwraith, W. and J.F. Fessler. 1978. Arthroscopy in the diagnosis of equine joint disease. J.A.V.M.A. 172(3):263.

McKay, A.G. and F.J. Milne. 1976. Observations on the intraarticular use of corticosteroids in the racing Thoroughbred. J.A.V.M.A. 168(11):1039.

Miller, R.M. 1972. Vet's corner-The diagnosis of lameness. The Western Horseman. (July):32.

Miller, R.M. 1975. Vet's corner-Common causes of lameness. The Western Horseman. (Feb.):7.

Milne, D.W. and A.S. Turner. 1979. An Atlas of Surgical Approaches to the Bones of the Horse. W.B. Saunders Co., Philadelphia.

Milne, F.J. 1967. Clinical examination and diagnosis of the diseased equine foot. J.A.V.M.A. 151(12):1599.

Morgan, J.P., S. Silverman, and W.J. Zontine. 1977. Techniques of Veterinary Radiography (2nd ed.). Veterinary Radiology Associates, Davis, CA.

Purohit, R.C. and M.D. McCoy. 1980. Thermography in the diagnosis of inflammatory processes in the horse. J.A.V.M.A. 41(8):1167.

Rendano, V.T. 1977. Radiographic interpretation-equine radiology-the fetlock. Mod. Vet. Practice. 58(10):871.

Rinedollar, D. 1975. Hoofprints. Welsh Pony Tales. (Autumn):19.

Roberts, E.J. 1967. Firing a horse: is it the best way? The Chronicle of the Horse. (Mar. 17):26.

Rooney, J.R. 1974. The Lame Horse. A.S. Barnes and Co., Cranbury, NJ.

Rooney, J.R. 1977. The Sick Horse. A.S. Barnes and Co., Cranbury, NJ.

Russell, W. 1887. Scientific Horseshoeing. Robert Clarke and Co., Cincinnati. p.xxv.

Siegmund, O.H. (Ed.) 1973. The Merck Veterinary Manual. Merck and Co., Inc., Rahway, NJ.

Simmons, H. 1963. Horseman's Veterinary Guide. The Western Horseman, Colorado Springs, CO.

Staff Report. 1976. Practicing without a license? Rodeo News. (Oct.):25.

Staff Report. 1977. Lasix can camouflage bute. Ill. Equine Mkt. (Apr.):1.

Staff Report. 1978. Checking vital functions. Saddle Action. (May):36.

Staff Report. 1980. Acupuncture in horses evaluated at University of Georgia. Norden News. Winter/Spring:39.

Staff Report. 1980. Getting the jump on the juice in the joint. Equus. 35:58.

Stromberg, B.R.G. and A.W. Norberg. 1971. Infra-red emission and ^{133}Xe-disappearance rate studies in the horse. Equine Vet. J. 3:7.

Swenson, M.J. (Ed.). 1977. Duke's Physiology of Domestic Animals (9th ed.). Comstock Publishing Associates, Ithaca, NY.

Szabuniewicz, M. 1969. Use of the hoof hammer and its handle in diagnosing lameness in horses. Vet. Med./S.A.C. (July):618.

Szabuniewicz, M. and J.M. Szabuniewicz, 1975. Use of the hoof tester in diagnosing lameness in horses. Vet. Med./S.A.C. (Feb.):205.

Turner, A.S. 1980. Courting risk with cortisone. Equus. 38:14.

Van Pelt, R.W. 1974. Interpretation of synovial fluid findings in the horse. J.A.V.M.A. 165(1):91.

Vaughan, J.T. 1980. Diagnosis of Lameness in the Horse. American Farriers' Assn. Conv. Jackson, MS.

Vaughan, J.T. et. al. 1965. Tips on managing equine lameness. Modern Vet. Practice. (Apr.):58.

Yeats, J.J. 1968. Incidence of Lameness. Vet. Rec. (Dec.):617.

Young, H.G. 1976. Acupuncture, a new modality. Vet. Econ. (Jan.):21.

Zoll, D. 1979. Are we asking too much of our horses? Equine Market and Horseman's Review. (Oct.):22.

NOTES:

Chapter 34

Lamenesses of the Foot

Lamenesses of the foot are classified as veterinary problems but all involve the horseshoer, directly or indirectly. The horseshoer is expected to take care of most foot problems and know when to call a veterinarian. When in doubt as to your ability to provide for a horse's needs, refer the owner to a veterinarian. The veterinarian will then be responsible for the treatment of the condition and request the horseshoer to support the medical treatment or surgery by regular shoeing.

Thrush

Thrush is a common disease of the frog. It is distinguished by its foul odor and cheesy appearance. There may be a black or gray discharge from a neglected infection. The condition is usually not serious, but may cause severe lameness if allowed to progress.

Pockets of infection develop in the frog or

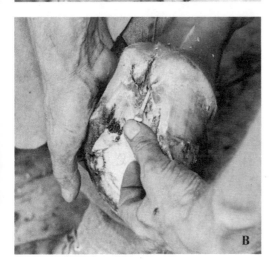

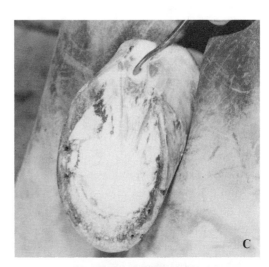

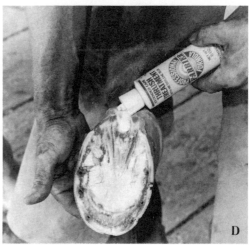

Fig. 34-1. Thrush treatment:
(A) Cut away the infected tissue.
(B) Determine the extent of the problem.
(C) Clean out the infection. Use cotton balls on the end of a hoof pick until they come out clean.
(D) Pack the foot with medication until it is thoroughly dried up. Photos by J. Graves.

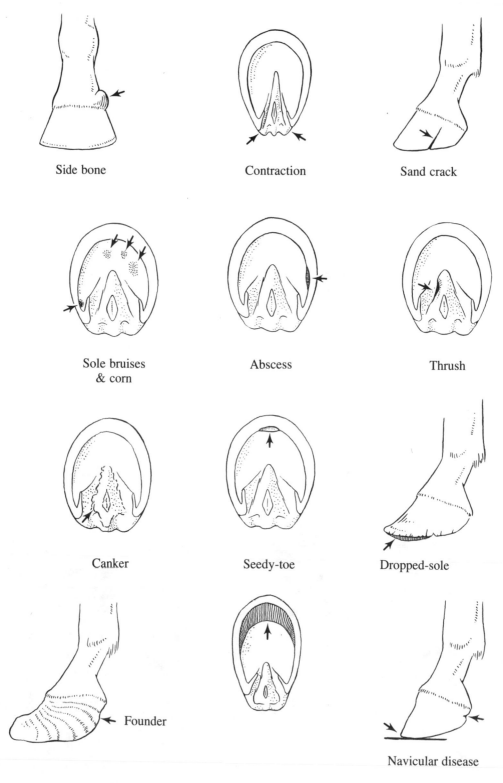

Fig. 34-2. Location of lamenesses of the foot. Drawing by L. Sadler.

between the frog and packed-in filth. Anaerobic conditions (no air present) are necessary for the disease to develop. Filthy stable conditions and lack of regular hoof cleaning and trimming are the most common causes. Thrush may be encouraged by hoof contraction, sudden climatic changes (wet seasons) or lack of exercise and frog stimulation.

The anaerobic bacteria primarily responsible for thrush are called *Spherophorus necrophorus*. These bacteria have recently been renamed *Fusobacterium necrophorum*. Aerobic bacteria of the *Staphylococcus* and *Streptococcus* type are often present as well. *Spherophorus necrophorus* are present in the manure of all domestic animals. The organisms are very concentrated in decomposing organic matter.

Thrush may be treated by trimming away the infected parts of the frog and washing the hoof with a scrub brush. Deep infections should be permitted to drain and then be irrigated with 7 percent iodine or copper sulfate solution (Kopertox). Other drying agents such as formalin solution, alum, copper sulfate (blue stone), clorox or turpentine may be used. However, these topical applications can be over emphasized. Regular hoof cleaning and frequent stable cleaning are the most effective preventions and treatments.

Severe cases may require padding of the hoof and packing with medication. Intravenous injections of sulfa solutions and sodium iodide have been reported effective in several cases. Tetanus immunization should be current if the condition reaches the sensitive tissues. An important part of treatment is to encourage the owner to prevent its reoccurrence.

Abscess

Abscess, gravel or pus pocket is an infection of the sensitive tissues of the foot. It is most common in the sensitive sole next to the white line. Often, a drainage hole or puncture entry hole can be seen after sole paring. It will appear as a black spot next to the white line. The digit will be hot and swollen. The horse may be moderately to severely (threelegged) lame. Abscess will follow a path of least resistance. It will migrate through soft tissue and may break out and drain from the coronary band. Once the abscess begins to drain, lameness usually subsides.

Abscesses can be located with a hoof tester. Paring the sole also helps. The sole may have a dryer, harder texture below the site of the infection due to the heat generated. As the sole is thinned over the infected area, it will become softer and spongy over the abscess.

Abscesses may result from puncture wounds or bacterial infection (*Spherophorus necrophorus*) entering the soft tissues of the foot through the white line. Alternate wet and dry conditions may be an indirect cause. The wall expands when wet causing the leaves at the white line to separate from the sole. This allows anaerobic bacteria present in mud and manure to enter the sensitive structures. Dryer conditions cause the bacteria to be trapped beneath the sole. Bacteria then form a fistulous tract(s) in the sensitive tissue following the path(s) of least resistance. Abscesses have been called gravels with the idea that a piece of gravel migrated up through the sensitive tissues and out through the coronary band. There is no evidence to indicate that such a thing takes place. However, occasionally a sharp rock will puncture the sole and introduce bacteria which in turn cause an abscess. Abscesses are most common during or immediately after the wet season of the year.

The quickest relief from an abscess can be obtained by paring until the pus pocket is reached and drainage is initiated. Gas forming bacteria (*Clostridia*) occasionally infect the foot along with *Spherophorus*. They cause extreme pain and the horse experiences immediate relief when they are opened. A salve poultice applied directly or soaking with Epsom salts is often necessary in persistent cases. Avoid cutting a large hole in the hoof. In most cases, the less hoof removed the better. The horse can then be returned to useful service as soon as it is sound. Solar abscesses usually heal in less than 2 weeks. Abscesses under the frog may take 4 weeks.

Affected horses should have current tetanus immunization. Injected antibiotics may be helpful. Establish drainage in the abscessed area and flush with hydrogen peroxide or other suitable solution. Irrigate with a germicide (7 percent iodine). Pack with a drawing agent (20 percent Ichthammol). Shoe with a pad. Cover pared area with a bar welded across the shoe. When frequent changing of dressing and/or soaking of the wound is necessary, a removable sole plate may be necessary. A rubber poultice boot may work best for a few days. Soon the infection will be walled off and normal work can resume when the horse shows no lameness.

Canker

Canker or hoof cancer is a chronic hypertrophy (vegetative growth) of the sensitive frog. Rarely, the sensitive sole is also affected. The frog has a ragged and oily appearance. The frog grows so out of shape that it appears tumorous. There is an unmistakable odor. *Spirochaeta* microorganisms have been isolated from diseased tissue. Draft horses are most commonly affected.

Hoof cancer is caused by constant contact of strong ammonia compounds. These substances irritate the sensitive structures and cause benign and possibly malignant growths to be produced. Prevention consists of regular stall and hoof cleaning.

The frog and sole should be trimmed to their normal shape and diseased material removed.

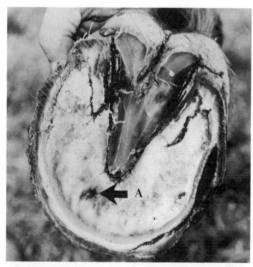

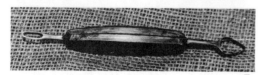

Fig. 34-3. (A) Abscess (arrow) resulting from puncture wound.
(B) Special hoof knife made by J. Peterka (called a searcher or groover) to dig out abscesses.

The bottom of the foot should be packed with a sulfa (furacin) salve. The foot should be shod with pressure from a bar shoe or metal plate on the affected area. The horse may be very tender in the bulbs and affected area. Lameness will gradually subside as the inflammation is treated and the horse is placed in a clean environment. The foot dressing should be changed regularly. A removable bolt-on sole plate is convenient.

Penicillin is often administered in chronic cases where systemic infection may be present. Penicillin may also be used on the bottom of the foot. Drying agents may be applied to toughen the softened hoof after the initial treatment of infection.

Yeast Infection

Yeast infection by *Candida albicans* is fairly common in the humid climate of Florida. It has been observed in other areas where horses are kept in damp and filthy conditions. These infections usually involve only the inner third of the hoof wall. However, the damage from the fungus may weaken the wall and indirectly cause lameness. The infected area is soft and appears like a granulated cheese mixture. The condition is commonly called seedy-toe. It may be related to a chronic progressive pododermatitis reported in Sweden.

Yeast infection seems to be related to thrush. The yeast may enter the wall below the bulbs

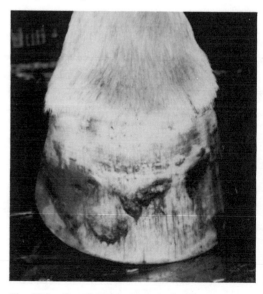

Fig. 34-4. Yeast infection. Photo by B. Laraway.

where the frog joins the wall or at the white line. Yeast may also travel around the wall under the periople before entering the hoof. Infections of this type may cause irregular wavy or crossed rings to be produced on the wall. Yeast prefer the inner layer of the hoof wall whereas thrush organisms prefer the frog. The wall surrounding a yeast infection will be a characteristic pale yellow. All of the infected material must be removed with a hoof knife or a motorized burr. Germicidal agents may be used but are not usually necessary if all yeast are removed. Large holes may be filled with hoof repair acrylic.

Filthy stabling conditions and wet, sandy soil encourage yeast infection. Frequently applied topical hoof dressings also encourage the condition. Hoof areas that contain yeast may be predisposed to abscesses or hoof cracks.

Sandcrack

Sandcrack is a vertical crack in the hoof wall. A sandcrack is referred to by location as a toe, quarter, heel or bar crack. Cracks are usually parallel to the hoof tubules. Cracks may be su-

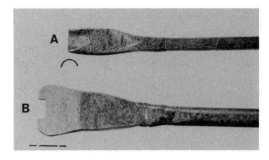

Fig. 34-6. Sandcrack irons.

perficial and harmless or deep and penetrating the sensitive structures.

Wall cracks may be caused by flares or unbalanced feet. Dry and brittle hoofs crack more easily than healthy hoofs. Large nails in proportion to hoof size and condition and driven near the outside edge will split even a healthy hoof wall.

Treatment of hoof cracks consists of various methods to immobilize the crack permitting sound horn to grow down from the coronary band. Shoe clips on each side of the crack may be sufficient.

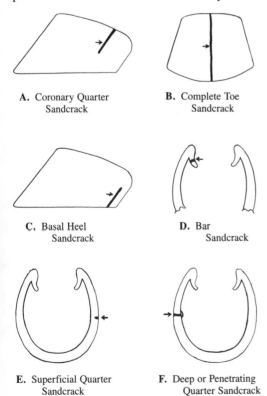

A. Coronary Quarter Sandcrack

B. Complete Toe Sandcrack

C. Basal Heel Sandcrack

D. Bar Sandcrack

E. Superficial Quarter Sandcrack

F. Deep or Penetrating Quarter Sandcrack

Fig. 34-5. Types of sandcracks.

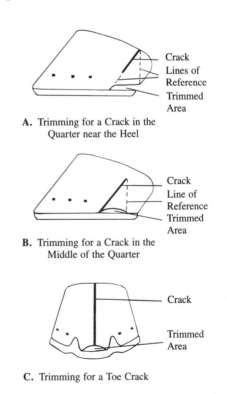

A. Trimming for a Crack in the Quarter near the Heel

B. Trimming for a Crack in the Middle of the Quarter

C. Trimming for a Toe Crack

Fig. 34-7. Trimming for sandcracks.

Cracks that originate from the base of the hoof or do not extend all the way through the wall may be contained by burning at the top with a half-moon or similar shaped iron. This has the effect of deflecting stress away from the wall above the crack. Long cracks of this type may be burned on each side of the crack and clinched with a small horseshoe nail. The burning should be about three-quarters of the way through the wall. Many other techniques have been invented (and patented) to treat sandcracks. Most are only a memory. Surgical excision (removal) is still practiced in some areas.

Cracks that move and cause pain with each step are best immobilized by binding and filling the crack with selfpolymerizing acrylic plastics or epoxy hoof repair materials[1]. These modern farrier aids have the advantage of decreasing the convalescing time by replacing the destroyed tissue and remaining a part of the hoof until they grow out. Pressure around the crack should be relieved.

The crack should be cleaned out and undercut with a motorized burr. Sensitive tissue should be protected by a seton of sterile cotton or other suitable material. Acrylics should be applied in layers no more than ⅜ inch thick to prevent the possibility of sensitive tissue injury from heat created by polymerization.

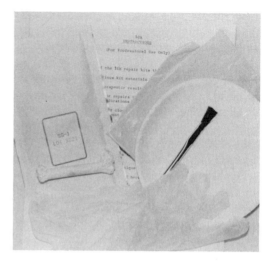

Fig. 34-9. 10X hoof repair material.

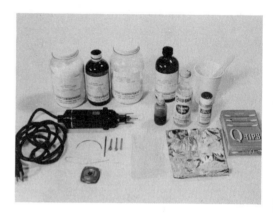

Fig. 34-10. Hoof repair drill and other accessories.

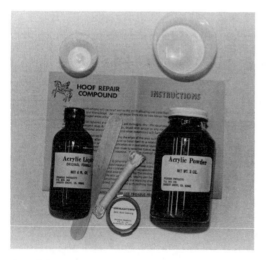

Fig. 34-8. Pegasus acrylic hoof repair material. Photos by J. Graves.

Centaur Forge, Ltd., Burlington, WI

Keratoma

Keratoma or keraphyllocele is a rare tumor of the horny laminae. It may be caused by an injury to the coronary band, hoof grooving, a sandcrack, a close nail or a large hammered-in clip. The white line will appear bent in toward the center of the sole. The horse may be lame due to pressure from the tumor against the coffin bone. Bone changes may be seen in radiographs.

The tumor mass must be surgically removed. This should be done by a veterinarian while the horse is under anesthesia. A motorized burr is required. Shoeing should protect the area while it is healing. Wire cuts or other injuries to the coronary band may cause deformities of the hoof wall. These are not tumors and may be safely rasped away.

Hoof Loss

Hoof loss or avulsion is usually due to trauma of some kind. Catching the foot in a tight spot (such as a cattle guard) when traveling at speed is the usual cause. However, hoofs can also be lost due to selenium poisoning, vitamin A deficiency, wire cut or puncture wound infection, laminitis or extremely long neglected feet shod with very heavy shoes.

Hoof loss cases must be carefully evaluated by the owner, veterinarian and horseshoer. A judgment must be made on the probable prognosis before treatment begins. Timing and future use are most important considerations. Results are often disappointing if the hoof has been gone for more than a few hours before treatment begins. At first, the foot is usually packed with Furacin ointment and bandaged.

A leather or rubber tie-on boot should be constructed to protect the coriums of the hoof and permit regular dressing of the wound. It takes several days for a protective horn scale to form and nearly a year to grow a new hoof. In the meantime, the opposite foot may founder or the tendons may bow due to the increased strain. A stall sling can be used, but they are rarely successful. They usually produce sores and most horses are poor patients when it comes to bed rest. (See Fig. 36-8.)

Protect the foot with a shoe as soon as enough hoof is present to permit shoe attachment at the heels. The rest of the hoof may be built up and protected with hoof repair acrylic as it grows out. The new hoof may never reach normal size and may always be weak. The horse may not even be sound enough to breed. Rarely, a horse with proper treatment will make a complete recovery.

Contraction

Contraction, hoof bound or atrophy of the hoof is a drawing together of the buttresses causing a constriction of the hoof. Contraction may affect one or both heels. There may or may not be lameness associated with the condition. A foot is said to be contracted when the buttresses are closer together than 1/4 inch inside of parallel lines extended back from the toe nail holes of keg shoes.

Contracted heels may be said to be a symptom

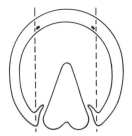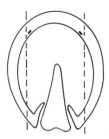

Fig. 34-11. Contraction: (left) normal hoof, (right) contracted hoof.

(sign of a disease) rather than a disease when it is associated with navicular disease. The heel halfway between the coronary band and buttress (navicular waist) and the sole (arched) are often contracted when navicular disease is present.

Contraction may be caused by a lack of moisture in the hoof. Lack of pressure or weight bearing on the heels and especially the frog is a common cause. Lack of use of a leg due to a fracture or other injury causes atrophy (withering away) of the hoof. Lack of exercise destroys the internal circulation of the hoof. Excessive hoof length and repeated fitting of too small a shoe also causes the hoof to contract.

Moisture can be restored to the hoof by turning the horse out barefoot in a damp pasture. Some veterinary clinics have special foot soaking stalls for treatment of contraction and infectious foot diseases. Moisture can also be restored to the hoof by the use of rubber poultice boots, packing the feet with clay and wrapping the foot with burlap sacks. Rasping or slippering the quarters to encourage expansion is not recommended. A bar shoe with frog pressure and/or bevel-edged shoe is a preferred supplement to moisture restoration. Several "expanding" shoes have been designed for treatment of contraction. Hoof springs may be used under pads. But, even then they are difficult to retain in position.

Corns

Corns start as bruises of the sensitive sole in the angle formed by the wall and bars. A dry corn is a red circular bruise in the seat of corn area. The redness is caused by ruptured blood vessels draining into the horn tubules. A dry corn may have had time to heal before it is observed at the ground surface. A moist corn is usually yellow and has serum present. A suppurating corn has become infected and turned into an abscess.

Corns are caused by unequal pressure and concussion created by a conformation defect(s), overtrimming of the heels, heel calks, short-heeled shoes or unlevel shoes. Neglect of the feet and leaving shoes on for extended periods of time is a common cause. The forefeet are most often affected since they carry more weight than the hind feet and the heels of front feet usually strike the ground first.

Corns can be prevented by removing or compensating for their causes. Trimming the sole between the bars and wall so that it is 1/8 inch lower than the wall will relieve the pressure on the seat of corn.

A bar shoe should be used to treat corns in cases where lameness is evident. The pressure of weight bearing at the heels should be transferred from the heels to the frog. A pad should be used to reduce concussion. A wide-heeled shoe fit full at the heels may be helpful. The mushroom shoe is occasionally used to transfer weight bearing from the heels to the frog. Infected corns which have been opened to facilitate draining must be protected by a rubber boot or pad. Pads also help hold medication in the wound(s).

Sole Bruises

Sole bruises are red spots or "strawberries" in the sole or frog of variable size. They appear as a mass of tiny red specks. Blood vessels in the sensitive structures rupture due to trauma and stain the horny sole. The white line or the hoof wall may also be red. The effects seen at the ground surface originated in the corium shortly after keratinization of the horn.

Sole bruises are caused by sharp trauma or excessive weight bearing by the sole due to balled up snow or rocky ground or shoe sole pressure. Shoes should be concaved or seated out away from the sole. Barefoot horses should be trimmed so that they walk on the wall. Hoofs that are trimmed too short are easily bruised in any terrain. Also, thin soles tend to dry out, contract and cause bruising of the coffin bone. A horse with a dropped or extremely flat sole is very susceptible to bruising. A horse with a persistent bruised (red) sole probably has pedal osteitis (inflammation of the coffin bone).

Horses that hit hind toe first, especially those that wear away the front of the toe, often develop redness in the white line and toe of the wall. Such horses are called toe-hitters or toe-stabbers. This condition may be a symptom of other problems such as bone spavin. Toe grabs or calks may also cause bruises by increasing the strain on the toe and white line junction between the wall and sole. Horses that hit hard heel first often develop bruises and eventually pedal osteitis.

Bruised soles can be protected by shoeing with a pad and flat concaved shoe. A wide-webbed seated out shoe may be helpful when dropped sole is present. A bar welded across the shoe will protect one bruised area. A solid plate welded across a bar shoe will protect the entire sole and frog. Hoof cushion (silicone) injected between a pad and the sole may be useful in preventing a severe sole bruise. It may be effective in treating some cases of pedal osteitis. Horses vary in their response to the application of hoof cushion. Sometimes it gives relief, in others its presence aggravates the lameness.

Pedal Osteitis

Pedal osteitis is an inflammation of the coffin bone. It is usually the result of a constant or serious bruising of the sole. The sole will consistently appear bruised. However, radiographs are necessary to substantiate the presence of the condition. Osteophytes (bone growths) lytic areas (decreased bone density) and a localized increased vascular pattern are often present. The commonly seen notch in the toe of the coffin bone should not be confused with bone demineralization. Most pedal osteitis may be treated as sole bruises. Heel lameness may require a tongue bar shoe. Some cases require stall rest for many months.

Sidebone

Sidebone or ossification of the lateral cartilage(s) is a loss of flexibility of the foot cartilages. Lameness may or may not be present. The affected side of the hoof is usually shorter and more contracted at one heel than the other. The lateral cartilage does not yield readily under thumb pressure. In long standing cases there will be a raised enlargement above the coronary band near

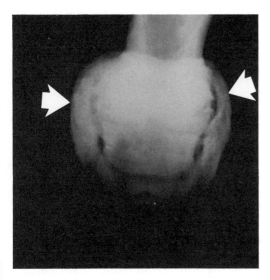

Fig. 34-12. Side bone (radiograph).

the heel. Severity of the condition depends upon the age of the horse, the stage of the ossification, the concussion produced by the terrain, horse's gait or conformation, and other complicating conditions. The condition seems to be a natural part of the ageing process in some horse breeds and families.

Sidebone is most common in toed-in draft horses and bulldog type Quarter Horses, especially in those that are also steep shouldered and short pasterned. Any use which creates concussion on one side of the foot such as barrel racing or jumping may further predispose a horse to sidebone. Wire cuts in the coronary region, excessively dry or contracted hoofs and small feet in proportion to the horse's weight are other possible causes.

Sidebone is difficult to treat. Trimming the foot so it lands flat is one of the most common recommendations. A wide web shoe and pad help distribute concussion over a wider area. Sometimes shifting weight to the sound side may temporarily help. A rocker-toed bar shoe with pad helps some hunters. Hoof cushion (silicone) may be injected under the pads. Hoof grooving and thinning or "slippering" the quarters has been recommended. Results are rarely positive. However, moistening the hoof and applying counterirritants to the coronary band may be helpful.

Quittor

Quittor or necrosis of the lateral cartilage(s) is an infection of the lateral cartilage(s). It is characterized by a pus discharge and severe lameness. The condition may result from an infected puncture wound or chronic sole abscess.

The affected area must be curetted (scraped clean) and persistently treated both topically and systemically with antibiotics and sulfa drugs. Removal of the lateral cartilage by surgery was once recommended. However, it is rarely successful due to the extensive venous circulation adjacent to the cartilage(s). Curetting (scraping) the cartilage is sometimes successful. The disease is best treated in its early stages. The prognosis (possibility of complete recovery) is poor for a horse with chronic lameness due to quittor.

Sheared Heels

Sheared heels are the result of unequal weight bearing by the foot. One heel is higher (and longer) than the other. The unequal weight causes a shearing to take place in the heel region above the cleft of the frog. This may be very painful and further aggravated by constant movement in this region. Occasionally, heel and quarter laminae are torn and inflamed by hoof imbalance.

Conformation or gait defects and attempts to correct them may cause the condition. The hoof wall twists as weight is distributed unevenly over it. The skin and cleft hoof between the heel bulbs tear at the weakest point.

The hoof must be balanced to allow equal weight bearing of both sides. This may be done with a combination of trimming and shoeing to place the center of the weight bearing surface (shoe) in the center of the leg and perpendicular to a plumb line from the horse's shoulder or hip. When the horse moves, the foot should land as flat as possible. Germicidal salve and bandaging of the heel above the cleft may be necessary until the corium heals and the pain subsides. A bar shoe is useful to reinforce and protect the sore area. An egg bar shoe is especially useful when the horse also has very sloping heels.

Coffin Bone Fracture

Coffin bone (third phalanx) fracture is most commonly of two types. A fracture through the center of the bone (intra-articular or mid-sagit-

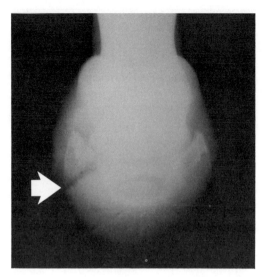

Fig. 34-13. Coffin bone fracture (radiograph).

tal) including the articular or joint surface is most serious and must be surgically repaired by the veterinarian using a compression bone screw. The horse is put under general anesthesia. A hole is cut in the wall with a trephine (round saw). A hole is drilled through one bone half and into the other. A compression bone screw is inserted. After healing begins, the hoof hole can be filled with acrylic.

A fracture of the wing of the coffin bone (extra-articular or alar) can usually be stabilized and treated with only a bar shoe. The shoe has three clips, one at the toe and one on each quar-

ter. A diagonal bar may be welded under the fracture line to further protect and stabilize the foot. The shoe acts as a cast to hold the bone in place until it heals and is sound again. Complete healing may take many months. Healing time is reduced when a screw is used. Abscesses sometimes complicate and extend healing time.

Rarely, the navicular bone or short pastern may fracture. Navicular bone fracture is treated similar to coffin bone fracture. In addition, the heels are elevated and the toe of the shoe is rocked. The short pastern bone must be surgically repaired by screws and a compression plate.

Laminitis

Laminitis or founder has been a problem associated with equine mismanagement for centuries. It is thought to be a metabolic disease that selectively affects the feet. Laminitis is associated with endotoxemia. Researchers are experimenting with anti-endotoxin serums and vaccines. The disease is not well understood and can be acute or chronic in severity. Overweight cresty-necked mares and stallions are most susceptible.

Laminitis is often caused by overfeeding and neglect. Feeding large amounts of grain to inactive horses is a leading cause of laminitis. Many horses fed this way need only a slight amount of stress to cause an attack. Spring grass affects some horses adversely after they have been on hay all winter. Fescue grass, especially when mature, may cause laminitis. Ergot toxicosis resulting from poisoning by toxic fungi may also be a problem. Horses are usually lame within one to two days after ingesting harmful feeds.

Various stress factors have also been known to cause laminitis. These include abnormal concussion or weight bearing, overwork for the level of conditioning, drinking cold water when hot, high fever for an extended period of time and toxic drugs (especially steroids) or poisonous feed stuffs. Postparturient laminitis in mares results from a retained placenta and subsequent metritis after foaling. High blood pressure may also be a cause.

The blood concentration of lactic acid increases when laminitis occurs. Apparently,

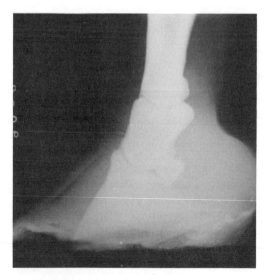

Fig. 34-14. Laminitis (radiograph).

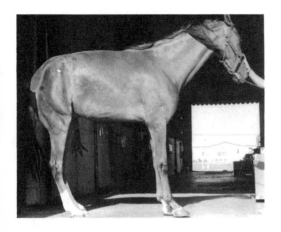

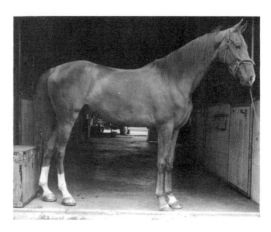

Fig. 34-15. (Left) Laminitis stance. Note that ears are back, hind legs are up under the body, flanks are tucked up, front legs are forward and weight is borne on the heels.

(Right) Normal stance. Same horse after one year of therapeutic shoeing and treatment.

endotoxins cause histamine formation and blood platelet function is impaired. Blood circulation to the sensitive laminae is disturbed and the process of cornification is disrupted. The secondary laminae eventually become necrotic and the coffin bone rotates or sinks (founders) as it pulls away from the hoof wall. The intense pain is due to the separation of the laminae and the absence of oxygen in the tissues. The initial pain experienced by the horse could be compared to a severe headache aggravated by a tight-fitting hat. First symptoms may be loss of appetite, elevated temperature, listlessness, colic and profuse sweating. The feet are warm to the touch. Bacteria invade and create abscesses in the necrotic areas.

The degree of lameness a foundered horse exhibits is related to the stage of the disease. Horses with acute laminitis are very lame and not usable. The acute condition generally progresses to the chronic condition in about 2 weeks. Horses with chronic laminitis are occasionally lame but may be usable for light work when shod properly. Horses with acute laminitis have a characteristic stance. They rock back on their hind legs and push their front feet forward. Fever may be present in the feet during the acute stage and the pulse will be stronger than normal. The front feet only or all four feet may be affected.

Horses with chronic laminitis are occasionally lame but may be usable for light work. Experience has shown that all pain must be gone

before a breeding mare will conceive and carry a foal to parturition (birth). Horses with chronic laminitis must be managed to avoid overeating and recurrence of the acute form. Horses with chronic laminitis have distorted hoofs that grow faster in the heel. This creates characteristic rings which are wider apart at the heel than at the toe. The toe may be dished or concave. The white line will be much wider than normal (1/8 in.) at the toe. Seedy-toe or hoof wall separation at the toe will often be evident. The sole will be flat or dropped in cases where there has been rotation of the third phalanx. The sole should not be pared between the point of the frog and the toe, except to drain abscesses that may form.

Treatment for laminitis must take into consideration the stage of the disease. Acute cases should be treated immediately by a veterinarian with a farrier's assistance. Chronic cases often can be treated by the horseshoer alone. Veterinary treatment may consist of a laxative such as mineral oil to purge the digestive tract, analgesics such as Bute (phenylbutazone) to reduce pain, nonsteroid anti-inflammation agents such as Banamine (flunixin meglumine) and antibiotics to treat systemic infection. Thyroid extract is sometimes prescribed for sluggish overweight horses. Antihistamines have been prescribed in the past. Recently, heparin (an anticlotting agent) has been used experimentally as a treatment. Anciently, foundered horses were bled from the jugular vein with a fleam. This

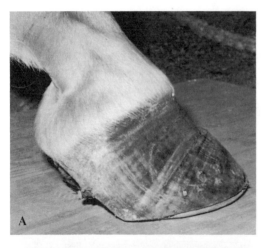

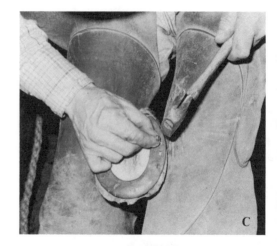

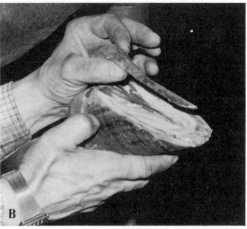

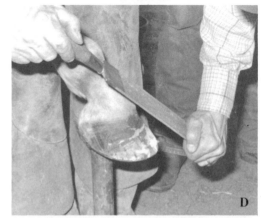

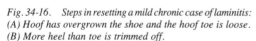

Fig. 34-16. Steps in resetting a mild chronic case of laminitis:
(A) Hoof has overgrown the shoe and the hoof toe is loose.
(B) More heel than toe is trimmed off.
(C) Shoe has been reshaped and fit to rear half of foot.
(D) Loose wall is rasped off.
(E) Most foundered horses need some sort of restraint to
take their mind off their feet during shoeing.

practice is still advocated by some using a large hypodermic needle.

Early treatment is crucial. A change in the horse's diet and management is usually necessary. Controlled exercise is helpful to promote circulation. Soaking the feet in cold water is said to slow the formation of necrotic tissue, but soaking in warm water improves circulation and helps abscesses to drain. Radiographs (x-rays) are useful to determine the degree of rotation, septic tracts and other complications.

Trimming of the hoof to a balanced angle and

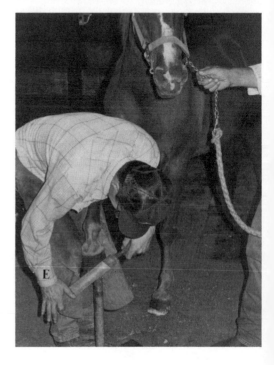

shape is important in the acute stages, especially if the horse has been neglected. Necrotic material must be removed. Soaking in a hot Epsom salt solution is recommended. Trimming usually involves lowering the heels and rasping back the toe to restore a balanced hoof shape and normal pastern angle. The point of the frog should not be trimmed and it should bear weight. Overlowering of the heels may cause the tip of the coffin bone to rotate more. In rare cases, raising the heel may make the horse more comfortable.

Shoeing foundered horses is based upon principles of relieving and applying pressure. Pressure is relieved from the sole and laminar region at the toe. Laminar scar tissue is removed. Abscesses are opened and irrigated with hydrogen peroxide or other suitable antiseptic. Pressure is applied slightly behind the point of the frog to relieve pressure from the wall and to stabilize and prevent further rotation of the coffin bone. This may be done by applying pressure with a heart bar shoe or flexible tapered frog pad. Shoes should have a rolled-toe and be nailed or screwed to sound hoof wall in the quarters. The pressure placed upon the frog must be the correct amount. Too much pressure may cause an increase in pain. Not enough pressure may cause pain in a few days as the bone continues to sink. Techniques of trimming and shoeing for founder were

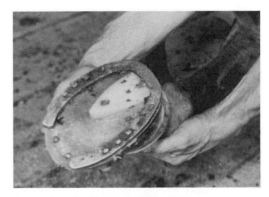

Fig. 34-18.   *Flexible frog pad for laminitis.*

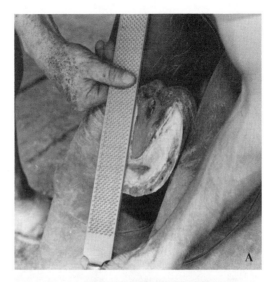

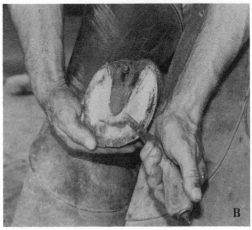

Fig. 34-19.   *Steps in trimming and shoeing a foundered horse with Morrison pads and a leather rim pad:*
(A) Trim down the heel wall and leave the toe wall—rasp back the toe to achieve desired angle.
(B) Trim sole uniformly thin and establish drainage of all abscesses.

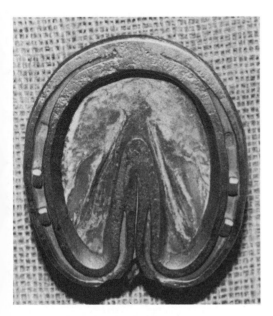

Fig. 34-17.   *Heart bar shoe for laminitis.*

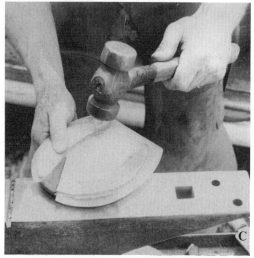

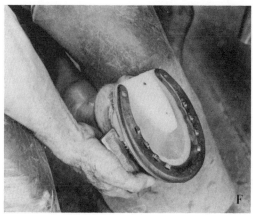

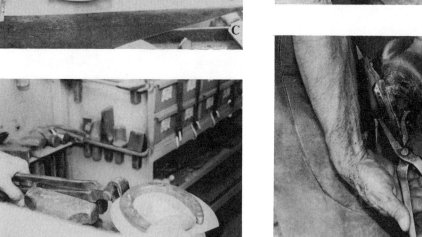

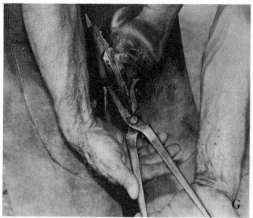

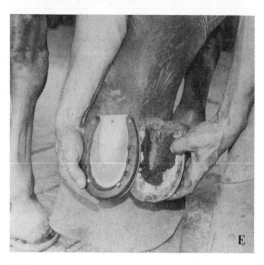

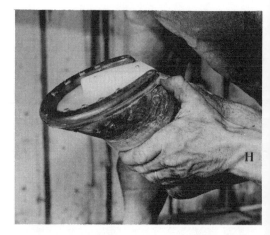

(C) Position tip of wedge near point of frog and rivet pads
to toe and heel of desired shoe.
(D) Trim away excess pad.
(E) Pack foot with packing.
(F) Block down nails evenly.
(G) Use clinchers, not hammer.
(H) The finished job—note wedge projects below the shoe.

developed by Burney Chapman of Lubbock, Texas, and Bobby Morrison of Braddyville, Iowa.

A firm sponge rubber pad, soft acrylic or silicone injected under a pad has been used to apply pressure on the sole. This is not as effective as the above procedure and may cause further abscesses and pain. Stalling a horse on sand or sawdust has been recommended. Pressure may be relieved from the sole of chronic non-sinking cases by concaving (seating out) a wide-webbed shoe away from the sole or applying a rim pad above a full pad between a shoe and the foot. Nails should be small and driven into the rear half of the hoof wall. Acrylic plastics can be used to reconstruct the hoof after pain has subsided and infections are dried up.

Once horses have foundered, they usually remain chronic for some time. The horse seems to be more susceptible to future acute attacks of the disease. At least a year of therapeutic shoeing is necessary in most cases, providing there are no recurring acute attacks.

Navicular Disease

For nearly two centuries navicular disease has been considered "the curse of good horseflesh." Navicular was reported to be "usually common" in English Thoroughbred horses around 1800. It was said to be a disease of well bred horses (meaning light horses) with high narrow feet. A small narrow foot with an arched sole was thought to be especially susceptible.

The effects of navicular disease were first recorded in 1752 by Bridges. The condition was accurately described, attributed to lack of exercise resulting in contraction of the foot, and appropriately named navicular lameness or disease in 1832 by Turner. The pathogenesis of navicular disease was completely described by numerous authors, including Fleming, in 1892. The treatments (shoeing, management changes and neurotomy) proposed by Fleming are still widely used today.

Navicular lameness may result from a bursitis or inflammation of the synovial fluid-filled sac located between the articular cartilage of the navicular bone and the deep flexor tendon. The initial pain experienced by the horse has been compared to that created by a grain of sand under an eyelid.

Lameness may also be caused by spraining of one or more of the several ligamentous attachments holding the navicular bone in place. Or, pain may be the result of thrombosis (arterial congestion) and ischemia (bone degeneration) due to circulation disturbances. These conditions cause osteochondrosis (subcartilage bone change) or osteolysis (bone destruction). Concussion or compression forces may produce the above conditions.

Navicular disease usually involves only the front feet. Occasionally, it may occur in the hind feet and very rarely in all four feet. Navicular disease may be arrested temporarily but often progresses to a destruction of the articular cartilage of the navicular bone, deep flexor tendon adhesions, navicular bone caries (cavities) and coffin joint arthritis. Most texts classify it as a bursitis and terminal arthritis.

The navicular bone is located above the middle of the frog between the widest part of the coronary band about 1/2 inch below the coronary border of the hoof. The navicular bone is held in place as part of the coffin joint by the suspensory ligament of the navicular bone and the distal navicular ligament. These ligaments may be sprained by concussion forces coming through an excessively upright pastern and unequal loading. The position of the navicular bone relative to the insertion of the deep flexor places it in a pivot-point subject to compression forces. The small bone maintains a constant angle of insertion for the deep flexor and thereby acts as a fulcrum and increases the leverage on the foot. The navicular bursa is located between the deep flexor tendon and the articular cartilage of the navicular bone. It lubricates the pulley-like surface of the bone. The deep flexor becomes wide and thin as it passes under the bursa and inserts on the semilunar arch of the coffin bone.

Concussion or compression forces may traumatize navicular blood vessels causing thrombosis and resulting ischemia. This condition is especially prevalent in stabled horses used only occasionally and then for very strenuous activity such as rodeo, jumping, etc. These horses are not properly conditioned, they are fed high quality feeds, and their feet are usually contracted due to lack of exercise and hard, dry stalls. Horses that have a quiet disposition and small

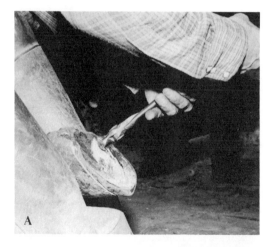

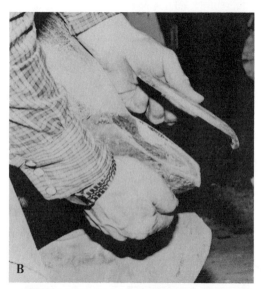

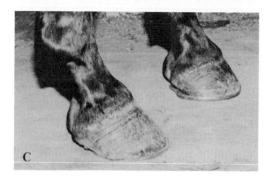

Fig. 34-20. Trimming and shoeing for navicular disease:
(A) More toe than heel is trimmed off.
(B) The full web of the bar shoe is rockered.
(C) The shoe extends behind the foot to support the sloping heel—left foot has been reset, right has not. Note axis of pasterns and hoofs.

feet in proportion to their body size are especially susceptible. The navicular bone is normally protected from injury by the frog and digital cushion. If these atrophy and become nonfunctional, damage to the navicular bursa or articular cartilage of the navicular bone may result.

Seventy-five percent of the intrinsic blood supply to the navicular bone enters through the distal navicular ligament. The remaining arteries enter through the suspensory ligament of the navicular bone. When the bone blood supply is disturbed, bone cells become necrotic and die. This condition is believed to be irreversible. However, it can be arrested. Bone that is absorbed from the area may be replaced with fibrous tissue. Remodeling of the bone is constantly going on in this as well as other parts of the body. Exercise is necessary for proper functioning of the blood circulation mechanism of the equine foot.

Horses with navicular disease at first show intermittent lameness in one or both front legs. The horse will point the painful foot when at rest. Pointing refers to placing one foot in front of the other when viewed from the side. Sometimes the horse will rest the toe on the ground and the heel off the ground. If both front feet are affected, it will point first one and then the other. The horse may lie down more than usual.

Navicular disease is most common in horses with steep shoulder/pastern conformation, low weak heel/long toe conformation, and/or small/contracted foot conformation. The hoofs are characteristically pinched in or "waisted" at the heels between the buttress and bulbs. The coronary band appears to bulge. The wall often appears rough, covered with uneven rings and brittle. The trimmed hoof may show redness at the junction of the wall and sole at the toe in the white line due to increased concussion on the toe.

Horses with navicular disease exhibit a stiff movement, especially after standing idle. They usually will warm out of the lameness, but it will be worse following hard work. Horses trotted out on the line, especially those lame in both feet, often hold their head up so high and rigid that no head nod can be observed. Trotting them in tight circles in alternating directions may be a useful aid in diagnosis.

Hoof testers are probably the most conclusive diagnostic tool for navicular disease. When applied with sensitivity they can reveal much about the location, type and clinical severity of the condition. Hoof testers should be applied in a systematic sequence, the same way and in the same order every time. This is important to distinguish navicular disease from other foot lameness (differential diagnosis) such as sheared heel(s), pedal osteitis, thrush, foot abscess(es) or fractured coffin bone.

Radiographs (x-rays) are said to be conclusive in only about one-half the cases. Even a perfect "lollipop" lesion must be confirmed clinically. Perhaps a major reason for discrepancies between radiographs and clinical lameness is the quality of the radiographs taken by clinicians. Another is the variation between horses in their individual response in pain. How extensive must observable bone changes be before the horse is noticeably uncomfortable? Also, fibrous healing that has taken place in the bone, as well as recent ligament damage, is not resolvable radiologically. Nerve blocks may be useful to confirm a diagnosis and to determine the probable result of neurectomy.

Breeders must receive much of the blame for the navicular disease problem. Bone and structural conformation are some of the most highly heritable traits. However, the traits many breeders are intent on selecting for—speed, color, intelligence, disposition—are some of the lowest. Some of our modern horse breeders seem to be breeding for everything except soundness. One result is the creation of horses with feet too small to adequately support a large body size. Another is the production of horses with relatively short cannons and long sloping pasterns creating excessive compression of the navicular bone. Still another is the trend toward tall horses with steep-angled shoulders and pasterns creating concussion on the navicular bone. There must be a return to breeding for balanced horses with sound feet and legs before the navicular disease problem will go away.

Owners and trainers may be blamed for management practices (or lack of them) which create conditions favoring navicular disease development. Lack of exercise is a major problem. Training with drugs and gimmicks rather than

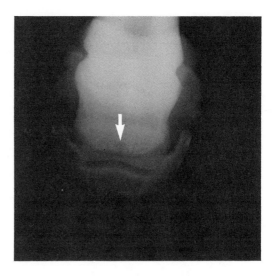

Fig. 34-21. Navicular disease lesion (radiograph).

sweat and time has become popular. Asking a horse to do more than it is capable of or conditioned for is the order of the day. It is not unusual for horses to be ridden strenuously for a few minutes and be retired to a stall for hours or even days and weeks. When the animals are worked, they fatigue quickly causing excessive vibration of tendons and joints. This interrupts and reduces the blood supply to bone tissues. When horses are idle for extended periods, navicular blood vessels atrophy or are smashed by standing compression. Sudden exertion creates thrombosis and pain and eventually ischemia.

Horses need access to constant exercise. They need to be conditioned slowly, avoiding the stress of running and jumping in unnatural ways until they are fit and hardened by daily conditioning. Horses should be stabled on a soft, moist surface. Peat litter or moss has been acclaimed as ideal. However, they are not available to most of us. If horses must be stabled on straw or saw dust, the floor under them should be clay or board (not cement) and the foot should be packed with clay each night. Ideally, horses should run out in a wet pasture with only an open shed for shelter. The pasture should be a safe area with no possibility of puncture to the navicular bursa. Unskilled riding may also contribute to the problem. Uncollected horses put more strain on their forehand. Nutrition of adequate quality and quantity to develop foot bones (and hoof) to their potential size and strength may be neglected. Rations should be balanced to National Research Council recommendations and overfeeding of idle horses should be avoided.

Shoeing fads have contributed greatly to the navicular disease problem. Trimming the foot to a "textbook" angle that is usually much lower than the horse's natural pastern angle creates more compression. Purposely lowering the heels adds strain to the deep flexor tendon and navicular bone. Raising the heels increases concussion on the navicular ligaments and bone. Changing lateral balance to improve the stance places uneven weight bearing on the bones of the foot. Reducing the hoof's size by excessive rasping of the hoof wall concentrates concussion forces into a smaller area and thus magnifies them. High toe grabs, jar calks, mud stickers, and rim shoes all create increased strain on the horse when it is working. However, this effect is not nearly as severe as that produced by the horse standing on the shoes in the stall, van or trailer for extended periods of time.

After the causes have been considered and dealt with in a preventative way, palliative (temporary) treatments for this irreversible condition may be implemented.

Treatments of a "band-aid" nature and of questionable value are drugs and neurectomy. Analgesic and anti-inflammatory drugs such as Bute (phenylbutazone) or Arquel (meclofenamic acid) mask the pain but fail to treat the cause of the problem. In addition, they are illegal in some circles of horse activity. Anticoagulant drugs such as warfarin or heparin have been reported successful in treating the ischemic type of navicular disease by Colles (1979). However, problems accompany its use. The proper dosage is difficult to determine: to little, no effect - too much, internal bleeding. Intolerance to other medication when needed is a major problem. One stage prothrombin times (blood clotting time) must be monitored twice a week when first placed on the medication, later once a week and finally once a month. There have been very limited studies. Exercise and diet regulation, as well as corrective trimming and shoeing, were major factors contributing to the success of the treatment in these studies. It is too early yet to call warfarin the panacea for navicular disease.

Posterior digital neurectomy or nerving has been a treatment for navicular for over 150 years. It has the advantage (if you are lucky) of relieving pain and allowing the horse to go sound for a while. If a horse that has severe navicular is kept alive, nerving is probably a most humane alternative. However, success in nerving is variable since nerve branching is unpredictable. Horse insurance becomes invalid. There is a good chance that the nerves will regenerate in 2 to 5 years, cancelling the operation. There is always a chance of a neuroma (inflammation of the severed nerve ends) that may produce more pain than the original condition. Sloughing of the hoof is a rare but possible result. Horses that have been nerved are susceptible to undetected foot punctures and abscesses. Finally, there is always a concern, however rare, that the horse may not be as safe for riding (especially on uneven ground) as it was before nerving.

Nerving has been so well accepted by the horse show community that a recent survey by the American Horse Show Association found that as many as 5 percent of Three Day Event horses, 10 percent of Dressage horses and 20 percent of Show Jumpers had been nerved one or more times. Neurectomy has been recommended as beneficial when accompanied by careful selection. Horses that are not advanced in the disease and have sound hoofs are the best candidates. The heels of nerved horses may not be as strong as those of a sound horse. Hoof toes grow more rapidly after posterior digital neurectomy. If careful selection is not made by a competent veterinary surgeon, nerving becomes a practice of the dishonest and brings upon itself condemnation.

Treatments of lasting value in slowing the progression of or preventing the disease consider hoof and horse management. Gradually condition horses for strenuous exercise and stable them with access to *ad libitum* (free choice) exercise. Feed a balanced diet both as to quantity and quality of nutrients. Trim the hoof so that it is balanced in relation to the horse's individual conformation. Shoe the horse with consideration of the physiology of the foot and pathology of navicular disease. Protect the injured and painful area with a bar shoe. The bar also prevents the heel from sinking into the ground. In dry seasons, retain moisture in the foot and further protect it with a pad. Reduce the strain on the deep flexor tendon at the moment of breaking over by using a full-web rocker-toe. Raise the angle of low heeled horses by using a degree-wedge pad or shoe. Heels or jar calks may be added to a bar shoe, but they are usually less effective than a wedge pad or shoe since they either sink on a soft surface or increase concussion on a hard surface. A bar shoe applied to balanced feet with a rocker-toe the full web of the shoe is a very effective treatment for the navicular lameness. Many horses will continue to be useful for several years when they are routinely shod in this manner. However, shoeing only complements changes in management in the most successful cases.

References

Adams, J.W. 1917. Diseases of the foot. Practitioner Short Course in Vet. Med. Iowa State U., Ames. 2:234.

Adams, O.R. 1974. Lameness in Horses (3rd ed.). Lea & Febiger, Philadelphia.

Anstey, W.J. 1910. Corns. The Farriers' Annual. 1:6.

Bane, W.R. 1964. Process of patching hoofs. United States Patent Number 3,118,449. U.S. Pat. Office. Washington, DC.

Becker, E. 1961. Experiments with acrylics on equine hoof (translation by V. Nowading). Berliner und Munchener Tierarztliche Wochenschrift. 74:123.

Bjorck, G. and G. Nilsson. 1971. Chronic progressive pododermatitis in the horse. Equine Vet. J. 3:65.

Bobylev, I., H. Gerber, J. Hickman, J.A. Wasowski, and R. Zeller. 1980. FEI Veterinary Committee Report on Neurectomy. Horse Show. (May): 13.

Bone, J.F. 1963. Special shoeing. Equine Medicine and Surgery. American Veterinary Publications, Inc. Santa Barbara.

Burr, C. Treatment for injured neglected feet. Amer. Farriers' J. 8(6):372.

Butler, K.D. 1967. The Application and Comparative Value of Acrylics and Other Synthetic Materials in the Repair of the Sandcrack Syndrome on the Equine Hoof. M.S. Thesis. The Pennsylvania State University, University Park.

Butler, K.D. 1968. Repairing sandcracks with synthetic materials. The Western Horseman. 33(2):38.

Callcott, M.V. and B. Chapman. 1983. Convention preview: Chapman Laminitis treatment. Amer. Farriers' J. 9(1):45.

Colles, C.M. 1979. A preliminary report on the use of warfarin in the treatment of navicular disease. Equine Vet. J. 11(3):187.

Colles, C.M., H.E. Garner, and J.R. Coffman, 1980. The blood supply of the horse's foot. Proceedings of Amer. Assoc. of Equine Practitioners. 25:385.

Colles, C.M. 1980. The pathology of navicular disease and its treatment using cumarin (warfarin). Proceedings of Amer. Assoc. of Equine Practitioners. 25:399.

Dollar, J.A.W. 1898. A Handbook of Horseshoeing. W.R. Jenkins, New York.

Emery, L., J. Miller, and N. Van Hoosen. 1977. Horseshoeing Theory and Hoof Care. Lea & Febiger, Philadelphia.

Fackelman, C.E. 1974. Screw fixation of sagittal fractures of the third phalanx in horses. Vet. Med./S.A.C. (Oct.):1317.

Fessler, J.F. 1971. Surgical management of equine foot injuries. Mod. Vet. Pract. 52:41.

Fleming, G. 1892. Navicular disease. Baily's Magazine. 58 (Dec.):405.

Fleming, G. 1893. Navicular disease. Baily's Magazine. 59 (Jan.):36.

Fleming, G. 1893. The treatment of navicular disease. Baily's Magazine. 59 (Feb.):100.

Frank, E.R. 1964. Veterinary Surgery (7th ed.). Burgess Publ. Co., Minneapolis.

Garner, H.E., J.R. Coffman, A.W. Hahn, N. Ackerman, and J.H. Johnson. 1975. Equine laminitis and associated hypertension: a review. J.A.V.M.A. 166(1):56.

Garner, H.E., R.F. Sprouse, and V.K. Ganjam. 1982. Proceedings of the first equine endotoxemia/laminitis symposium. Newsletter of Amer. Assn. of Equine Pract. (June)2:29.

Graham, C.W. 1965. Care of the horse's foot. Vet. Med./ S.A.C. (Mar.):255.

Hickman, J. 1977. Farriery. J.A. Allen & Co., London.

Jenny, J. and L.H. Evans. 1964. The use of self-curing acrylic plastics for repairing the hoof. Pa. Vet. 6:6.

Jenny, J., L.H. Evans, and C.W. Raker. 1965. Hoof repair with plastics. J. Am. Vet. Med. Assn. 147:1340.

Johnson, J.H. 1970. Puncture wounds of the foot. Vet. Med./S.A.C. (Feb.):147.

Johnson, J.H. 1972. Septic conditions of the equine foot. J.A.V.M.A. 161(11):1276.

Keown, G.H. 1962. Method of treating a quarter crack. Proc. Ann. Am. Assn. Equine Practitioners Mtg. 8:144.

Kilby, E. 1983. Laminitis: the lowest blow. Equus 44:66.

Laraway, R 1981. Yeast infections of the hoof wall. Amer. Farriers' J. 7(4):184.

Layton, E.W. 1965. Care of the horse's foot. Vet. Med./ S.A.C. (Mar.):248.

Mackay-Smith, M. 1980. The nerving dilemma. Equus. 31:56.

Manning, D.C. 1981. Two centuries of shoeing foundered horses. Amer. Farriers' J. 7(5):258.

Mason, J.H. 1962. Penicillin treatment of foot canker of the horse. J.S. Afr. Vet. Med. Assoc. 33(2):223.

McKibbin, L.S. 1977. Horse Owner's Handbook. W.B. Sanders Co., Philadelphia.

Moller, H. and J.A.W. Dollar. 1911. Regional veterinary surgery. W.R. Jenkins Co., New York.

Moyer, W. and J. Anderson. 1975. Lameness caused by improper shoeing. J.A.V.M.A. 166(1):47.

Moyer, W. and J. Anderson. 1975. Sheared heels: diagnosis and treatment. J.A.V.M.A. 166(1):53.

Navicular. 1980. Equus. 31:56.

Pires, A. 1949. Fractures de la una o casco. Tratado De Las Enfermedades Del Pie Del Caballo. Kraft. Buenos Aires, ARGENTINA.

Prescott, C.W. 1970. Canker in the hoof of a horse. Austral. Vet. J. 46:449.

Reeks, H.C. 1925. Diseases of the Horse's Foot (2nd ed.). Alex Eger, Chicago.

Reeves, L. 1980. A shoe for a fractured coffin bone. Amer. Farriers' J. 6(3):95.

Roberge, D. 1919. The Foot of the Horse. American Veterinary Publishing Co., Chicago.

Rubano, A.R. 1964. Acrylic repair technique. Proc. Ann. Am. Assn. Equine Practitioners Mtg. 10:272.

Smalley, A. 1983. Medical update: the shot heard 'round the world. Equus. 68:62.

Smith, F. 1976. The Early History of Veterinary Literature. (4 vols). J.A. Allen & Co., London. 4:4.

Smith, H.A., T.C. Jones, and R.D. Hunt. 1972. Veterinary Pathology. Lea and Febiger, Philadelphia. p. 1083.

Sutton, B. and D. Butler. 1980. Selenium toxicity in horses. Amer. Farriers' J. 6(2):44.

Swanstrom, O.G. 1978. Septic conditions of the equine foot part I. Equine Market and Horseman's Review. (Dec.):20.

Swanstrom, O.G. 1979. Septic conditions of the equine foot part II. Equine Market and Horseman's Review. (Jan.):21.

White, N.A. and N. Baggett. 1983. A method of corrective shoeing for laminitis in horses. Vet. Med./S.A.C. 78(5):775.

Youatt, W. and J.S. Skinner. 1843. The Horse, Ass and Mule. Porter and Coates, Philadelphia.

NOTES:

Chapter 35

Lamenesses of the Forelimb

Lamenesses of the forelimb are more common than lamenesses of the hindlimb. The horse bears a greater proportion of his weight on his front limbs. Trimming and/or shoeing alone rarely can improve lamenesses located in the upper limb. Treatment of limb lamenesses is usually combined with veterinary medical treatment. The horseshoer's role may be as simple as balancing the foot and distributing weight more evenly over its ground surface to relieve strain. However, the horseshoer may be asked to build intricate shoes and/or braces to support and protect the unsound limb. Experimentation is often necessary to fabricate exactly the best appliance for each individual horse.

Shoulder Lameness

Shoulder lamenesses are often confused with navicular lameness. After navicular lameness is ruled out then look for shoulder lameness.

Causes of shoulder lameness may include bicipital bursitis, arthritis, sweeny, fistula withers, radial nerve paralysis, fracture(s) and pressure from improperly fitting saddles or collars.

Bicipital bursitis is an inflammation of a bursa underneath the tendon of the biceps on the lateral side of the shoulder joint. Afflicted animals will point the entire limb laterally as well as forward when standing. They attempt to shift their weight onto the hind limbs by raising the head as they walk. Shoulder flexion is decreased and the front feet are not elevated to the same height when the horse is viewed from the side. A bump and occasionally a depression may be observed on the side of the shoulder joint. Rarely, a popping noise may be heard as the animal walks. Bicipital bursitis is usually the result of trauma. Rest and corticosteroid injection is usually prescribed as treatment.

Arthritis of the shoulder or elbow joint may occur in older horses that have very steep joint angles. However, horses with the predisposing conformation that are also worked hard enough to become lame in the shoulder will probably break down in the lower limb first. Horses with upper limb arthritis will show swinging leg lameness (hurt when the limb is moved but not supporting weight) and have an overall stiff action. Lameness is usually more pronounced as the horse moves up hill.

Sweeny is atrophy of the supraspinatus and infraspinatus muscles of the shoulder behind the spine of the scapula bone. Sweeny results from trauma to the suprascapular nerve where it passes over the front of the lower border of the scapula. Nerve injuries may be caused by poorly fitting collars, wild spurring, trailer accidents, kicks and slippage. Both shoulders should be observed and compared to determine how much atrophy has taken place. The elbow will rotate away from the body as the horse walks. Counterirritants can be applied to the area, but these are rarely effective. Occasionally, a piece of scapula is removed from under the nerve. Rest and muscle massage are the most effective treatments. Horses with extensive nerve damage will not become sound.

Fistula withers, sometimes called thisalow, results from an infection in the supraspinous bursa located under the highest part of the withers. *Brucella* organisms may be found in fistula withers and poll evil (behind the ears). This infection is transmittable to man in the form of undulant fever. Fistula tracts may gravitate between the layers of muscle in the shoulder making it very difficult for the veterinarian to treat. Fistula withers may be caused by an injury or by a collar or saddle that rubs the top of the withers.

Radial nerve paralysis is caused by trauma to the radial nerve. The nerve may be injured when a horse is kicked, thrown on its side or run into an immovable object. The radial nerve controls the extensor muscles. In severe cases, the horse drags the limb on the coronary band. Some injuries heal quickly; others take months to recover. Exercise, especially swimming, has been reported as beneficial.

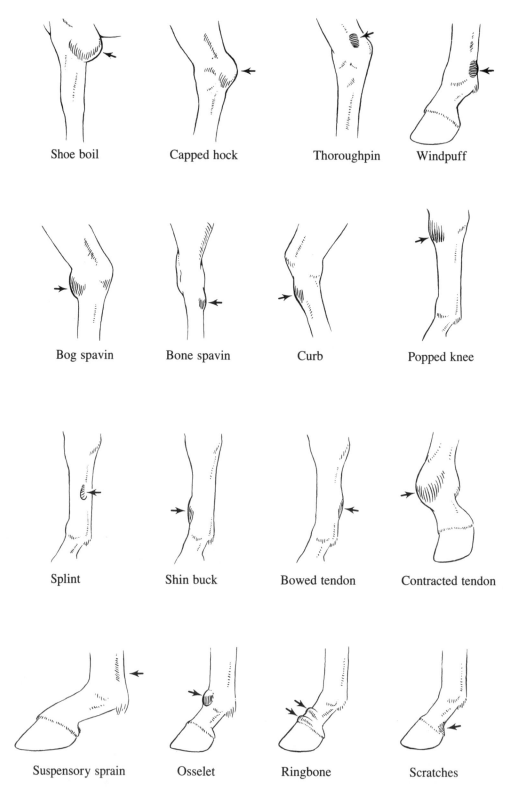

Fig. 35-1. Location of lamenesses of the leg. Drawing by L. Sadler.

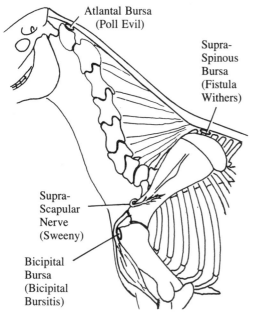

Fig. 35-2. Location of bicipital bursitis, sweeny, fistula withers and poll evil.

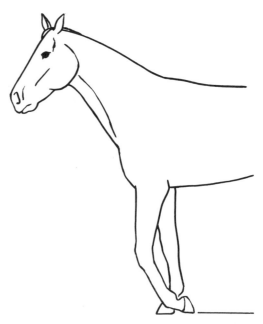

Fig. 35-3. Radial nerve paralysis stance.

Fractures in the upper limb are difficult to treat. Usually, the most humane and economical thing to do is to destroy the horse. The humerus is the most frequently broken bone. Most fractures of the lower limb may be repaired with bone screws and compression plates. However, the economics of repair and horse's suitability as a patient must be carefully evaluated.

Pressure from improperly fitting saddles or collars will cause horses to be lame only when they are being ridden or worked. After an initial examination, have the rider or driver work the horse for you under tack or harness. Inadequate padding and poorly constructed equipment will make a horse sore. Pressure from your hand will also help you detect the site of lameness.

Capped Elbow

Capped elbow or shoe boil is a subcutaneous bursitis on the point of the elbow (olecranon). Horses with this condition are rarely lame. However, it can be an extremely noticeable blemish.

The point of the elbow is irritated when the horse gets up after lying on a hard surface. The horse extends its front feet and rocks back. Then it pushes itself up with its hind feet. The elbows are frequently irritated in this process. The point of the elbow can also be irritated by the sharp heel of a shoe. The injury may occur as the horse lies down with its feet under its body or when it is moving at speed.

Sometimes fluid buildup in these subcutaneous bursas is best removed by needle. Deeper bedding of stalls often helps. The shoe heel(s) may be shortened and rounded smooth. Removable studs can be used in place of permanent calks or stickers.

The shoe boil or sausage boot is a doughnut shaped collar that may be buckled around the pastern. The padding rests against the point of the elbow and prevents injury. This is especially useful when shoes cannot be shortened or removed as on gaited show horses with hoof buildup and extended heel shoes.

Popped Knee

Popped knee is a general term for inflammation of the knee. It may also be called hygroma, capped knee or big knee. It may be like capped elbow if a subcutaneous bursa is present. However, the swelling could also be due to a hernia of one of the knee joint capsules or a distention of the sheath of the lateral extensor tendon. Poor conformation and lack of conditioning are common causes. Rest, counterirritation and pressure bandaging are recommended treatments. Injection of corticoids should be a last resort.

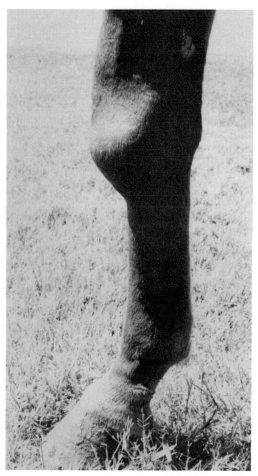

Fig. 35-4. Popped knee.

Knee Spavin

Knee spavin, carpitis or arthritis of the knee is a more serious condition than popped knee. Ligament sprain, bone bruising or fracture, and joint damage may each or all be involved. Poor conformation, especially calf knees, predispose a horse to this condition. Concussion causing compression of the knee bones and trauma bring on the condition. The knee is swollen and warm. It most commonly occurs in horses that are raced before they are properly conditioned. Kicks and accidents of various kinds also are a common cause. Lameness may be of a supporting or swinging leg type or both. Radiographs are necessary to distinguish between arthritis inflammation and fracture. Most fractures can be surgically removed or repaired with screws if discovered before excessive scar tissue forms.

The cost and future prognosis must be carefully considered. The prognosis for arthritic conditions is poor.

Splints

Splints are abnormal bony growths between the splint bone(s) and the cannon bone. They are most common on the inside of the front legs. The interosseous ligament between the splint and cannon bone may be torn by uneven weight bearing. Splints may also be caused by limb interference, unbalanced feet, kicks or concussion from hard working surfaces. Occasionally, high levels of phosphorus in the diet cause splint development.

The bony growth produced by the body is an effort to repair the weakened area. Horses with toed-out or base-wide conformation are predisposed to inside splints. Horses with toe-in or base-narrow conformation may develop splints on the outside of the legs. A horse will usually not develop splints unless it is overstressed when underconditioned at a young age. Splints are rare in older horses. Splints that are high and near the knee are more serious than low splints since there is more chance of interference with ligaments or tendons. Peg splints located behind the cannon bone and next to the suspensory ligament may be hidden but cause lameness. Splints are common in two and three year old race horses. Affected horses will often walk sound but jog or gallop lame.

Splints are usually considered a blemish. There may be lameness when they first appear, but when they quit actively growing or set, the horse will be sound. Various counterirritant treatments have been used. The condition can be prevented by gradual conditioning and wearing protective shin or splint boots. Animals should not be subjected to intensive training until their skeleton is mature enough to withstand stress. Interfering boots, sometimes called splint boots, should be worn on horses that travel close and/or may be uncoordinated. The feet must be balanced regularly as the young horse grows.

Shin Buck

Shin buck or shin splints is a periostitis of the front surface of the cannon bone. The pain is produced by a hairline (incomplete or surface)

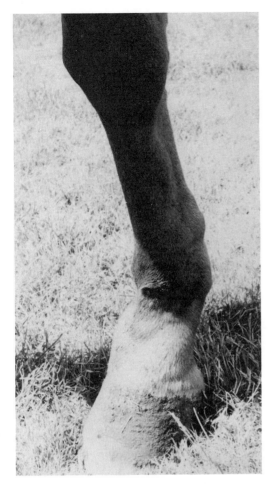

Fig. 35-5. Splint, bowed tendon and ringbone on the same leg.

fracture of the cannon bone. The swelling and bony growth are the body's effort to repair the damaged bone. Lack of gradual conditioning for racing and uneven track surfaces are most often blamed for this condition. High toe grabs on racing plates may also be responsible. The feet should be balanced and the fracture be given a chance to heal. Blistering, firing, radiation and ultrasound therapy have all been tried as treatments.

Bowed Tendon

Bowed tendon may also be called tendosynovitis, peritendinitis, tendinitis, or tendovaginitis. These injuries usually occur to the flexor tendons of the front legs. The superficial flexor is most often affected. A bow in its early stages is usually soft and involves only the tendon sheath. These can be treated by astringent preparations and wrapping the sprained area when stressing the animal. Most horses will heal with rest. A bow in a late stage will be hard and have scar tissue. These will not go away completely. Complete tendon rupture is rare, although the flexor muscles may be strained and the check ligaments may be affected. Bows may be classified as high (near knee) or low bows (near fetlock). Rarely are bows seen below the fetlock.

Bowed tendon is the most common lameness of race horses. It may be caused by overexertion and fatigue, unequal weight distribution on the foot and leg due to unbalanced trimming or high grabs on racing plates. In addition, an uneven track surface, racing around a flat track in one direction, runaways due to lack of training and control and, of course, lack of conditioning may also cause bowed tendons.

There are several surgical procedures that have been used to reduce scar tissue and increase mobility. Shoeing consists of transferring pressure to the uninjured flexor or suspensory ligament. Superficial tendon bows are most common. The feet should be balanced. Wrapping the leg is most beneficial. The opposite leg(s) should also be wrapped to allow the horse to rest the injured leg without stressing it. A rocker-toe shoe should be applied to relieve the stress of breakover. The heels should be raised when the deep flexor is injured. The heels should be lowered when the suspensory ligament is injured. Massage and mild exercise will help the circulation in injured areas at first. Later rest is necessary for bows to heal. Swimming is beneficial to maintain a horse's muscle condition without subjecting the tendons to concussion.

Contracted Tendons

Contracted tendons in foals and weanlings were once thought to be inherited. There are some cases that may be due to faulty positioning of the fetus in the womb. Others may be due to post natal infection such as navel ill. However, the majority of the cases one sees today are due to overfeeding and under exercising. Contraction may be complicated by epiphysitis due to calcium and phosphorus mineral imbalance and feeding excess energy and protein. The bones seem to lengthen faster than the tendons lengthen. The traits encouraging fast and nonuniform growth may be inherited. Pain in the feet can also cause contracture in older horses.

Tendon contractures are usually one of two types and vary in severity. Deep flexor tendon contractures are due to abnormal growth of the cannon bone. They cause the hoof to be deformed. The fetlock appears nearly normal. At first the toe may be dished, later it may become bull nosed as the horse bears weight on the toe of the hoof. The coffin joint will appear luxated (dislocated). Stretching the toe of the foot will reveal inflexibility in the coffin joint.

Superficial flexor contractures are due to abnormal growth of the radius. They can be recognized by the horse's straight fetlocks, normal but atrophied hoofs and lack of flexion in the fetlock joint.

Treatment consists of removing the nutritional cause and providing exercise. This is all that is necessary if the fetlock or pastern has not luxated or knuckled over. Bone growth will then slow down and allow the tendons to catch up. After the joint has become luxated, desmotomy (cutting) of the check ligament of the affected tendon is necessary. The check ligament is part of the stay apparatus and prevents the muscle(s) from stretching and thus, the tendon from lengthening. A shoe with an extended toe assists the leg to regain a normal stance. Bracing may be necessary for a week or so until the muscle belly stretches. Cutting the flexor tendons was formerly recommended. This should never be done as horses will not become sound after such an operation.

Suspensory Sprain

Suspensory sprain (may be called desmitis or breaking down) is a tearing or spraining of the suspensory ligament. The branches of the ligament are usually affected where they join the proximal points of the sesamoid bones. Frequently, the point of the bone fractures producing sesamoiditis. Rarely, the superficial sesamoidean ligament is sprained and the distal portion or base of the sesamoid bones fracture. Other injuries usually occur to the leg when strain is serious enough to affect the suspensory ligament. A horse with suspensory sprain will

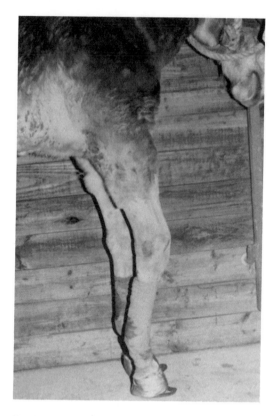

Fig. 35-6.   *Belgian foal with contracted tendons shod after subcarpal check ligament desmotomy.*

stand with its knee and fetlock bent forward after the injury first occurs. Later it will place pressure on the heels to transfer pressure from the suspensory to the flexor tendons.

Sprains are caused by fatigue due to lack of conditioning, racing on an uneven or soft track, foot trimmed out of balance, or leg conformation defects that concentrate forces in this area of the limb.

Veterinary treatment consists of elastic bandages and rest for mild cases to surgical repair and pinning of broken bones. Firing is not as helpful as it is with the more superficial tendons. Shoeing prescribed by the veterinarian may include a brace support or extended egg bar. A chronic case will usually get along best with a flat-heeled rocker-toed shoe applied to a foot with the axis broken back. This transfers strain to the flexor tendons.

Sesamoiditis

Sesamoiditis or popped sesamoids is an inflammation of the sesamoid bone(s). It may be due to a fracture of the bone and spraining of the suspensory or superficial sesamoidean ligament due to uneven weight bearing. Trauma to the bone(s) due to interfering or other injury may also cause the condition. These may be related to fatigue and poor track surfaces. Radiographs are necessary to detect the bone changes that separate sesamoiditis from other swellings that may occur at the back of the fetlock. However, sesamoiditis swelling is usually firmer than other conditions that may occur in the same area.

Treatment of sesamoiditis may require injections or surgery. Sesamoiditis can be prevented by protecting a horse with elastic wrap, run down patches, interfering or overreaching boots.

Osselets

Osselets is the common name for traumatic arthritis of the fetlock joint. The hard swellings will be on the front or side of the fetlock joint. Most osselets are caused by hyperflexion, sometimes called dorsiflexion (sinking), of the fetlock joint. Fatigue of ligaments and tendons allows the fetlock to overbend and irritate or fracture the front proximal edge of the long pastern bone.

Osselets may be prevented by proper conditioning of horses and using an extended egg bar shoe on horses with very low underslung heels.

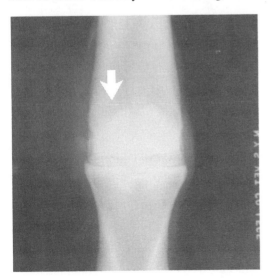

Fig. 35-7. Fractured sesamoid (radiograph).

Horses with osselets may or may not be lame even with obvious radiographic bone changes. Support of the fetlock with elastic bandages may be most beneficial in preventing and avoiding further damage. Rest is most advantageous. However, many other treatments including firing are usually tried. Few horses can stay sound after osteophyte production begins.

Windpuff

Windpuff, windgall, road puff, popped ankle, or hygromata is a soft puffy swelling occurring on the side(s) of the fetlock area. Windpuffs are caused by severe strain due to overexertion. Excess synovial fluid is produced and the joint capsule or tendon sheath distends (stretches). Windpuffs are considered a blemish, but they indicate excessive strain which may create an unsoundness.

There are two types of windpuffs. These can be distinguished by their location. Articular windpuffs are distentions of the fetlock joint. The soft swelling(s) appear next to the cannon bone. The joint capsule pushes out between the suspensory ligament and the cannon bone. Tendinous windpuffs are distentions of the sheath of the deep flexor tendon. The swelling is farther back between the suspensory ligament and flexor tendons.

Windpuffs will usually go down if a mild counterirritant or skin tightener is applied and the ankle is wrapped. Very large and unsightly swellings are sometimes drained with a needle. However, there is always danger of introducing infection into the joint when performing this procedure.

Ringbone

Ringbone or phalangeal exostosis refers to a bony growth on any part of the pastern area. High ringbone occurs around the pastern joint, low ringbone at the coffin joint. Both of these types are called articular or periarticular. Ringbone between the joints on the pastern bone(s) is called nonarticular or false ringbone. Ringbone is caused by trauma due to concussion from conformation defects such as short and steep pasterns, severe toed-in or toed-out conformation, and prolonged shoeing out of balance. Vitamin and mineral deficiencies and imbalance

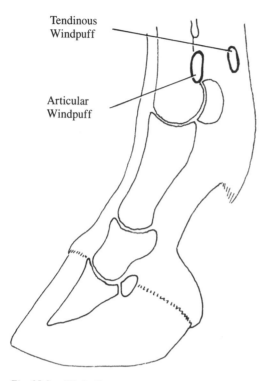

Tendinous
Windpuff

Articular
Windpuff

Fig. 35-8.   Windpuff types.

also may cause a type of rachitic ringbone at the epiphyseal plates in fast growing horses.

Articular ringbone usually results in lameness and is difficult to treat. A roller-motion shoe is usually prescribed. Horses can often tolerate the condition at rest but usually go lame when they are worked. Ankylosis of the pastern joint may improve soundness. When this is done surgically it is called arthrodesis. Low ringbone is difficult to arrest due to the extensive range of joint movement. The hoof may be distorted due to low ringbone, especially when it results from a fractured extensor process of the coffin bone. Counterirritant treatments are rarely successful except to encourage the owner to rest the horse.

Scratches

Scratches or grease heel is a dermatitis of the pastern area. Lameness may result in severe cases. There will be extensive skin chapping and scab formation on the back of the pastern below the fetlocks and above the inflamed bulbs of the heels. Sometimes a distinction is made between the chapped skin condition called scratches and inflammation in the sebaceous glands of the skin called grease heel or eczema.

Grease heel is usually caused by mud due to wet weather or damp and filthy stabling condi-

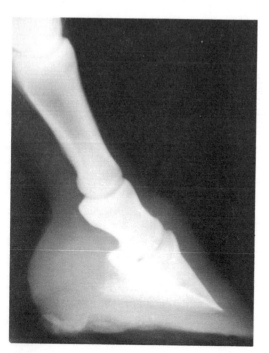

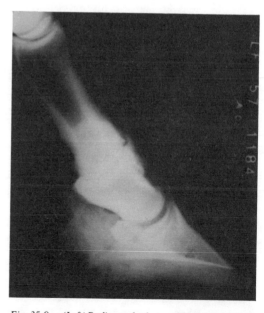

Fig. 35-9.   (Left) Radiograph of normal digit. (Right) Digit with high ringbone at the pastern joint, low ringbone at the coffin joint and sidebone at the rear of the foot.

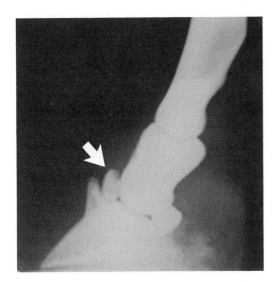

Fig. 35-10. Fractured extensor process of the third phalanx (radiograph).

tions. Clipping of leg hair on show horses destroys the protective function of the fetlock hair (feather). However, a long unclean feather holds filth in this area. Excessive irritation of the pastern by deep track surfaces and stretching of skin may be a cause. The pastern may be purposely sored by action devices and irritants added to lubricants on the gaited show horses. Rarely mite or fungae infestation may be involved. Sudden appearance may be due to metabolic disturbances, fever or overfeeding.

Scratches may be treated by cleaning the affected area thoroughly and stabling in a clean, dry environment. Sulfa urea cream or an astringent dressing is most effective. Severe cases may need to be bandaged to hold medication in place.

References

Adams, O.R. 1974. Lameness in Horses (3rd ed.). Lea and Febiger, Philadelphia.

Frank, E.R. 1964. Veterinary Surgery (7th ed.). Burgess, Minneapolis.

Gillette, E.L., D.E. Thrall and J.L. Lebel. 1977. Carlson's Veterinary Radiology. Lea and Febiger, Philadelphia.

Mackay-Smith, M. 1978. Contracted tendons. Equus 14:60.

McIlwraith, C.W. and J.F. Fessler. 1978. Evaluation of inferior check ligament desmotomy for treatment of acquired flexor tendon contracture in the horse. J.A.V.M.A. 172(3):293.

McKibbin, L.S. 1977. Horse Owner's Handbook. W.B. Saunders Co., Philadelphia.

Miller, R.M. 1981. Epiphysitis and contracted tendons. The Western Horseman. (Jan):62.

Myers and Lundvall. 1966. Corrective trimming for weak flexor tendons in a foal. J.A.V.M.A. 148(12):1523.

Rooney, J.R. 1969. Biomechanics of Lameness in Horses. Williams and Wilkins, Baltimore.

Rooney, J.R. 1974. The Lame Horse. A.S. Barnes and Co., Cranbury, NJ.

Siegmund, O.H. (Ed.). 1979. The Merck Veterinary Manual (5th ed.). Merck and Co., Inc., Rahway, NJ.

Sonnichsen, H.V. 1977. Desmotomia carpitis tendinei. Veterinary Annual. 17:133.

Stehsel, D.L. 1974. Farrier's Orthopedics Handbook. Geddes Press, Pasadena, CA.

NOTES:

Chapter 36

Lamenesses of the Hindlimb

Lamenesses of the hindlimb are often more difficult to detect than those of the frontlimb. Fortunately, lameness is less frequent in the hindlimbs than in the front. Standardbred harness race horses are an exception. Due to the balanced nature of their gaits and the speed at which they perform, they have a higher percentage of hindlimb lamenesses than other horses. Hunters and jumpers also have a comparatively high percentage of hindlimb and back problems due to the stress of their activity. Back problems are comparatively high in pacers due to the twisting (side-rolling) nature of their gait.

Hip Lameness

Hip, high hindlimb or back lamenesses are often difficult for even experienced clinicians to diagnose. One can tell the horse is off, but pinpointing the site may be difficult. Frequently, lamenesses are subtle and vary in intensity. The horseshoer's role may be only to state that the lameness appears to be located in the upper hindlimb. Make it a habit to check the foot thor-

oughly before making such a statement. Obvious causes may be overlooked and later cause embarrassment.

Sacroiliac luxation, knocked down hip or hunter bump is most common on hunters and jumpers. The iliac portion of the pelvis and the sacral portion of the spine separate. The resulting bump is due to the new position of the tuber sacrale portion of the pelvis. Horses may do this moving through crowded or narrow gates and when they fall or are thrown down. Many good ranch, rodeo and jumping horses have suffered from an accident causing this condition. Horses can return to work after sufficient rest to strengthen the torn area. The resulting bump should be considered a blemish after the injury heals.

Trochanteric bursitis or whirlbone lameness is an inflammation of the trochanteric bursa where the gluteus medius muscle passes over the major trochanter on the proximal end of the femur bone. Racing trotters and pacers are most commonly afflicted with this condition. It is due to the strain of reaching for long strides when racing.

A horse with whirlbone lameness has a charac-

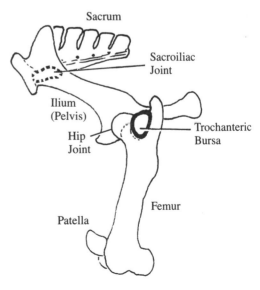

Fig. 36-1. Limbs with multiple blemishes and unsoundnesses.

Fig. 36-2. Location of sacroiliac joint and trochanteric bursa.

teristic dog gait. The hind legs do not track directly behind the fronts. Instead, the afflicted horse carries its hindquarters toward the sound side when viewed from the rear. The inside wall of the hind hoof is worn excessively as the lame leg is rotated inward. The stride of the lame leg will be shorter when viewed from the side. Veterinary treatments by injection of corticoids are not always promising. Shoe to protect the hind hoofs from uneven wear.

Stifle Lameness

Stifle lameness or gonitis may be due to concussion resulting from straight hind leg conformation, sprains due to lack of conditioning, cruciate ligament or meniscus (cartilage) damage, dislocation or fracture of the patella. Fortunately, these conditions are all rare. Injuries are most likely to occur in the stifle joint of unconditioned Standardbred race horses. They also are sometimes seen in unconditioned Quarter Horses used for roping events in rodeo.

The most commonly fractured bone in the upper rear limb is the tibia. Occasionally, a young horse will break this bone or the femur when being thrown or tied up for shoeing. Rarely, a horse will tear the semitendinous muscle (fibrotic myopathy) when fighting restraint. It is best to avoid such situations by insisting that horses be trained before trimming or shoeing is attempted.

Stifled

Stifled or upward fixation of the patella is an abnormal locking of the patella over the medial trochlea of the femur. The horse normally locks the patella while standing. The medial patellar ligament runs from the tibia to the patellar fibrocartilage. It holds the patella in place over the medial trochlea. This arrangement is part of the reciprocal or stay apparatus of the hind limb. When the stifle is locked, the hock cannot flex. (See Chapter 12.)

Horses with straight hind legs are especially prone to abnormal locking or upward fixation. Animals that are not sufficiently conditioned for the work they are asked to do are especially predisposed to being stifled. It also may occur more frequently when it is cold and animals have been inactive for long periods.

A stifled horse will hold its leg back and to the side and drag its foot. The fixation may be partial and intermittently released every few steps or be complete with the horse helplessly dragging the foot. Startling the horse in a backward or forward direction may be all that is necessary to release the patella. Other times the leg may be pulled forward with a scotch hobble and the patella manually released by pushing the patella up and forward. Once a horse stretches the ligament and acquires the habit of locking the patella, it is difficult to return to a normal situation.

Formerly, horses with upward fixation were

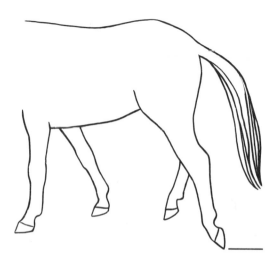

Fig. 36-3. Stifled posture.

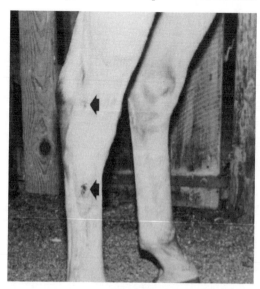

Fig. 36-4. Stringhalt operation scars (arrows).

blistered around the stifle joint, and shod with the stifled or rest shoe. The horse was tied and made to stand with its weight on the injured leg. The object was to lengthen the medial patellar ligament. Others recommended shoeing the stifled leg with the rest shoe. The object was to shorten the ligament.

Now, the veterinarian performs a simple operation cutting (called desmotomy) the medial patellar ligament at its base. This prevents the patella from locking over the trochlea. The horse can return to work in a few days. The only adverse effect is that the horse can no longer completely relax or sleep standing up.

Stringhalt

Stringhalt or springhalt is a sudden spastic flexion of one or both hind legs. It is more noticeable when the horse is backed from his stall, turned on the affected leg or suddenly frightened. The condition appears to be a nervous condition. However, there is evidence to indicate it may be due to a nutritional deficiency (pantothenic acid) or ingestion of poisonous plants. Other researchers have concluded that the stringhalt gait is learned as a habit and that it is not easily broken.

Stringhalt has been treated by feeding a balanced diet and surgery. The tendon of the lateral digital extensor is often removed where it passes over the outside of the hock to stop this annoying condition.

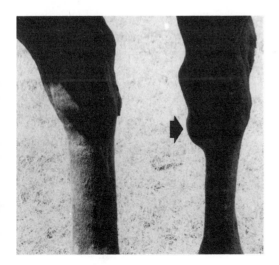

Fig. 36-5. Bog spavin (arrow).

Capped Hock

Capped hock is similar to capped elbow. It is a subcutaneous or false bursitis on the calcanean process or point of the hock. The swelling is usually firm and can be as large as an apple or so small it is unnoticed. Horses are rarely lame and the condition may be classified as a blemish. Large fluid filled swellings may be drained by a needle and the skin tightened by astringents. Old injuries will often have scar tissue that will not go away. Horses that constantly kick the stall wall or trailer door will develop capped hocks. Other sources of irritation are in poorly designed roping boxes and starting gates.

Thoroughpin

Thoroughpin or hollows is a soft puffy swelling on one or both sides and in front of the tendons above the point of the hock. The swelling may be pushed from one side to the other. The condition is usually considered a blemish as afflicted horses are seldom lame. The swelling is actually an expansion or distention of the deep flexor (Achilles) tendon sheath. It is also called the tarsal sheath. The swelling is more prominent when weight is placed on the foot. The skin over the area may be tightened by using a counterirritant. Thoroughpins are a sign of excessive stress in the hock region.

Bog Spavin

Bog spavin is a large soft swelling on the front and inside of the hock. It is similar to articular windpuff of the fetlock. Bog spavin is usually considered a blemish. However, bog spavin is an indication of severe strain or concussion to the hocks. Bone spavin may develop due to the original injury. Horses with excessively straight or sickle hocks and that are subject to hard stops are especially susceptible.

Blood spavin is sometimes mistaken for bog spavin. Blood spavin is a harmless swelling of the subcutaneous saphenous vein in approximately the same location as one would expect to find a bog spavin. The condition may be compared to varicose veins in man. There is never any lameness and no treatment necessary.

Bone Spavin

Bone spavin is a hard swelling on the inside of the hock. It is an exostosis that may occur on any of the tarsal bones. The central tarsal bone is most commonly involved. In fact, the central tarsal bone may become fused to the other bones. Large spavins, sometimes called jacks are easily seen by standing behind or in front and a little to one side of the horse. Occult or blind spavins must be located on a radiograph. Prognosis is poor when bone spavin of any type is located in the hock. Spavin is most common in crooked-legged, weak-hocked, young horses that are subjected to excessive strain.

Spavin lameness should be suspected when a horse has a stiff gait behind, wears the toes of its shoes excessively, drags its rear toes, or stabs the ground with the rear toes. Blood stains in the white line at the toe are symptoms of upper limb lameness. A horse will often work out of spavin lameness, but it will return after rest.

The spavin test is performed by flexing the rear leg and holding it up by the cannon bone for at least two minutes, dropping the leg and immediately trotting the horse. Lameness will be noticeable in the first few steps if the horse has spavin or stifle lameness.

Spavin is difficult to treat and should be considered a serious and permanent unsoundness. Bone surgery, cunean tenectomy and pin firing may be tried in an effort to remove a source of pain or to cause the irritated area to stop growing. Horses with spavin that are still serviceable are shod with a spavin shoe. It has high wedge-type heels and a rocker-toe. These are usually put on in pairs. A patten or rest shoe may be used on one leg when an animal is confined to a stall after surgery.

Curb

Curb is a hard swelling on the back surface of the hind leg about a hand's width (3 to 4 in.) below the point of the hock. The horse may stand at rest with the heel elevated.

A curb is caused by a sprain of the plantar ligament. Jumping horses commonly have a curb on one or both hocks. Horses with sickle hocks are most susceptible to curb. A hard blow as a result of stall kicking or fighting with another horse may also cause curb. Horses with curb can often be helped with heel calks or by trimming the foot to a steep angle. A horse with an old curb that is set or noninflamed is usually said to be serviceably sound.

Cocked Ankles

Cocked ankles or knuckling over is a dislocation of the fetlock joints of the hind legs. Some cases may be due to poor nourishment or lack of exercise. Overexertion of immature horses may also be a cause. There is some evidence that this condition may be related to a copper deficiency.

Most cases of knuckling over that are seen today are the result of too rapid growth of the bones relative to the growth of the tendons. The pain resulting from epiphysitis caused by a calcium/phosphorus imbalance causes a knuckling effect. The superficial flexor is always involved. It is attached at the point of the hock and is unyielding if the bones grow too fast. Corrective shoeing with an extended-toe and wedged-heel may be all that is necessary until the superficial flexor tendons catch up. Handmade aluminum shoes punched for the smallest size nails work very well. The deep flexors are usually not involved on the hind feet because the check ligament below the hock is small (or absent) and subject to stretching.

Epiphysitis can be recognized before the horse is lame by swellings above the knees or fetlocks of the front legs and the fetlocks and hocks of the hind legs. Reducing the animal's feed intake and allowing it to exercise will usually help. Large swellings above (or below) the fetlocks may not be completely reabsorbed. Laminitis may accompany some cases.

Run Down

Run down or suspensory sprain is a breaking down of the suspensory ligaments of the hind limbs. The fetlock sinks and there is usually damage to the flexor tendons. Fatigue due to overexertion and under conditioning is the most common cause of tearing of one or both of the sesamoid branches of the suspensory ligament.

Elastic bandages will support the limb while the horse is resting. Surgery may be effective in the few cases where a large enough portion of the bone is broken off to make screw fixation possible.

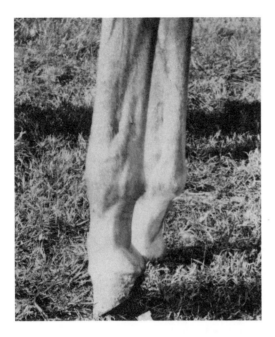

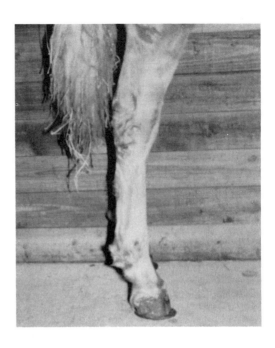

Fig. 36-6. (Left) Cocked ankles. (Right) Shoes for knuckling over.

A run down shoe has an extended base like an egg bar shoe with the heel turned down for traction. Prevention by wrapping the legs firmly is more practical than trying to treat the condition. A leg brace may be applied in severe cases. Lowering the heels will transfer some strain from the suspensory ligament to the flexor tendons.

Weak Flexor Tendons

Foals are occasionally born with weak flexor tendons. Most of those afflicted will grow out of the condition within 14 to 30 days. Those that don't may need to have an extended-heel shoe taped or nailed to the foot. Horses that don't improve may need special surgery and bracing.

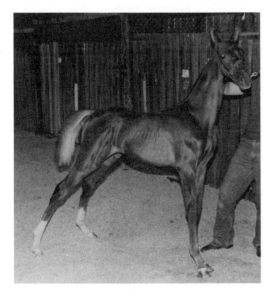

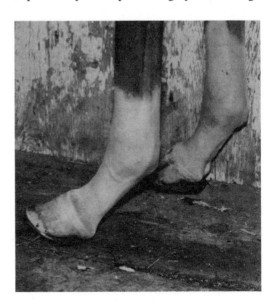

Fig. 36-7. (Left) weak flexor tendons behind, (right) right foot shod with an extended egg bar shoe and wedge.

Severed Tendons

Severed tendons are difficult to treat. The veterinarian should examine the wound immediately and perform surgery if practical. He will often request a shoe brace of some type to support the limb until the tendon(s) heals. There are many types. The best are light but strong as well as functional. The horseshoer must work closely with the veterinarian in designing and applying limb braces.

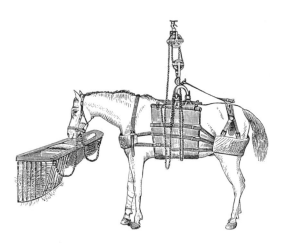

*Fig. 36-8. Slinging a horse may be useful for some injuries providing that the recovering animal will stand quietly. A sling can be made from sailcloth. Slings shold be avoided when an animal has complete paralysis since the abdomen becomes dangerously compressed. (*The Veterinarian, *1870).*

Conditions Common to Front and Hind Legs

Splints and other exostoses are found less frequently in the hind limb than the front. The conformation and use of the horse will usually determine the location of the lameness. Jumping horses are especially susceptible to shin splints on the hind legs. Cutting and reining horses are more susceptible to windpuffs on the hind legs than the front. Many of the lower leg lamenesses may occur on the hind legs. However, they rarely do because of the increased weight and strain on the front limbs of most horses.

References

Adams, O.R. 1974. Lameness in Horses (3rd ed.) Lea and Febiger, Philadelphia.

Daniels, B. 1982. Tips on shoeing youngsters. Amer. Farriers' J. 8(6):350.

Finocchio, E.J., J. Merriam, and B. Chase. 1982. Contracted tendons. Amer. Farriers' J. 8(6):334.

Frank, E.R. 1964. Veterinary Surgery (7th ed.). Burgess, Minneapolis.

Manning, D.C. 1983. Making and using the patten shoe. Amer. Farriers' J. 9(1):24.

Metcalf, S., P. Wagner and O. Balch-Burnett. 1983. Tendon disorders in young horses. Amer. Farriers' J. 9(1):17.

Rooney, J.R. 1974. The Lame Horse. A.J. Barnes and Co., Cranbury, NJ.

Siegmund, O.H. (Ed.). 1979. The Merck Veterinary Manual (5th ed.). Merck and Co., Inc., Rahway, NJ.

Staff. 1870. The Veterinarian. 43:802.

Yovich, J.V., T.S. Stashak and C.W. McIlwraith. 1984. Rupture of the common digital extensor tendon in foals. The Compendium. 6(7):S373.

NOTES:

Chapter 37

Forging and Applying Therapeutic Shoes

Therapeutic shoes, sometimes called pathological or surgical shoes, are usually handmade. The stock size must be appropriate to the size and use of the horse. They are applied in conjunction with veterinary medical treatment and instructions. Horses requiring these shoes would only rarely be shod without consultation with the veterinarian. An exception would be chronic cases where a diagnosis had been previously made and treatment prescribed. Veterinarians appreciate a courteous and knowledgeable horseshoer who can accurately make and apply therapeutic shoes.

Clips

Clips may be used to stabilize therapeutic shoes on the foot, especially when the wall is damaged or diseased. Clips may also be used to stabilize the foot in cases of quarter and sandcracks. Clips are used to prevent hoof movement in coffin bone fractures. Clips should be made at the angle of the wall and then fit into the hoof. They should not fit perpendicular and then be hammered into the hoof. Making and fitting clips is covered in Chapter 32.

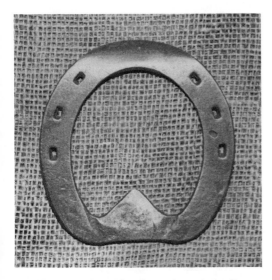

Fig. 37-1. Bar shoe with rocker toe for navicular disease.

Bar Shoe

The bar shoe is probably the most frequently used of all therapeutic shoes. It is also the hardest for most shoers to make and fit, especially in pairs. Bar shoes are more frequently forged from bar stock than any other type of corrective shoe.

The bar shoe is used whenever it is advantageous to apply pressure to, or relieve pressure from, one part of the foot. An example of a case to apply pressure would be shoeing for contracted heels. One to relieve pressure would be shoeing for quarter crack. It may also be desirable for cases in which the wall is broken, or weak, and nails cannot be placed in the machine-made nail holes which will securely hold the shoe on, and thus additional holes must be punched in the toe and heel of the shoe.

Bar shoes which are designed to apply pressure are usually fit so that 1/16 to 1/8 inch of daylight can be seen between the heels of the shoe and the heels of the hoof wall, when the bar is resting on the frog. A larger gap can be dangerous, possibly causing splitting of the hoof, especially if the foot is not moist and very flexible. This pressure can be created by rasping the wall or frog when preparing the foot. Or, it can be created when making the shoe by bending the bar of the shoe.

Steps in making a bar shoe:
1. Measure the foot as in making a plate shoe. Add the distance between the buttresses (across the frog) plus the thickness of the stock to make a handmade shoe. Or, select a keg hot shoe a size larger than the one ordinarily used on the foot in order to obtain the heel length necessary in a keg shoe. It is possible to draw out the heel of a hot shoe that is the regular size for the foot. However, it is difficult to make a functional, strong and lightweight bar shoe from most keg shoes.
2. Turn and punch the handmade shoe. Note the condition of the wall before selecting the position of the nail holes. Fit the shoe to the foot and mark the heels on the edge of the anvil or straight hardy as though they

were going to be cut. (See "Marking the Heels" in Chapter 24.)

3. "Scarf" the white hot heel of the shoe by holding the shoe on the face of the anvil and striking the upper edge of the extremity of the heel with the hammer face at a 45 degree angle. Strike in this manner until the tip of the heel is sharp. This should make a bevel about 3/8 inch long.

4. Turn the shoe over and scarf the other heel in the same manner. Shape the bevels on the horn so that their edges are flat or slightly pointed. This will aid the welding process when the heels are turned and welded. A right-handed person should scarf the shoe with the scarf of the upper heel pointing right when the shoe is held by the toe. A left-handed person should scarf the opposite surfaces so they point left. This is done for convenience in welding. When welding, you can "pull" the sharp point of the bevel into the other heel and make a fast, solid weld.

5. Place the white hot heel of the shoe on the point of the horn or off edge of the anvil. Hold the shoe at the toe or above with the tongs, and place the inside end of the heel mark on the point of the horn. Strike down once directly over the heel mark. This makes it easier to get the metal to bend at that point.

6. Strike on the upper edge of the portion of the heel projecting over the horn, and rotate the shoe downward as the bend progresses until the turned-in heel is at nearly a right angle to the branch.

7. Turn the other heel in the same manner. Usually one branch must be moved one way or the other to allow the two heels to pass each other.

8. Close the shoe and line up the heels on the horn or heel of the anvil preparatory to welding them. Hammer the points until they fit closely so that no coal dust will accumulate between them. The bevels should be aligned as shown.

9. Place the shoe in a clean reducing fire. You must have a hot, clean fire to forge weld. The area to be welded should be positioned over the hottest point of the fire. Cover the bar with coke. *Slowly* bring the metal of the bar to a welding heat. Turn the shoe over periodically to insure an even heat on both sides and through the metal. Clean the face of the anvil and set the hammer in position on it so that the handle may be easily grasped.

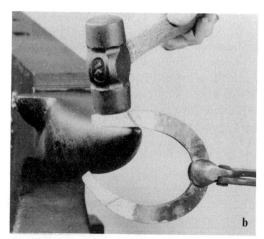

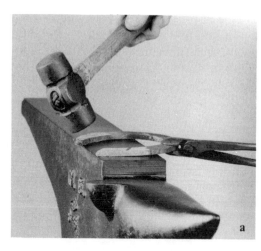

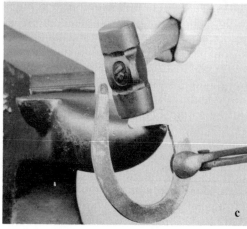

Fig. 37-2. *Steps in making a bar shoe from a keg or long heeled shoe:*
(a) *Scarf the heels.*
(b) *Notch and turn the heels over the point of the horn at the inside of the heel mark.*
(c) *Turn the heels nearly to a right angle.*
(d) *Overlap the heels and align them for welding.*
(e) *Position of the overlapped and scarfed heels before welding.*
(f) *Position of hammer when starting the weld with light blows.*
(g) *Finish the weld with heavier blows and shape the bar until it is the thickness of the shoe.*
(h) *Finished long heeled (A) or keg (B) bar shoes.*

10. Flux the area to be welded and continue heating. When the flux runs and the metal is the same color as the fire, remove the shoe from the fire and quickly take it to the anvil.

11. Tap the shoe lightly on the edge of the anvil to remove the loose scale and dirt that may have formed and collected on and between the heels of the bar. Quickly strike *light* blows on the scarf points. This must be done very quickly while the metal is still sparking and at optimum welding temperature. As soon as one side is welded, quickly turn the shoe over and weld the other. Follow with heavier blows to weld the center and flatten out the weld. Stop hammering when the metal gets orange.

12. Reheat the bar to a welding heat and complete the weld, if necessary, using light blows at first on the ends of the scarf, and then heavier blows in the middle. The ends or points of the heels must be welded first. Beginners should take two heats to complete the welding of a bar shoe.

13. Smash the bar down flat to the thickness of the shoe or thinner. Shape the bar while it is at a white heat by holding one corner on the point of the horn or corner of the heel of the anvil and striking on the center of the bar. Reverse the shoe and repeat the shaping of the other corner. This will set the center of the bar forward and give the shoe the correct shape at the heels.

14. Bevel and draw the ground surface of the

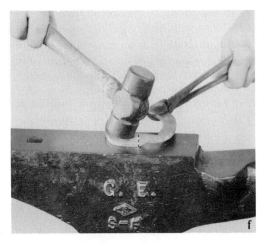

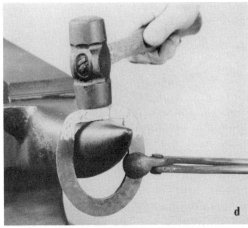

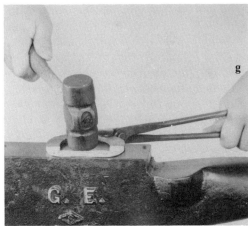

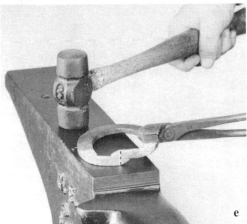

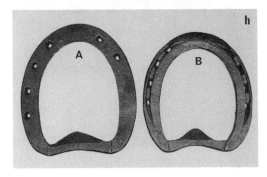

bar toward the center of the shoe with the rounded face of the hammer to form a "cradle" for the frog. Hot rasp the bar smooth.

15. Carry the shoe to the foot and check the fit. Make minor adjustments. Note and mark the nail hole positions if they have not previously been punched. Punch the nail holes.

Many horseshoers can guess fairly accurately the measurements for a bar shoe and prefer to form the shoe first and then fit it to the foot. This is more difficult for beginners but the procedure should be well understood since it is often necessary to change a shoe, even one that was measured carefully, in order to get it to fit the foot. A handmade shoe made from stock of the correct length is easier to fit to a foot than an altered keg shoe.

Basic principles for shaping a bar shoe:

1. **To Open the Toe:** Heat the shoe throughout to a red heat and hold it upright with the bar on the face of the anvil. Strike along the toe. This opens the toe and quarters without changing the bar. Or the toe may be opened over the horn as a plate shoe.

2. **To Widen the Heels: When the quarters are too long,** the bar must be lengthened to widen the heels. Heat the bar and heels to a white heat. Hold the shoe at the toe and place the inside edge of the heel on the point of the horn at the point from which it is desired to turn the heel into the bar. Strike the end of the heel projecting over the horn. Then reverse the shoe and in the same manner, turn the heel in.

3. **To Widen the Heels: When the quarters are the correct length,** the bar must be drawn out to widen the heels. Heat the bar to a white heat and draw it out by flattening

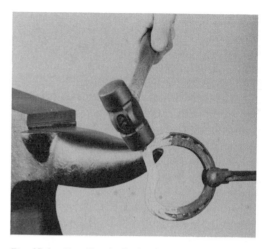

Fig. 37-4. *To widen the heels when the quarters are too long.*

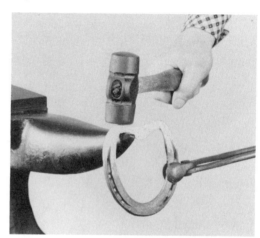

Fig. 37-5. *To widen the heels when the quarters are the correct length.*

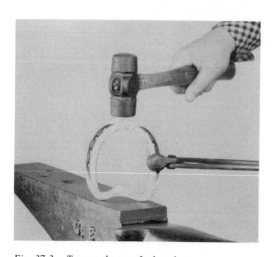

Fig. 37-3. *To open the toe of a bar shoe.*

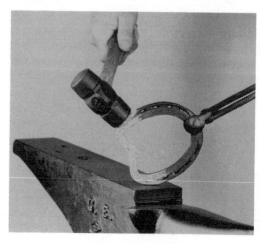

Fig. 37-6. *To close the heels when the quarters are the correct length.*

it on the face of the anvil. This will lengthen the bar and at the same time reduce its thickness. After drawing out the bar, it must be made to correspond to the foot surface to produce the desired frog pressure.

It may be desirable to draw out the bar on the point of the horn, working one-half, and then reversing the shoe. This method lengthens and thickens the bar.

4. **To Close the Heels: When the quarters are the correct length,** the heels may be closed by shortening the bar. Heat the bar and heels and hold one heel on the face of the anvil with the shoe perpendicular to it. Strike the elevated heel. This will shorten the bar by upsetting it and narrow and straighten the quarters.

5. **To Close the Heels: When the quarters are too short,** part of the bar must be turned into the heel to close the heels of the shoe. Heat the heels and bar and place the inside edge of the triangular part of the bar on the point of the horn. Strike the part projecting over it. This will turn part of the bar into the heel.

6. **To Close the Heels: When the quarters are too long,** and the shoe needs to be closed at the heels, the bar must be pushed in toward the center. Heat the rear half of the shoe and hold it upright, the center of the bar on the point of the horn of the anvil. Strike the toe. This will push the bar toward the toe and shorten the shoe, thus bringing the heels closer together.

7. **To Lengthen the Quarters:** Heat and draw out the heels on the horn as on a plate or weighted shoe.

8. **To Shorten One Branch:** Heat the shoe throughout and hold it upright with the point of the longer heel on the face of the anvil.

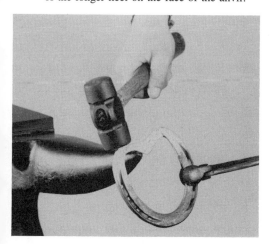

Fig. 37-7. To close the heels when the quarters are too short.

Strike the upper edge of the shoe directly over the point resting on the anvil. This will push the heel toward the toe and slightly round the quarter and toe on the same side.

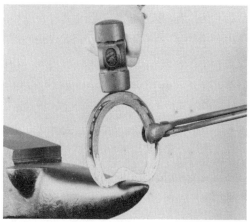

Fig. 37-8. To close the heels when the quarters are too long.

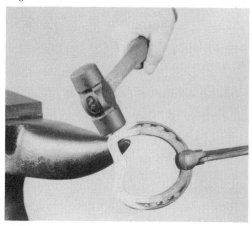

Fig. 37-9. To lengthen the quarters.

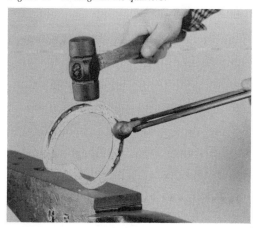

Fig. 37-10. To shorten one branch.

405

Bar Shoe Types

Curved bar shoes are curved above or below the ground surface of the shoe. They are used to apply or to relieve frog pressure, especially when a frog is small and atrophied or large and protruding. The shoe is held so that one end of the bar rests on the edge of the anvil face and the other on the horn. The center of the foot or ground surface of the bar is curved as the case may require. Raised (toward the frog) bar shoes may be used when treating contraction. Dropped (away from the frog) bars may be used when treating thrush, corns, or sheared heels.

Heart bar shoes are shaped like hearts. The larger bar area covering the frog may be added and arc welded between the heels, or an extra long piece of stock can be cut and the heels folded toward the toe and forge welded. Heart bar shoes are used in some cases of navicular and founder. They are used to relieve pressure from horses that have navicular disease and are sensitive to pressure on the center of the frog. They are used to apply pressure slightly behind the point of the frog to prevent further coffin bone rotation resulting from founder.

Mushroom bar shoes are shaped like mushrooms. The shoe is bent in at the quarters and then over the frog. The edges are welded together. A hole(s) is punched in the stem to rivet pads or leather wedges to the bar. The mushroom shoe is used to apply pressure to the frog and relieve pressure from the heels, especially on a horse that has corns or sore heels.

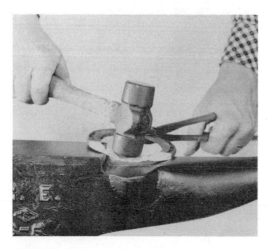

Fig. 37-11. To curve or drop the bar.

Egg bar shoes are shaped like eggs. They are used on horses with flexor tendon trouble and horses with low, sloping heels. They may be used on horses with either founder or navicular disease if their conformation warrants it. The joining of the shoe branches into a bar gives more support at the heels and prevents possible interference with the opposite limb.

Tongue bar shoes are a combination of a heart bar shoe and an egg bar. The egg bar is squared to give lateral support and bent down to raise the heel angle without putting pressure on the heel wall or rear of the frog. The tongue is welded to the center of the bar and distributes weight over the front third of the frog. A strong toe clip is essential to the success of this shoe. It is most effective on a horse with sore heels due to pedal osteitis.

Jumped-in bars are welded between the heels of an open keg shoe or a shoe with calks or other projections on both heels. These may be created in various patterns. For example, jumped-in bars are called butterfly bars or diamond bars depending upon their shape. The shape of these bars often becomes the trademark of an individual horseshoer. Jumped-in bars are usually welded on the foot surface. Bars of assorted sizes and shapes may be made up ahead of time. This type of bar can also be welded with an oxy-acetylene or electric arc welder.

Whip-across bars or **Canadian bars** are made when a trailer and/or calk is on one heel. They require a very sound weld since a calk must be made and a trailer turned next to the welded area. Whip-across bars are probably the most difficult of all bar shoes to make. They are used most on the rear feet of pacing harness horses. Bars are frequently used on the light shoes of harness horses to keep them from spreading when they become worn.

Fig. 37-12. Steps in making a creased bar shoe from a straight bar:
(a) Start the toe bend with the tongs perpendicular to the stock.
(b) Finish the toe bend with the tongs perpendicular to the stock.
(c) Completed toe bend.
(d) Turn the outside heel in over the anvil face or the point of the horn.
(e) Scarf the heel.
(f) Turn the outside branch.

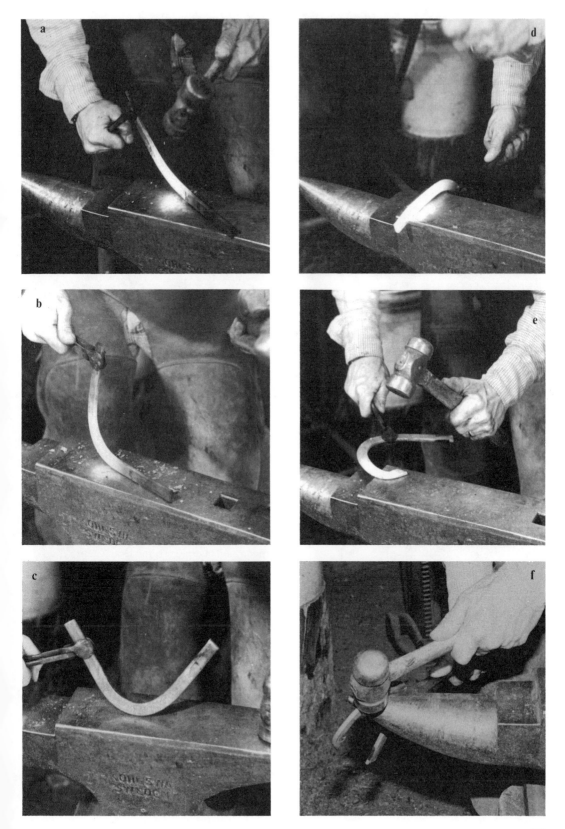

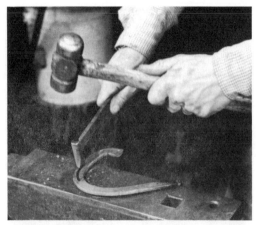

(g) Crease the outside branch moving the creaser with a rocking motion.

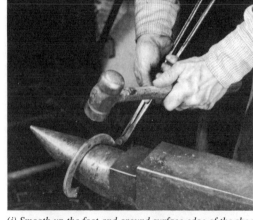

(j) Smooth up the foot and ground surface edge of the shoe with the hammer.

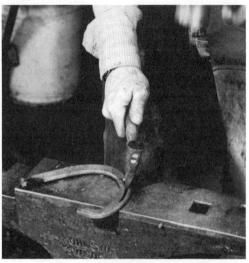

(h) Stamp the nail holes in the crease.

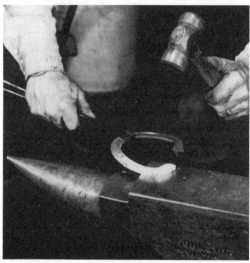

(k) Turn the inside heel and scarf it.

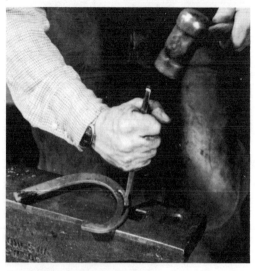

(i) Pritchel out the nail holes.

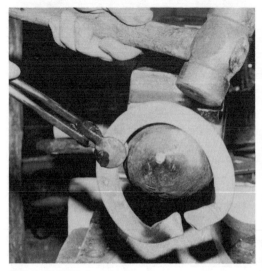

(l) Turn the inside branch.

408

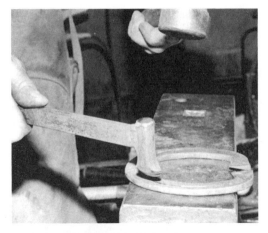

(m) Crease and punch the inside branch.

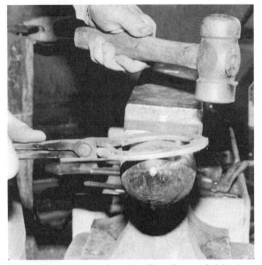

(n) Bend one branch down to allow the scarfed heels to overlap.

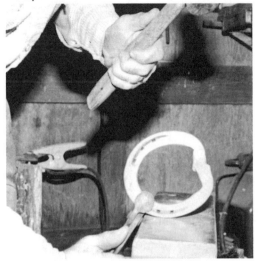

(o) Close the heels and align them for welding.

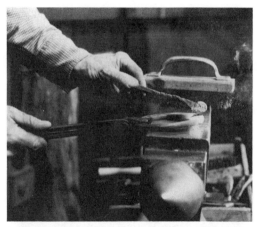

(p) Heat and brush the area to be welded before applying welding flux.

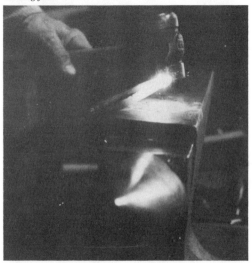

(q) Don't touch the area to be welded on the anvil until you are ready to hammer it.

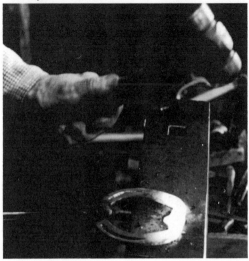

(r) Weld the bar on both sides and draw the frog cradle.

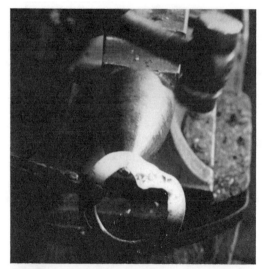

(s) Shape the bar on the anvil horn . . .

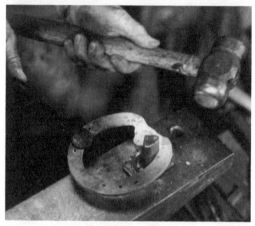

(t) . . . or a tool in the hardy hole.

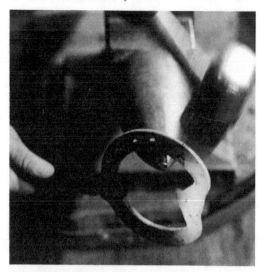

(u) Round and shape the quarters of the shoe as the bar is shaped.

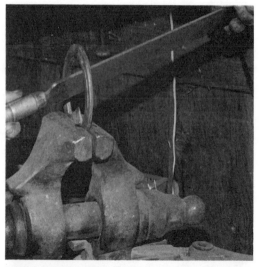

(v) Finish the bar with a file.

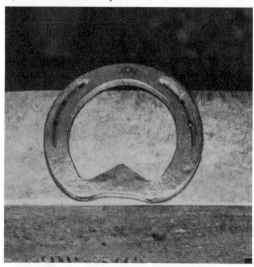

(w) The finished shoe.

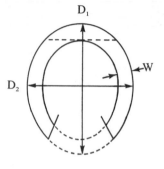

$$3\left(\frac{D_1 + D_2}{2}\right) - 1W = \text{Stock}$$

(x) Formula for determining the amount of stock needed to make an egg bar shoe. Subtract 2W (instead of 1W) for regular bar shoes.

Cross Bars and Sole Plates

Cross bars and sole plates are welded across or bolted to shoes at various points to protect the bottom of the foot from pressure. Bruises and abscesses can often be treated best this way. Bars are usually relatively flat and wide. Bars or plates may be bent away from the sole when it is very flat. A plastic pad is often used next to the foot and riveted to the bar. The pad holds in medication and protects the sole. Bars and plates are sometimes bolted to a shoe when a dressing must be frequently changed. The shoe can be drilled and tapped or nuts can be welded on the inside edge of the shoe.

Rocker-Shoe

The rocker-shoe can be made of 5/8 inch thick square or round stock. The foot surface is left flat. The shoe is left thick in the quarters and beveled or rolled from the center third to the toe and heels. It is an interesting forging exercise. The shoe may be made in a bar shoe pattern. Turn and weld the stock into a ring and then bevel it and shape it to fit the foot.

The rocker-shoe is most useful to treat arthritic conditions of the front legs. It may be used in some founder cases. A simple version of the rocker-shoe may be made from a keg shoe by rocking the toe the full web of the shoe and

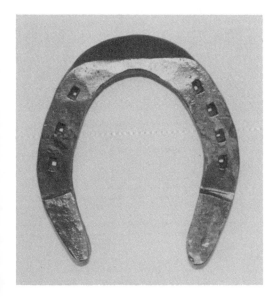

Fig. 37-13. Spavin shoe made by C. Swan from 1 x ½ inch stock.

by beveling and thinning the heels. Another form of this shoe, called the Roberge shoe, is a flat plate hammered into a convex pattern with a flattened outer rim for nailing. A rocker-shoe can also be made by welding a curved (convex) bar to the toe and bar of a bar shoe. This also gives a horse a rocker motion.

Rocker-Toe and Swelled Heels

The rocker-toe and swelled heel shoe, sometimes called a roller-motion shoe, is used on horses that have chronic bowed tendons. It may also be used with success on some arthritic cases and is much easier to make than a rocker-shoe. Making and fitting a rocker-toe and swelled heel is covered in Chapter 32.

Spavin Shoe

The spavin or wedge-heeled shoe is used on horses that are spavined. The toe is rolled to prevent the hoof toe from stabbing into the ground. The heels are high to relieve stress on the joint and sloping to prevent catching in the ground.

The spavin shoe can be made from ⅜ x ¾ inch stock. For heavy horses, ½ x 1 inch stock may be appropriate. The heels are upset and thickened to a height of about 1 inch. The tip of the toe is thinned and rolled. The stock should be at least 2 inches longer than the hoof measurement to allow for upsetting. Swelled heels made on a keg shoe can be substituted for a handmade wedge-heeled shoe.

Horses that are spavined sometimes work better when they are left high on the inside and trimmed lower on the outside of the hoof. Horses that are shod with extremely high wedge heels should be stall rested. Horses that get no relief from this kind of shoeing should be considered candidates for surgery.

Patten Shoe

The Patten or rest shoe is used to treat damaged flexor tendons. It raises the heels of the foot and prevents the heel from sinking into the ground. It features high heels and a solid bar connecting them at the base. As the cut flexor tendon or other injury heals, the heels of the shoe can be lowered by heating and smashing them down. When the heel lift is no longer needed, the heel can be cut out of the shoe.

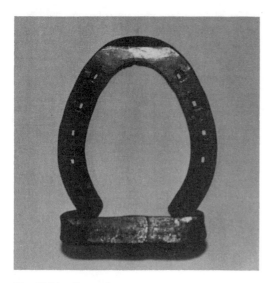

Fig. 37-14. Patten shoe.

Patten shoes should be made from ⅝ x ¼ or ¾ x ¼ inch stock. Light stock is best due to the extra weight in the heel lift. This shoe will show little wear since it is worn while the horse is resting. Patten shoes are not put on in pairs.

Steps in making a Patten shoe:

1. Measure the foot as you would when making a handmade plate shoe. Add 1 inch to each heel, add twice the desired height of the heels, and add the width of the bar between the heels. Cut the stock.

2. Make a center punch mark in the center of the stock. Make center punch marks where the end of each heel would be on a plate shoe.

3. Turn and punch the shoe leaving the heels extending straight back.

4. Heat the area of the heel center punch marks. Place the shoe in the vise with the heels projecting up. The heel center punch marks should be even with the top of the vise jaw.

5. Place an adjustable wrench about 1 inch above the vise jaws and twist each of the

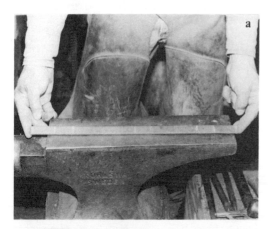

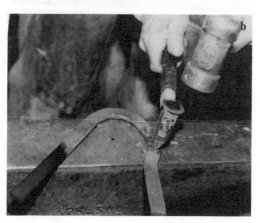

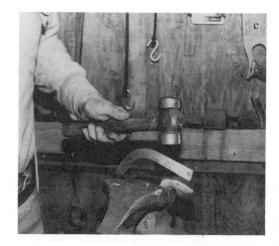

Fig. 37-15. Steps in making a patten shoe:
(a) Measure the foot and lay out the stock and mark with a center punch.
(b) Turn and punch the shoe.
(c) Bend the heels down in a vise . . .
(d) . . . until they are both extending perpendicular to the shoe.
(e) Scarf the heel ends and bend them in.
(f) Align the heels for welding.
(g) Weld the ends on the off heel corner of the anvil, first on the foot surface . . .
(h) . . . and then on the ground surface.
(i) Smooth up the edges of the weld with the hammer.
(j) Level the bar with a flatter.
(k) Heat and rock the toe.
(l) The finished shoe.

heels 90 degrees toward the center. Bend the extended heels over until they are 90 degrees to the ground surface of the shoe.
6. Heat the ends and prepare them for welding by scarfing them.

7. Heat and turn in the end to form the bar making the height of both the heels the same. Overlap the scarfed ends for welding.
8. Heat and flux the area to be welded.
9. Weld the bar by striking the first blows with the shoe up on the anvil face. Quickly turn

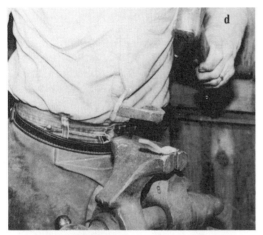

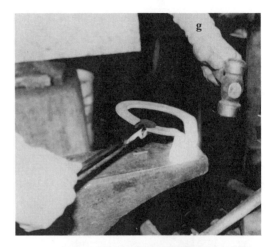

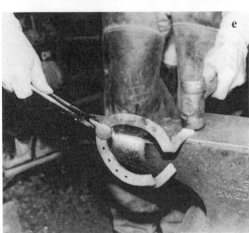

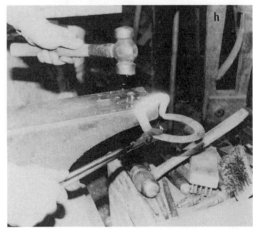

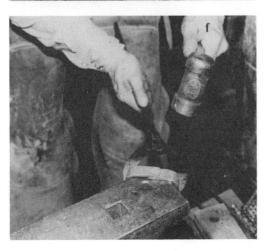

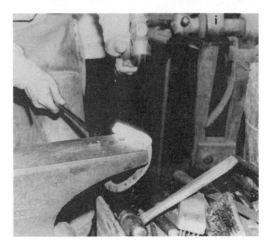

the shoe over a corner of the heel of the anvil and strike the second welding hammer blows.

10. Heat and rock the tip of the toe (⅓ to ½ the web) of the shoe.
11. Make a final fitting of the shoe to the foot.

12. Heat up the heel lift apparatus. Cool the shoe in water. Align the heel and flatten the ground bar so that it lines up with the rocker-toe and the shoe rests flat on the anvil. A flatter struck by a helper with a sledgehammer is ideal.

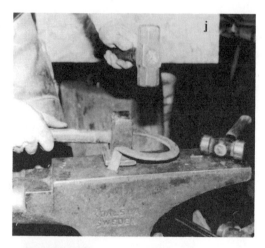

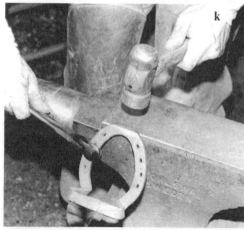

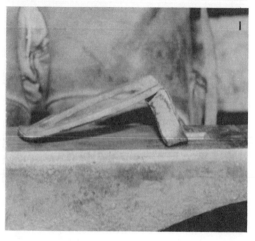

Extended-Toe Shoe

The extended-toe or beaked shoe is used on the feet of clubfooted horses or horses with contracted tendons. The shoe can be fit forward of the natural toe of the foot exposing the ground surface of the wall at the toe. Or, the shoe can have a projection welded in the center of the toe. The object is to slow the breakover of the foot and prevent the foot from knuckling over. The space between the shoe tip and front of the hoof can be filled in with acrylic plastic on show horses. When feet are of unequal size, both shoes are made the same size. The shoe for the largest foot is fit and nailed on. The matching shoe for the smaller foot is placed on the foot and nail hole location is marked. The shoe is punched and nailed to compensate for the missing hoof base. If an extra long toe extension is needed, the metal may be extended forward and bent back against the front of the hoof to prevent injury of other limbs or premature pulling of the shoe.

Surgical Leg Braces

Braces can be constructed to assist in supporting surgical or trauma damaged sites while they heal. Most braces are built using a shoe as a base. Braces are often unique due to the variation in location and extent of limb injuries. Many are made with hinged or bolt-on portions to make the changing of wound dressings easier.

Bowed Tendon Shoe

The bowed tendon shoe (sometimes called a run down shoe) is used to help a horse rest sprained or bowed tendons. The simplest form of this shoe would be a keg shoe fit longer than the foot with plastic wedge pads inserted between the shoe and hoof. An egg bar shoe with a wedge effect is excellent. Another form is a ½ web rocker-toe with swelled heels. These

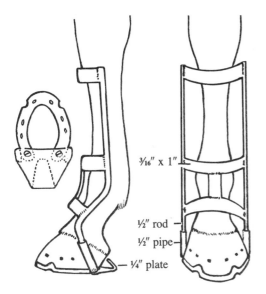
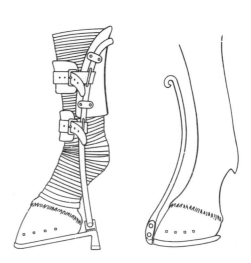

3/16" x 1"

1/2" rod

1/2" pipe

1/4" plate

Fig. 37-16. (Left) Surgical leg brace that supports the fetlock but can be removed when treating. Brace designed by J. Dienlin. (Right) Other types of leg braces.

shoes should be placed on each foot of a pair even if only one is injured. The heels of bowed tendon shoes are let down gradually as the horse heals. Horses that have old scars and are subject to recurrent bows should continue to be shod with some sort of heel elevation.

Navicular Shoe

The navicular shoe is used to treat chronic navicular disease. Many of these horses have low heels and should be shod on their natural pastern angle. The shoe is made from a stock appropriate to the size and use of the horse. It

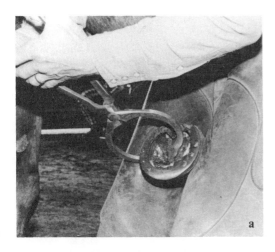
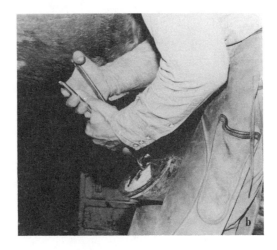

a

b

Fig. 37-17. Shoeing for navicular disease:
(a) Check for pain response with hoof testers.
(b) Trim more toe than heel and balance the foot.

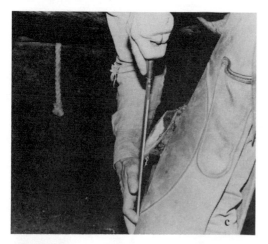

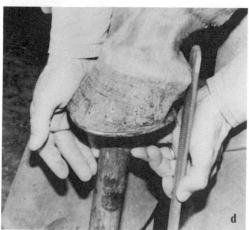

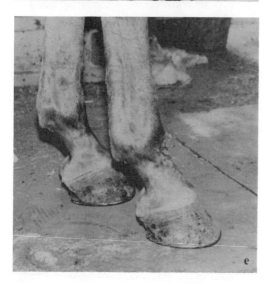

has a full web rocker-toe. The bar protects the navicular bone from injury and keeps the heel from sinking in soft ground. A heart bar gives more surface area coverage to the frog and bone especially in horses with low underslung heels. The back of the bar should extend behind the buttresses, especially when the heels are low and sloping, to give an egg bar effect. The nail holes are punched in the front half of the shoe. A hole is usually punched in the bar so that a full pad can be riveted to the shoe. Bar wedge pads should be used when the pastern angle cannot be obtained by trimming.

Founder Shoe

Acutely foundered horses should be shod with bar shoes of the heart or tongue type to stabilize and prevent further rotation of the coffin bone. Burney Chapman of Lubbock, Texas, has recommended putting pressure slightly behind the point of the frog equal to one-fourth the distance from the inner border of the wall to the tip of the coffin bone. A convex steel cover or bar across the center of the shoe may also be used to make the shoe work as a rocker-shoe.

Shoes for chronically foundered horses are usually made from ¼ x 1 inch stock or a wide-

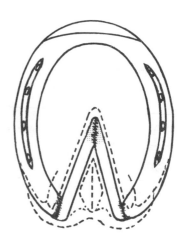

Fig. 37-18. Keg heart bar shoe for founder. Use a size larger creased shoe. Roll or rock the toe. Turn the heels in toward the frog. Make the legs of the bar narrow so they won't touch the sole. Put about ¼ inch of pressure (gap at the heels when nailing) slightly behind the point of the frog. Adjust pressure by placing an open shoe between the heart bar shoe and the anvil. Strike the bar.

(c) Rasp the hoof toe to match the rocker-toe of the shoe.
(d) Fit the bar shoe so that it extends back to support the deep flexor tendon.
(e) Completed job.

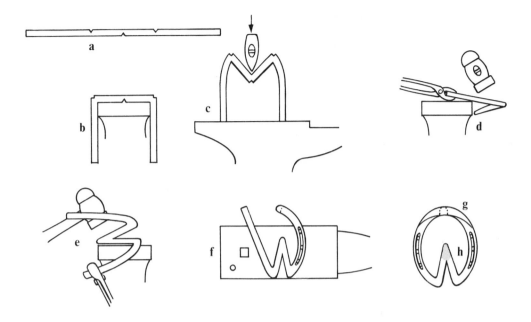

Fig. 37-19. Steps in making a handmade heart bar shoe:
(a) Measure and mark stock on sharp hardy.
(b) Bend ends over the edges of the anvil.
(c) Drive center down with straight pein or fuller to form point.
(d) Hold over edge of anvil and drive point down.

(e) Shape point to correspond to width of frog.
(f) Turn each branch, crease and punch the nail holes.
(g) Adjust and weld at the toe.
(h) Roll the toe and concave the foot surface. Adjust the pressure on the bar.

webbed stock appropriate to the size and use of the horse. The shoe is seated out or strongly concaved on the inner rim to prevent sole pressure. A rolled-toe is desirable. A rocker-toe may be used if it does not put pressure on the toe. The nail holes are punched in the rear half of the shoe to prevent pressure at the toe. Often, feed regulation and light exercise are as important as shoeing in the treatment of chronic founder.

Contraction Shoe

The contraction shoe (slipper heeled or bevel heeled shoe) is used to encourage a contracted hoof to spread. The shoe should not be used unless the foot is in a moist environment. A dropped bar may be used in conjunction with the beveled heels. The heels can be beveled with a hammer or a rasp. The shoe is beveled to the outside from zero at the last nail hole (at the widest part of the quarters) to ⅛ inch at the heel.

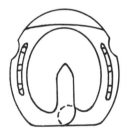

Fig. 37-20. A variation of the heart bar shoe designed by J.W. Huws. The shoe is forge welded at the site within the dotted lines.

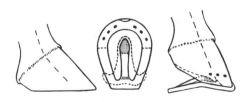

Fig. 37-21. A tongue bar shoe for pedal osteitis or sheared heels. The tongue is welded to the egg bar shoe with an oxyacetylene or electric arc welder.

417

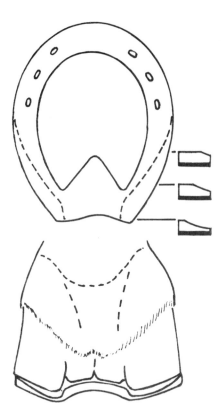

Fig. 37-22. Bevel heeled shoe.

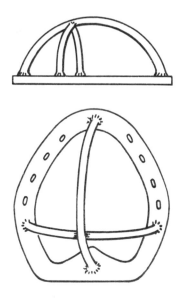

Fig. 37-23. Stifled shoe. Also see Fig. 31-8, No. 43.

Stifled Shoe

The stifle shoe is a relic of the past. Modern surgical procedure (medial patellar desmotomy) has taken its place. The idea behind the shoe was to prevent the horse locking its patella by always keeping the leg bent. It could also be used on an uninjured leg to make the horse keep weight or "traction" on an injury. It was made by arching ⁵⁄₁₆ to ⅜ inch round or square stock about 3 inches above the center of the foot. An open shoe was made with a three-legged arch. A bar shoe was made with a four-legged arch.

References

Adams, O.R. 1974. Lameness in Horses (3rd ed.). Lea and Febiger, Philadelphia.

Asmus, H. 1946. Horseshoes of Interest to Veterinarians. Ken Kimbel, Plant City, FL.

Chapman, B. 1983. Personal communication. Lubbock, TX.

Daniels, B.B. 1984. Bar shoes. Amer. Farriers' J. 10(4):348.

Dienlin, J.A. 1973. Balance of the Equine Foot and Gait and Therapeutic Shoeing. Auburn Univ., Auburn, AL.

Dollar, J.A.W. and A. Wheatley. 1898. A Handbook of Horseshoeing. David Douglas, Edinburgh.

Hickman, J. 1977. Farriery. J.A. Allen and Co., London.

Holmes, C.M. 1949. The Principles and Practice of Horse Shoeing. The Farrier's Journal Publ. Co. Ltd., Leeds, ENGLAND.

Manning, D. 1983. Making and using the patten shoe. Amer. Farriers' J. 9(1):24.

Manning, D. 1984. A steel plate held with studs. Amer. Farriers' J. 10(5):406.

Reeks, H.C. 1925. Diseases of the Horse's Foot (2nd ed.). Alex Eger, Chicago.

Richardson, C. 1950. Practical Farriery. Pitman and Sons, London.

Roberge, D. 1894. The Foot of the Horse. William R. Jenkins, New York.

Stehsel, D.L. 1974. Farrier's Orthopedics Handbook. Geddes Press, Pasadena, CA.

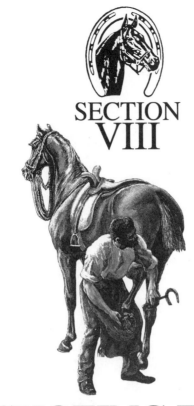

SECTION
VIII

SHOEING THE
SPECIALIZED
HORSE

Chapter 38

Performance Horses

Performance horses are athletic horses used for work or sport. They may be ridden Western or English in an arena or cross country. They may be shown in equitation classes or pleasure and performance classes. The rider is judged in equitation classes. The horse is judged in pleasure and performance classes.

The most popular breed of horse in America is the Quarter Horse. The next is the Thoroughbred followed by the Arabian and Appaloosa. These breeds are also the most common in the performance events.

The type of tack (riding equipment) used on performance horses differs according to event and tradition. Many of the basic maneuvers, speed of travel and ground conditions are similar for both Western and English style performance events.

Western riding style performance uses include ranch work, western riding, rodeo events, gymkhana games, cutting, reining and stock horse classes.

English riding style performance uses include polo playing, dressage, hunting, jumping and eventing (3-day). Combined training events include competition in dressage, endurance (steeplechase and cross country), and stadium jumping.

Ranch Work

Western ranch or stock working horses are used to help gather, move, separate and doctor livestock. Ranch raised livestock are often ranged in very rough terrain. Most ranch horses are shod with plain keg shoes as are western pleasure horses. However, toe and heeled shoes are preferred in some areas. The sole and frog are not trimmed. Rock bruises are common. Plastic or leather pads are necessary to prevent sole injury in the roughest areas. The heels of front and hind shoes may be bent up behind the buttresses to protect the bulbs from rock bruising. Self-cleaning or concave shoe patterns are very desirable.

Ranch horses used in the winter are shod with calks or borium treated shoes. Snow shoe or self-cleaning mud patterns are desirable. Screw calks (formerly called never-slips) used to be very popular to create traction for horses used during the winter. They are still used in some areas. Methods of shoeing horses for winter are described in Chapter 43.

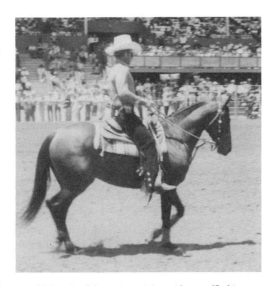

Fig. 38-1. Stock horse in training with a snaffle bit.

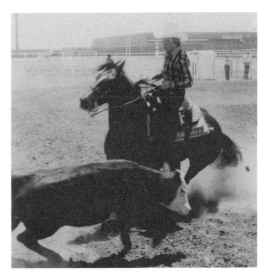

Fig. 38-2. Finished stock horse with a spade bit.

Western Riding

Western riding is a horse show class to demonstrate the performance and characteristics of an ideal ranch horse. The horse is ridden through a pattern made by plastic cone markers. The class is judged much like an English riding dressage test with form and position being more important than speed. It is very popular in some parts of the country.

Rodeo

Rodeo is America's own exciting sport. Rodeos are more popular than horse shows in most of America. Only horse racing outdraws rodeo as a horse spectator sport. Rodeo events were originally contests of skill between ranch cowboys. Now they are highly specialized competitive sports contests. The winners are professional athletes who have specialized in mastering each of the various events.

Rodeo horses are powerful athletes that perform in deep ground at high speed in runs that last only a few seconds. Some rodeo horses are dual purpose animals that are also used for ranch work. They are usually shod with plain keg shoes. However, horses that are used strictly in the arena should be shod with lighter shoes. An extra light pattern (saddle-lite) is preferable to a heavier plain pattern.

A heavy steel training plate, which is still lighter than an extra light keg shoe, is a better choice. The training plate provides more traction

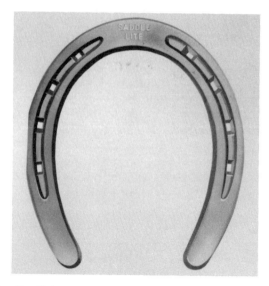

Fig. 38-4. Extra light (saddle-lite) shoe.

and has a self-cleaning design. Grabs can be added if desired. Grabs are not desirable, except under special ground conditions because of the stress they put on a horse's legs when it is hauled. Many contestants put foam rubber under their trailer mats to insulate and protect the feet from concussion.

A flat shoe is preferred. One company makes an extra heavy swedged training plate that it calls a roping horse shoe. Another company makes a swedged pattern with a high outer rim that it calls a barrel racing shoe. In addition to being hard to level, barrel racing shoes can be hard on a horse's knees and may cause severe damage if a horse accidentally treads on itself.

The best all around shoe for rodeo horses is the so-called rim shoe. It is a full swedge (creased or fullered) self-cleaning (concave) pattern with the substance of a heavier plain shoe. The steel size of the rim shoe should be in proportion to the body size of the horse. The rim shoe is a desirable shoe for all timed event horses that are used in and out of the arena. This would include horses used for barrel racing, calf roping, team roping, steer wrestling and bronc riding pickup horses.

Some calf ropers prefer a conventional plain or slick shoe on the hind feet of their young horses to encourage them to slide. In the rare case where a rodeo is held on grass (turf), a polo

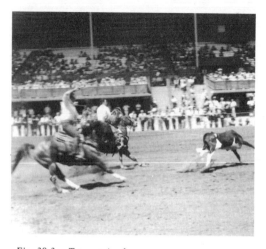

Fig. 38-3. Team roping horses.

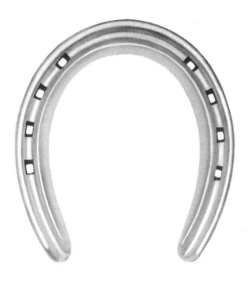

Fig. 38-5. Rim shoe for roping and other performance horses.

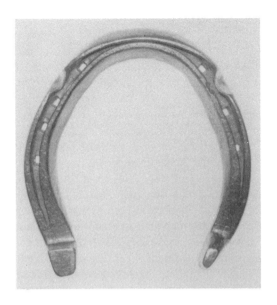

Fig. 38-7. A hind rim shoe "safed" to prevent damage from overreaching made by A.Calvert. Photos by J. Graves.

plate (high inner rim) or barrel racing shoe (high outer rim) is preferred.

Rodeo horses should be fit very close, especially in the front feet. Deep plowed arenas make overreaching and missteps very common. A horse that is bumped or jerked during a run may tread on itself or an exposed heel of a shoe. Shoe heels

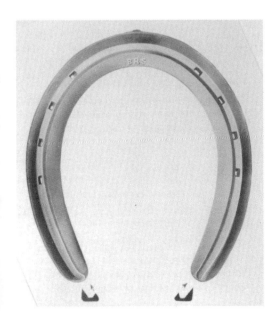

Fig. 38-6. Barrel racing shoe.

should be fit to end exactly at the buttress of the front feet. Overreach boots or heel and bulb protecting bell boots should be worn on the front feet of rodeo horses. Fetlock protecting skid boots should also be worn on the back feet of calf roping horses.

Some calf roping horses must be protected from overreaching by squaring the toe of the shoe and setting it under the toe of the hoof. Rim shoe toes can be hammered back under the toe (called a safe toe) to prevent damage from accidental overreaching. Shoes should be clipped: hind shoes with side clips, front shoes with toe clips.

Gymkhana

Gymkhana horses are game horses. In some areas, events where games on horseback are played are called playdays. Gymkhana events include various types of races run against a clock. They provide recreation and competition for many younger horsemen. However, the quick starts and stops and turns required by these predominantly heavy handed riders cause many of these horses to sour. Shoeing will not change this. Gymkhana horses are shod like rodeo horses. A few specialized horses are shod like race horses with aluminum racing plates and toe grabs.

Cutting

Cutting horses are cow horses. They are used to separate (cut) individual cattle from a herd on a ranch. Cutting horses are shown with a time limit for their work of 2½ minutes. They are aided by turnback men. Their performance is scored from 60 to 80 points.

Cutting horses are shod much like rodeo horses. Some cutting horse trainers request polo plates on the hind feet. Side clips are a necessity on horses shod with shoes that provide much traction. Horses that are especially hard on their joints because they turn so hard should be shod with flat shoes that provide little traction. The horse will stay sound longer. The inside edge of front and hind shoes should be hot rasped smooth to prevent the chance of injury to opposite limbs by treading. Splint boots (interfering boots) should be worn on the front legs of young horses.

Reining

Reining horses are trained to slide to a stop and to roll back over their hocks and spin. They are shown performing one of several approved patterns. Ideally, a horse used for any type of stock work is a reining horse. The reining patterns demonstrate the horse's collection and suitability for stock work.

The front feet of reining horses can be shod with steel training plates, rim shoes or half-round shoes. The selection of shoe type depends upon the trainer's preference, the ground condition and other uses of the horse.

During the training process, and to some extent when showing, sliding plates are preferred by many trainers. A sliding plate is a wide-

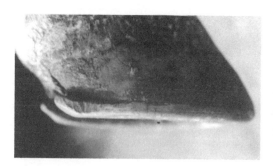

Fig. 38-9. Fit of spooned heels on a foot.

webbed shoe with the nail holes recessed, the heels spooned (bent up) and the toe rolled. The object is to create a slick surface that helps the horse collect its hind legs up under its body when it is reined to a stop. The rolled-toe and spooned heels prevent any dragging action on the shoe.

Steps for making sliding plates:

1. Measure the hind feet and cut off the desired width and calculated length. One-fourth x 1 to 1¼ inch stock makes a nice shoe.
2. Heat and bend the toe more than 90 degrees.
3. Turn and punch the branches. Stamp the nail holes so a nail of appropriate size will fit in the hole with the head almost flush.
4. Taper and draw the heels to one-half the width of the stock. Trailer the extended heels. This may be done before each shoe branch is turned. Sometimes the heels are left wide and trailered until parallel with the line of motion.
5. Roll the toe from one toe nail to the other. Pull a short wide clip from the roll. Or, side clips may be added. However, side clips are not usually needed since the slick surface places little strain on the nails.
6. Fit the clip or roll to the foot and mark the end of the heels with a chalk line perpendicular to the trailer on the ground surface.
7. Make a center punch mark on the outside edge of the chalk mark. Turn the shoe over and make a mark on the foot surface in the middle of the shoe web about ½ inch toward the end of the heel from the previous mark.
8. Heat each heel and cut it in the center of the half-round hardy by striking on the mark.
9. Hold the shoe with the heels perpendicular to the off edge of the anvil. Line up the outside center punch mark. Strike the outside edge (mark) of the heel and bend the end of the shoe to an angle less than the angle of the hoof heel bevel. Sometimes one heel is turned up and the other is left flat. Or, wide heels may not be spooned at all.

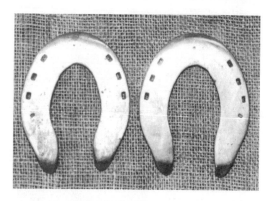

Fig. 38-8. Sliding plates.

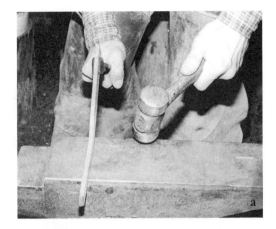

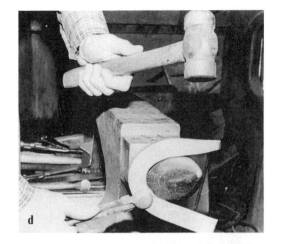

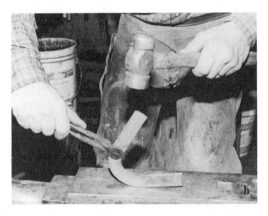

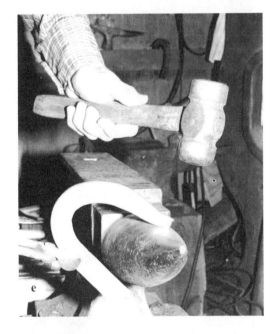

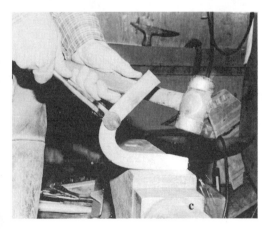

Fig. 38-10. Steps in making a sliding plate:
(a) Start the toe bend in the conventional manner.
(b) Point the toe of the shoe to correspond to the radius of
the toe of the hoof.
(c) Taper the inside of the heel.
(d) Turn the branch.
(e) Lift up on the tongs and trailer the heel.
(f) Stamp and pritchel out the nail holes in the branch.

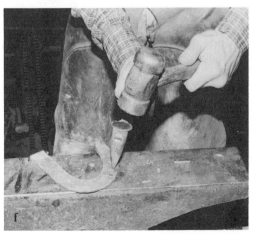

10. Turn the shoe around and hold it down from the off side of the anvil and taper the heel. Hot rasp it smooth. The spooned heel should fit about flush with the buttress at its base but about ¼ inch away from the hoof at its end. Hot rasp the inside edges of the heels to prevent drag.

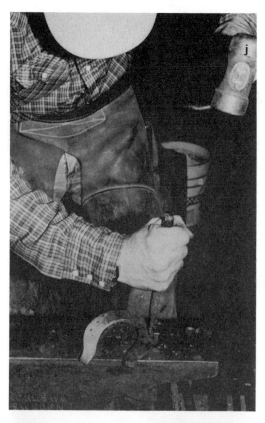

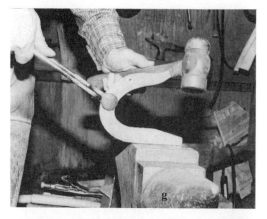

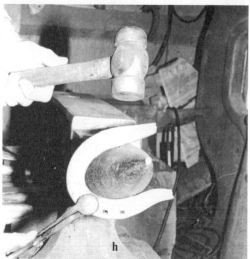

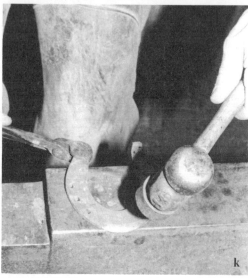

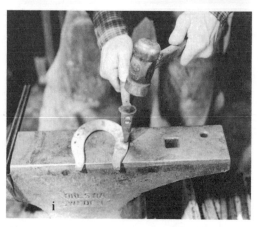

(g) Taper the inside branch.
(h) Turn and trailer the inside branch.
(i) Stamp the inside branch.
(j) Pritchel the inside branch.
(k) Roll the toe.

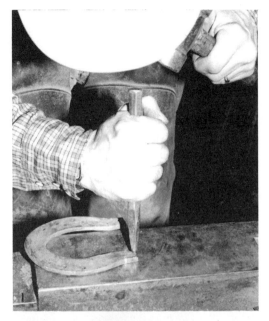

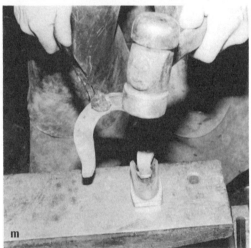

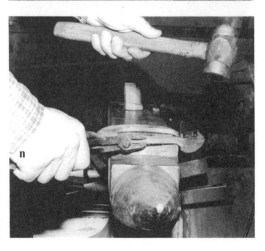

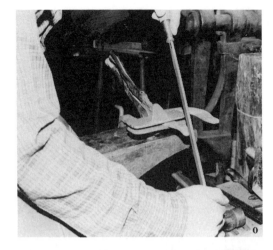

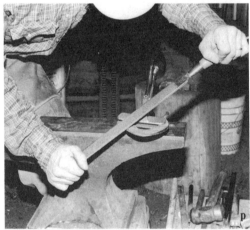

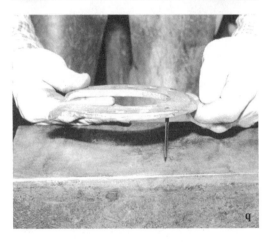

(l) After checking the fit—locate and center punch the end of the foot (buttress) and the end of the shoe on each heel.
(m) Cut off each heel in the center of the hardy.
(n) Bend or spoon each heel by striking on its outside edge.
(o) Smooth the heels with the hot rasp.
(p) File the sharp ground surface edges smooth.
(q) The finished shoe showing the fit of the nail head.

Stock Horses

Stock horses are a combination between cutting and reining horses. The horse is shown in a specified reining pattern (called dry work). Then a cow is released into the arena and the horse must turn the cow at least twice each way against the fence. The cow must then be circled each way in the center of the arena. There are no turnback men as in the cutting. The dry work and cow work portion are each scored from 60 to 80 points and totaled. The stock horse must be shifty and smooth, work at reasonable speed, but be under control. Stock horses are shod like reining horses. They are the most highly trained of the western performance horses.

Polo

Polo horses are ridden hard during six 7 minute chukkers. They turn, stop and run with quick bursts of speed. Horses must be very fit and handy. Polo horses are ridden with English tack but are neck reined and maneuvered like Western reining horses. Polo matches may be played on turf or in the soft ground of an indoor riding arena. The rules vary according to the arena.

Polo horses are shod according to the type of arena they are used in. Polo plates are recommended in turf or grass arenas. Rim shoes or self-cleaning extra light shoes or swedged training plates are recommended in dirt arenas. The rim shoe is a good all around shoe. The hind shoes are often calked. The inside heel may be formed into a diamond calk or wedge heel. This permits the outside calk to hold as the horse pivots over his hocks, while the inside can slide along the ground as it maintains lateral stability.

Dressage

Dressage horses are the ballet dancers of the horse world. They demonstrate their skill and fitness by performing tests at various levels. There are currently 13 dressage tests at eight levels. They vary in complexity and are timed. They each require from four to nine minutes to complete.

The object of dressage tests is to encourage the harmonious development of the physique and ability of the horse. The extensive training required makes the horse calm, supple, loose and flexible. The goal is a confident, attentive and keen horse that achieves perfect understanding with its rider. The horse must be light and submissive, showing no resistance to the rider.

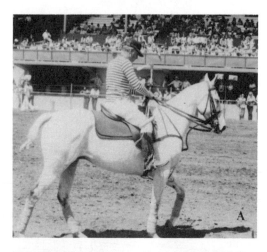

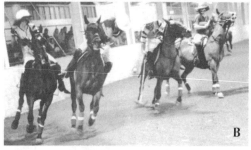

Fig. 38-11. (A) Outdoor polo pony, (B) Indoor polo ponies.

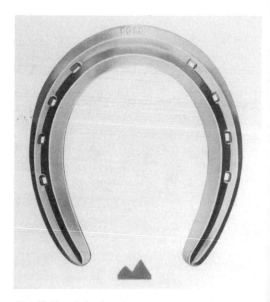

Fig. 38-12. Polo plate.

The horse should give the impression that it is voluntarily doing what is required of it.

Dressage horses are shod like English pleasure horses. Flat light shoes are preferred. However, dressage horses that are also used for eventing (combined training) are shod with rim or concave fullered iron. This gives the horse a strong base of support, but also provides traction over cross country courses. Shoes are often drilled or punched for studs (screw-in or drive-in calks). The type of stud can be varied according to the ground encountered and the type of performance desired. Horses wearing studs are said to be more confident in their performances.

Dressage horses must be balanced and free movers. Coordination and gait may occasionally be improved by changing hoof angles, shoe weight or design. However, the effect of aids is usually not as great as a change in rein or leg pressure by an experienced dressage rider. Upper level (Grand Prix) dressage riders must be the most skilled of all equestrians.

Hunters and Jumpers

Hunting and jumping classes are the most popular classes at many of the nation's largest horse shows. They are even more favored in the British Isles and on the Continent of Europe.

Hunters must move smoothly at an even pace over relatively low fences. They must be sound. They are judged on their conformation, form when jumping and manners. Hunters must be easy to control as well as pretty to look at. Hunters are heavier than jumpers. Tack appointments and riding attire count considerably when judging hunters. Hunters are shown in Breeding, Conformation and Working classes. They are further divided by experience into Green and Regular classes. A green horse is one of any age that has not been shown for more than one or two years.

Jumpers must have the ability and courage to jump high obstacles. Form and style are not as important as speed and ability. Soundness is not critical unless it is considered cruelty to ride the horse. Jumpers may be of any age or breed. They are usually more difficult to control than hunters. They are classified by the amount of money they have won and the type of jumps. Jumps may be wide (spread) or high and be made

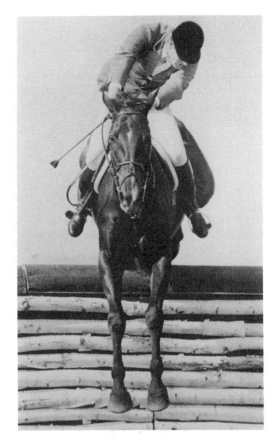

Fig. 38-13. Jumper ridden by Rodney Jenkins. Photo from the Devon Horse Show.

solid, of poles or of brush. Penalties are awarded for the various faults a horse may make in a round. Horses may be off course, run out, refuse to jump, touch or knockdown a jump. Many rounds of jumping are timed. Faults are converted to seconds in some classes. Knock down and out is one type of class. The puissance (high jump) class is a favorite. Several jumps start at 4 feet 6 inches and become progressively higher in eliminations. They may reach nearly 7 feet in height. Horses have jumped fences over 8 feet in height. Grand Prix jumping is considered the most difficult class and is patterned after the Olympic games competition. There are only about 15 Grand Prix jumping courses in the U.S.

Hunters and jumpers put a great deal of stress on their feet and legs. Their shoes must be substantial enough to support the foot during the stress of jumping and conditioning (road work), yet light enough to prevent fatigue. Clips are a necessity on these horses.

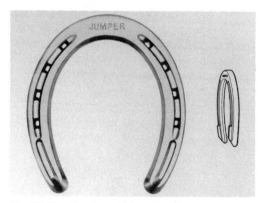

Fig. 38-14. Keg shoe with jumping calks.

In America, jumping calks have been traditionally used to provide traction on the front feet of jumping and hunting horses. These calks are set under the foot at an angle of 30 to 45 degrees, and are made so that the shoe does not extend past the buttresses. This degree of slope prevents a horse from touching the shoe, if he happens to overreach in the process of landing after taking a fence.

Steps in making a jumping calk:
1. Prepare the shoe as though you were going to make a regular heel calk, i.e., fit the shoe the same, square the heel if needed, and trailer about an inch of metal.
2. Turn the white hot heel over the edge of the anvil as in making a heel calk.
3. Turn the shoe over and with the turned heel up, strike down on the end of the heel. As you strike, the heel will tilt forward. Do not make any attempt to prevent this and don't place the heel back over the edge of the anvil to straighten it.
4. Place the inside edge of the calk on the heel of the anvil and taper the heel to follow the natural outline of the wall of the foot.
5. Hot rasp the calk smooth. Further slope the back of the calk as you rasp.

In some areas copper-brazed and welded-on jar (jumping) calks are preferred to turned jumping calks.

Welded jar calks can be drawn from the heel of the shoe, folded back on to its ground surface and welded. Or, they can be added by jump welding. Very thin jar calks should be brazed on. Brazing is covered in Chapter 32.

In Great Britain, the wedge heel has been traditionally used on the inside heel of hind shoes. The outside heel is a wide, thick and low calkin (calk). The shoe is referred to as a calk and a wedge. The toe of the shoe is usually knocked

back creating a safe toe to prevent overreaching. The toe of the shoe is fit under the toe of the hoof. The wedge heel or diamond calk may be occasionally used on the inside heel of the hind shoes of polo horses.

The wedge heel can be used any time height and lateral traction are desired but some degree of slippage is advantageous. The wedge combined with a calk on the outside heel tends to make the shoe stationary from side to side in soft ground or on turf but allows forward and backward movement. On jumping horses, the inside heel sinks in on soft ground but creates a level bearing surface when working on hard surfaces. On polo horses a standard calk on the outside heel of the leg in the direction the horse is turning tends to anchor that foot, and a diamond calk on the inside tends to slide as the foot rotates about the calk.

Steps in making a wedge heel:
1. Upset the white hot end of the bar stock by striking it against the anvil face. Allow the end to bend toward the ground surface.
2. Hold the stock against the anvil face and slightly toward you. Strike the end of the heel toward you to further upset it.
3. Turn the heel on its side (left for left heel, right for right heel) and bevel it against the anvil face.
4. Place ½ to ¾ inches of the wedge over a round edge of the anvil and hold at about a 30 degree angle. Strike the foot surface with half-face hammer blows. Turn it over on the anvil face and strike the tip of the calk to flatten the foot surface against the anvil.
5. True (bevel again) the inside edge making it safe from interference.
6. Heat up and hot rasp the calk smooth.

Steps in turning an outside heel calk (calkin):
1. Upset the end to be calked if the steel is under ⅜ inch in thickness.
2. Hold the end perpendicular to the off edge of the anvil with about 1¼ inches projecting. The ground surface of the shoe should be *up*.
3. Crease the stock by striking it twice with half-face hammer blows over the edge of the anvil.
4. Turn the stock over and bend the calk over the horn or rounded edge of the anvil (prevent marking the inside of the stock on the sharp edge).
5. Upset the end forming it perpendicular to the shoe at the desired height. Straighten the calk as necessary while upsetting it.
6. Hammer finish the calk by striking on the outside edges. Angle it slightly away from the frog.
7. Rasp the calk smooth.

Steps in making a diamond calk from a swelled heel:

1. Turn about ¾ inch of a white hot heel over the edge of the anvil. The ground surface should be up. Taper the end as it is hammered back against the foot surface of the branch.
2. Bring the heel to a welding heat and weld the swelled heel by striking the scarfed edge into the branch.
3. Level the foot surface by quickly striking the shoe on the ground surface adjacent to the point of the welded heel.
4. Place the inside edge of the welded heel, while it is still white hot, flat against the horn of the anvil.
5. Bevel the heel and draw it to a point by holding the hammer on an angle and striking the outside edge of the heel.
6. Hold the calk against the step of the anvil face at the base of the horn (or on the heel), with the ground surface of the shoe toward the point of the horn, and shape the end of the calk as much as possible by striking it on an angle.

Hot rasp the calk to its final diamond shape.

Screw calks or studs are used extensively on hunters and jumpers. The type and height of the studs are changed to permit maximum traction and confidence on the performance surface. (See Combined Training.)

Pads may be used to absorb concussion as well as protect the foot. Silicone rubber may be injected with a calking gun between the pad and foot after the shoe has been nailed on. Or, it may be placed on the pad or in the hoof space before the shoe is nailed in place. Silicone will set up faster when mixed with a small dab of body putty hardener. The horse should be standing on the foot when the material hardens. There is a possibility that unnatural weight bearing on the sole instead of the wall could contribute to pedal osteitis or coffin bone fracture. However, when used properly, hoof cushion elastomer combined with a pad may reduce concussion by 20 percent. New Sorbothane[1] hoof pads are said to absorb even more concussion.

Combined Training or Eventing

Combined training includes tests or trials to demonstrate the level of training and fitness of horse and rider. They were once military competitions for cavalry mounts. Courses are designed for three levels of rider skill: Preliminary, Intermediate and Advanced. A 3-day event includes three tests, each held on a different day.

The first day is a dressage test. The nature and level of the test is determined by the degree of difficulty of the whole competition. Tests are conducted in a standard arena 60 meters long and 20 meters wide. Dressage tests must be ridden from memory. Errors of the course are penalized. The jury (Judges) awards marks to the contestant for each movement and for each of the general impressions.

The second day is an endurance test of four parts. The first and third phases are called Roads and Tracks. These are considered warm-up and rest phases. The rider must pace the horse, usually at a trot or slow canter to complete the distance required near the optimum time posted. The contestant is penalized when he goes over the optimum time and eliminated if he exceeds the time limit. The second phase is a Steeplechase. A steeplechase is a race run at the gallop with obstacles including water jumps. The name steeplechase originated with 18th century fox hunters who ran impromptu cross country races to the nearest church steeple. In addition to an optimum time and time limit, penalties are incurred for mistakes at obstacles. Roads and Tracks are then trotted and slow cantered over for the third phase. A ten minute halt is required before the fourth phase. The fourth phase is a longer cross-country race against the clock with difficult obstacles. When this portion is conducted alone it is called a Horse Trial.

The third day is a jumping competition, often called stadium jumping. It is not an ordinary show jumping competition or test of endurance. Its object is to show that the horses have retained suppleness, energy and obedience after a severe endurance test.

The shoes on combined training horses are almost always fitted with studs. Borium may be applied. Borium may be applied directly to steel shoes and to small bolts, rivets or worn studs to be riveted or screwed into thick, wide-webbed aluminum shoes. Shoes should be of a self-cleaning or concave design.

Studs are drive-in or screw-in calks with hardened centers. They stay sharp as they wear. The screw type may be added or removed from the shoe. This is very convenient for hauling when a flat shoe is desired and for studding up to allow for the ground surface differences.

[1] *Sterivet Labs., Inc., Strongsville, OH*

There are at least three patterns of screw calks or studs. Road studs are low and most suitable for hard ground and roads. They are a good substitute for borium spots and if only this type is needed, the drive-in type will suffice. Bullets[2] are used when the ground is fairly firm but soft on top. Blocks[3] are used when the ground is soft and muddy. The largest screw-in calk is called an Olympic stud[2].

Most studs come in at least two thread diameters, some come in four—from 5/16 to 1/2 inch. The thread diameter must be related to the width of the shoe and the weight of the horse. The larger the shoe and the horse, the heavier the calk. Often, a larger diameter stud will be put on the outside of the shoe. Many hind shoes only have one low stud on the outside heel.

Steps in applying drive-in calks (studs):
1. Fit the shoe to the foot. Shoes with a wide web are preferred (3/4 in. or more) due to the size of the hole necessary for the calk.
2. Heat one heel of the shoe. Stamp the *ground surface* of the heel with a round flat-tipped punch down to the anvil. The diameter of the end of the punch should be smaller than the drive calk stem. Practice on an old shoe before hot punching on the job. Drive calk holes can also be drilled.
3. Turn the shoe over and punch the burr of metal out from the hoof surface. The center of the hole will not be difficult to locate if this is done immediately. Eventually, you will be able to do both heels in one heat.
4. Hot rasp the bulging metal (frog eye) away from the outside edge of the shoe. Less bulge is formed if the punch is placed toward the inner edge of the shoe.
5. After the shoe has cooled, drive in the appropriate Morris taper punch from the ground surface. The punch must be the correct size for the calk used and it must be well oiled with cutting oil.
6. Wipe the oil from the shoe and hole.
7. Drive-in calks are best installed after the shoe is nailed on. A tool with a recessed end to fit over the calk is needed to protect the tungsten pin. Place the calk in the hole and drive it to within 1/8 to 1/16 inch of the ground surface of the shoe. Do not drive it down against the shoe as it will not hold tight.
8. To remove drive-in calks, use a forked chisel and strike from the side. Hold your thumb on the extracted calk to prevent it from flying. You sometimes see calk extractors at auction

sales. You can make a tool that incorporates both features from high carbon steel (Daniels, 1983).

Steps in applying screw-in calks (studs):
1. Fit the shoe to the foot. The web of the shoe must be wide enough to support the size of calk to be used.
2. Heat one (or both) heels of the shoe. Stamp the *foot surface* of the heel with a round flat-tipped punch down to the anvil. The diameter of the punch should be slightly smaller than the size of the screw-in calk. Holes can also be drilled.
3. Turn the shoe over and punch the burr of metal out from the ground surface. This procedure will fill the crease of fullered shoes with metal. This makes tap starting easier and makes more threads to hold the calk.

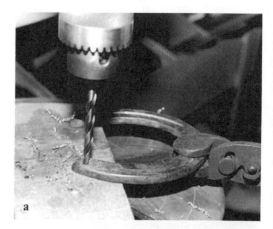

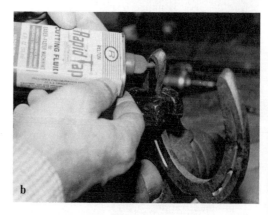

Fig. 38-15. Steps in applying a screw-in calk:
(a) Drill a hole with a drill bit 1/32 to 1/64 inch under the calk thread size.
(b) Lubricate the hole with Rapid Tap or cutting fluid.
(c) Thread the hole using the proper tap and a carpenter's brace.
(d) Tighten the stud with a crescent wrench.
(e) The completed job.

[2] *Mordax studs, Centaur Forge, Ltd., Burlington, WI*
[3] *Stromsholm studs, Centaur Forge, Ltd., Burlington, WI*

4. Hot rasp the bulging metal (frog eye) from the outside edge of the shoe.
5. Let the shoe cool slowly after both heels have been punched. This anneals the shoe and makes tapping easier.
6. Tap (thread) the holes with a well oiled tap. Tapping can be done most accurately and rapidly by placing the tap in a carpenter's brace. A slow RPM (revolutions per minute) reversible electric drill may also be used. Compact hand-held taps and wrenches are available from the screw calk companies.

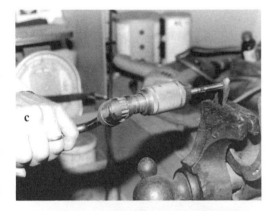

c

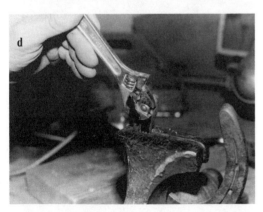

d

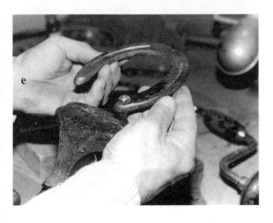

e

However, these are only useful for cleaning out the threads or changing calks. Self-threading (tapping) calks are also available[4].

7. Screw-in calks are easiest to install after the shoe is nailed on. A small crescent wrench or a rachet drive wrench can be used to install or change the calks.

Studs are not always needed. They should not be used when the footing is firm or when the horse is hauled. There is always danger of damaging the coronary band (called calking) when studs are worn. Studs are removed with a wrench and the holes are filled with special plugs, oiled cotton, cork or foam pieces. Special plugs with recessed allen screw heads are necessary to protect the threads in aluminum shoes. Steel shoe threads can be protected adequately with one of the three materials mentioned. A tap should be available to ream holes when the threads become damaged.

Aluminum racing plates have been manufactured for many years. Recently, manufactured aluminum shoes made of wider and thicker stock have become very popular for performance horses, especially for hunters, jumpers and three-day event horses. These shoes are substantial enough that they must be heated to clip or make major changes in them. They can be drilled and tapped for studs. Aluminum shoes are desirable when a light shoe is needed to prevent fatigue and encourage front leg folding when jumping, but support and protection or cover of the foot is also essential. Aluminum is an ideal material since when combined with alloys it is reasonably strong but weighs only one-third as much as steel per cubic measurement. However, aluminum shoes are not considered as good for the foot as those of steel. Also, they wear out quickly and do not hold a screw-in calk as well as steel.

Occasionally, a handmade aluminum shoe will be needed. They can be turned cold in a mechanical bender or heated and turned in the conventional manner. Bars can be welded in with an oxy-acetylene welder. A handmade wedge-heeled shoe can be made from ½ x 1 inch aluminum stock. This shoe is used to elevate a low heeled horse without adding pads, weight or traction. The ends of the stock are upset and the toe is drawn and flattened. The nail holes may be drilled or stamped.

[4] *Centaur Forge, Ltd., Burlington, WI*

Aluminum is considered difficult to forge. It does not change color when heated. However, a few tricks of the trade make forging aluminum a simple exercise. Some farriers dip the shoes in crankcase oil and heat the shoes in a low coal fire or gas forge until the oil burns off. When oil is sizzling or bubbling, the shoes are ready to forge. Others warm the aluminum in the fire and every few seconds take it out and strike it with the hammer. The metal is ready when it gives under the hammer. Another method is to

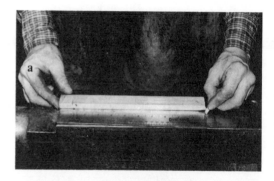

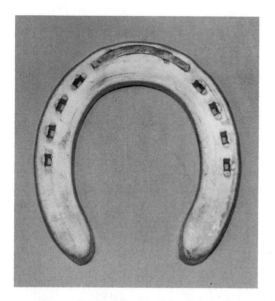

Fig. 38-16.   Flat aluminum shoe with steel wear insert.

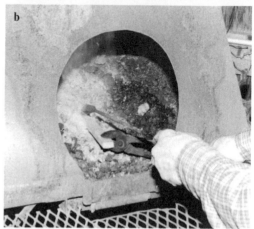

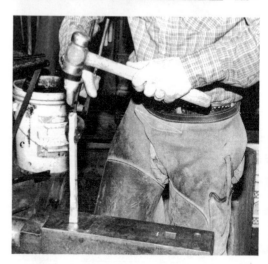

Fig. 38-18.   Steps in making a wedge-heeled (two-degree) aluminum shoe:
(a) Measure the stock and mark its length on the anvil.
(b) Heat until the fire poker drags or sticks on the aluminum.
(c) Upset the end against the anvil face.

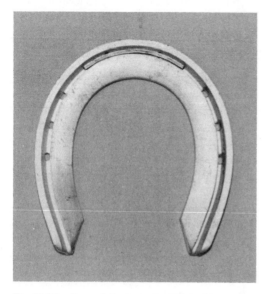

Fig. 38-17.   Creased aluminum shoe with steel wear insert.

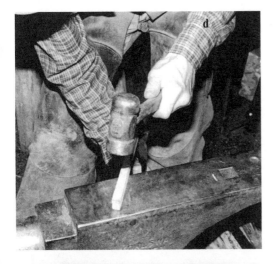

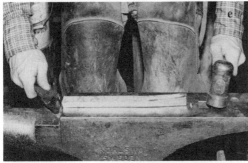

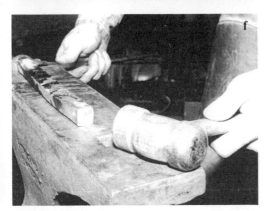

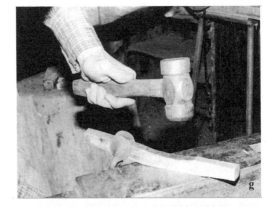

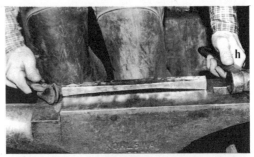

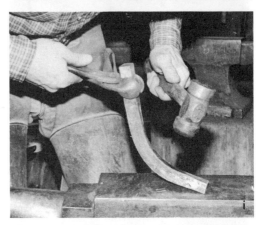

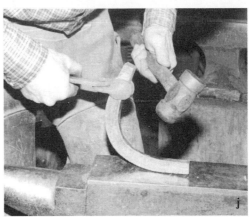

(d) Square and true it as needed.

(e) Check against the anvil mark—the stock should be ½ inch shorter.

(f) Upset the other heel until it is square and the stock is 1 inch shorter overall.

(g) Heat and flatten the center portion of the stock—then draw it to its original width.

(h) The stock should now be the original length.

(i) Turn the one branch from the inside edge on the anvil face.

(j) Turn the other branch.

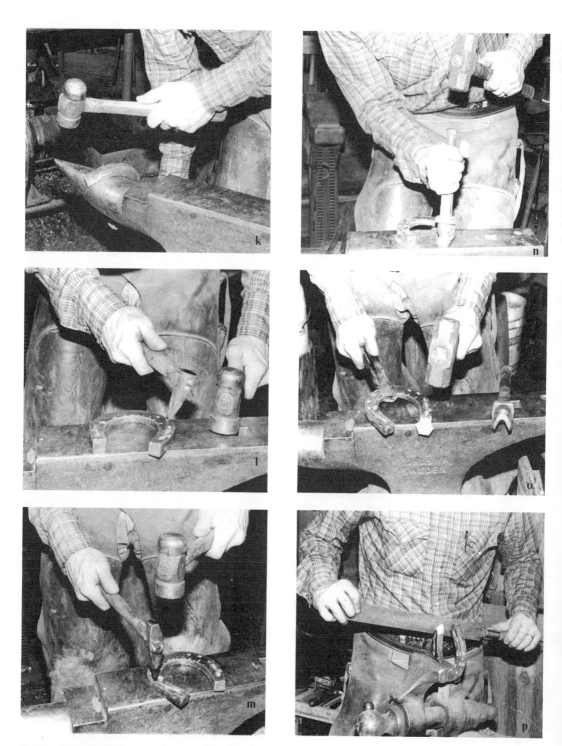

(k) Turn the heel over the horn.
(l) Stamp the nail holes.
(m) Drive in a stem punch—especially in the heel nail hole
so that the fore-punching goes the full depth of the stock.
(n) Cut the heels from above with a hand-held hardy.
(o) Knock the cut heels off over the edge of the anvil.
(p) Rasp and finish the heels.

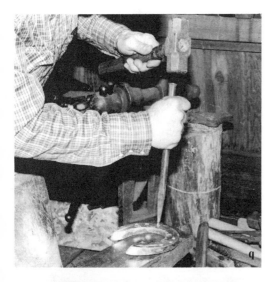

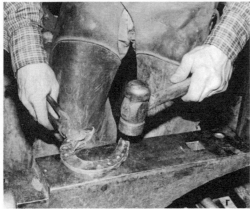

rub the hammer handle across the metal. If it is sticky or the wood sparks, the aluminum is ready to forge. It is soon easy to tell the correct forging temperature.

Aluminum holds heat longer than steel. It can be punched cold. However, many horseshoers drill their holes first and then shape them with punches. Aluminum welding is covered in Chapter 40.

Some shoers heat aluminum shoes by laying them on a steel plate over the forge fire. This is not necessary. Aluminum can be placed directly in the fire. However, it must be monitored closely. If a shoe does get too hot, shake it in the air before striking it. This will chill it. Aluminum will crumble if struck after being overheated. Do not cool aluminum in water. Let it air cool. Clips should be made over a rounded edge of the anvil with a ball pein hammer to prevent weakening of the shoe.

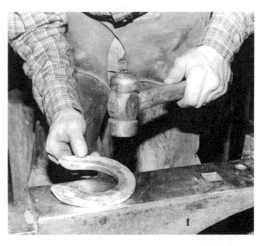

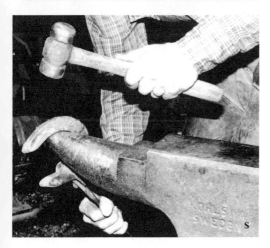

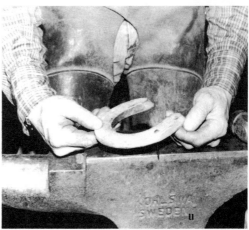

(q) Pritchel out the holes when the shoe is cold.
(r) Level the raised areas around the nail holes.
(s) True the edges and repritchel the holes.
(t) Concave the inside bearing surface of the shoe.
(u) The finished shoe showing the fit of the nail head.

Steel toe inserts (wear plates) to prevent wear and/or toe grabs or heel jar calks to create traction and absorb concussion are available from shoe suppliers. These may be attached to aluminum shoes. The insert or grab is shaped to the curvature of the shoe over the hardy hole. The calk or insert is held on the shoe in the position desired with pliers or tongs and struck with a hammer. This marks the position of the holes to be drilled. The holes are drilled and the insert is driven down and riveted in place. Drive the insert down on first one side and then the other. It will rivet against the anvil face. You can make your own grabs and fasten them in the shoe using a grab set. This procedure has been described by Daniels (1978).

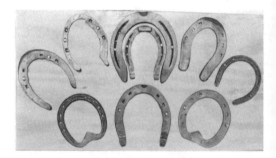

Fig. 38-20. Specialty horseshoes handmade by Northwest Missouri State University farrier craftsmanship student Jim Littrel.

References

Carter, W.H. 1923. The Story of the Horse. The National Geographic. 44(5):455.

Close, P. 1980. Tips for shoeing when you ride 'em and slide 'em. The Western Horseman (Apr):22.

Daniels, B. 1978. Shop talk (Aluminum shoes). Amer. Farriers' J. 4(4): 101.

Daniels, B.B. 1983. Replaceable calks. Amer. Farriers' J. 9(3):213.

Davis, R. Shoes for barrel racing horses. The Western Horseman. :62.

DeHaan, C. 1967. The big stop and how to apply it. Western Riders' Yearbook. Horseman. Cordovan, Houston.

Ingram, P. 1982. Pointers on hoof pads. The Chronicle of the Horse. (May 21):72.

Juell, A. 1982. Shoeing the combined training horse. The Chronicle of the Horse. (May 21):12.

Leitschuh, J. and J. Potter. 1982. Studding up. Horse Play. (June):32.

Marks, D., M.P. Mackay-Smith, L.S. Cushing and J.A. Leslie. 1971. Use of elastomer to reduce concussion to horse's feet. J.A.V.M.A. 158(8):1361.

Pieh, B. 1983. Calks, studs and borium information sheet. Centaur Forge, Ltd., Burlington, WI.

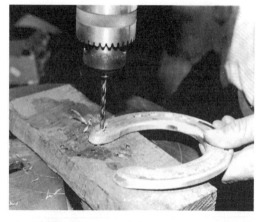

Fig. 38-19. Borium coated rivets or screw-in calks may be applied to aluminum shoes.

NOTES:

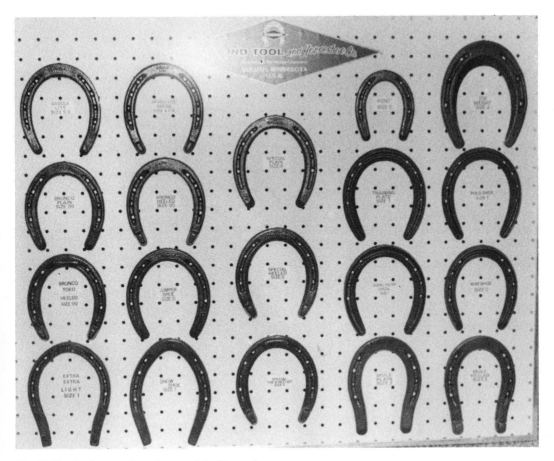

Fig. 38-21. Performance horseshoes made by Diamond.

Chapter 39

Running Race Horses

Racing is America's most popular spectator sport. It has been number one since 1952. For several years it was more popular than football and baseball combined. Over 80 million people attend horse races each year. About 50 million attend running horse races and about 30 million attend harness horse races. New York is the number one racing state. It has the most racing days, the highest attendance and the greatest revenue from racing. California is second. Both states have breeder's incentive awards.

Types of Running Horses

Runners are generally of two breeds—Quarter Horse or Thoroughbred. Thoroughbred racing has been popular for centuries and has been called the Sport of Kings. The Thoroughbred has been recognized as a breed since 1750. All U.S. Thoroughbreds are registered in The Jockey Club, established since 1894. The English Jockey Club is responsible for changing the official birth date of Thoroughbreds from May 1 to January 1 in 1833. Other horse breeds have adopted the January 1 birthday. This has been one cause of racing immature animals. Another has been the relatively large purses offered for younger horses. (The universal birthday rule is also responsible for many equine reproductive problems.)

Most Thoroughbred races are from a mile to a mile and one-half or more in length (8 or more furlongs). A furlong is one-eighth mile or 220 yards. Thoroughbred racing's prestigious Triple Crown is bestowed upon the consecutive winner of the following races for three-year olds: The Kentucky Derby (1¼ mi.), The Preakness (1³⁄₁₆ mi.), and The Belmont Stakes (1½ mi.).

Quarter Horses were selected and developed from imported Thoroughbreds and native stock in colonial America. They were selected for their ability to run a short race of under one-quarter mile. The Quarter Horse breed registry was formed in 1940. Purses for Quarter Horse races have multiplied over 20 times in the past 20 years. Today, the world's richest horse race is

the All-American Futurity run at Ruidoso, New Mexico.

Types of Races

A **flat track** race is a race with no obstacles. The track surface may be dirt consisting of a base covered by a cushion of several inches of loose soil. These tracks must be regularly maintained and deteriorate rapidly in inclement weather. Flat track races may be run with one or two turns in them depending upon the size of the track and the length of the race. Turns are always dangerous to negotiate and slow down a race. Many Quarter Horse races are run with no turns and rails on both sides.

A **steeplechase** race is a race over obstacles or jumps. The track surface is usually turf. Turf consists of a rolled and mowed grass surface. At several major tracks the steeplechase or turf course is inside of the dirt track course. Many Thoroughbred races in Europe are run on turf tracks. A well maintained turf surface is known to be less damaging to a horse's legs than dirt. However, the turf surface is more difficult to maintain and repair if heavily used and damaged.

A **sprint** is a short race of several hundred yards. Quarter Horses excel at these. Sprints are run from 220 yards to 440 yards. Recently, Quarter Horse races have been added between 440 and 880 yards or one-half mile. Sprints are not as popular as longer races for spectators in most areas because they are over so fast. A good time for a 2 furlong race is 22 seconds.

A **chariot** race is a one-quarter mile (2 furlong) race between two teams of Quarter Horses. It is most popular in the northern Rocky Mountain states. The ability to stride in harmony is as important as speed. A team is said to be able to go no faster than seven-eighths the speed of its slowest horse. Driver and chariot must weigh less than 275 pounds. Many young race horses learn to run and can be conditioned at an earlier age pulling a light chariot. There are said to be fewer risks in chariot racing than flat track racing. Chariot races started as cutter racing in the early 1940's with ski runners attached to the chariot. The sport has grown with the Quarter Horse breed. It is still traditionally called cutter racing in some areas. Today, chariots are made of welded pipe tubing, cut down oil drums, and bicycle tires.

Modern breeding trends have concentrated even more Thoroughbred blood (percentage of ancestry) into the Quarter Horse breed. Two common conformation defects that have been a problem are feet too small for the body size and weak, underslung heels. In their effort to increase speed, breeders have ignored the consequences of conformation faults in the legs and feet.

Fatigue is the greatest enemy of the race horse. Tired legs don't load evenly and are more subject to tendon, ligament and bone failure. Lack of conditioning is the most common cause of fatigue. Fatigued horses may change leads as often as 35 times in a long distance race. They are more subject to limb interference as well as breakdowns.

Trimming Foals

Race horse foals should be trimmed soon after they are halter broken. Ideally, the first trimming should be completed by the time the foal is 1 month of age. Some farms wait until the foal is 2 months old. Others synchronize the first trimming with the halter breaking lesson. Racing prospects should be trimmed once a month after the first trim until they are shod for training.

Some large farms have a special stall with padded sides for trimming and halterbreaking foals. A padded bonnet under the poll strap of the halter is also a good idea. Manners developed during these first few contacts with the foal will probably stay with it throughout its life. Be calm and work rapidly. Review Chapter 9.

Most foals will be a little splay-footed immediately after birth. This is their way of achieving stability. If the condition persists and becomes a habit, foals will wear down the inside of the foot more than the outside. Trimming must be done to remove the excess horn at the toe and on the outside. The outside edge of the wall should be rounded and shaped. The frog and sole should not be trimmed. The object of regular trimming is to allow the leg and foot to grow

straight by maintaining a uniform distribution of weight over the foot. It's much easier to keep a leg straight than to try and correct or change the conformation of a crooked hoof or leg. Furthermore, regular handling of the legs and feet will establish the habit of standing for trimming and eventually shoeing. Running horses are very high strung (nervous). They must be taught to stand still. It is easier to teach them when they are small.

First Shoes

Foals and weanlings should not be shod unless they have a special problem that needs correction. Shoes limit the natural expansion and spreading of the feet.

Customarily, light steel training plates are applied to the front feet of horses sold as yearlings. These shoes should be removed immediately after the sale unless the horse is going into training.

Horses are shod with flat training plates when they begin training. These are light swedged steel shoes. They are usually sized from 3 to 9 and come in several weights.

Some trainers insist on felt or foam plastic rim pads between the shoe and hoof. Manufactured shoe styles are available with rim pads bonded to the shoe. These are said to cushion the shock to the foot and legs from the track that may cause young horses to fear running.

Young horses may resist the pounding of nails into the hoof the first time. The lead chain may have to be placed in the mouth or under the upper lip against the gum to divert their attention. It is best to try to get by the horse as fast as possible with patient firmness. High-strung horses in training get on the fight easily. Also, many trainers resent any discipline by the shoer of a horse in their care. Know your trainer before you attempt to discipline a yearling. Ideally, the teaching of proper manners for shoeing should be done at the farm before the horse goes into training.

Racing Plates

There are several manufacturers of racing plates. Quality, convenience, and cost should determine your source. Training plates and racing plates are made up in three basic styles (with variations) in each.

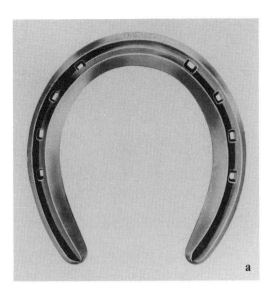

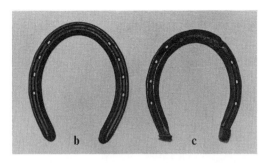

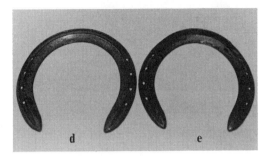

Fig. 39-1. Training (steel) plates: (a) Diamond keg, (b) flat, (c) light with block and sticker, (d) heavy flat, and (e) heavy with toe grab.

Training plates are made of swedged steel. They are sized from 3 to 9. The plates that are swedged rather than dropped forged seem to last longer and have more resistance to springing at the heel(s). Those made of a higher carbon steel last the longest. Flat plates are used on young horses to avoid strains on the legs. Flat plates are used on turf courses to prevent destruction of the racing surface. Regular toe grabs (5/16 in.) are copper-brazed into the toes of steel training plates to add traction on deep tracks. High toe grabs (7/16 in.), often called Louisiana toe grabs, are added along with block(s) or an inside block and outside sticker for deeper tracks and ice racing with chariots. Training plates come in several widths of light patterns and a heavy pattern. Heavy swedged pattern shoes are sometimes called roping or performance horse shoes.

Racing plates are made of drop forged aluminum with high carbon steel grabs molded into the toes. Aluminum race plates are available in many styles and are sized from 3 to 7. Aluminum weighs one-third the weight of steel. However, it is widely believed that aluminum does not absorb as much shock as steel.

The regular toe grab style racing plate is used mostly on Thoroughbreds. A low toe and level grip style are available. These create less strain on the horse's leg and are desirable on hard tracks. Standard hind shoes include the plain heel, outside sticker, block and sticker, and double block. Jar calks can be added to front or hind shoes by riveting them on the heel or branch of the shoe when tracks are muddy. Shoes with the calks already molded into the shoe are available. The Queen's plate style has no grabs. They were designed for use on turf tracks and make a good therapeutic shoe for a horse with sore legs. They have the disadvantage of wearing out quickly. They are definitely the best racing plate for the horse's legs.

The Quarter Horse racing plate (Louisiana toe style) has very high toe grabs. These shoes are hard on a horse's legs in all but the softest tracks. Hind shoes are available in plain, sticker, and blocked style heels. Some platers use the high toe grabs on the hind feet of larger Thoroughbreds. The power drive for speed comes from the hind limbs.

Shoeing Running Horses

Shoes are shaped on a portable anvil called a stall jack. This tool is driven into the ground near the horse so the shoe can be shaped while the plater is holding the foot between his legs.

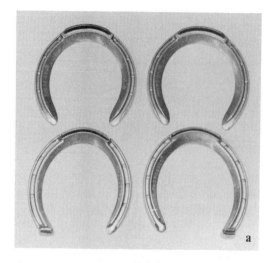

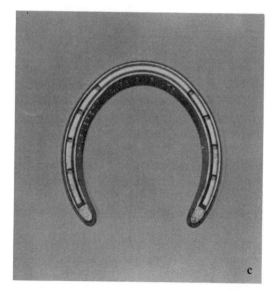

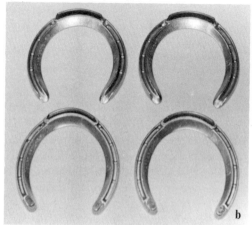

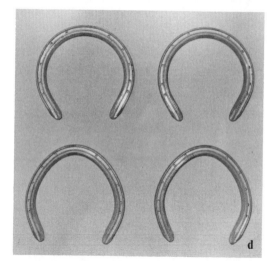

Fig. 39-2. Racing (aluminum) plates: (a) regular toe and sticker (Thoroughbred), (b) Louisiana toe and block (Quarter Horse), (c) flat Queen's plate, and (d) imported double grip turf plate.

Some platers attach the stall jack to their shoeing box. The heels of racing plates should not be fit level. They should be bent slightly toward the heel creating a gap between hoof and shoe at the last nail hole. When the shoe is clinched down it will then remain flat and tight. If thin racing plates are fit flat, the heels will spring when the shoe is clinched.

Racing plates are nailed on with No. 3 or 3½ city head nails. Training plates are nailed on with No. 3½ or 4 city head nails. Heavier training plates with a deeper swedge may be nailed on with No. 4½ regular or even No. 5 city head

nails. A light driving hammer of 6 to 10 ounces is preferred. Nails may be wrung or clipped off. Goose neck clinchers are needed to turn over the low, small nails. The clinches are usually rasped flush with the wall on race horses. This is done to allow a shoe to come off all at once in a race if it is stepped on or somehow pulled loose.

Race horses are shod frequently. Aluminum shoes wear out quickly. There are few resets. Horses that are racing are reshod every 3 to 4 weeks. Horses in training may go 4 to 6 weeks between shoeings. The hoof should be brought into alignment with the pastern at each shoeing.

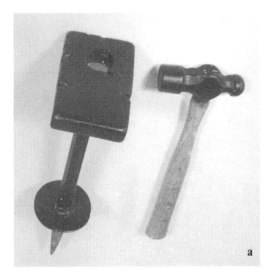

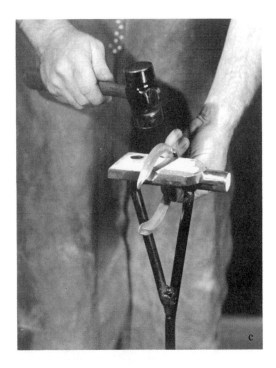

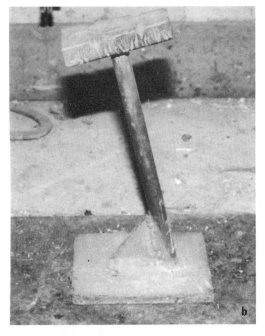

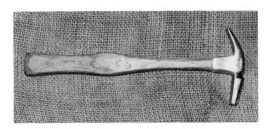

Fig. 39-4.   *Handmade 6 oz. driving hammer for race horse nails made by Paul Brewer. Photo by J. Graves.*

Fig. 39-3.   Stall jacks: (a) for use in a shed row, (b) for use on concrete floor, and (c) for shaping racing plates at the foot. Photos by Poellot and McLain.

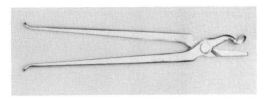

Fig. 39-5.   *Gooseneck clinchers used for plating race horses. Photo by McLain.*

The wall should be trimmed level with the sole at the toe. A minimum amount should be trimmed from the bottom of the foot. The frog and bars should be left intact. Many Thoroughbreds have weak heels. This condition is aggravated by over trimming these structures. Racing plates should be concaved away from the sole on short hoofs.

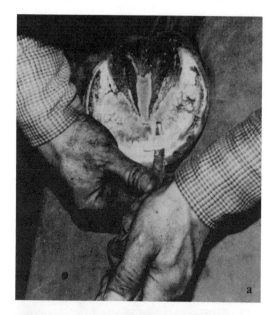

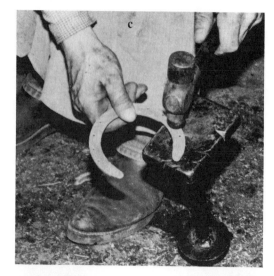

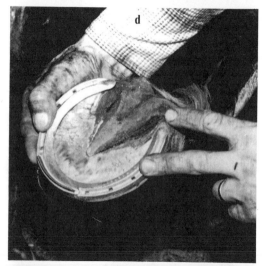

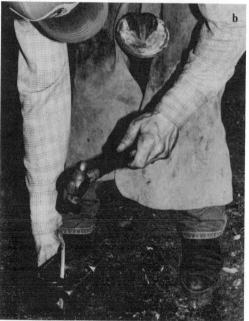

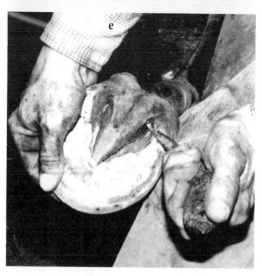

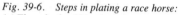

Fig. 39-6.   Steps in plating a race horse:
(a) The sole should be shaved away next to the white line to prevent sole pressure. The frog and bars should not be trimmed away.
(b) Turning the plate heel on a stall jack.
(c) Bending the heel of the shoe up against the foot.
(d) Fitting the toe grab in the center of the foot.
(e) Trimming the heel of the hoof to make the short shoe heel fit.
(f) A long shoe heel may be rasped to make it fit.
(g) The clinches should be rasped flush with the wall.
(h) The shoe should follow the edge of the wall and end at the buttresses.

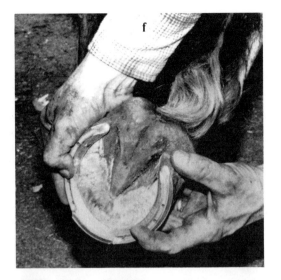

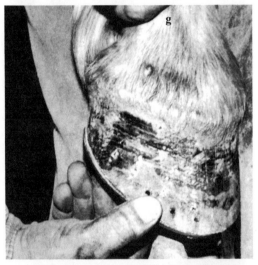

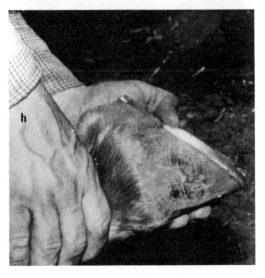

Pads

Rim pads cover only the wall and part of the sole. They are cut out slightly larger than the web of the shoe and are riveted to the shoe at the heels to prevent spreading. Rim pads may be used to absorb concussion to the wall or to give a foot length without weight. They have the advantage of being open over most of the sole and frog.

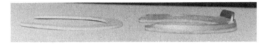

Fig. 39-7.   Rim pads: (left) foam plastic, and (right) bonded.

Full pads cover the bottom of the foot. They are cut out slightly larger than the outline of the shoe and are held in place for nailing by two bent over nails. Full pads may be used to absorb concussion and/or to protect the bottom of the foot from injury. Hoof packing is required under full pads to prevent bacterial growth and filling in with dirt. A piece of sponge rubber may be glued to the foot surface of the pad between the bars to keep dirt out. Pads are rasped flush with the shoe after nailing.

Felt has been used as a rim pad to pad young horses. It is riveted at the heels to prevent spreading. A foam plastic rim pad can be purchased bonded to the shoe. Or, they can be purchased separately[1] and be glued to the shoe.

Plastic pads made of wear resistant plastic are used to protect the bottom of the foot and to dissipate or spread out concussion. These are usually applied as full pads and riveted at the heels of open shoes or in the center of the bar on bar shoes. They come in a thin (3/32 in.) and thick (3/16 in.) weight. Plastic lasts longer than leather and is not affected by moisture. However, some types crack in subfreezing temperatures.

Leather pads are still preferred by some trainers. They seem to be better for the foot and can be trimmed easier than plastic. They don't crack in freezing weather. However, they are affected by moisture. They increase in weight and sink and spread when wet.

[1] *Cliff Carroll's Horseshoers Supplies, Inc., Boynton Beach, FL*

447

Aluminum pads are occasionally welded to the bottom of a racing plate to protect a very sensitive and flexible sole. Thick aluminum bar stock may also be used under the aluminum pad at the heel to prevent its collapse.

Sorbothane and other soft top pads[2] have been successful in absorbing shock and reducing tenderness of sensitive structures due to various clinical problems.

Swedging Steel Plates

Straight or turned swedge molds are available to make bar shoes for race horses. However, those who shoe race horses will want to learn to use a swedge block and make shoes for special cases. Twelve patterns of swedge blocks are available[3]. Some shoers make their own blocks from die steel. Swedge block tie downs can be purchased[4] or handmade to suit the individual plater.

Swedging special racing plates is an essential skill for treating many of the serious hoof ailments and gait defects that afflict race horses. The swedging of light racing shoes is required for passing examination into the International Union of Journeymen Horseshoers (JHU). This skill of plate swedging was once possessed by most platers as they had to make many of their own shoes. Today, it is rarely practiced due to the availability and variety of ready-made horseshoe patterns. Swedging has become a forging exercise for most horseshoers. Still, there are occasions when having the skill allows the horseshoer to do more for the horse than could be done with the manufactured shoes immediately available.

The most important thing to know about swedging is what the block(s) does(do) to the metal. Each block fills a little differently. You must know how much the metal will stretch when it is driven down into your block.

Take, for example, a block made for ¼ x ⅜ inch stock and a 12⅜ inch foot. For a foot of this size, the block stretches the swedged metal 2⅜ inches. The metal is laid out before swedging with a ruler and a center punch. The area to be swedged and stretched is given the measurement

of the foot. In this case, if the foot measures 12⅜ inches, the distance between the center punch marks should be 10 inches. When making a bar shoe, add 1½ inches to each heel beyond the swedged portion. The punch marks are placed up so you can see them. They will be on the foot surface of the shoe. Both shoes of a pair should be swedged before shearing the stock in the middle. This way you have a handle that helps you hold the work in the block.

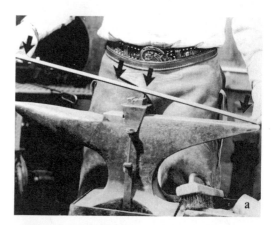

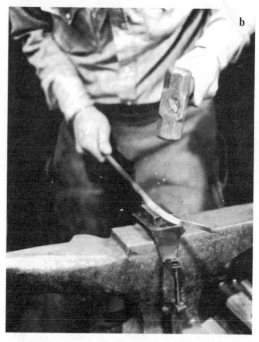

Fig. 39-8. Steps in swedging a light steel racing plate bar shoe:
(a) Center punch the beginning and ending points of the swedged plate after calculating how much metal it will take.
(b) Drive the hot metal into the swedge block by pulling it toward you.

[2] *Sterivet Labs., Inc., Strongsville, OH*
[3] *Thoro'bred Racing Plate Co., Inc., Anaheim, CA*
[4] *Jay Sharp Farrier Tools, Salmon, ID*

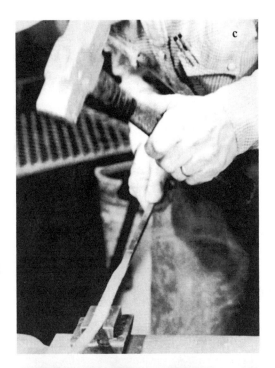

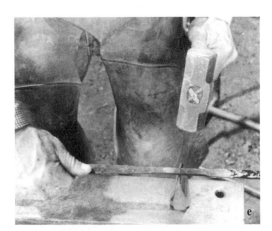

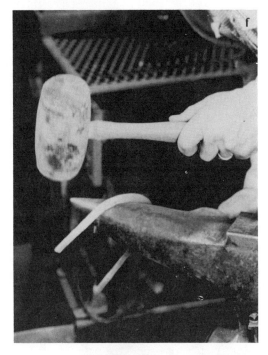

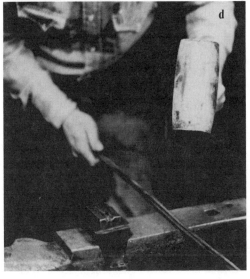

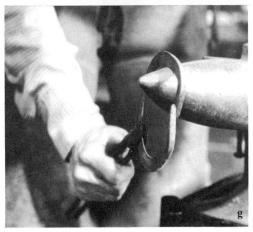

(c) Uniformly fill the block until flashing may be seen (this is ground off before turning the shoe).

(d) Periodically level the swedged stock with a wooden hammer.

(e) After swedging both shoes of a pair cut the stock in half.

(f) Turn the swedged portion of the shoe with a wooden hammer.

(g) Turn the unswedged portion of the shoe with a light hammer.

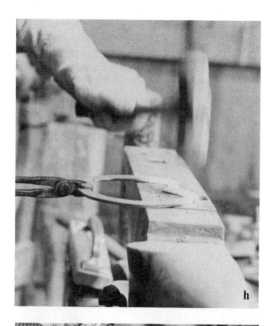

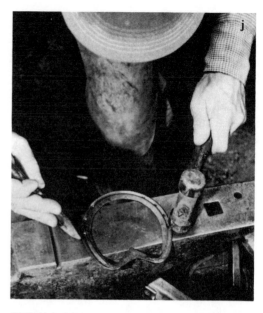

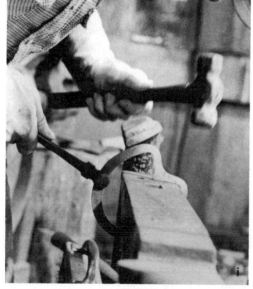

(h) Weld the bar.
(i) Shape the bar.
(j) Punch the nail holes when the shoe is a dull red to a black heat. Light shoes are easily distorted when punching.

Blocks and Stickers

Blocked heels can be made on swedged steel training plates by folding the end of stock over and rolling it over again. Most blocks are made square. However, they can be made as high as desired. Hind shoes may be made with a block on each heel, or more commonly, with a block on the inside and a sticker on the outside heel. A horse with very low heels or flexor tendon trouble may be shod with blocked heels in front, especially if a toe grab is necessary due to soft track conditions.

Stickers are made on the outside heels of hind shoes to create traction. They help stabilize a running horse in a turn. They are bent over and hammer-sharpened in a vise. Stickers are flared to the outside and may be sharpened with a grinder or rasp.

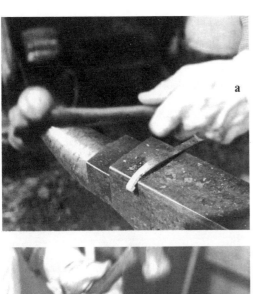
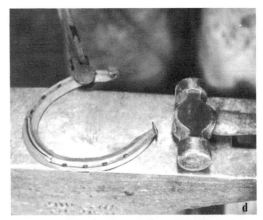
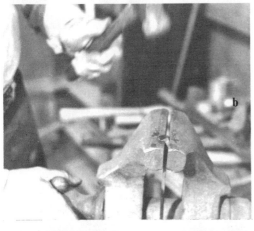
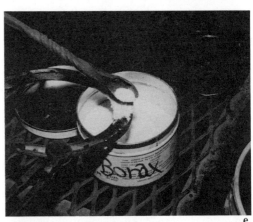
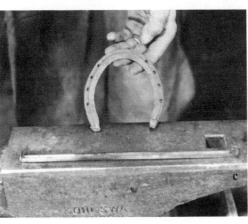
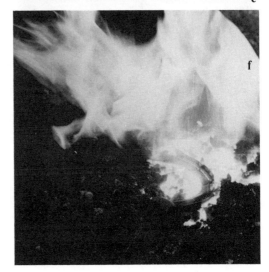

Fig. 39-9.   Steps in turning a blocked heel and sticker and copper brazing a toe grab onto a racing plate:
(a) Turn the blocked heel over twice, roll it up and square it.
(b) Turn the sticker over and bevel it in a vise.
(c) Turned and unturned swedged shoe with block and sticker.
(d) Toe grab with copper wire in place for brazing.
(e) Applying borax to the heated toe.
(f) Remove the shoe from the fire when the copper begins to melt (run).

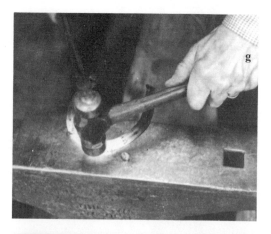

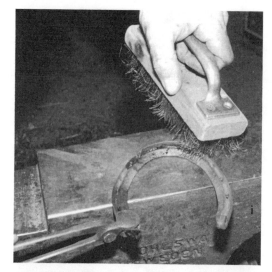

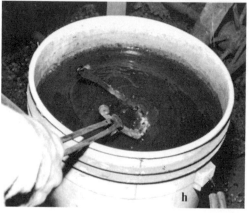

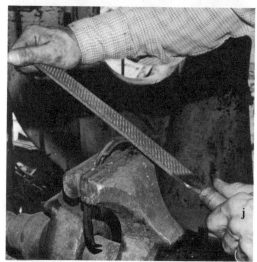

(g) Hold the hammer on the grab against the anvil until the copper sets up.
(h) Quickly dip the shoe in water to loosen the scale.
(i) Brush off the scale.
(j) Finish with a file.

Jar Calks

Racing or training plate jar calks machine-made from high carbon steel and ready to install can be purchased or they can be made from used farm implement springs. Machine-made jar calks are riveted to the shoe. They may be placed in the swedge or across the swedge. Jar calks are usually attached ¾ to 1 inch from each heel on front shoes. However, they may be placed anywhere along the branches to create the effect desired. Jar calks may be brazed into the swedge with copper.

Grabs

Toe grabs may be purchased or swedged from any high carbon or spring steel. Grabs are usually copper brazed into the toes of shoes. However, special limb interference or traction problems may require long or short grabs brazed on another part of the shoe or branch. Old copper wiring of heavy gauge is the most desirable brazing material. Brass brazing rod will work but usually requires two passes. Borax or commercial brazing flux is necessary to clean the metal when it is hot and create a strong bond.

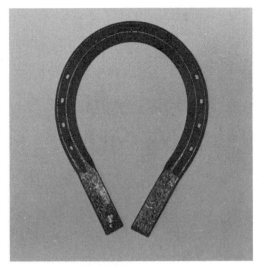

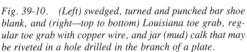

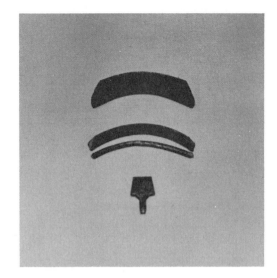

Fig. 39-10.   (Left) swedged, turned and punched bar shoe blank, and (right—top to bottom) Louisiana toe grab, regular toe grab with copper wire, and jar (mud) calk that may be riveted in a hole drilled in the branch of a plate.

References

Butler, D. 1982. Swedging racing plates. Amer. Farriers' J. 8(4):225.

Garvan, F. 1982. Jockey club racing conference—leg injuries. Amer. Farriers' J. 8(5):290.

Kenney, R.M., V.K. Ganjam and R.V. Bergman. 1975. Noninfectious breeding problems in mares. Scope 14(1):16.

Leach, D. 1981. Factors influencing horse locomotion. Amer. Farriers' J. 7(1):22.

Moyer, W. 1982. Commentary on racehorse shoeing. Amer. Farriers' J. 8(4):232.

Simpson, S. 1982. How to make a stall jack. Amer. Farriers' J. 8(4):229.

NOTES:

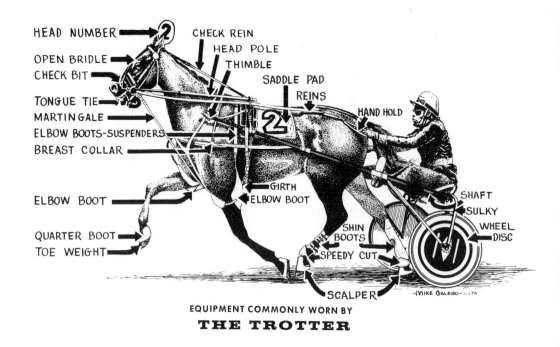

EQUIPMENT COMMONLY WORN BY
THE TROTTER

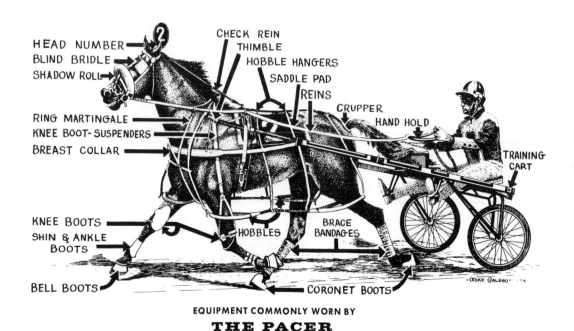

EQUIPMENT COMMONLY WORN BY
THE PACER

Fig. 40-1. Harness race horse terms. Drawings from the United States Trotting Association.

Chapter 40

Harness Race Horses

Harness horse racing is a popular and uniquely American sport. Standardbred (harness) racing is more popular than flat track racing along the East Coast and in parts of the Midwest and is the most popular type of night racing in America. In 1982 there were about 500,000 Standardbreds racing for over 200 million dollars in purses at nearly 500 United States Trotting Association (USTA) sanctioned tracks. Many race meets are at county and state fairs.

Unlike Thoroughbreds, Standardbreds are often raced (driven) by their trainers. Owners may train and race their horses at fair races. Standardbreds are usually more thoroughly conditioned and trained than Thoroughbreds. They go at nearly as fast a gait but weight and stress are borne equally by both front and hind limbs. There is more hind limb lameness in Standardbreds. Harness horses start from a moving starting gait that folds forward when they reach the starting line. Runners start from a stationary chute. Standardbreds may trot or pace a mile in under 1:55 (1 min. 55 sec.), while Thoroughbreds may run a mile in 1:35.

Harness horses race coast to coast in the U.S. and Canada. Some follow the Grand Circuit; others compete in local regions. The Grand Circuit consists of about 20 rich races scheduled to make travel convenient for the top horses in any one year. The trotting "Triple Crown" consists of The Yonkers Trot, The Kentucky Futurity and The Hambletonian. Corresponding races for pacers are The Messenger Pace at Roosevelt, The Cane Pace at Yonkers, and The Little Brown Jug at Delaware, Ohio. All races are 1 mile in length.

Finely tuned and balanced harness horses require specialized horseshoeing. Shoers of harness horses were some of the last to adopt modern machine-made shoes. As a result, some of the best craftsmen in the trade are still practicing this specialty. The specialized skill necessary to keep horses balanced and "on gait" makes shoeing Standardbreds a special challenge.

Types of Harness Horses

Standardbred race horses are either trotters or pacers. Today, there are far more pacers than trotters. Pacers are easier to gait and train than

Leading Money Earning Racehorses of 1983

Rank	Horse's Name	Horse's Breed	Money Earned
1.	All Along	Thoroughbred	$2,138,963
2.	Ralph Hanover	Pacer	1,711,990
3.	Cam Fella	Pacer	1,144,056
4.	On A High	Quarter Horse	1,085,852
5.	Sunny's Halo	Thoroughbred	1,011,962
6.	Joie De Vie	Trotter	1,007,705
7.	Duenna	Trotter	966,709
8.	Dashingly	Quarter Horse	916,877
9.	Carls Bird	Pacer	901,760
10.	Slew O'Gold	Thoroughbred	883,390
11.	Trinycarol	Thoroughbred	877,896
12.	Tolltac	Quarter Horse	847,218
13.	Trutone Lobell	Pacer	805,130
14.	Bates Motel	Thoroughbred	783,000
15.	Sangue	Thoroughbred	764,600

Fig. 40-2. Leading money earning race horses of 1983.
Statistics by Patrick Premo from The Horse Digest.

trotters. Pacers are a few seconds faster than trotters over a mile. Over a longer distance trotters are faster. The name Standardbred was adopted in 1879 to describe a horse that met a time standard for trotting one mile in 2:30 or pacing a mile in 2:25. There were more trotters than pacers then. Standardbreds have been intensively selected for speed. As a result, today's race horses have exceptionally efficient and correct gaits.

In parts of the Northeast and Midwestern United States, pony harness racing is popular. Shetland ponies with trotting ancestry are raced on small tracks or in show rings. They are shod similar to Standardbred race horses. Ponies may be raced as trotters or pacers.

There are two types of trotting bred horses. They are called passing-gaited and line-gaited. Fortunately, most trotters are passing-gaited. They are wider behind than in front. Their hind feet land outside the tracks of the front feet. Line-gaited trotters are wider in the chest than they are behind. They carry their hind feet in a direct line with their front feet. These horses tend to interfere and potential speed may be decreased. The amount of forward extension is relatively the same for either type.

There are two types of pacing bred horses. They are either hobbled or free-legged. Most pacers are hobbled. Their lateral legs are tied together by the hobbles or hopples.

Free-legged pacers will pace without hobbles. Even so, most race horses wear the hobbles when racing. Hobbles must be adjusted to prevent chafing.

Harness Horse Shoeing

An efficient round stroke (stride) is highly desirable on both trotters and pacers. To encourage this, trotters are traditionally shod with a relatively long toe and a heavy, low traction shoe in front. Pacers traditionally are shod with a short toe and a light, high traction shoe in front. Trotters are usually shod with at least two degrees less angle in front than pacers. Both are shod fairly short and steep with light shoes behind.

Trotters are more difficult to shoe than pacers. Trotters require more weight to balance their gait. Trotters don't wear hobbles to help steady them at speed. Trotters hit the ground harder, causing more concussion and creating a need to break the feet over quickly. Trotters are more likely to interfere behind and may hit their knees in front. Pacers often hit their knees. Protective boots of various styles are worn to prevent limb interference.

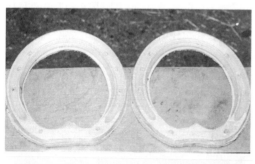
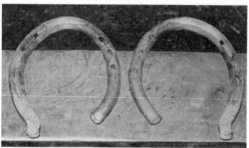

Fig. 40-3. Shoes for a pacer made by Joe Brandau. Front are oxy-acetylene welded aluminum bar shoes with leather rim pads. Hind are half-round half-swedge with a trailer.

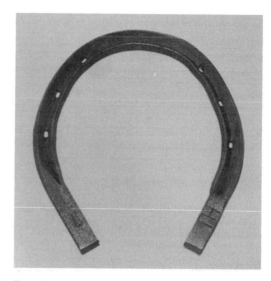

Fig. 40-4. Full swedged front shoe made by Bruce Daniels.

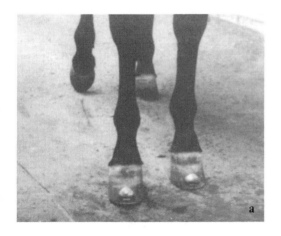

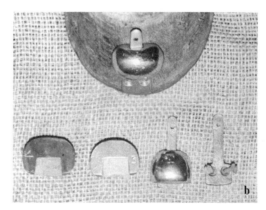

Fig. 40-5. a) Brock toe weights, b) Williams toe weights.

Weight is necessary to balance the gait of many trotters. A simple way to add or subtract weight is to use Brock or Williams toe weights. These are attached to a 2 ounce base plate that is screwed to the outside border of the hoof wall, usually at the toe. Weights of 1, 2, or 3 ounces may be experimented with until the desired gait is achieved. Then the weights are removed and the weight desired is incorporated into the shoe. Weighted bell boots are also available.

Pacing horses are shod with a relatively short foot and a very light (aluminum) shoe, much like a running plate. Freelegged pacers may be shod with a longer foot and heavier shoe (especially behind) than a horse that must be hobbled.

Trimming harness horses usually consists of removing less than a month's hoof growth. Some horses may be reset in two weeks. Only light rasping or "brushing" of the foot is necessary in many cases. It is considered very important to keep a race horse at a specified toe length and angle shod with a sharp shoe of specified weight. Frequent shoeing requires placing the nails back in the old nail holes on resets and moving the hole position on new shoes. Frequent shoeing, along with the variation in wall thickness, caused manufacturers of harness horse shoes to market their shoes without nail holes.

Horses with flexible soles should not be overtrimmed. Light weight plastic racing pads should be used on horses subject to bruising as a preventative measure. The soles and frogs of most harness race horses are packed with clay mud each night. This makes their feet very soft and flexible.

Harness horse trainers usually insist that a foot be trimmed so that it lands flat. They want the horse to stand and go as naturally as possible. As a rule, trainers insist that the side of the foot be trimmed that shows the most wear. They want a horse shod with as short a foot as possible. To a point, a short hoof creates less stress and encourages more speed. The goal of shoeing should be to aid the horse achieve maximum speed on gait. Changes should be made gradually. For example, as a rule, there should be no more than two degrees change in hoof angle at each shoeing.

Shoe Types, Styles and Application

There are many types and styles of shoes used on harness horses. Some are favorites of particular trainers. Others have been fads and are no longer popular.

At one time, it was essential that a harness horse shoer have a forge and know how to make shoes. Machine-made shoes were made with long heels and unpunched. The shoer had to at least know how to make bars and punch nail holes. Today, nearly any shoe style desired can be purchased. Many owners are shoeing their own horses. The faster and better bred (specialized for speed) horses are less complicated to shoe. The trend is toward simple shoeing with just enough material to cover the hoof and prevent hoof breakage and uneven wear. However, there are still many cases where only an expert blacksmith can fashion the special shoes needed to keep a potentially great horse on gait and sound.

Modern front steel shoes are of three basic

types with variations of weight and style in each. They are half-round, flat and swedged (sometimes spelled swaged).

Half-round shoes create the fastest breakover and hold the foot on the ground the shortest time. They sink in and stabilize the foot without holding it. They are self-cleaning due to the concave inner edge. They are comparatively easy on joints and tendons.

Swedged shoes slow the breakover, increase the traction, and hold the foot on the ground the longest. A toe grab further increases this effect.

Flat shoes or flats are half-way in between half-round and swedged shoes. A shoe between a half-round and a flat can be made by flattening a half-round or by running a flat bar through a larger than stock size half-round swedge block. More holding effect can be created in a half-round or flat by creasing the toe or heel(s).

Trotters are usually started in a heavier half-round shoe in front than pacers. A trotter that is a little pacy may need even more weight in front. A pacer that wants to trot may need less weight in front and more weight behind. Most trotters race in a light **full-swedge shoe** behind. They usually train in flats.

Most pacers race in a **half-round half-swedge shoe** behind with the swedge on the outside. This tends to widen the horse and prevents injury due to crossfiring. However, these shoes are hard on a horse's hocks and stifles and overemphasize

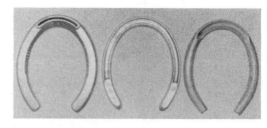

Fig. 40-7. Aluminum harness horse shoes: (left) flat with toe grab, (middle) full-swedge, and (right) half-round with creased or swedged toe.

the pacer's natural rolling gait. Half-round half-swedge shoes may be reversed and applied to problem trotters to narrow them up. This may also shorten the stride. Rarely, half-swedge shoes are used in front to prevent knee knocking.

Aluminum shoes have been tried with some success on harness race horses. They are worn mostly by pacers in front. Nail holes may be drilled and shaped with punches or made in the conventional manner. Aluminum bar shoes may be required. They must be welded with an oxy-acetylene torch or TIG electric arc welder. However, TIG welders are nonportable and uneconomical for welding aluminum over 1/8 inch thick.

The edges to be welded should be beveled slightly. This can be done with a hammer and chisel. Notching is recommended. The area to be welded should be wire brushed in hot water to remove grease and oxide that naturally coats aluminum. Powdered flux mixed with water to form a paste should be applied to the edges. A size larger tip than would be used for similar size steel should be used. Aluminum conducts heat faster than steel. A slight excess acetylene feather (1 1/2 X) is recommended. (See Chapter 43.) Always use a back up plate or anvil face when welding aluminum. Stir the puddle vigorously and try to complete the weld in one pass. Wire brush the cooled shoe in hot water to remove flux.

Aluminum welding requires some practice. Most horseshoers have difficulty, at first, recognizing when the molten puddle is ready for filler rod. The backup plate or anvil face allows you to make mistakes and still make an acceptable weld. Aluminum bars can also be drilled or punched and riveted. Aluminum can be ham-

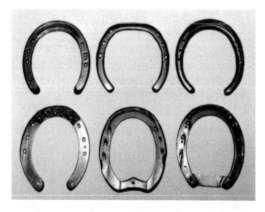

Fig. 40-6. Steel harness horse shoes: (Top left) flat with creased-toe, (top middle) flattened half-round with square-toe, (top right) toe-weighted half-round with creased-toe, (bottom left) flat drilled for rim pad with borium-toe, (bottom middle) forge welded bar shoe with creased-toe and quarter clips, (bottom right) riveted bar shoe drilled for rim pad with low toe grab.

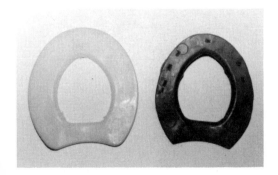

Fig. 40-8.   Plastic shoes before and after fitting.

mered cold or hot. It shows no color when hot and is ready to work as it becomes sticky when rubbed with a hammer or fire poker. Aluminum shoes should be allowed to air cool.

Plastic shoes are used on some horses. They are cut to fit to a hoof tracing. They may be cut with nippers or a band or saber saw. Plastic shoes may be superior on a few horses under some track conditions. However, plastic shoes are difficult to keep from moving on the foot. They do not have the rigidity of steel shoes. Dirt may ball up under the heel. One nail must be put at the toe to hold it down. Clips may be attached by heating and burning them into the shoe. Plastic shoes can be made to create traction by inserting borium coated rivets or steel grabs. A washer is placed over the rivet on the foot surface before riveting.

Steel bar shoes are used extensively on harness horses. Sometimes they are used to prevent or treat hoof ailments by applying pressure to or relieving pressure from a part of the foot. More commonly, bar shoes are applied to prevent spreading of the shoe when the toe wears thin. Pads are commonly riveted to the center of the bar. Rivet holes may be hot punched or drilled. Pads may be riveted to the heels of open shoes. A riveted pad acts like a bar to prevent spreading of thin open shoes.

The **egg bar shoe** is used on the hind feet of harness horses instead of double trailers. Its object is to extend the surface of the foot. It relieves stress on the tendons of the leg. It is especially useful on horses with sloping heels. It also may be used on the front feet to prevent the toe from turning up on a horse with very limber joints or

an old tendon injury. The egg bar shoe is also said to help a trotter with excessive hock action extend by holding the hind foot and creating more backward extension.

The **mushroom shoe** is a bar shoe that has been acclaimed as being useful in preventing and curing corns or sore heels on horses that hit the ground hard. It has helped some cases of sidebone. A mushroom shoe is usually applied with a pad riveted at the heels. It may be forge welded. Or, it may have the open ends bent in and then back and be welded to a plate that covers the frog. Shoes and plates may be made of steel or aluminum.

The **double trailer bar shoe** requires a jump welded bar when heel calks or trailers are desired on both heels. The added stock is cut part way through, welded on one side, twisted off and then welded on the other. The calks may be turned first. This bar is sometimes called a butterfly bar because the added stock may spread out (like wings) where it joins the branches and be narrow in the center. Another way of making this shoe is to upset and split the heels. The inner halves are welded and calks are turned on the outer halves.

The **whip-across bar shoe** is used on the hind feet of harness horses when a calk and trailer are desired in conjunction with a bar shoe. A common application is on a pacer that is going narrow and has a tendency to crossfire. A half-round half-swedge shoe is usually used. The half-round pattern on the inside encourages breakover on the inside of the foot and prevents possible damage from limb interference. The half-swedge pattern on the outside and toe provides traction and holds the foot on the ground an instant longer. This separates the horse's foot flight patterns. The height of the calk and its position lateral to the heel of the foot on the trailer encourages a wider stance. The calk also helps hold the foot and discourages twisting at the moment of breakover.

The whip-across bar shoe is said to be the most difficult of all harness horse shoes to make. The bar must be welded on light stock without burning off the trailer. If the trailer is long enough to allow for a calk, the chances of the trailer burning off during the welding heat may be increased. The weld is severely strained when

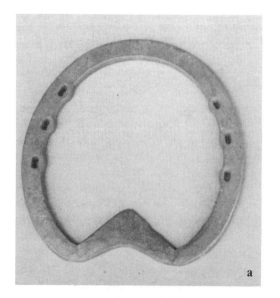
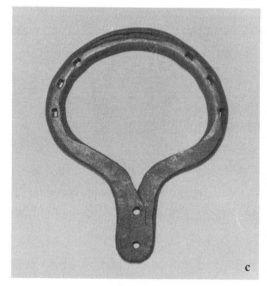
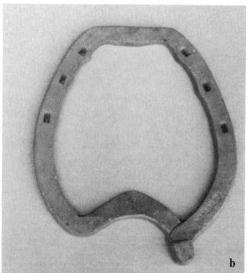
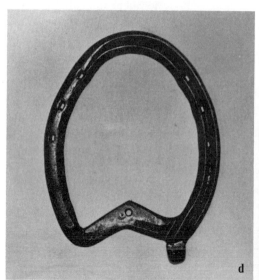

Fig. 40-9. Steel bar shoes: (a) flat bar shoe, (b) flat square-toe whip-across bar shoe with calk or trailer, (c) half-round mushroom shoe with creased toe, and (d) half-round half-swedge whip-across bar shoe with calk on trailer.

Fig. 40-10. Steps in making a whip-across bar shoe: (a) Slope one side of the stock to correspond to the deep side of the swedge block. (b) Run the outside of the shoe stock through the rim swedge block across the toe to the first nail hole. (c) Run the inside of the stock through the half-round swedge block leaving enough for the bar and weld. (d) Turn the toe using the eye portion of the wooden hammer. (e) Turn the branches to correspond to the hoof wall with the inside bar extending. (f) Upset and shape the end of the bar.

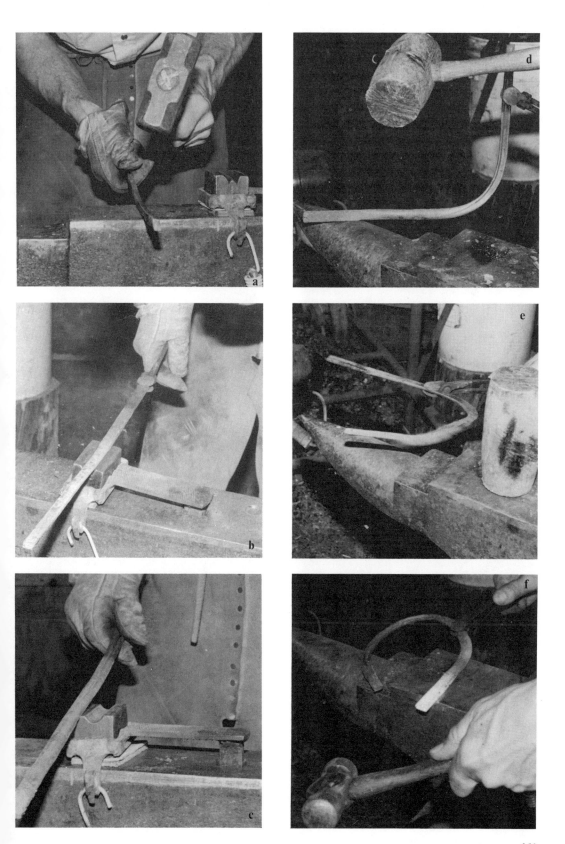

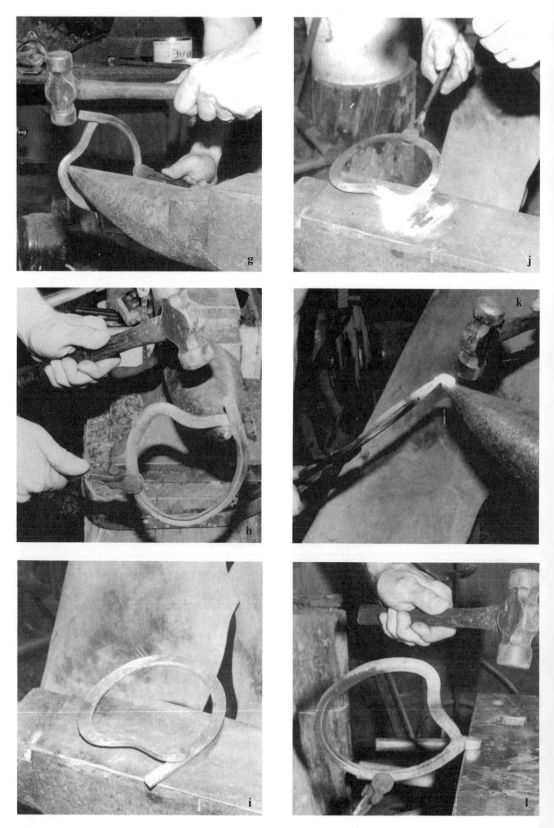

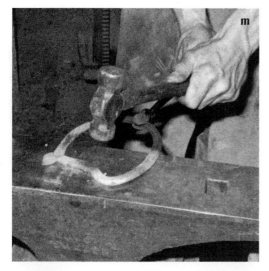

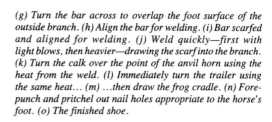

(g) Turn the bar across to overlap the foot surface of the outside branch. (h) Align the bar for welding. (i) Bar scarfed and aligned for welding. (j) Weld quickly—first with light blows, then heavier—drawing the scarf into the branch. (k) Turn the calk over the point of the anvil horn using the heat from the weld. (l) Immediately turn the trailer using the same heat… (m) …then draw the frog cradle. (n) Forepunch and pritchel out nail holes appropriate to the horse's foot. (o) The finished shoe.

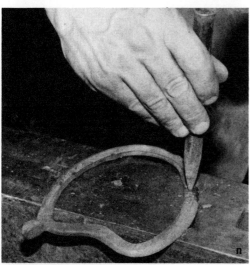

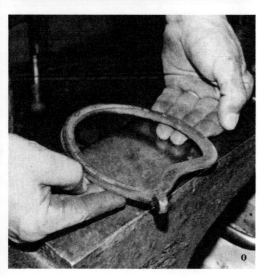

turning the calk and trailer. Only a long weld made at exactly the right temperature will take this sort of abuse.

Challoner (1983) has suggested lap welding the ends so that they turn together when making the calk. This is a preferable method when there is enough stock available from the inside branch.

The **crossfiring shoe** is usually made from a half-round half-swedge shoe. The inside branch from mid-toe to mid-quarter is flattened and fit under the hoof. This prevents shoe caused injury. A trailer with a calk on it is turned at the end of the outside branch. The toe of a crossfiring shoe is sometimes called an oblique or diamond-toe.

The **square-toed shoe** is commonly used on both front and hind shoes of Standardbreds. It is normally set under the foot and the exposed hoof is rounded. The object is to shorten the foot surface and speed up breakover. It may also be used to prevent lateral limb interference. In severe cases (e.g., scalping or crossfiring), a bar shoe can be made and a portion of the shoe cut out (e.g., toe or inside) to prevent interference.

Weighted shoes are no longer common on race horses. Toe-weights may be used to get a trotter on gait. Side-weights are rarely used now except to create lateral support to the foot. They were once a popular prescription for crossfiring horses.

Memphis nub and **Memphis bar shoes** were used to create a rolling motion when gaiting trotting colts. These were a replacement for weighted shoes. They placed a lot of strain on joints, tendons and ligaments. They are no longer popular for trotters. Memphis bars are still used on the hind feet of gaited horses.

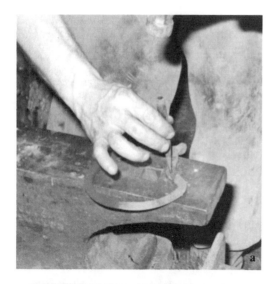

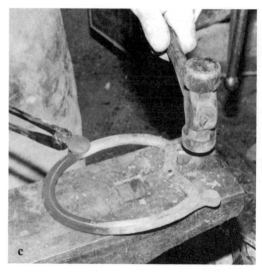

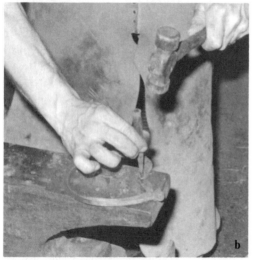

Fig. 40-11. Steps in punching a rivet hole for full or rim pads: (a) Using the same heat that was used for finishing the heels, drive the punch into foot surface until you can feel it stop, (b) Turn the shoe over and place punch in center of "rose" formed on the opposite side—drive it through pritchel hole. (c) Smooth hole with hammer.

NOTES:

Rim shoes were once popular for pacers. They gave a grab effect all the way around the shoe. They were hard on the knee, hock, and stifle joints and difficult to level. The swedge shoe has replaced them.

The **four-calk shoe** was a widely used shoe to prevent knee hitting. The calks were to prevent the foot from twisting as it left the ground. Calks or grabs have been placed in various ways on shoes to increase traction and change the action of the foot. A rim shoe was a full grab or full calk shoe.

Scooped-rolled toe shoes were once used extensively on the front feet of trotters. This was a self-cleaning shoe that allowed an easy breakover while the ridge between the scoop and roll prevented the shoe from slipping. The half-round shoe has replaced it.

Shoes are nailed on with No. 4 or 4 1/2 city head nails. Occasionally, No. 4 1/2 regular or No. 5 special nails may be necessary (especially when pads are used). Nails may be driven into the same hoof holes due to the frequency of shoeing.

Limb Interference

Common limb interference problems are discussed in Chapter 31. Modern breeding has eliminated many problems that were commonplace just a few years ago. However, a shoer of harness horses will occasionally see the following defects in gait: knee hitting, speedy cutting (high interference of lateral legs), hind leg interference (high interference of opposite legs),

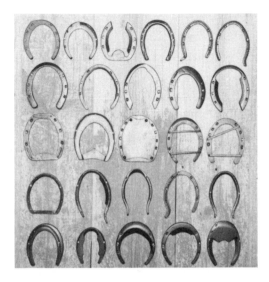

Fig. 40-12. Old harness horse shoes (circa 1900) made by Carl (Mike) Wiles of Maryville, MO.

crossfiring, elbow hitting, forging, and scalping. Changes in gait may require various methods to change the elevation, forward extension, or lateral distance of the feet in flight. The least severe measure to stop the interference is usually recommended.

Occasional limb interference should be prevented by boots and protective devices of various types. These are applied as insurance by many trainers. Severe changes in foot balance and shoe design should be avoided. Horses with legs of unequal length or stride show dramatic improvement when opposite feet are shod with unequal toe length, angle, weight, or shoe style.

References

Brandau, J. 1982. How to make an aluminum bar shoe. Amer. Farriers' J. 8(5):288.

Butler, D. 1982. How to make a whip across bar shoe. Amer. Farriers' J. 8(5): 292.

Canfield, D.M. 1968. Elements of Farrier Science (2nd ed.). Enderes Tool Co., Inc., Albert Lea, MN.

Challoner, T. 1983. Whip across bar shoe, British style. Amer. Farriers' J. 9(2):105.

Clark, J. 1916. Shoeing and Balancing the Light Harness Horse. The Horse World Co., Buffalo, NY.

Daniels, B. 1982. An introduction to Standardbred shoeing. Amer. Farriers' J. 8(5):277.

Daniels, B. 1982. Tips on shoeing youngsters. Amer. Farriers' J. 8(6):350.

Dunkin, T.E. 1964. Standardbred equipment and its importance to the veterinary clinician. Proc. of Amer. Assoc. of Eq. Practit. 10:73.

Evans, D.P. 1976. This is Harness Racing. United States Trotting Assoc., Columbus, OH.

Harrison, J.C. 1968. Care and Training of the Trotter and Pacer. United States Trotting Assoc., Columbus, OH.

Jordan, R. 1910. The Gait of the American Trotter and Pacer. William R. Jenkins Co., New York.

McLellan, C.A. 1927. The Art of Shoeing and Balancing the Trotter. The Trotter and Pacer, New York.

Miller, B. 1982. Journeyman horseshoers union: myths and realities. Amer. Farriers' J. 8(5):285.

Moore, W.J. Balancing and Shoeing Trotting and Pacing Horses. Francis McGovern, North Adams, MA.

United States Trotting Association. 1983. The world of the Standardbred. Equus 69:75.

Wall, M. 1977. A growing interest in mushroom shoes. Hoof Beats. (Nov):28.

Chapter 41

Gaited Show Horses

Gaited horses are the elegant show horses of the equine world. They are often referred to as society or high tailed horses. Most of these highly trained aristocrats require a special style of shoeing in order to execute their gaits in proper form. The role of the gaited horse farrier is primarily that of a technician who makes and applies shoes and hoof buildups as instructed by knowledgeable trainers.

There are several divisions of gaited show horses and many classes within each division. The major divisions recognized by the American Horse Shows Association (AHSA) are divided according to breed or type.

The AHSA is the rule making body of the show horse world. There are many rules governing the shoeing of show horses. These have changed often in recent years and may be different for each division. Horseshoers who shoe show horses or intend to be employed as show farriers should belong to the AHSA and receive its annual rulebook[1].

Every show that offers a division or section with an "A" rating must have a farrier who is qualified in those divisions or sections available during all performances. "B" and "C" rated shows should also have a farrier available at all

[1] American Horse Shows Assn., 598 Madison Ave., New York, NY 10022

times. A farrier is classified as a show employee—not as an official.

The show farrier has 5 minutes to replace a shoe lost in competition. No more than two time-outs per class may be called for shoe loss or broken equipment and time is not to exceed 5 minutes total. Time starts when the farrier enters the ring or touches the shoe. After the time limit has been reached, the horse must proceed or be eliminated. Black duct tape may be used to temporarily hold on a thrown shoe. A means of conveniently transporting tools into the ring and a rapid work sequence have been developed by show farriers (See Liles and Akers, 1980).

The following AHSA divisions have classes for horses that may be considered gaited: Fox Trotting Horse, Hackney and Harness Pony, Morgan, Parade, Paso Fino, Roadster, Saddle Horse, Shetland Pony, and Tennessee Walking Horse.

Arabian English Pleasure and Park horses are trained to trot in a way that may be considered gaited. However, the use of weight and action devices in training and showing is prohibited. Paso Finos are true gaited horses, performing a broken pace at three speeds. But, they also have strict natural foot and unweighted shoe requirements. The Racking Horse is also a type of gaited horse. Its popularity is regional and there is no separate division in the AHSA for it at this time.

Principles of Shoeing Gaited Horses

The shoeing and balancing of gaited horses may be considered a fine art. Many of the techniques for shoeing each of the types are the same. However, there are variations in rules and traditions. A champion horse is a combination of breeding, training, riding and shoeing.

There are five factors that may be regulated by the shoer: 1) the length of the hoof, 2) the angle of the hoof, 3) the weight of the shoe, 4) the position of weight on the foot, and 5) the position of weight on the horse. These factors,

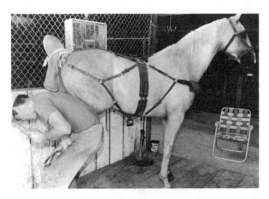

Fig. 41-1. Show horses require special shoeing to execute their gaits in proper form. Photos by J. Graves.

together with the horse's natural ability, training and performance speed determine the type of action displayed in the show ring. One factor may limit or cancel another. Excessive length of hoof (over 5 to 5 1/2 in.) may cancel the effect of other factors. Hoof angle and weight are closely related. The position and pull of the trainer's hands when riding influence the effect of weight and angle. Position of weight on the shoe has little effect unless the horse is very limber. Speed of performance affects all of the factors.

The length of the hoof may be increased naturally by allowing the wall to grow, or artificially by building it up with pads. Increased hoof length places more weight and creates more leverage on the end of the leg. A short hoof breaks over quickly and is raised slowly. A long hoof breaks over slowly but is raised quickly and folds higher than a short foot. A long hoof helps to create a snappy, animated gait.

The length of hoof may be measured in three ways: 1) natural length (from the hair line at the coronary band to the base of the natural hoof); 2) overall length (from the hair line to top of hoof surface of the shoe); and 3) official length (from the hair line to the ground). Length of hoof is usually measured at the center of the toe; the hoof gauge automatically figures in the heel length. However, in some cases the heel length is measured. It is officially measured from the hair line at the bulbs to the ground by a line perpendicular to the ground.

The angle of the hoof is normally the same as that of the axis of the pastern. It may be changed by trimming. An accurate hoof gauge is essential. Check your gauge for accuracy with a protractor or square. Trainers will usually specify the hoof angle and will often want to check the angle with their own hoof gauge.

Trimming more off the toe and leaving the heel will increase the angle. In general, this causes the foot to breakover relatively more quickly and reach forward more. Trimming more off the heel and leaving the toe will decrease the angle. In general, this causes the foot to breakover more slowly, and fold up more. The effect of angle on the action of the feet will often differ between the front and hind limbs.

Horses with unsymmetrical feet (one dished [club] and one bull-nosed) should be studied from the side. The perpendicular distance between the ground surface at the toe and coronary band should be made the same by rasping the front of the dished foot. The toe-lengths should be equal. The shoes should be equal in length and weight. The low, sloping-heeled foot will need a heel wedge to make the hoof angles equal. A piece of lead equal to the weight of the wedge can be added to the pad stack of the opposite foot if the difference in weight is significant.

The weight of the shoe affects the flight pattern of the foot. Weight increases the momentum of the foot causing it to make a faster, higher and longer flight arc than an unweighted foot. Weight, no matter how added, increases the foot flight arc. It also decreases agility and endurance, slows down breakover and increases fatigue. Since show horses are highly trained and

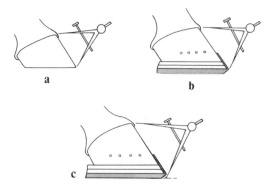

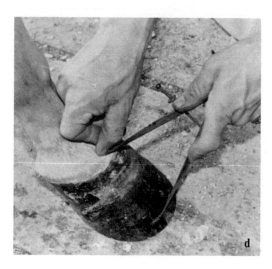

Fig. 41-2. The length of hoof on a show horse may be measured in three ways: (a) natural length, (b) overall length, and (c) official length. Calipers (d) are used to mark the amount to be trimmed off.

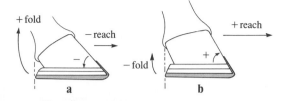

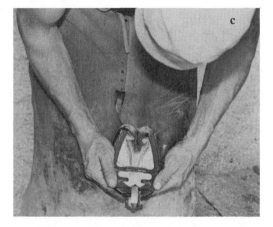

Fig. 41-3. Hoof angle affects leg fold and reach: (a) decrease in toe angle creates more fold and less reach, (b) increase in toe angle creates less fold and more reach. A hoof protractor (c) is used to measure toe angle.

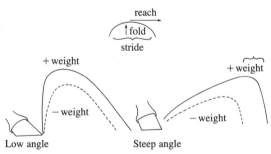

Fig. 41-4. Weight increases the momentum of the foot regardless of the toe angle.

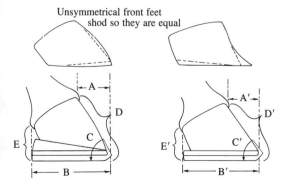

A, B, C, D & E should equal A′, B′, C′, D′ & E′.

Fig. 41-5. Unsymmetrical feet may be balanced by close attention to detail.

conditioned, and worked very hard for very short periods of time, the exaggerated but graceful foot flight arc outweighs the negative factors of applying weight for this type of horse.

The position of weight on the shoe mostly affects the position of the suspended hoof. A limber horse with flexible joints is more affected by weight position than one with stiff joints. Any effect weight position may have on the foot flight arc can be cancelled by an overall increase in weight, change in hoof angle or hoof length. However, toe weights are usually given credit for improving fold, heel weights for improving reach, and side weights for widening or narrowing the distance between the feet in flight.

There are many differences of opinion on what these shoes and weight do. A lot of the differences can be accounted for in the way a horse is trimmed and ridden. Weight may be experimentally positioned on the sides or bottom of the pads by using pieces of lead that have been poured into molds and nailed or screwed on at various sites. After the best position is determined, the weight can be incorporated into the next pair of shoes or pad build-up.

The position of weight on the horse affects the gait of the horse. As a rule, weight in front causes a horse to trot, weight behind causes a horse to pace. A natural gaited or "pacy" horse will usually need heavy weighted shoes in front to show at the trot in Walk Trot or Fine Harness classes. A horse that prefers to trot but is trained to be a Gaited Horse usually needs to be shod with comparatively heavy shoes behind. Weight tends to hold the foot on the ground longer, slowing breakover but increasing the flight arc (fold and reach) of the foot. The true pace is a two-beat gait. The slow gait, rack and running walk are four-beat gaits that are broken paces. The position and amount of weight on the horse help to create the desired smoothness of gait.

Skill and judgment are required to properly balance and maintain a highly pampered show horse. Fortunately, the horseshoer is not totally responsible. However, even good trainers need scapegoats to justify why a horse doesn't always win. Horseshoers should be prepared for and accept this. Advise (when requested) against asking a horse for more than he is capable of delivering. It may help keep you out of trouble.

Techniques of Shoeing Gaited Horses

Pads must be used on hoofs of unnatural length to retain and protect the sole from flaking away. Hoofs that readily shed the sole must be filled and braced to prevent wall collapse. Silicone rubber may be used. It can be mixed with body filler putty cream hardener to make it set up faster. Scrap ends of retread rubber may also be used. They are cut into pieces, warmed (in coal shovel over fire or hot sun) and packed into the foot before nailing. The excess will squeeze out the back and may be trimmed off after the horse stands on the foot for a few minutes. Thick foam rubber and pieces of used pads may also be used. Used plastic pads may be cut into small pieces and melted in a tin can over the forge fire. The liquid may be used to fill in missing areas of the hoof wall or support the bottom of the foot.

Pads should follow the angle of the foot from one quarter to the other. The dimensions of the shoe for a built-up foot can be determined approximately by viewing the hoof from above with the ground surface of the shoe extended. The rounded toe of the shoe should extend forward from the toe a little less than the thickness of the pads. Allow the branches of the shoe to extend from the widest part of the hoof a little more than one-half the thickness of the pads on each side. The shoe heels should extend back with a smooth curve but be wide enough to prevent instability. The heels of the shoe usually should extend beyond the buttresses to a plumb line dropped from the base of the bulbs.

Exact shoe dimensions can be determined using the charts in this Chapter. They have been developed using mathematical formulas (See Luikart, 1980). These can be used until you learn to estimate dimensions accurately. The horseshoer's job is to build and fit a shoe with the correct dimensions. The weight, style of the shoe and hoof length are supplied by the trainer.

Pads can be stacked and fastened together with corrugated-roofing, ring-shank, or cement-coated nails. Stacked pads can be attached to the shoe and cut using a band saw or saber saw. Plastic pads are difficult to cut with a knife unless the blade is hot. Sawing works much better. The pads can then be roughly beveled and shaped to conform to the shape of the hoof with a rasp or electric sander before nailing.

It is usually best to put a leather pad next to the foot. Leather holds up better under the heels than many plastics and allows the foot to "breathe" or fluctuate in moisture content. Plastics have the advantage of not absorbing moisture and remaining at a constant weight and consistency. They are unaffected by manure acids. Polyurethane, neolite, and neoprene plastics are commonly used as padding materials for degree and wedge pads. A full pad should be next to the shoe to prevent dirt from getting between the pads. Plastic against the foot may cause slippage and increase the chance of nail sheer and hoof distortion.

Any time the foot is padded, an antiseptic hoof packing material must be applied next to the hoof to prevent thrush infection. Pine tar and oakum are commonly used between the pads and hoof. The pine tar can be brushed or poured on. The oakum holds it in the foot and prevents foreign matter from entering. Pine tar is brushed on and used without oakum when the foot is filled with retread rubber. Pine tar soaked peat moss packing (Forshner's) is a favorite to fill small spaces in short hoofs. Foam rubber glued to the back of the pad between the buttresses will help keep the packing in and dirt out. Silicone injected with a calking gun is the most popular way to fill large spaces in long hoofs. Duct tape may be used to hold the silicone in place while it cures. Use only 100 percent silicone rubber.

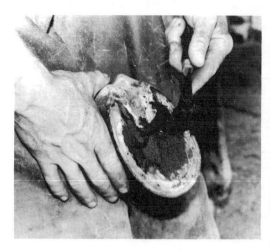

Fig. 41-6.   Antiseptic hoof packing material must be placed next to the hoof under pads.

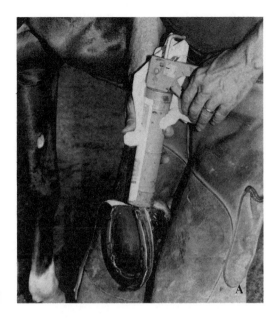
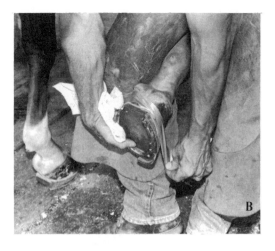

Fig. 41-7. *Silicone rubber can be used to fill and support long hoofs. (A) Stick duct tape on one side and fill hoof space with silicone, (B) Pull tape around against heel and stick down to hold silicone in until it sets.*

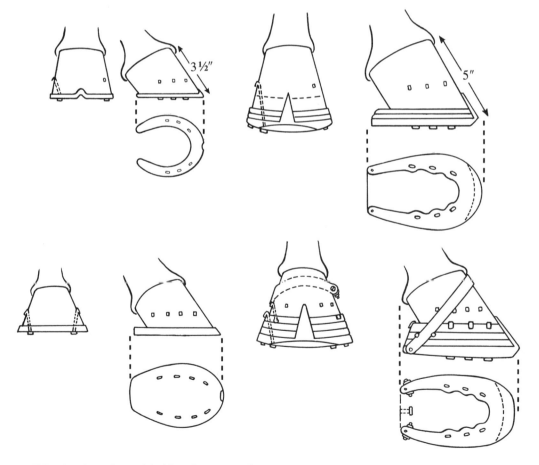

Fig. 41-8. *Regular nailing and double nailing compared.*

471

Regular nailing of weighted shoes and one or more pads is routinely done on long footed Saddlebred horses. The shoe is sized to match the ground surface at the desired length of hoof. The heels of the shoe are extended back and kept wide to provide lateral stability to the foot.

Toe clips on front shoes and side clips on hind shoes help to stabilize the shoe and prevent shearing forces on the nails. They should be used on all shoes that are put on with a pad build-up. The clips must reach above the pads and contact the hoof. Toe clips look especially good if, when viewed from the front, they are in the center of the toe and the sides of the clip are parallel with the sides of the hoof. Weld-on clips of various sizes are available from suppliers. Clips should be adjusted to the angle of the wall before fitting pads.

One or more pads are cut to the size of the shoe and attached to it by nails (rivets) through holes drilled at the heels. Or, pads may be attached by two horseshoe nails driven in the middle nail hole of each branch and then cut off flush with the foot surface of the pads. The foot should be placed on the package and viewed from above. When the hoof and shoe are lined up, trace the hoof on the pads. Shape the pads in the vise with a rasp or grinder back to 1/8 inch from the line.

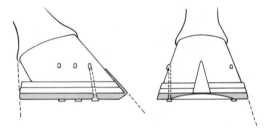

Fig. 41-10. The build-up (shoe and pads) should follow the angle of the hoof at the toe when viewed from the side and from widest point to widest point when viewed from in front.

Pad next to shoe pinned with nail

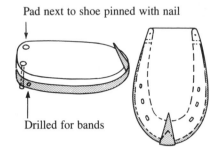

Drilled for bands

Fig. 41-11. Pads next to the shoe are pinned with roofing nails. Shoes may also be drilled for bands.

A = Shoe-toe to foot-toe distance
B = Shoe-quarter to foot-quarter distance
C = Shoe-heel to foot-bulb distance

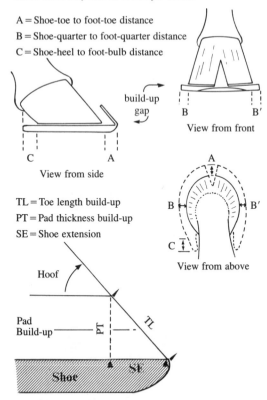

build-up gap

View from front

View from side

TL = Toe length build-up
PT = Pad thickness build-up
SE = Shoe extension

View from above

Fig. 41-12. Determining shoe dimensions (fit) with a build-up. Distance A is slightly less than build-up thickness. Distance B is slightly less than one-half build-up thickness. Exact distances can be determined by measurements and use of the charts.

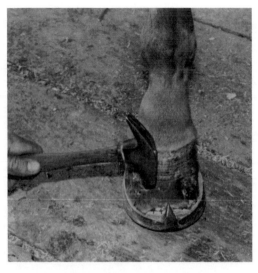

Fig. 41-9. Holes in the hoof may be patched with nailed-in leather, melted-in plastic pads or plastic wood.

The bottom of the foot is filled with hoof packing before applying the pad and shoe package. If the hoof is exceptionally long and the sole has deteriorated and fallen out, the sole cavity should be filled with rubber before or after nailing to prevent wall collapse.

The nails should be driven up into sound hoof

just below the height that small nails would be driven into a natural short foot. The nails used are large in diameter (#8 to #16) and the possibility of close nailing (causing pressure on the sensitive structures) is greater when these nails are driven too high into the foot. However, they must be driven high enough to hold the shoe to

SHOE EXTENSION (in.)

Beyond Base of Natural Hoof

Cos of Angle x Toe Length = Shoe Extension

Toe Length Build-up in Inches	Angle of Natural Hoof (Toe or Mid-Quarter) in Degrees									
	45	48	50	52	55	58	60	62	65	70
0.25	0.18	0.17	0.16	0.15	0.14	0.14	0.13	0.12	0.11	0.09
0.50	0.36	0.33	0.32	0.31	0.29	0.27	0.25	0.24	0.21	0.17
0.75	0.53	0.50	0.48	0.46	0.43	0.41	0.38	0.35	0.32	0.26
1.00	0.71	0.67	0.64	0.62	0.57	0.55	0.50	0.47	0.42	0.34
1.25	0.89	0.84	0.80	0.77	0.72	0.68	0.63	0.59	0.53	0.43
1.50	1.07	1.00	0.96	0.92	0.86	0.82	0.75	0.71	0.63	0.51
1.75	1.24	1.17	1.13	1.08	1.00	0.95	0.88	0.82	0.74	0.60
2.00	1.42	1.34	1.29	1.23	1.15	1.09	1.00	0.94	0.85	0.68

PAD THICKNESS BUILD-UP (in.)

Between Shoe and Hoof

Sin of Angle x Toe Length = Pad Thickness Build-up

Toe Length Build-up in Inches	Angle of Natural Hoof (Toe or Mid-Quarter) in Degrees									
	45	48	50	52	55	58	60	62	65	70
0.25	0.18	0.19	0.19	0.20	0.21	0.21	0.22	0.22	0.23	0.24
0.50	0.36	0.37	0.39	0.40	0.41	0.43	0.44	0.44	0.46	0.47
0.75	0.53	0.56	0.58	0.59	0.62	0.64	0.65	0.66	0.68	0.71
1.00	0.71	0.74	0.77	0.79	0.82	0.85	0.87	0.88	0.91	0.94
1.25	0.89	0.93	0.96	0.99	1.03	1.06	1.09	1.10	1.14	1.18
1.50	1.07	1.11	1.16	1.19	1.23	1.28	1.31	1.32	1.37	1.41
1.75	1.24	1.30	1.35	1.38	1.44	1.49	1.52	1.54	1.59	1.65
2.00	1.42	1.48	1.54	1.58	1.64	1.70	1.74	1.76	1.82	1.88

DECIMAL EQUIVALENTS (in.)

1/16	0.063	9/16	0.563	1 1/16	1.063	1 9/16	1.563
1/8	0.125	5/8	0.625	1 1/8	1.125	1 5/8	1.625
3/16	0.188	11/16	0.688	1 3/16	1.188	1 11/16	1.688
1/4	0.250	3/4	0.750	1 1/4	1.250	1 3/4	1.750
5/16	0.313	13/16	0.813	1 5/16	1.313	1 13/16	1.813
3/8	0.375	7/8	0.875	1 3/8	1.375	1 7/8	1.875
7/16	0.438	15/16	0.938	1 7/16	1.438	1 15/16	1.938
1/2	0.500	1	1.000	1 1/2	1.500	2	2.000

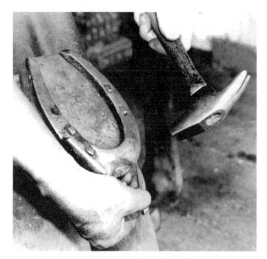

Fig. 41-13.   Nailing with long nails through several pads may require shaping the end of a nail to change its direction.

the hoof for at least 8 weeks. After two nails are driven, check the position of the package with the hoof on the ground. Pull the nails and realign the package if necessary.

Regular clinchers do not work well on large nails that exit a great distance from the shoe. Clinches must be formed with the driving hammer unless you make a special tool. Most shoers bend over the nails after driving them rather than wringing them off. After blocking and tightening the nails, the ends are cut off and a clinch is formed. The clinches are made longer than they are wide. They are flattened against the hoof with the hammer. The head of the nail is backed up with the block while the clinch is being formed with the hammer.

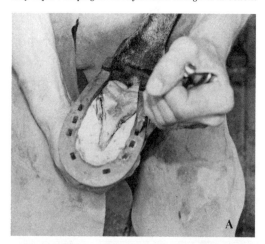

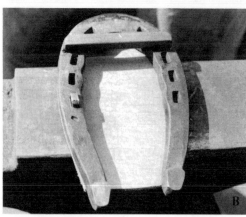

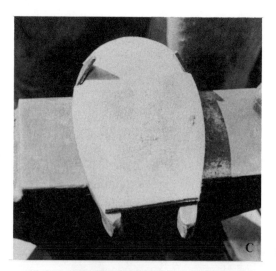

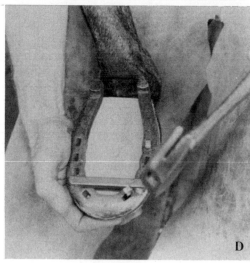

Fig. 41-14.   Steps in regular nailing with one pad:
(A) Fit the shoe.
(B) Cut out the pad.
(C) Notch for clip(s) and attach the pad to the shoe.
(D) Pack the foot and nail the shoe and pad on.

Double nailing is a technique for increasing the hoof length of gaited horses. It is especially popular with Walking Horse shoers. A 1/2 inch thick, tough plastic pad called a double nail pad is nailed to the hoof with eight or ten small (#5 or #6) regular head nails. DNPs (double nail pads) are available with leather bonded to the foot surface[2]. The pads making up the artificial length of the foot and the shoe, which have been previously attached together, are nailed to the double nail pad. The shoe and pad package are nailed or screwed to the double nail pad from above in extremely large buildups.

Before the advent of double nailing, hoofs had to be kept unnaturally long and nails had to reach all the way from the shoe to the sound hoof.

[2] *Curtis Hamilton, Easley, SC*

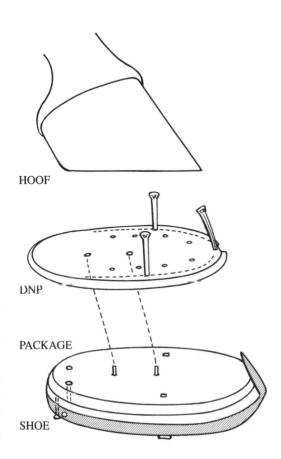

HOOF

DNP

PACKAGE

SHOE

Fig. 41-15. Double nail pad and package assembly.

Some of the advantages of double nailing on long-footed show horses include:
1. Immediate increase in toe-length.
2. Foot remains short, strong, and natural.
3. Less chance of splitting the hoof wall with smaller size nails.
4. Shoes can be wider at the heels, providing more lateral stability.
5. Feet of unequal size can be shod with the same size shoe.
6. Less thrown shoes. When shoes are thrown, they are easier to replace.
7. Greater length of foot can be obtained with conventional large nails (#12 or #16). Triple nailing is possible to create extremely large buildups. Of course, this is rarely desirable.

Steps in using the double nailing technique:
1. Trim foot to specified angle and length.
2. Decide on build-up (desired toe-length or thickness).
3. Figure foot-toe to shoe-toe distance. Measure the angle of the toe. Decide how far back the shoe will extend. Using the Shoe Extension chart, figure the amount to be added to the overall length of the shoe. Figure the lateral and medial edge of the hoof at the mid-quarter to edge of shoe branch distance. Measure the angle(s) of the wall at mid-quarter. Using the Shoe Extension chart, figure the amount to be added to the overall width of the shoe. The number in the chart must be multiplied by two if only one side is measured. The Pad Build-Up Thickness chart is used when the trainer specifies toe length but not build-up thickness. Place chalk marks on anvil (write numbers on the side, mark lines on the horn).
4. Figure shoe stock length for specified weight and design (See steps in making toe-weighted shoes).
5. Make and fit or adjust old shoe and clip(s) at hoof angle. *Fit is critical* (toe around to quarters, width and length of heels). Heels should be wide enough to provide lateral stability but narrow enough to prevent limb interference. Toe may be wider than hoof outline to provide lateral stability.
6. Drill holes in shoe for heel pins and bands, if required.
7. Pin (rivet with shingle nails) the pad next to the shoe at the heels. Or, temporarily nail the pad to the shoe with horseshoe nails of correct head size. Cut or twist off horseshoe nails flush with the top pad after driving through the pad.
8. Notch pads (V) with a saber or band saw a little wider than the base of the clip. Or, notch each pad to fit the clip with hoof nippers starting with the bottom. Stack and

nail the pads together. If no clip, cut out each pad the shape of the shoe. Cut each individually on a pad cutter or with hoof nippers. The top pad or the DNP is the only one that must fit tight at the clip. It may need final shaping with a knife.

9. Stack pads to specified height (including DNP), fit tight against the clip and nail together and to the bottom pad with one or two nails from the ground surface. Cut the nails off flush with the foot surface.

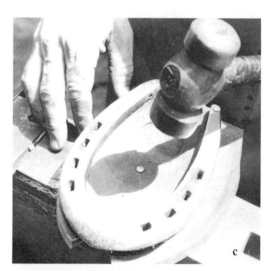

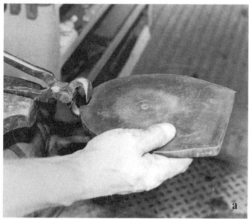

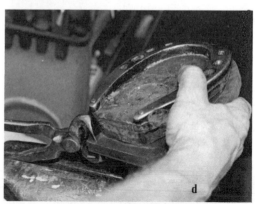

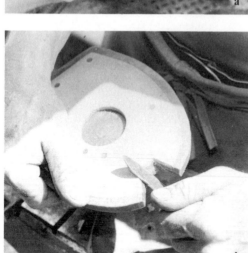

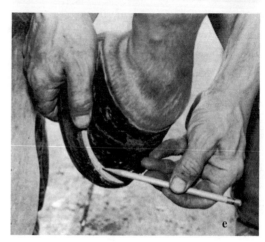

Fig. 41-16.   Steps in double nailing:
(a) The DNP (double nail pad) must be notched out for the shoe clip with nippers or saw.
(b) Final trimming with a knife may be necessary to get the DNP to fit tightly against the clip.
(c) Nail the pad (or stack) that is attached to the shoe to the DNP. Cut the nail(s) off flush with the foot surface of the DNP.
(d) Trim the DNP to roughly the same size as the shoe.
(e) Center the package on the foot (in relation to the shoe) and trace around the outer border of the wall. Mark the position of the nail holes so that nails enter sound wall.

10. Saw, nip, grind and/or rasp stack *perpendicular* to outside edge of shoe. Nip with shoe up and pad down. Hold saber saw next to foot surface of package. Place foot surface down on band saw table.

11. Go to foot with package and take the foot forward on your knee. Line up shoe with bottom of foot and trace on DNP or top pad. Use pen or pencil and trace perpendicular to foot. Mark nail position on edge of trace line of DNP. If the hoof is weak or broken, an irregular nail pattern may be required. If the hoof is sound, make hoof nail marks on DNP between shoe nail holes. Sketch in the

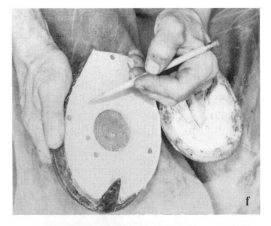

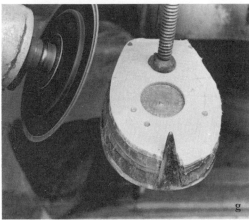

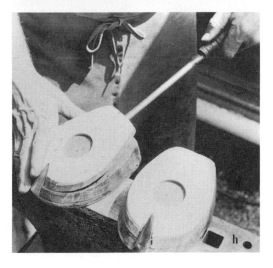

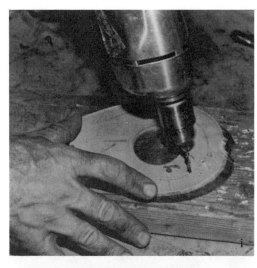

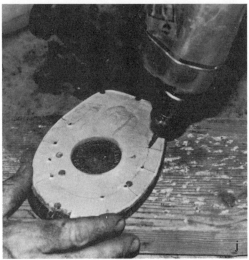

(f) *Estimate and sketch the white line on the DNP. Extend the lines marking the nail holes into the interior line.*
(g) *Grind the pads to within 1/8 inch of the wall outline.*
(h) *Separate the DNP from the package with a screwdriver.*
(i) *Drill holes on the inner line of the foot surface of the DNP.*
(j) *Drill holes at the angle of the wall. Ream out the center hole(s) from the build-up side.*

477

white line and make round marks where
hoof nail holes are to be drilled in DNP.
12. Grind the stack so you can see the hoof
outline (leave 1/8 inch between line and
edge of DNP). Pilot holes for the large shoe
nails may be drilled through the shoe nail
holes to the DNP with a long 5/32 inch drill
bit. This is optional.
13. Separate DNP from package with large screw
driver.
14. Drill holes with 1/8 inch bit from foot surface at the angle nail will be in the hoof.
(Not necessary if hoof wall is thick and 4
in. or more in length.) Ream the one or two
plug-in holes in center of DNP.

15. Put three (or four) positioning nails into DNP;
one at the center of the toe inside and touching the trace line (or two—one on each side
of the clip), one on each side inside the trace
line. Use small horse nails. Place with side
of nail against side of foot. Angle them in
slightly so they will hold the pad tight against
the foot.
16. Place DNP on foot while it is resting on
your knee to check centering. Bend nails to
center pad if necessary.
17. Pack the foot with hoof packing (medicated
peat moss[3] or pine tar and oakum).

[3] *Forshner's Medicated Hoof Packing, Foxboro, MA*

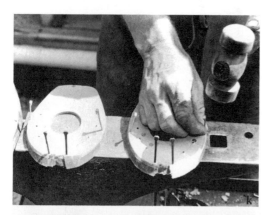
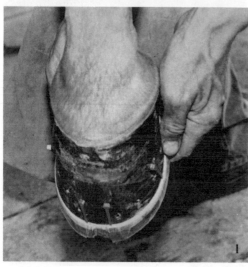
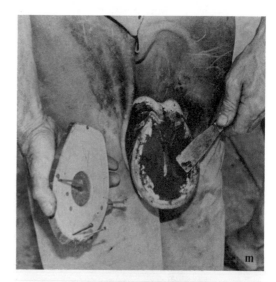
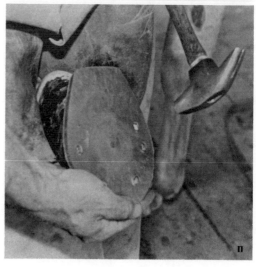

(k) Drive small positioning nails on each side of the clip
notch and at the mid-quarter to hold the DNP in place when
nailing on.
(l) Take the foot forward and check the alignment of
the DNP.
(m) Pack the foot with hoof packing.
(n) Center and nail on the DNP with No. 6 regular head
nails.

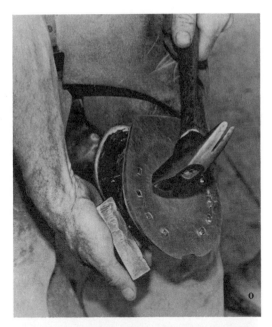

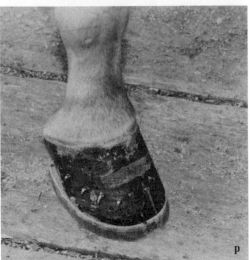

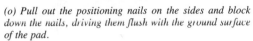

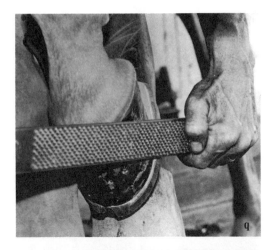

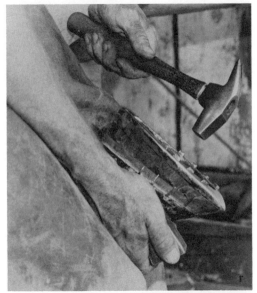

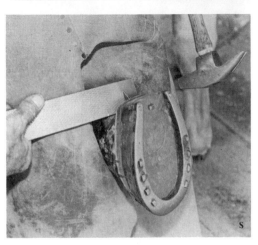

(o) Pull out the positioning nails on the sides and block down the nails, driving them flush with the ground surface of the pad.

(p) DNP ready for clinching.

(q) Clinch and finish the set of nails in the DNP before nailing the shoe on.

(r) Drive the nails into the shoe and through the package so they come out on the hoof edge of the DNP. Block them down.

(s) Drive a nail in between the shoe heels to hold down the back of the DNP and further secure the job.

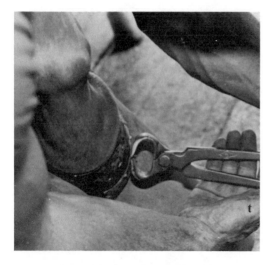

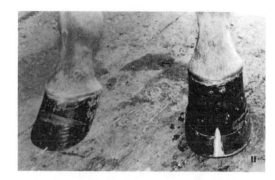

(t) Cut off the nail ends and clinch the shoe nails.
(u) Finish the foot with the smooth side of the rasp.

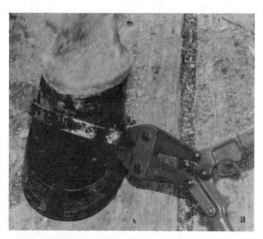

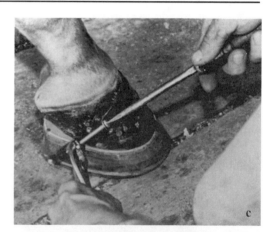

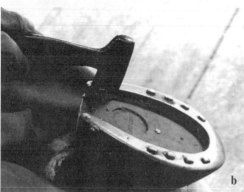

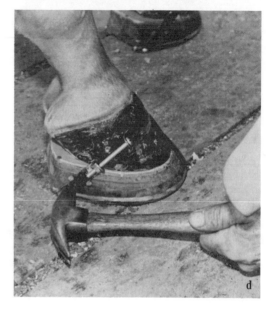

Fig. 41-17.   Bands: (a) Bands may be removed quickly by cutting the old bolt. (b) Band shoe bolts may be cut from the shoe with a clinch cutter. (c) Bands should be adjusted so they are about 3/4 inch below the coronary border of the hoof. Bands can be tightened when the horse is worked and loosened when it is in the stall. (d) Small screw shank nails may be used on each side to prevent the band from moving.

18. Line up heel of DNP with bulbs and nail DNP to hoof with eight to ten No. 6 regular nails. Pull out the three positioning nails. To pull nails set in DNP, use crease nail pullers.
19. Clinch hoof nails. Set the nails so that heads are flush with the DNP.
20. Line up and plug in the one or two center nails in the package.
21. Nail package to DNP with No. 8 to No. 16 nails. Larger nails are required in heel nail holes if wedges are used. Nails should exit next to the hoof through the leather on top of the DNP. Bend the nails over. Drive an appropriate length (#6 or #8) regular head horseshoe nail(s) into pads between the heels. Angle the nail(s) to come out on the edge of the DNP. A nail can be forced out and down against the DNP as it is driven by holding the clinch block flat against the hoof surface of the pad.
22. Clinch the shoe down to the DNP using a block and hammer. Cut clinches so they are longer than the width of the nail (1/4 in. or more in length).
23. Take the foot forward on your knee or a stand. Hold the clinch block under the nail heads in the shoe and drive the clinches into the edge of the DNP.
24. Rasp clinches lightly. Use the fine side of the rasp and rasp in a rotary motion to polish the hoof and pads and achieve a smooth edge all around the pads.

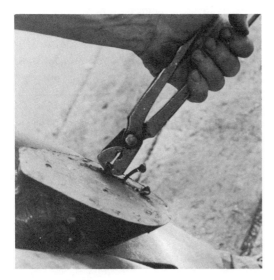

Fig. 41-18. Crease nail pullers are used to remove nails from the DNP when resetting shoes. New DNP's are used at each shoeing.

25. Put on bands (if used). Place ring shank nails in front and behind bands to hold bands in place and prevent pressure on the coronary band. Bands should be adjusted so they are 1/2 to 3/4 inch below the hair line at the toe. The bands should be bolted to holes drilled in the side of the heels of the shoe on shorter build-ups. Bands may be attached by screw type nails driven into wedges near the shoe on higher build-ups containing thick heel wedges. Fill in broken spaces around the hoof with plastic wood mixed with contact cement.

A double nail job can be taken off the foot by following the steps in reverse order. Crease nail pullers are necessary to pull nails from the DNP. Or, the clinches may be cut on the nails in the hoof and a long screwdriver inserted under the heel and the entire package may be pried from the foot. It then may be secured in a vise and taken apart.

Shoes for gaited horses are usually heavier than conventional horseshoes. They are called weighted shoes and their names describe the position of the weight in the shoe: shoes may be toe-weighted, side-weighted, or heel-weighted. Shoes may be purchased ready-made or drawn from 3/8 x 1 or 1/2 x 1 or 1 1/4 inch bar stock. Shoes are also made from 5/8 and 3/4 inch round stock. Occasionally, a trainer will call for a shoe of heavier dimensions. Standard toe-weighted shoes can be used, even in cases where more weight is called for, if lead weight is inserted in between the pads at the toe or wherever desired.

The toes are usually rolled (beveled from the foot surface back under the toe) from one toe nail to the other on Saddlebred horseshoes. Toes are usually not rolled on Walking Horse shoes. Shoe style influences the action of the limbs according to the following principles:

1. **Flat toe-weighted shoes** with no roll extend the leg's reach. They make a horse use its forearm muscles. The momentum created by the weight makes the horse carry its foot forward.
2. **Half-round weighted shoes** or toe-weights with rolled toes increase the leg's fold. This is often referred to as snap, animation, or motion. The roll makes a horse use its shoulder muscles. The faster a horse goes (at the rack), the more roll is needed to maintain motion and avoid limb interference. The roll extends from one side of the toe to the other.

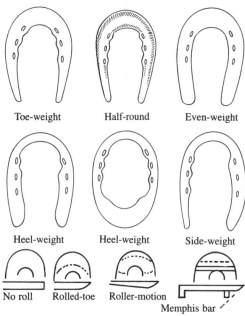

| Toe-weight | Half-round | Even-weight |
| Heel-weight | Heel-weight | Side-weight |

No roll   Rolled-toe   Roller-motion

Memphis bar

Fig. 41-19. Shoe design for gaited horses: (top) types of weighted shoes, (bottom) types of shoe toes.

3. **Even-weighted shoes** prevent over folding. Over folding may be caused by toe-weights. A horse that over folds may get off in its timing at speed. Even-weighted shoes support the heels, prevent sinking, thus increasing breakover speed. An even-weighted shoe allows more weight for a given stock size and is therefore used on Walking Horses.

4. **Roller-motion shoes** are toe-weighted shoes, often made from round stock, with a combination of flatness and roundness that both extend the reach and increase the snap and fold of the legs. The horse lands flat on the heel and rolls off the bulge. This requires increased effort and the use of the forearm muscles. The roll makes the horse use the shoulder muscles.

5. **Heel-weighted shoes** cause a horse to reach forward. The momentum created by the weight causes the foot to go forward. However, changing the angle of the foot usually has more effect on action than heel weights. Thus, heel-weighted shoes are rarely used. Heel-weighted shoes may be open-heeled or bar shoes. The bar is usually welded where the stock is the smallest dimension (at the toe).

6. **Side-weighted shoes** are sometimes used on the hind feet of racking horses to prevent crossfiring. They may also be used to throw a horse off balance when training a horse to rack. Rarely, a side-weighted shoe may be used to stabilize a foot (front or hind) in

flight. Side weights are most often applied to the outside of hind feet and the inside of front feet. The side weight is only effective on horses with very limber or flexible joints.

Position of weight and type of roll are cancelled when the horse's weight limit is reached. The horse then has an undesirable laboring action that is no longer beautiful. Fatigue from lack of conditioning and overwork can also create a laboring action, even when the correct weight and roll are used.

A heavy duty postage scale is a necessity for gaited-horse farriers. A chart showing the ounces per inch of the various stock sizes is useful. A draw chart is also helpful. Of course, many experienced shoers are able to accurately estimate the weight of a completed shoe. Stock can be cut up ahead of time and the length and weight of each piece can be written on the blanks with chalk. You can also make up turned and punched shoes for adaptation on the job. Or, you can buy turned and tapered blanks or punched shoes from a supplier.

You must learn how much to draw a piece of stock to get it to look and weigh the way you want it to. You can usually figure on losing 2 or 3 ounces per shoe due to scaling, punching, and finishing the heels. Most weight loss is from scaling since less than one ounce is lost when punching nail holes. A welded-on toe clip or jar calk will add about 1 ounce each. A Memphis bar will add 2 to 3 ounces.

Weighted shoes must be punched relatively coarse (nail holes close to the inside edge) in order to prevent splitting the wall when doing a regular nailing job and to get the nails to come out in the DNP next to the hoof when double nailing.

Steps in making a *handmade toe-weight* shoe with a rolled-toe:

1. Measure the foot to determine the length and width of the shoe. This may be calculated using the Shoe Extension chart in this chapter. You must know the desired length of hoof from coronary band to the shoe and the hoof angle at the toe and midquarter.

2. Write the shoe length and width measurements on the side of your anvil with chalk. Make two chalk marks on the horn of your anvil at these distances from the step between the horn and face. These will be points of reference while making and shaping the shoe.

3. Twice the length of the shoe plus two times the stock width (e.g., 1 in.) will give a rough estimate of the length of a tapered blank. Two times the length of the shoe minus the stock width (e.g., 1 in.) will give a rough estimate of the untapered stock length.

ESTIMATED INCREASE IN STOCK LENGTH (DRAW) AND WEIGHT LOSS OF TOE-WEIGHT TAPERED SHOE BLANKS

	Width of Stock (Web) in Inches			
	¾	1	1¼	1½
Subtracted from tapered blank to get stock size (in.)	1½	2	2½	3
Added to stock on each branch to get anvil mark (in.)	¾	1	1¼	1½
Subtract from stock weight as forging weight loss (oz.) (varies with thickness —⅜ or ½ in.)	1 or 2	2 or 3	2 or 3	3 or 4

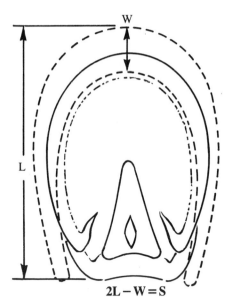

$$2L - W = S$$

L = Toe to heel distance of the finished shoe
W = Width of stock
S = Undrawn length of stock

Fig. 41-20. Steps in making a toe-weighted shoe with a rolled-toe:
(a) Figure the shoe stock size and draw.
(b) Figure the draw and mark the anvil.
(c) Estimate the weight of the finished shoe.

Draw stock to at least twice its width

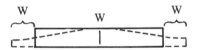

a

b

ESTIMATED DRAW CHART FOR TOE-WEIGHTED SHOES

1. Length of Tapered Blank (in.)
2. Distance from Center to End of Blank (in.)

	Width of Stock (Web) in Inches							
	¾		1		1¼		1½	
Length of Stock (in.)	1	2	1	2	1	2	1	2
10	11.50	5.75	12.00	6.00	12.50	6.25	13.00	6.50
11	12.50	6.25	13.00	6.50	13.50	6.75	14.00	7.00
12	13.50	6.75	14.00	7.00	14.50	7.25	15.00	7.50
13	14.50	7.25	15.00	7.50	15.50	7.75	16.00	8.00
14	15.50	7.75	16.00	8.00	16.50	8.25	17.00	8.50
15	16.50	8.25	17.00	8.50	17.50	8.75	18.00	9.00

ESTIMATED WEIGHT CHART FOR TOE-WEIGHTED SHOES

c

1. Approximate Finished Shoe Weight (oz.) ⅜ in. stock thickness
2. Approximate Finished Shoe Weight (oz.) ½ in. stock thickness

	Width of Stock (Web) in Inches							
	¾		1		1¼		1½	
Length of Stock (in.)	1	2	1	2	1	2	1	2
10	10.00	15.00	15.00	19.75	19.25	25.50	22.50	30.00
11	13.00	16.75	16.75	22.00	21.25	28.25	25.00	33.50
12	14.25	18.50	18.50	25.25	23.50	31.00	27.50	36.75
13	15.50	20.25	20.25	26.50	25.50	34.00	30.25	40.25
14	16.75	22.00	22.00	28.75	27.75	36.75	32.75	43.50
15	18.00	23.75	23.75	31.00	29.75	39.50	35.25	47.00

4. Figure the weight of the finished shoe. The size of bar stock that requires the least drawing and tapering to get the required weight is usually the most desirable. Estimate the amount the finished shoe will weigh. Allow about 2 ounces for 3/8 inch and 3 ounces for 1/2 inch more weight in a piece of stock than requested to allow for weight loss from scaling, nail hole punching, and hot rasping the heels. Weight of shoe accessories can be estimated by the use of the charts found in Chapter 25. Welded on clips weigh about 1 ounce each; Memphis bars about 3 ounces. Soon you will be able to estimate the weight of the various steel sizes without the chart(s).

WEIGHT OF FLAT MILD STEEL IN OUNCES PER LINEAR INCH

Thickness in Inches	Width (web) in Inches			
	¾	1	1¼	1½
⅜	1.27	1.71	2.12	2.55
½	1.71	2.27	2.84	3.40

5. Cut the stock the appropriate length with a shear, torch or sledge and handled cold cutter. Make a center punch mark in the middle of the stock.

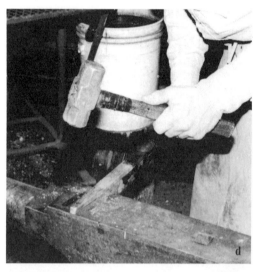

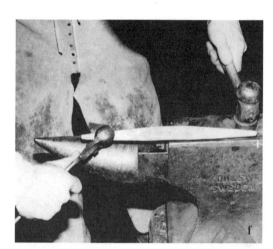

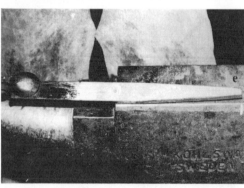

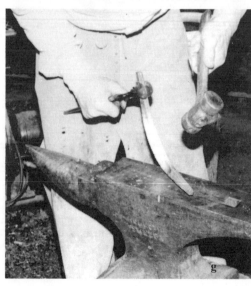

(d) Draw out one branch of the shoe by alternately striking each side of the stock until the end is square.
(e) Periodically check the length against the chalk mark showing the desired draw.
(f) Draw the other branch until it is the correct length.

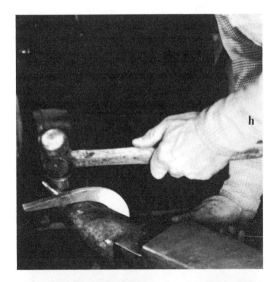

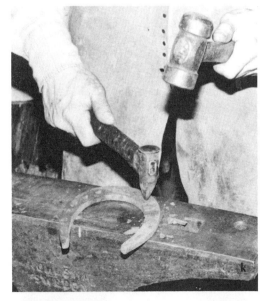

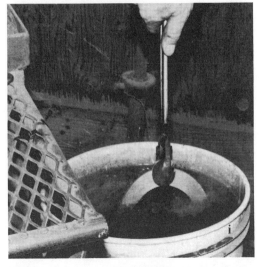

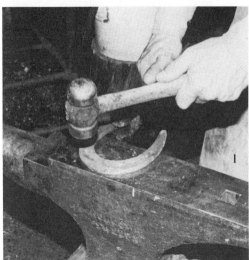

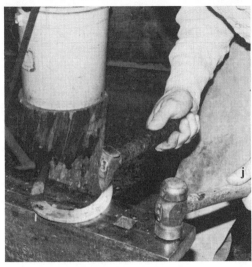

(g) Turn the toe as round as possible.

(h) Finish the toe bend over the horn. Be sure it is centered and round.

(i) Uneven heating can be centered by quenching both branches.

(j) Turn and punch the outside branch.

(k) Turn and punch the inside branch.

(l) Hold the shoe near the edge of the anvil and roll the toe from one toe nail hole to the other.

6. Heat the stock with the web facing the fire for half its length. Stagger the heating time so that one shoe of a pair is being worked while the other is heating. Use box tongs to hold the stock firmly by one end.

7. Draw out the entire branch from about 1 to 2 inches (this varies with the length of the stock) away from the center punch mark to the end. The stock should be struck the same number of times on one edge as the other to avoid distortion. Work toward a goal of drawing each branch on a heavy shoe in two or three heats. The ends should be the thickness of the stock square when you are finished. The edges of the stock should be slightly rounded with the hammer. The distance from the center punch mark to the end should be marked on your anvil for quick reference (See Step 2). Note that the amount the stock is lengthened by the tapering varies with the width of the stock web. Estimated weights can be figured using figures estimating the weight loss per shoe due to forging and finishing.

8. Taper and draw the other branch. You may desire to use smaller box tongs to hold the drawn end of the stock.

9. Heat the middle two-thirds of the shoe.

10. Turn the toe. Make the toe very round. This will give the horse lots of lateral support and it will make it easier to keep the toe the proper shape after you roll it. Some shoers use a toe bender to help them "break the toe" or start the bend in shoes made of heavy stock. However, a toe bender tends to make the toe too narrow.

11. Heat the branch from the center of the stock to the heel.

12. Finish turning the branch. The branch will straighten slightly when the nail holes are punched coarse (toward the inside edge). Punch three or four nail holes on a side, depending upon the size of the shoe. Mark the outside branch.

13. Heat, finish turning and punch the other branch.

14. Heat the toe and roll the toe of the shoe. The roll should extend from one side of the toe to the other. Start with a broad, almost square toe, as rolling the toe tends to point it.

15. A toe clip should be welded on. This may be done in the forge or with a welder. Many shoers use sheared clips and a portable welder.

16. Check the heel length and cut the heels if necessary.

17. Heat and finish both heels. Work toward a goal of completing a pair of shoes in 1 hour.

Steps in *forge welding a toe clip* onto a toe-weighted shoe:

1. Heat the toe and place it over the off corner of the anvil with the ground surface up. Smash the toe over the corner and draw out a short ear from the center of the toe. This ear can also be made on an anvil clip horn, if available.

2. Prepare the clip stock. Heat one end of an 18 inch piece of 1/4 x 3/4 inch bar stock. Upset, round and bevel the end.

3. Flux the foot surface of the shoe toe and place it back in the fire.

4. Flux the clip stock end while at a yellow heat and place back in the fire.

5. Adjust the two pieces in the fire until the flux is melting on both. The clip will usually be placed higher in the fire.

6. Remove both pieces from the fire when they simultaneously reach a welding heat. The shoe will be held in the tongs with the heels away from you and the foot surface up. Place the end of the clip stock fluxed side down on the edge and in the middle of the

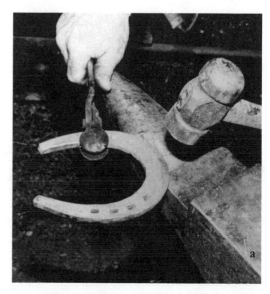

Fig. 41-21. *Steps in forge welding a toe clip onto a toe-weighted shoe.*
(a) Smash the center of the toe over the off corner of the anvil.
(b) Draw a small ear or clip from this area.
(c) Taper and point the clip stock.
(d) Flux the shoe and clip and adjust them in the fire.
(e) Place the shoe and clip together on the anvil and hold the shoe in place with the clip stock.
(f) Drop the tongs and smash the clip into the shoe.
(g) Flip the shoe over and smash the shoe into the clip.

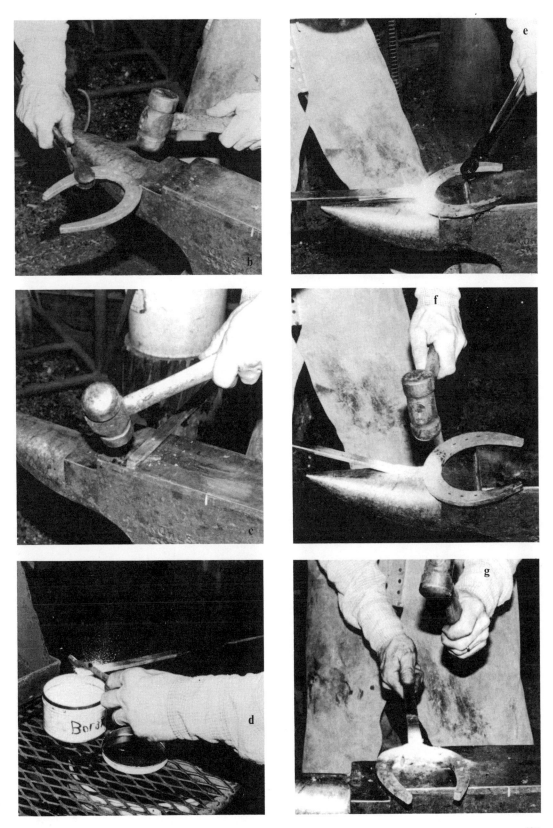

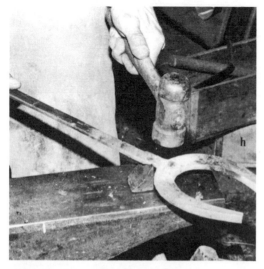

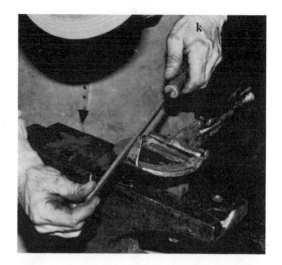

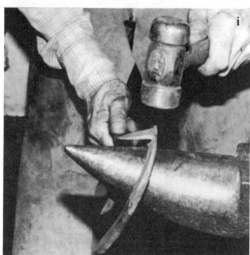

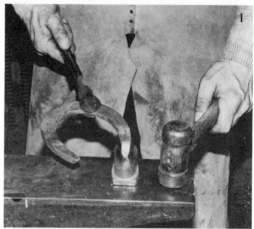

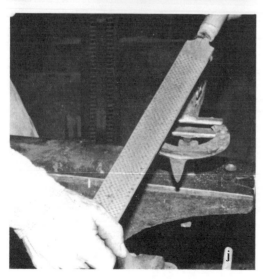

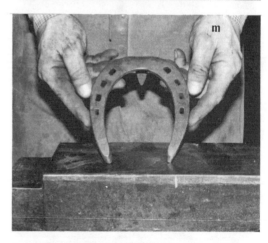

(h) Cut the clip off on the hardy.
(i) Weld, draw and shape the clip.
(j) Rasp the rolled-toe smooth.
(k) File the clip smooth.
(l) Mark and cut the heels.
(m) The finished shoe.

shoe toe with about 1/2 inch or more projecting over it. Push down against the shoe with the clip stock holding the shoe in place. Drop your shoe tongs and pick up your hammer. Strike softly in the middle of the area to be welded. Quickly strike several more harder blows on the edges of the weld until it sticks. Flip the shoe over by rolling the clipping stock in your tong hand. Try to get the metal stuck on the edges only on the ground surface. Stop striking when the flux quits running and the metal stops sparking.

7. While the metal is still hot, cut the clip off on the hardy. Cut it about 3/8 to 1/2 inch from the shoe and the full length of the hardy.

8. Straighten the clip and bend it over the edge of the anvil toward the foot surface. This will open the ground surface of the weld. Shape the clip edges with the hammer.

9. Reflux and heat the shoe to a welding heat with the clip up in the fire.

10. Weld the clip with the shoe against the off side of the anvil and the clip on the anvil face. Draw the clip. The heel of the anvil may work best for this operation. Immediately move to the horn and round the toe smoothing and angling in the clip to coincide with the angle of the hoof. Straighten the clip if necessary. Leave it at least 1/8 inch thick at the base. These shoes have to be reset many times.

11. Rasp the roll of the toe smooth. File and finish the clip half-round so it follows the contour of the foot.

12. Check the fit, mark and cut the shoe heels.

Shoe accessories such as Memphis bars, jar calks and spooned heels may be brazed on with an oxy-acetylene torch or in the forge. This way they can be easily removed by reheating the shoe if the horse's requirements change and they are no longer needed. Some shoers prefer to weld on accessories due to the difficulty of heating and adjusting shoes that have been brazed. Memphis bars are pieces of small diameter (1/4 in. to 3/8 in.) round or square stock that extend the width of the shoe an inch or so back off the toe of the hind shoes. They create a snappy roller motion effect. They are mostly used to improve hock action and occasionally to shorten stride and prevent limb interference. Jar calks stabilize a foot and prevent it from twisting at the moment of breaking over. Spooned heels prevent a horse that occasionally crossfires at the rack from tearing shoes off the front feet.

Heel calks are used to hold a front foot from going forward, to add more weight for length of steel and to elevate and stabilize the hind legs. Calks may be turned at a right angle and upset (usually on the hind feet of Saddlebreds) or turned over against the shoe (usually on the front shoes of Walking Horses). A sharp bar drawn and turned in from a heel, or added (like a Memphis bar) and welded across the heel calks, shortens the stride even more than calks. This accessory may be necessary to prevent crossfiring of some gaited horses.

Toe clips stabilize shoes on long-footed horses. There is a tendency for shoes to slip back and portions of the foot to break away when using large nails driven into long hoofs and through several pads. Double nailing is a great improvement when a big build-up is required. But, for most Saddlebreds, only two or three pads are used. Clips help stabilize these shoes. Side clips are used on hind shoes because of the strain on the nails created by calks or Memphis bars and the lateral twisting of the feet.

Lead truck-tire weights or molded weights can be moved around on a foot by nailing or screwing to the side or bottom of a pad stack. Once the desired position is determined, the weight can be incorporated into the next set of shoes or put in between cut-out pads. Exposed lead is no longer acceptable in most horse show classes. Aluminum molds for making several different weights of lead inserts are available[4].

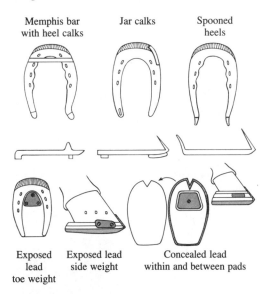

Memphis bar with heel calks   Jar calks   Spooned heels

Exposed lead toe weight   Exposed lead side weight   Concealed lead within and between pads

[4] *Curtis Hamilton, Easley, SC*

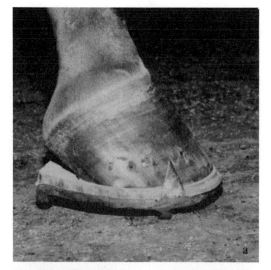

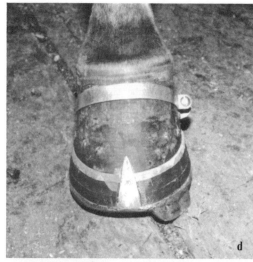

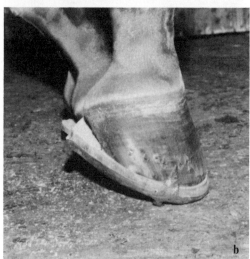

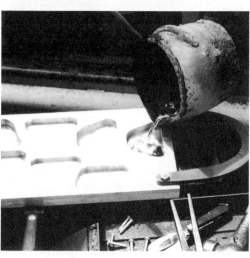

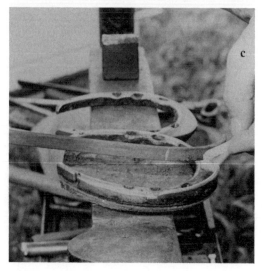

Fig. 41-22. Shoe accessories:
(a) Memphis bar with heel calks and welded-on side clips on a hind foot.
(b) Memphis bars create extra snap or hock action when a horse is moving, yet provide stability when it is standing.
(c) Jar calks prevent a foot from twisting at the moment of breakover.
(d) Left front foot shod with forge-welded clip, jar calk and band.
(e) Molten lead that has been heated in the forge being poured into the mold.
(f) Lead is dumped out and allowed to air cool.
(g) Lead weight being drilled for screws.
(h) Pilot holes being drilled into the pad.
(i) Lead weight being attached to the toe with screws.
(j) Lead weight attached in the heel.
(k) Lead weight nailed to the inside of a rear pad.

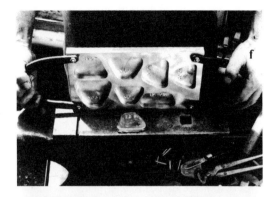

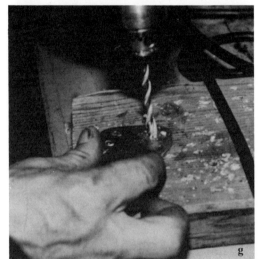

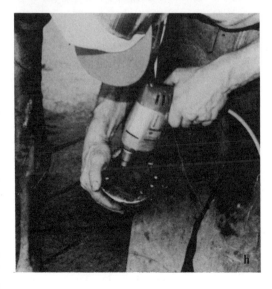

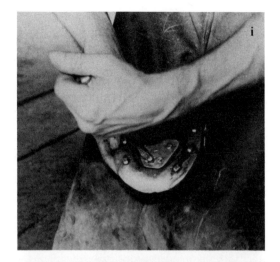

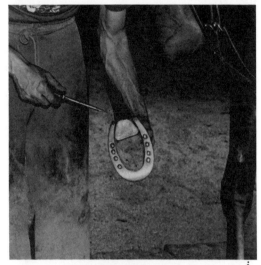

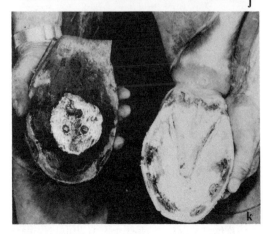

Gaited Horse Divisions

The breeds, types and horse show divisions of gaited horses may be grouped to consider information of interest to shoers of show horses: 1) Hackney, Harness, and Shetland Ponies, 2) Roadsters, 3) Saddle, Parade and Morgan horses, and 4) Tennessee Walking Horses. The least shoe weight (excluding nails) and toe length (hair line to ground) is allowed on Paso Finos (10 oz., 4 1/2 in.) and Arabians (12 oz., 4 1/2 in.). The most shoe weight and toe length is usually found on the Tennessee Walking Horse (no shoe weight or toe length limit). The gaited horse shoer should carefully study outstanding horses in the various horse show classes in order to fix in his mind the ideal way of going for each type.

Hackney, Harness, and Shetland Ponies

Hackney ponies have the snappiest action of the gaited breeds. They naturally show extreme knee fold and hock action when compared to the other horse breeds. However, training and shoeing by adding weight and toe length accentuates this action. Many types of artificial appliances or action creating devices are employed to create the animated effect. Knee and hock action and brilliance are more important than speed in this type.

Hackney ponies are shod with small heavy shoes. They are very straight in the branches. The hind shoes are usually calked. They may or may not have a rolled toe. Hackneys have so much action that it is difficult to keep them from hitting their elbows. Increasing the angle of the foot may prevent elbow hitting.

Hackney or harness ponies may be shown in various hitch combinations at the park pace and smart trot ("show your pony"). Speed is not a consideration. A few classes require walking and backing. Ponies may be shown in light harness (breast strap pulling a light vehicle or viceroy) or heavy harness (neck collar pulling a heavy vehicle or park drag) depending on the type of vehicle they are shown to. Hackney and harness ponies are shown to various vehicles including a viceroy, miniature side rail buggy, gig, park drag and road coach.

Harness ponies may or may not be purebred Hackney. Hackney ponies are exhibited with a short mane braided and short (docked) tail. Harness ponies are exhibited with a long mane and undocked tail. Ponies cannot be cross entered. Harness ponies are smaller Hackney or crossbred ponies and cannot be over 12.2 hands. Hackney ponies must be under 14.2 hands and may be divided into two groups, above and below 13 hands. Hackney horses are over 14.2 hands and are used for pulling road vehicles of various types.

Shetland harness ponies are trained and shod similar to harness ponies. Shetlands are smaller than Hackneys and cannot exceed 11.2 hands. Shetlands and Hackneys are frequently crossed to produce Harness ponies.

Shetland ponies shown in the junior exhibitors pleasure driving class must be shown with unweighted keg shoes (no pads or weight) or barefoot. Ponies shown in Draft Harness pony classes must be shown with a natural barefoot or a light show plate or draft type shoe with toe and heel calks. Pads are allowed but additional weight is prohibited. Ponies one year of age and older should be shod when shown in breeding classes.

Welsh ponies may be shown as harness ponies. However, if they are also to be shown in breed classes (within the AHSA Welsh division) they must conform to AHSA Shoeing rules. Toe-length cannot be longer than 4 inches, and the shoe (excluding nails but including the pad) must not weight more than 10 ounces for Section A ponies. Section B ponies may not have more than a 4 1/2 inch toe and a 12 ounce shoe. Ponies shown in Breeding classes must be shown barefoot or shod with foot natural, no weight or pads allowed.

Roadsters

Roadsters are of standard (Standardbred) or trotting type. There are roadster horses and roadster ponies. Recently, the Saddlebred division has designated its own roadster type without Standardbred influence. There are two horse types: those suitable for a bike (two-wheeled cart) and those suitable for a road wagon. Those suitable for a wagon are generally the largest of the two, but cross entering is allowed. Both horse and pony roadsters have a full mane and tail. Roadsters trot at three different speeds: 1) the slow jog trot, 2) the fast road gait, and 3) at full speed ("drive on"). Occasionally, they may be asked to walk as a rest. At all speeds they should work in an animated and collected form. They are trained and shod to enhance their natural action or form, but not in a way to sacrifice speed.

Saddle, Parade and Morgan Horses

American Saddlebred Horses have been referred to as the "peacocks of the show ring" and the "most beautiful horse in the world". They possess a very high head carriage on a finely arched neck and have a straight croup. The Saddle Horse breed was developed in Kentucky for the use of the Southern pioneers. These highly refined animals later became the society horse of the plantation owners. They were unique in their ability to do the rack and show brilliant showing presence. They became *the* show horse.

Saddle Horses are shown in four sections: 1) Three-gaited, 2) Five-gaited, 3) Fine Harness, and 4) Pleasure Horse. These are distinct types of horses and are not shown in more than one division at any one time.

The Three-Gaited Saddle Horse is also referred to as a Walk, Trot horse. They are shown at three gaits: 1) an animated walk, 2) a graceful collected trot, and 3) a slow, easy, collected canter. Three-gaited horses are shown with a roached mane and trimmed tail. They are shod

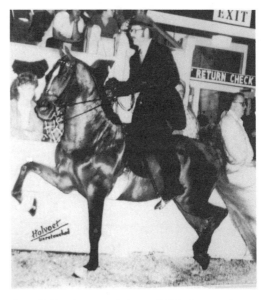

Fig. 41-24. Five-gaited horse. Folly's Supreme Dream ridden by Bobby Morrison. Photo by Holvoet.

with comparatively heavy shoes and do not wear quarter boots.

The Five-Gaited Saddle Horse does the three gaits of the Three-Gaited horse plus an additional two gaits: 4) the slow gait (a slow, high, animated, collected gait) and 5) the rack (a four-beat speed gait done in form). They are true gaited horses. Trainers often make this distinction by calling only five-gaited horses: "gaited horses". Five-Gaited horses are shown with a full mane and tail. They are shod with comparatively light shoes and may wear quarter boots to prevent crossfiring injury at speed.

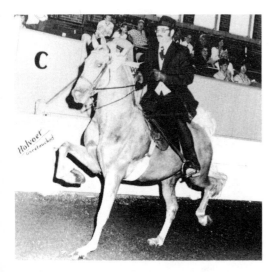

Fig. 41-23. Three-gaited horse. McClure's Super Star ridden by Bobby Morrison. Photo by Holvoet.

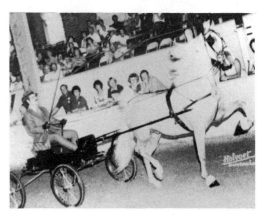

Fig. 41-25. Fine harness horse. McClure's Super Supreme driven by Bobby Morrison. Photo by Holvoet.

493

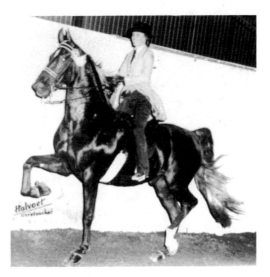

Fig. 41-26. Saddlebred pleasure horse. Elegant Example ridden by Lynn Morrison. Photo by Holvoet.

The Fine Harness Saddlebred Horse is shown to an appropriate viceroy type vehicle (a small buggy with four wire wheels and no top) at two gaits: 1) an animated and graceful walk, and 2) an animated Park Trot. The command "Show Your Horse" may be given in some classes. This implies a faster gait than a Park Trot. Fine Harness horses are shown with full manes and tails. They must stand quietly.

The Saddlebred Pleasure Horse may be shown as a Three-Gaited (English or Western tack), Five-Gaited or Fine Harness driving horse. The jog trot (free moving and slow) and lope (slow, smooth and straight) are substituted for the trot and canter in the Western class. Seventy-five percent of the score in a pleasure class is determined by the quality of performance (ground covering action) and apparent ability to give a good pleasure ride. Pleasure horses are shown with a full mane and tail. Tails must be carried naturally.

Weighted shoes, shoe bands and pads are permitted on most pleasure horses. However, Country Pleasure horses must be plain shod without pads or bands. Toe-weight keg shoes are often used on these horses.

Each of the sections for Saddlebreds is also offered for ponies under 14.2 hands at many shows. They do the same things as the large animals and are usually ridden by junior exhibitors. Shetland or Shetland-Saddlebred crossed are most popular for these classes.

Saddlebred Horses (as well as other breeds) may be shown in the Saddle Type, Western Equipment class. Colorful appearance, animated and collected action are stressed. Animals may be divided by color. Pinto and palomino horses are popular for this class. It is similar to the Parade class, except the saddles and clothing are not as elaborate and the horses are shown at

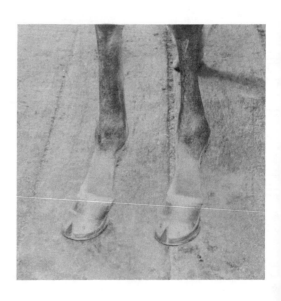

Fig. 41-27. Saddlebred weanlings are frequently shod when they are shown. (Left) Weanling trained to stretch, (right) weanling shoes. Photos by J. Graves.

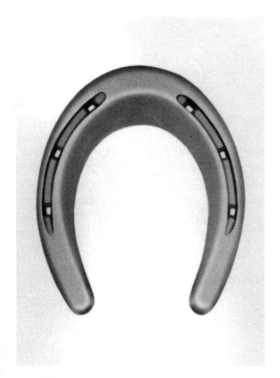

Fig. 41-28. Machine-made toe-weighted shoe for pleasure and trail horses. Photo from Diamond.

three gaits instead of two for Parade horses. The three gaits are: 1) a flat-footed and elastic walk, 2) a collected, high action, balanced trot, and 3) a smooth, easy, collected and straight canter.

The Parade Horse must be a beautiful and stylish animal that is sound and free from blemish. Horses may be of any color or breed, but Palomino Saddlebred type is preferred. Parade horses are shown with a full mane and tail at two gaits: 1) an animated walk, and 2) a high prancing parade gait. The parade gait cannot be faster than 5 mph (miles per hour). The walk must be slow enough to differentiate between the walk and the parade gait. Manners, standing quietly and staying in the required gaits are stressed because of their obvious importance in a parade. Elaborate and expensive saddles, tack and costumes are traditional in this class. Since parade horses go so slow, they are often shod with very heavy shoes and long toes. Shoes, of whatever type, may be treated with borium to prevent slipping on paved roads.

The Morgan Horse originated in Vermont from one horse, Justin Morgan. It has been one of the most versatile breeds from its beginning. The Morgan division offers several unique classes to demonstrate the breed's versatility. In recent years Morgans have been trained and shown in much the same way as the three-gaited and fine harness American Saddlebred. However, emphasis is on natural breed type and movement. Morgans are increasing in popularity as carriage horses. They have always been good endurance horses.

Long toes and heavily weighted shoes are penalized in Pleasure, Natural Park and Stock classes. Shoes including pads (excluding nails; no allowance made for wet leather pads) must not weigh more than 18 ounces (Lead shot is sometimes mixed with the hoof packing). Toe length cannot be more than 4 3/4 inches (hair line to ground). In other classes, toe length cannot exceed 5 3/4 inches but weight of shoe and pads has no specific weight limits.

All Morgans must be shod open heeled without bars, turnbuckles or bands. Weight attached to the exterior of the hoof or pad is prohibited. At all Morgan shows, all champions and reserve champions must have one foot measured immediately upon leaving the ring.

Tennessee Walking Horses

Walking Horses are very popular in some areas as a show or a pleasure horse. One of the best attended horseshows in the U.S. is the Annual Walking Horse Celebration at Shelbyville, Tennessee.

The Walking Horse breed was developed from several breeds. The Thoroughbred contributed strength and stamina; the Saddlebred, a quiet disposition and aptitude for the running walk; the Morgan, a stout handsome look; and the Standardbred, long stride and speed. The result is a rugged horse that is heavier boned than the other light breeds.

Walking Horses were originally bred as Southern plantation horses and called Tennessee Pacers. They were selected for their ability to smoothly travel down straight crop rows for many miles each day. Today's show horse is highly selected and trained. Tennessee Walking Horses are distinguished from any other breed by the nodding of the head and walking up under themselves behind.

The running walk is a four-beat gait in which all four feet strike the ground at separate intervals with the hind foot overstriding the footprint of the lateral front foot by 2 to 4 feet.

Walking Horses are shown at three gaits: 1) the flat walk (true, square and flat with a cadenced head motion), 2) the running walk (free, easy, smooth, overstepping, four-beat gait with stride length and head motion) and 3) the canter (smooth, straight, rolling motion).

Two and three year old horses and those shown by junior exhibitors are not required to do the canter. Plantation walking horses are shown at the plantation gait (an extended but relaxed flat walk) instead of the running walk. In the two wheel bike class, horses are shown at an extended running walk instead of the canter.

Hoof bands are allowed to assist in holding onto the hoof the heavy shoes and "pad packages, set ups or platforms" in all classes except the Plantation class. Most Walking horses are shod using the double nailing process due to the excessive hoof length required.

Exposed lead or other similar weight attached to the outside of hoof pad or shoe is prohibited in all classes. Added weight (lead, lead shot, ball bearings in oil, mercury or mercury block)

is permitted inside the pads or hollow shoes (Instant Walkin' Shoe[5]).

The height of the heel must be at least 1 inch less than the length of the toe. Boots and action devices (chains, etc.) are permitted in Park Pleasure but prohibited in Show Pleasure classes. Plantation Walking Horses must be plain shod as for trail riding (no pads, boots or action devices), and shoes cannot be made from metal larger than 1/2 inch in thickness or 1 1/2 inches in width (web). The shoe must be open with no other added weight inside. However, calks are allowed.

Walking ponies are under 14.2 hands and are ridden by a junior exhibitor (11 years and under).

Soring and the Horse Protection Act

The Walking Horse division is now regulated by the (Federal) Horse Protection Act of 1979 as amended. Visual inspections and thermovision examinations are made by designated officials to reduce the incidence of soring in the pastern and foot areas of these horses. Owners, trainers, riders and horseshoers may be subject to penalty for cruel practices.

Soring is the use of pain to accentuate a horse's

[5] Joe Webb, Searcy, AR

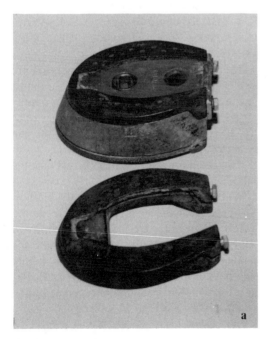

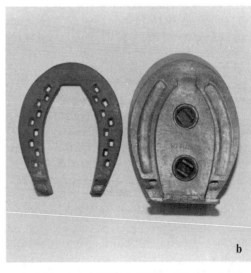

Fig. 41-29. Instant Walkin' shoes for Tennessee Walking Horses. Side view (a) and top view (b). Photos by J. Graves.

gait. Sored horses began to appear in the show ring in the early 1950's and reached their peak in the late 1960's. Soring is a short cut to the patient hard work of extensive training it takes to make a champion Walking Horse. Sored horses imitate the performance (called the Big Lick) of a sound, well trained horse.

Soring causes the front pastern and hoof area to be so sore that movement and the bearing of weight causes pain. The horse compensates by placing the hind feet farther forward and under himself to get the weight off the front feet. When the front feet come in contact with the ground, they are folded and snapped forward quickly. Combined with long hoofs and weighted shoes, the result is a high, far reaching action with the front feet and a long stretching stride with the hind feet. When done in proper rhythm, the action produced is called the Big Lick.

Chemical irritants (mustard oil or mercury blisters better known as scootin' juice, creepin' cream or Reach) or mechanical irritants (chain, wood, or metal bracelets and heavy knocker boots) are applied in the coronary region to create the sored horse. Tacks or nails may be driven in the sole or acid injected into the sensitive sole and frog. A technique known as "pressure shoeing" has also been used to sore horses.

Fierce competition causes many in the business to adopt soring practices. Unscrupulous individuals were known to engage in excessively cruel practices and make mediocre horses beat sound well trained horses. This brought the press and finally the public down on the Walking Horse industry in the late 1960's. Soring has also been practiced to a limited extent by Saddlebred and Racking horse trainers.

The (Federal) Horse Protection act was passed by Congress in 1970 and has been amended several times. It calls for inspection of horses at horse shows by DQP's (designated qualified persons) and the barring from competition by the show management of sored horses. Sponsors and managers may not hold shows that include sored horses, drivers may not haul sored horses across state lines, and owners, trainers or riders may not ride sored horses. Horses exhibiting signs of soreness must be immmediately excused from the ring. Horses foaled after Oct. 1, 1971, with any bilateral scar, callous or granulated tissue on the pastern or coronet areas indicative of soring are not eligible to be shown in any Walking Horse Performance Class.

DQP's must be fully aware of how a sored horse travels in comparison to a sound horse at the various gaits. Persons seeing a Walking Horse class for the first time may think that all the horses are sore and uncoordinated.

Clinical signs of soring when the horse is *at rest* are (after Nelson and Osheim, 1975):

1. Horse is reluctant to move in stall or truck, even to eat. Requires one person behind to force movement when leading.
2. Shows depressed attitude and minimal reaction to external stimuli.
3. Rear feet are placed up under the body as in acute laminitis.
4. Sensitivity (may be extreme) to palpation in the affected pastern or coronary band area.
5. Edema in the flexor tendon sheaths and around the fetlocks.
6. Reddening of light-skinned horses including exudation from blistering effect.
7. Visible sores or scars.

Clinical signs of soring when a horse is *moving* are:

1. Movement is very slow at first with most of weight carried on hindquarters as in acute laminitis.
2. Slightly uneven ground causes stumbling at slow speeds. Rider has to hold horse up with reins.
3. After standing, stiffness when starting and extreme lateral twisting of the hocks.
4. When the rider mounts, the hindquarters go down and the hind legs go under the horse.
5. When moving, there is a definite slope from the withers to the croup with extremely high action with the front feet and extreme overstride of the hind feet.
6. Labored and jerky gaits requiring constant urging to keep moving.
7. Move slower than other horses in the class, tire rapidly, sweat excessively, have rapid respiration rate and stop rapidly by dropping down on to the hind legs.
8. Pained expression in eye, oblivious to surroundings.

Article 11.2 (Prohibitions concerning exhibitors) of the Horse Protection Act 1979 specifically prohibits the following:

1. Any horseshoe that weighs in excess of 16 ounces or pads thicker than 1 inch at the heel on yearling horses (up to 2 yr. of age).
2. Official heel length more than 1 inch less than official toe length. Heel length is not to include normal heel calks that are under 3/4

inch in height. Excess height of calk (over 3/4 in.) must be added to official heel measurement in figuring heel-toe ratio.

3. Artificial extension of toe length by any means beyond the natural angle of the toe of the hoof wall and pastern, except when necessary to repair a broken hoof.

4. Single or double Memphis (rocker) bars on the bottom of horseshoes which are placed back more than 1 1/2 inches from the point of the toe, or which will cause unsteady stance with resulting muscle and tendon strain.

5. Metal hoof bands, such as used to anchor pads and shoes, placed less than ½ inch below the coronary band.

6. Metal hoof band that can be easily and quickly loosened by the hand (no wing nuts, etc.).

7. Shoeing or trimming a hoof in a way that will cause pain to a horse when moving.

8. Shoeing a horse with a device such as a lateral extension that might cause the horse to strike himself on the coronary band.

9. Lead or other weights attached to the outside surface of the hoof wall, pad or outside surface of the horseshoe.

More regulations have been proposed. The government is serious about reducing cruel treatment to show horses. Horseshoers can be implicated. You should know the current law and obey it.

The Fox Trotter

The original Fox Trotters came from the old American Saddlebred type and included Arabian, Morgan, Standardbred and Walking Horse blood. Farmers and ranchers in the rugged Ozarks of Missouri used these horses for cattle work and traveling long distances more than 100 years ago.

Fox Trotters have the ability to travel long distances at 5 to 8 mph. They are shown naturally and with a full mane and tail under Western tack at three gaits: 1) the flat-foot walk, 2) the fox trot, and 3) the canter. Fox Trotters are most famous as pleasure, trail and endurance horses. They are shod appropriate to their use. Fox trotters are used extensively by the U.S. Forest Service.

Fox Trotters range from 14.2 hands to 16 hands and weigh 950 to 1,200 pounds. Sorrel or chestnuts with white markings are most common, palominos and other colors including pinto and albino are accepted for registration.

The fox trot is a relaxed sort of shuffle with the horse doing a fast walk with the front feet and a slow trot with the hind feet. The hind foot on each side disfigures or caps the track made by the front foot by touching the front track and sliding forward over it. The sliding action of the hind feet makes these horses more sure-footed and comfortable for riding long distances. The head and tail exhibit a characteristic bobbing rhythm without high stepping animation.

The fox walk is sometimes used for distance traveling. The hind feet jog rather than trot, making it an intermediate gait.

A fox trot used to be an optional gait for American Saddlebred horses. It could be used in place of the slow gait. The modern fox trot is more relaxed, less animated, and more ground covering than today's slow gait. A modern Fox Trotter can do the fox trot all day.

Walking Horses used to look like the trail and cow horse type Fox Trotters of today before the unnatural, artificial appliances and heavy shoe weight became popular. Show Fox Trotters are becoming more and more like Walking Horses.

Horses are trained to fox trot by collecting (pushing forward while holding back) the horse at a flat footed walk and preventing them from trotting.

The use of other than standard or natural horse shoes is discouraged. The weight for each shoe must not exceed 21 ounces. No extra weight on the shoes or feet is allowed. Horse Protection Act antisoring and shoeing regulations also apply to Fox Trotters.

The Racking Horse

The Racking Horse is a Saddlebred type that has been popular in the Southeast since Colonial times. It was originally bred as a versatile horse in Alabama, similar to the Morgan in New England. The Racking Horse was designated the official horse of the state of Alabama in 1975. A Racking Horse must naturally do the distinctive four-beat gait from which it gets its name. No artificial training devices other than weighted shoes and pads are allowed. Animated hock action is undesirable. These horses are shown with English tack at three natural gaits: 1) the pleasure or show walk, 2) the slow rack and 3) the fast rack. In the trail pleasure division only two gaits are shown: 1) the trail pleasure walk and 2) the trail pleasure rack (without speed or collection).

Racking horses average 15.2 hands and 1,000 pounds. They may be sorrel, chestnut, black, roan, white, bay, brown, grey and sometimes yellow. They occasionally have white markings on the body as well as the face and legs.

Racking horses are shown either flat or open shod. Flat shod prohibits a pad between the hoof and shoe, but weighted shoes are allowed. Open shod permits the use of flat or wedge pads and weighted shoes. Trail Pleasure horses are flat shod. Show Pleasure and Open Show horses are shown open shod. There is also a flat shod division, due to the lack of qualified farriers.

The show farrier is considered a show official representing the show management. In cases when a horse loses a shoe the 5 minute rule is observed as in the AHSA, except timing shall begin when the farrier reaches the horse or touches the shoe (whichever occurs first), instead of when he enters the ring. Horse Protection Act shoeing regulations apply to Racking Horses.

Arabian

The Arabian is probably the oldest breed of light horses. All other breeds of light horses have developed from the original Arab lines.

The purebred Arabian is distinctive in its looks. Its comparatively short, dish face, long arching neck, and short back with a horizontal croup make it easy to recognize.

Arabians are solid in color except for white markings on the head and legs. They may be between 800 to 1,000 pounds and are from 14.1 to 15.1 hands in height.

Arabians are increasing in popularity due to their tremendous adaptability and versatility. Arabs entered in English Pleasure, Park and Driving classes may be considered uniquely gaited. Arabians are shown in their own division under AHSA rules.

The English Pleasure horse is shown at five gaits: 1) flat-footed walk, 2) normal trot, 3) strong trot, 4) canter, and 5) hand gallop. During the strong trot, the well trained horse holds each front leg forward and straight for a moment. This creates a dwelling or prancing effect. Manners are stressed in a pleasure class.

The Park Horse is shown in formal attire at three gaits: 1) an animated walk, 2) trot, and 3) canter. The park horse trot is a very precise and balanced gait.

The Arabian is shown in three types of driving classes. Pleasure Driving is done at the same gaits as the English Pleasure class without the canter and gallop. Formal Driving is the same as the Park Horse class without the canter. In Combination classes the horse is first shown in harness and then stripped in the ring and shown again under saddle.

The Arabian division of the AHSA has adopted rules which prohibit the use of pads and bars on the shoe and any action devices during or before the show. Maximum official toe length (measured from hair line to ground) is 4 1/2 inches. Maximum shoe weight is 12 ounces. In some areas, toe-weighted scooped-toed shoes are requested. The scoop picks up and holds dirt in the foot, increasing its weight and the action of the horse. In the event of a protest, only the shoe is weighed. Half-round shoes are popular on the front feet of Arabians. Square-toed shoes set back under the toe are popular on the hind feet. Toe-weighted shoes must be made from lightweight stock to stay under the weight limit.

Paso Fino

The Paso Fino and Peruvian Paso are gaited somewhat alike but differ in historical development, way of going, training methods and equipment. Although they average 14 hands in height, they are considered horses since they have no pony ancestry.

Paso Finos developed from the horses brought to the Caribbean from Spain by Columbus. While the original Paso Fino of the Caribbean was spread around and mixed with other types, the Peruvian Paso was isolated and remained pure for four centuries after they were brought to Peru by Pizarro.

Paso Finos are shown in a very collected manner with a short stride. An outward swimming motion of the front legs called termino is rare and undesirable. The Peruvian Pasos, however, have a long stride, are shown at greater speed and are encouraged to show termino in their gait. Peruvian Pasos may reach speeds of 18 mph at the andedura or running pace.

The Paso Fino gait is a four-beat lateral gait or broken pace with the hind foot on each side touching the ground a fraction of a second before the forefoot of the same side. The paso fino gait is performed at three speeds: 1) classic (paso) fino—fully collected, slow forward movement with an unbroken rhythm of hoofs hitting the ground rapidly (once every 1/10 of a second), 2) paso corto—medium collection, moderate speed, same steady rhythm, and 3) paso largo—less collection, more speed, same rhythm resulting in a fast, but smooth gait.

The Paso Finos may also walk or canter, but are not shown at these gaits. Pasos are born with their unique gait. They do not naturally bob their head. They are trained in a natural manner and are often trained and shown bare foot.

The ASHA rules state that a Paso Fino shown unshod must not have hoofs that exceed 4 inches. The shoes must not exceed 10 ounces, and official toe length of shod horses must not exceed 4 1/2 inches. They also state that characteristically the hoofs of these horses are small, well rounded, and have little heel.

References

Agony of the walking horse. 1969. Life (Oct. 3):77.

American Horse Shows Assn. 1982. 1982-1983 Rule Book. A.H.S.A., New York.

Armistead, W.W. 1955. Horseshoeing—Part 2. Southwestern Vet. 9(4):324.

Bright, J. 1978. Rules and Regulations. Racking Horse Breeders' Assn. of Amer., Helena, AL.

Canfield, D.M. 1968. Elements of Farrier Science. Enders Tool Co., Inc. Albert Lea, MN.

Daniels, B.B. 1977. Shop talk-rolled toes. Amer. Farriers' J. 3(4):65.

Edgington, D. 1969. Custom shoer. The Western Horseman. (Jan):67.

Edwards, E.H. 1979. Horses and Ponies of the World. Larousse, New York.

Evans, J.W. 1981. Horses. W.H. Freeman and Co., San Francisco.

Liles, L. and J. Akers. 1980. The show ring farrier. Amer. Farriers' J. 6(2):48.

Liles, L. and J. Akers. 1978. Lee Liles professional farrier. Voice. 17(1):28.

Liles, L. and J. Akers. 1978. The plantation shoe. Voice. 17(2):28.

Liles, L. and J. Akers. 1978. Trimming the hoof. Voice. 17(3):16.

Liles, L. and J. Akers. 1978. Pads. Voice. 17(4):24.

Liles, L. and J. Akers. 1978. Double nailed pads. Voice. 17(5):24.

Liles, L. and J. Akers. 1978. Repairing the broken toe. Voice 17(6):92.

Liles, L. and J. Akers. 1978. Rear shoes. Voice. 17(7):22.

Liles, L. and J. Akers. 1978. Crossing and knee knocking. Voice. 17(8):128.

Liles, L. and J. Akers. 1978. Quarter crack on the rear hoof. Voice. 17(9):10.

Luikart, R. 1980. Building up show horses: mathematics vs. rules of thumb. Amer. Farriers' J. 6(4):141.

Morrison, B. 1983. Personal communication. Braddyville, IA.

Nelson, H.A. and D.L. Osheim. 1975. Soring in Tennessee Walking Horses: Detection by Thermography. USDA—APHIS, Ames, IA.

Rinedollar, D. 1975. Hoofprints. Welsh Pony Tales. (Autumn):19.

Simpson, J.S. 1979. The Mechanics of Shoeing Gaited Horses. Published by the author.

Staff. 1972. The horse protection act. Southwestern Vet. (Fall):35.

USDA. 1979a. The Horse Protection Act and You. APHIS, Washington, DC.

USDA. 1979b. Horse protection; final rule. Federal Register. 44(83—Fri. Apr. 27):25172.

Ward, D.D. 1977. One pad—the first step to shoeing long footed horses. Amer. Farriers' J. 3(1).7.

NOTES:

Chapter 42

Draft Horses

The draft or cart horse type is the traditional heavy or work horse. They are of such size, form and substance that they are ideal for farm and city use requiring pulling power. They reached their peak numbers in the U.S. and abroad in the late teens and early twenties of this century. Draft horse numbers declined steadily until the mid sixties. Draft horse breeders kept only the best. This puts them in the unique position of possessing a type that has undergone an extensive selection process.

Draft horses are making a strong comeback on today's small farm because of their economy and flexibility. They can be maintained by farm grown feeds, requiring no fossil fuel. Two pairs of horses are equivalent to a medium tractor. However, they have the flexibility of being used as a single, double, or multiple hitch. And, they replace themselves, enrich the soil and require no repairs.

In England, draft horses continue to be popular as a short haul cart horse in many cities. The most well known examples of the draft type in America are the Budweiser Clydesdales shown by the Anheuser-Busch Brewery of St. Louis, Missouri.

Draft horses are used for farming, logging, packing, plowing matches, pulling contests, pulling heavy wagons or carts on farms or in cities and parades, circuses and horse shows.

A pair of draft horses is called a team. A draft horse hitch is made up of three sections. The lead horses must have the best action and be lively as they create the first impression and travel the farthest in the turns. The wheel horses are closest to the wagon and must be the heaviest as they pull the most. The swing horses are in between and must stay clear of the wagon tongue in turns and follow the leaders. Most hitches are six or eight pairs. However, there have been at least two 40 horse hitches in America. A random is three horses hitched in single file, a tandem is two horses hitched in single file, and a trandem is three horses hitched abreast.

The largest numbers of draft horses are in the Midwest, the Northwest and the Mid-Atlantic states. There are enthusiasts in all states.

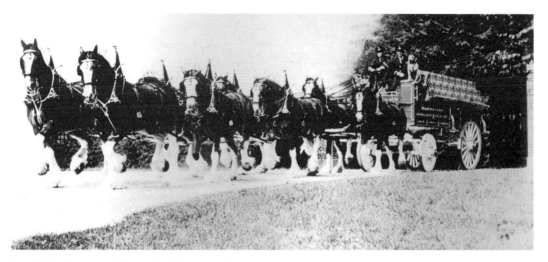

Fig. 42-1. The most well known hitch horses in the U.S. are the Budweiser Clydesdales. Photo from the Devon Horse Show.

Breeds

There are five principal breeds of draft horses in the United States.

The Belgian breed is currently the most popular breed of draft horse in the U.S. Its registry records more foals each year than all other draft breeds combined. Indiana, Ohio and Iowa are the leading states in Belgian numbers.

This ancient breed has descended from the Flemish horses of what was once northern France and is now Belgium. The Belgian is the state horse of Belgium and its production has been state subsidized. The farm plow horse in Belgium looks different from the American type. The European horse is coarser and not as stylish and upstanding as those preferred in the U.S. A brown type of bay or roan with dark heavy feathering (long hair below the fetlocks) is the most popular. One of the chief uses of the European horses is the production of edible horse meat.

Belgians were first imported into the U.S. as a sire breed. They became very popular in the 1930's due to their reputation as easy keepers and shippers. Belgians are coming back. One modern farmer figured that horses cost 25 percent less to maintain than tractors. The breed was and still is preferred by farmers for plowing and teamsters for the big hitch because of the Belgian's docile temperament and ease of cleaning (less white hair and feather). They are said to be the most sluggish and docile of the draft breeds. Belgians are preferred for horse pulling contests because of their low set heavy weight.

American breeders prefer the sorrel color with a flaxen (white) mane and tail. Principal colors of Belgians are sorrels (chestnut) and roans. They may be bay, brown, gray and occasionally black. Belgians have a more sloping croup and shorter neck than most of the draft breeds. Their manes are usually roached and tails docked (shortened to 6 in.) for ease of harnessing.

The Belgian is known as the thickest and heaviest of the drafters. Today, they are even heavier on the average than they have been in the past. There is a trend toward the short backed, short necked type of earlier years. Belgians may be shorter than some Shires, but usually weigh more. They average 1900 to 2200 pounds and may weight 2600 pounds or more. Their height ranges from 15.2 to 17 hands, average 16.1.

Some notable giants of the breed:

Brooklyn Supreme (Iowa, *circa* 1940) stallion, 19.2 hands, 3200 lb., 10 ft. 2 in. girth, 30 in. shoe.

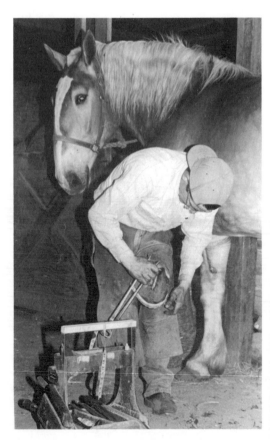

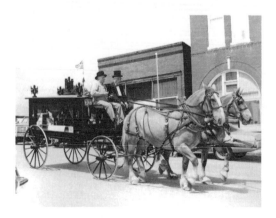

Fig. 42-2. A Belgian farm team pulling a hearse in a parade. Photo from Leo Baumli.

Fig. 42-3. Trimming a Belgian pulling horse. Photos by J. Graves.

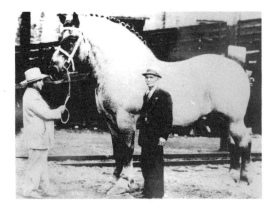

Fig. 42-4. Brooklyn Supreme, a giant draft horse. Photo from a postcard.

Wilma (Nevada, *circa* 1973) mare, 18.2 hands, 3200 lb.

Big John (New Jersey, *circa* 1974) gelding, 19.2 hands, 2560 lb.

Goliath (New Jersey, *circa* 1968) gelding, 20 hands, 2800 lb., 10 ft. long, no. 10 shoe, 33 in. collar.

The Percheron breed once was the most popular breed of draft horse in the U.S. Percherons were the number one draft breed for the first three decades of this century. In the 1930 farm census, two-thirds of all registered U.S. draft horses were Percherons. Until recently, more Percherons were registered than all the other draft horse breeds combined. The breed is now the second most popular breed in the U.S. Ohio, Wisconsin, Pennsylvania and Indiana are the leading states in Percheron numbers.

The breed originated in the small province of Perche, France (70 mi. southwest of Paris). The government maintained a stud at Hares du Pin. Most French farmers had only mares. A requirement for registration was that the animal foaled in La Perche and both parents had to be registered. These horses were formally used as battle chargers and saddle horses, as were all the early draft horse breeds. The French were more interested in style than the people of Belgium. Arab blood was periodically introduced from the 8th to the 19th Century. This produced a finer head, smaller ears, more endurance, more speed and more stylish action than that of other draft breeds.

Percherons are known to withstand hot weather better than other draft breeds. The Percheron breed gradually changed from a favorite diligence (stage coach) or omnibus horse, where these horses could trot for hours at 10 mph, to the preferred American draft horse.

The first imported horses were called Norman horses. Later the name was changed to Percheron to distinguish these horses from other French draft horses of lesser quality. The greatest number of Percherons were imported in the 1880's when the pioneers were settling the West. They were desirable because of their versatility. Early imports were crossed with native mustangs of the Northwest in an effort to create an all purpose horse. The undesirable result was called a Puddingfoot. Similar disappointment with Clydesdale mustang crosses created the Lummox. During the First World War, the Percheron was the favorite military horse and was exported by the U.S. to Europe for this purpose.

Percherons are still very popular on many small farms, especially in the Pennsylvania Dutch or Amish regions of the U.S. They are popular in parade hitches, particularly those connected with the circus. They are used almost exclusively by circus or vaulting riders because their broad white backs don't show the layer of rosin used for traction.

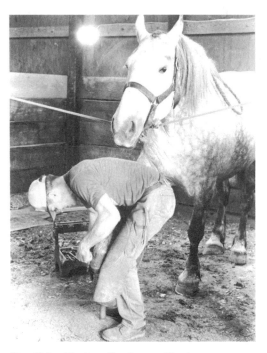

Fig. 42-5. Shoeing a Percheron pulling horse.

Percherons are the most refined of the draft horses. Their heads and gait show Arabian influence. They are not as heavy as the Belgian. They are known to be long lived, have high resistance to disease and hard sound hoofs. The tail may be docked. They are a combination of size, action, spirit and tractability. Average weight is 1900 to 2100 pounds. Height ranges between 16 and 17 hands, average 16.2. About 90 percent of Percherons are black or dappled gray (about 50% of each today); others are roan, sorrel, or bay. They have limited white markings and very little feather (but more than the Belgian).

A giant of the breed was Dr. LeGear (St. Louis, *circa* 1915), 21 hands, 2995 pounds, 33 inch collar, 31 inches around the fore arm, No. 10 shoe.

The Clydesdale breed is the best known of all draft horses in the U.S. because of its presence in the big hitch made famous by the advertising of the Anheuser-Busch brewery. Clydesdales are the third most popular draft breed in the U.S., behind the Belgian and Percheron. Wisconsin and Michigan are the leading states in Clydesdale numbers.

Clydesdales originated in the valley of the River Clyde in the Lanark shire (county) of Scotland. The Scots bred English and Flemish horses to obtain a horse with color, flashy white markings, silky white feather and most of all superb action. It is a Scottish adage, "No foot, no horse,—tops may go, but bottoms never." It is a great compliment to a draft horse to say, "He moves like a Clydesdale." They possess the longest and springiest stride of the draft horses. They are also the most energetic of the draft horses and require expert training and care to keep them in top shape. This made them unpopular with the American farmer. Clydesdales also have a finer (lighter, less coarse) build than the other draft breeds. For these reasons, the first imported Clydesdales were principally used for city wagon or street horses. Their showy style made them ideal for an advertising and show horse. Clydesdales are preferred for farm horses in Ireland as well as Scotland.

Clydesdales have longer necks and are more upstanding than other draft horses, except the taller Shire. They have sharper withers and less depth to their chest than other drafters. They are usually quite cow hocked and to be so is not considered a fault. Clydesdales are unusually broad between the eyes and have a flat face unlike the Shire. They usually weigh between 1700 and 1900 pounds and are 16 to 17 hands high. The tallest recorded was 21 hands. Their tails are usually docked to about 6 inches. The mane is plaited in 8 to 12 knobs when they are shown.

Clydesdales have more white than other breeds. It may be as high as the stifle, belly or chest. White markings are extensive on the legs and face. They have long, fine, silky feathering around, above and below the fetlocks. This white hair must be groomed daily. The feathering is desirable for showing since it flows when the legs move. It is undesirable for farming since it is easily tangled with mud and burrs. The dominant color is bay, but also seen are browns, blacks, chestnuts, grays and roans.

The Shire breed is the fourth most popular draft breed in the U.S. Most are in Idaho, Washington and Illinois. However, the Shire dominates the pulling of large vehicles in England such as coal carts, brewers' drays, wagons and vans as well as the hitch competitions. Shires descended from the medieval war horses (called the Great Horse) that carried knights and pulled chariots into battle. A knight in full armor (protecting man and horse) weighed over 400 pounds.

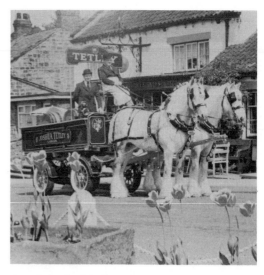

Fig. 42-6. English Shire cart (hitch) horses. Photo from a Tetley calendar.

The Shire may be said to be a cousin of the Clydesdale. They have similar type ancestry, only each was developed in different regions. Some of this difference was due to a law passed by Henry VIII that forbid the export of Great Horses to Scotland. The Shire was originally developed in the low Fen (marsh) country of England. Breeders worked toward size and substance, not action and style as did Scottish Clydesdale breeders. Robert Blakewell (1726-1795) was chiefly responsible for improving and establishing the Shire as a breed.

The Shire is often called the biggest (tallest) breed. However, there are big and little horses in every breed. Once, Shires were very massive and their legs had very heavy, coarse feathering. They were considered very sluggish. They used to have hair tuffs on the knee, hock and muzzle. Now, they are more refined, but still are very tall, show more draftiness, depth and coarseness than the Clydesdale. They have very large feet measuring up to 10 inches across. Shires average 2000 or more pounds (equaled in weight only by the Belgian) and are 16 to 18 hands in height. They have a characteristic Roman nose and a long lean head with long pointed ears. Their mane, tail, and feather hair is usually coarser and their pasterns shorter than the Clydesdales. Black is the dominant color in the U.S., but Shires may be bay, brown, roan or gray. White markings on the legs and face are common. An extra large Shire was Eufyl Lady Grey, (London, *circa* 1925) mare, 2500 pounds.

The English Cart Horse Society was formed in 1878 and had records going back to 1770. It later changed its name to the Shire Horse Society. The American Shire Horse Assn. was formed in 1885. Both the Shire and the Suffolk associations nearly ceased to exist in the 1950's, but they were revived in the 1960's.

The Suffolk breed is the least (fifth) popular of the draft horse breeds in the U.S. Most Suffolks are located in Pennsylvania, but there are very few and they are dispersed throughout the U.S. They are still popular in England as a plow horse.

The Suffolk can be traced back to the 16th Century as a distinct breed. All registered Suffolks can be traced to Crip's Horse, a stallion foaled in 1768. The breed was developed for farm work in the heavy soil of the Norwich and Suffolk shires (counties) of England. It is the purest of all the draft breeds. They were originally called Suffolk Punches due to their round, compact appearance.

Suffolks are short-legged, barrel-girthed, low shouldered, have no feather and are powerful pullers for their size. They are limited to one color (chestnut or sorrel). Seven shades from pale sorrel to dark copper are recognized. They have very little white except an occasional star on the face. The conformation of the Suffolk resembles the old Belgian type. They are known as easy keepers, willing to work, fast walkers, durable and long lived. They are criticized for their lack of size and action and frequently have sickle (set) hocks and short pasterns. Their hoofs are sometimes flat and flaring and may lack strength. Suffolks have straighter croups and smaller ears than other draft horses. Tails are generally docked. Sometimes these horses are called chunks, as are small drafters of any breed.

Suffolks used to average 1600 to 1800 pounds, but are somewhat heavier now. They range from 15.2 to 16.2 hands in height. A notable giant of the breed was Kirk Patrick (Pat) (upstate New York, *circa* 1935). He weighed 2810 pounds, was 21 hands high, and was 9 feet long. This size was rare for any breed, but especially the Suffolk.

The Suffolk Horse Society of Great Britain established its stud book in 1880. The breed never became very popular in the U.S. mostly because there was such a great demand for them in their native country. The American Suffolk Horse Assn. was established in 1911. In the 1960's registrations in America were less than 10 a year.

Draft Horse Types and Shoeing Styles

There are four general types of work draft horses do. They are shod according to the type of work required of them.

1. Farm work in the spring, summer and fall.
2. Logging or feeding in the winter.
3. Pulling stone boats or sleds in pulling contests.
4. Pulling heavy freight wagons or carts on the road or in the show ring.

Farm horses doing work such as plowing and pulling farm implements require only flat shoes.

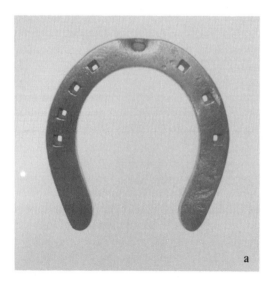

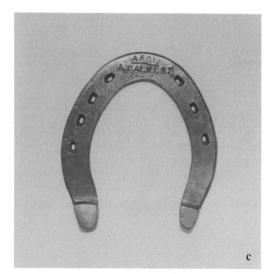

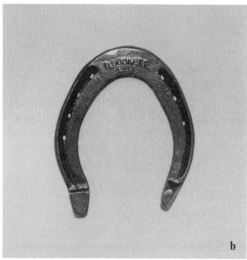

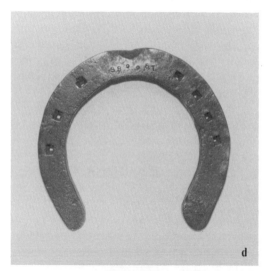

Fig. 42-7. Draft horse shoes from the British Isles: a) stamped front shoe made by Dave Duckett, b) fullered hind roadster shoe made by Dave Duckett, c) stamped hind agricultural shoe made by Alan Calvert, d) front Shire cart horse shoe made by Cyril Cooper, and e) hind Clydesdale farm horse shoe made by Edward Martin.

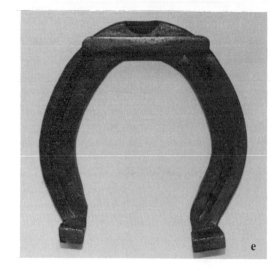

However, many farmers want toe and heel calks due to tradition. A number of horses are worked barefoot. Most need shoeing to preserve hoof shape and soundness. Clips are usually drawn on all draft horse shoes due to the stress placed on the nails by pulling and the heavy weight of the shoes. Shoeing farm horses is a challenge since so many are not trained to stand for shoeing and their feet are severely neglected.

Drop forged keg shoes may be applied by farmers. Keg shoes require only the heels be cropped or calked (turned down) to match hoof size. Clips should be drawn or welded on. Flat draft horse shoes with forged clips sizes 3 to 9 made by Werkman of Holland are now available in the U.S.[1] Cast steel keg shoes[2], available in many patterns, are also used on farm (and show) horses.

Logging horses work in the woods in the winter. They may require sharp shoeing. Sharp drive-on toe calks are forge welded or arc welded on a self-cleaning pattern (beveled inner edge) shoe. Heel calks are turned and beveled to a sharp edge. Shoes may be made from relatively light ⅜ x 1 or 1¼ inch stock. Screw calks or drive calks may also be used for winter logging or livestock feeding. Coarse borium, drill tech or hi-carb[3] may be used in place of or on the toe and heel calks. Logging horses are not shod as full or as long in the heels as other types of draft horses due to the risk of pulling shoes.

Pulling teams must pull a loaded stone boat or sled 15 or more feet in a deep arena. Some contests allow lunging (jerking) to move the load; others do not. The weight on the sled for the first pull usually equals the weight of the team. Weight is added until the horses can no longer pull the load the required distance in three attempts. Most teams can pull twice their weight and a few can pull three times their weight. The best pulling horses prance in time and squat to pull in unison. There is great strain on both front and hind legs. Pulling horses can exert a force of 20 horsepower (550 foot pounds per second) each for a short time. Champion pulling horses are highly trained and conditioned athletes.

[1] Mankel Blacksmith Shop, Cannonsburg, MI
[2] Russelloy Foundry, Durant, IA
[3] Postle Industries, Inc., Cleveland, OH

Pulling teams are shod with extremely high calks, sometimes 1 inch or more in height. The toe calks are often tilted forward on pulling shoes to allow more purchase on the ground at the point of break over. Sometimes the heel calks are made broad and flat to prevent their sinking in as the toe. Often, the heel calks are higher than the toe calks and bent backward. The shoe is usually set back and the toe is dubbed off. Shoes are usually made from ½ x 1 inch stock.

It has been scientifically proven by Bjorck (1958) that a horse exerts the greater proportion of the pulling force on the toes of the shoes. Also, the heavier the load, the more force exerted by the hind limbs. Light loads are resisted about equally with front and hind legs. Heavier horses have greater muscle mass and increased friction between the hoof and ground and therefore can pull more. Heavy front quarters and adding a rider also increases draft ability. Pulling tends to raise the front quarters. Increased weight increases ground friction.

Show draft horses or hitch horses pull heavy wagons or carts on the road or in the show ring. A flat or low heel calked shoe (no toe calks) is most popular. A full crease or fullering is often added (especially in England). Borium is more commonly used in the U.S. Rubber shoes with steel liners are popular for horses used exclusively on pavement. Drive calks (blunt or sharp) were once the most popular for all weather use. The rising cost of borium may cause them to be popular once again, especially for farm work under icy or other slippery conditions. Short studs (drive or screw type calks) are used in Europe in place of borium.

Show horse shoes for Clydesdales and Shires are frequently beveled on the outside edge (scotched) more than they would be for conventional draft work. This, along with a boxy square-toe creates the appearance of a wider, squarer foot than the horse naturally has. Originally, this type of foot was selected to prevent the sinking of the heavy horse in the boggy fields of Scotland and England. Today, this characteristic is enhanced by the shoers of show horses of all draft breeds.

A good shoeing job can earn a placing or two higher in a horse show class. Show draft horse shoeing often requires exaggeration of an individual animal's natural characteristics. The square-toe is supposed to speed up the breakover and increase the horse's action. Enough weight should be in the shoe to create momentum as the foot is lifted. When the horse flexes his front legs, you should see the bottom of his feet. Normally, extra weight in the shoe is thought to be detrimental since it increases fatigue and concussion. However, the object here is to enhance action, much like it's done when shoeing the gaited horse. Many show draft horses are shod with several pounds of iron per foot. For example, a Budweiser Clydesdale may be shod with 22 inches of ½ x 1½ inch iron weighing nearly 5 pounds per shoe.

It takes a long time to grow a show foot on a draft horse. The process must be started at least by January to have the horse ready to show in July. The shoes should be fit full and reset every six weeks. Leather pads packed with shredded newspaper soaked in water are applied to keep the hoofs moist and spreading. The last two shoeings before the show, only one-half the usual amount is trimmed off. The object is to create a long foot that has no nail holes in it. The long flaring foot enhances the horse's action and more iron (weight) is needed to cover it.

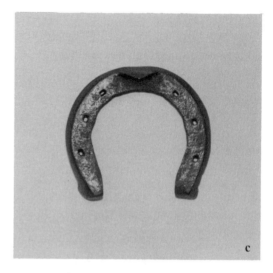

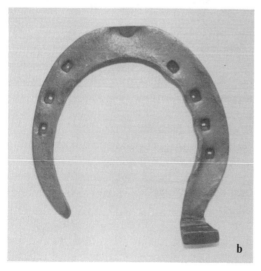

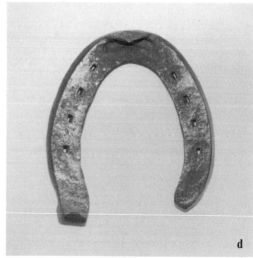

Fig. 42-8. American made show shoes: (a) Scotch bottom front and (b) hind Clydesdale show shoes made by Steve Kraus. (c) Foot surface of beveled front yearling show shoe, and (d) foot surface of Percheron beveled hind show shoe.

The shoes are made as long as possible (perhaps as much as 24 in. long including calks). They are made from ½ x 1¼ to 1½ inch iron. The sides of the shoes are beveled and they are creased or fullered. The fullering helps to increase the shoe width and ground surface. Shoes are usually calked and clipped.

The shoes should be fit wider than the foot all around at least the width of a dime so the edge of the shoe can be polished with a mill file before entering the show ring. The hoof is also highly polished with wax.

It is customary to force the hocks in on many show horses. This is done by trimming down the inside half of the hind foot until the sole gives under thumb pressure. The outside of the hoof is left longer and allowed to flare out. The inside branch of the hind shoe is drawn and thinned. The inside nail holes are punched fine and the inside edge of the shoe is fit close. The outside branch is punched coarse and fit very full (so it extends beyond the ground surface of the wall at least ¼ in.). A low calk is turned on the outside branch. The outside branch is extended behind the buttress of the foot at least an inch.

Foals and yearlings may be shown shod. They are usually shod with ⅜ x 1 inch stock punched for a No. 6 nail.

Nail sizes used on draft horse shoes will vary from a No. 6 to a No. 12, average is a No. 8 for Belgians and Percherons and a No. 9 for Clydesdales and Shires. It is best not to punch for larger than a No. 9 since No. 10 and 12 have the same head size and will not work for resets when the nail holes become larger.

At least eight and sometimes ten nail holes are punched in draft horse shoes. Hoof size varies a lot between and within breeds according to the type of ground the horse is worked in and the care of the feet. Belgians and Percherons may have front feet 7 to 8 inches wide, Clydesdales and Shires 8 to 10 inches wide. The hind feet may be ¼ to ¾ inch narrower than the fronts.

Traditionally, the Percheron and Belgian have a reputation for having the soundest hoofs and the Clydesdale and Shire have one for the poorest. The feet of Belgians and especially Percherons are round-toed, comparatively upright-heeled and straight side-walled. The feet of Shires and especially Clydesdales are square-toed, shallow-heeled, sloping side-walled and often shelly or weak. Belgians with light underlines (blonde) may have poor quality white feet. Cracked, shelly feet are filled with wood putty or hoof acrylic for showing.

Draft Horse Shoe Fitting Techniques

Ideally, all draft breeds have rather steep, dubbed toes. This trait is desirable for pulling or leg action. Massive frogs are also common especially in those horses with low or weak heels. Large feet are desirable and necessary to support a large horse.

Sidebones are a common occurrence in older draft horses due to toed-in or base-narrow conformation combined with short, straight pasterns and extreme concussion. Base-narrow conformation behind sometimes causes interfering.

Hoofs must be shaped *before* the shoe is fit. Draft horses are so heavy they spread the foot more than light horses. Shoes are fit full to the outside in order to shift the center of weight bearing to the center of the shoe and to help the horse break over straight.

It is desirable for the hocks of a draft horse to be close together. However, they should not be extremely cow hocked. When the hocks are close (with the cannons parallel) the horse is said to have more pulling power. The reasoning is that because the hocks go apart as the horse pulls, the closer together they are, the less outward twisting and strain will be on them.

Many draft horse shoe patterns are available[4]. Others can be handmade from heavy iron. Draft horse shoers use great quantities of coal or other forging fuel. The work is time consuming and difficult. They charge accordingly. Fortunately, most draft horses are gentle. However, they are heavy. Many shoers use foot stands. One type is used to support the feet for trimming and nailing. Another type is used for clinching and finishing. Homemade or Barcus shoeing stocks are often used for shoeing colts. Modern tranquilizing drugs are sometimes necessary.

[4] *Anvil Brand Shoe Co., Lexington, IL*

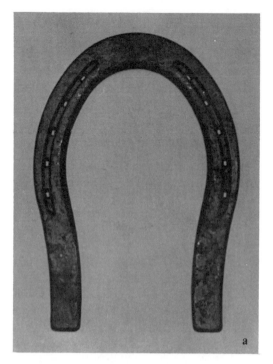

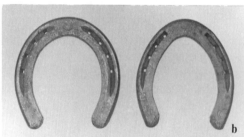

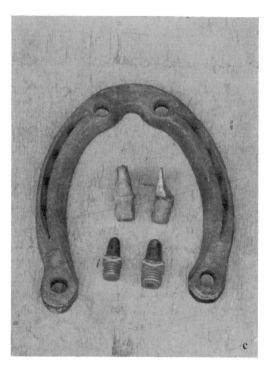

Fig. 42-9.   Draft horse keg shoes: (A) Diamond long heeled (hot) shoe, (B) Werkman front and hind short heeled (cold) shoes, (C) Phoenix keg shoe with blunt and sharp drive calks or cogs and screw calks or neverslips.

Special hand tools are required for draft horse shoeing. Large pull offs, clinchers and hoof knives are helpful. Heavy tongs, hammers and punches shaped for the larger sized nails are necessary. A striker to swing a sledge and tend the forge fire is most valuable. It is convenient to use a heavier anvil with a wide face and horn for making heavy shoes. Shoe shaping techniques are similar to those used for smaller shoes except draft horse shoes must be shaped when hot. Cold heavy iron is very unyielding.

Draft horse shoes are fit very full and with lots of expansion at the heels. These animals work at slow speed and the chance of interference or overreaching is minimal. The heels are extended beyond the buttresses ½ inch or more to give support to the foot and leg.

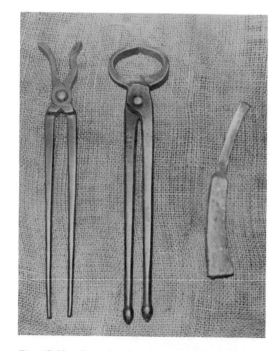

Fig. 42-10.   Special tools are required for draft horse shoeing. (Left) clinchers with larger teeth and longer jaws, (middle) large pull offs, (right) long bladed hoof knife.

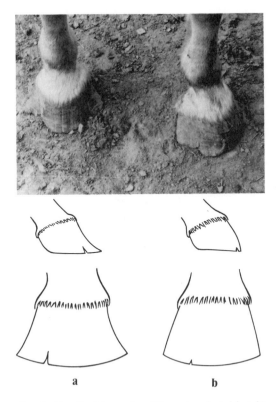

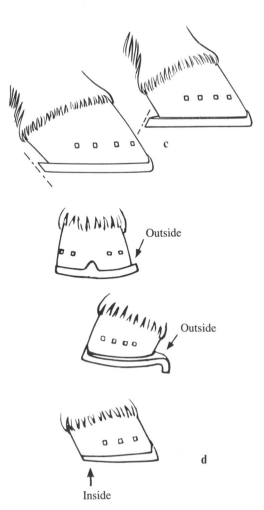

Fig. 42-11. Draft horse shoe fitting; a) neglected feet, b) flares should be removed before fitting the shoe, c) heels may be beveled from the ground side or the foot side, and d) Scotch bottom shoes are fit full and square in front and shifted to the outside behind.

The Daniels' method of hoof measuring for shoe stock size (see Chapter 26) can be used effectively on draft horses. However, some experienced draft horseshoers add to the width plus the length of the foot 1¼ to 1½ inches for flat shoes or 2¾ to 3 inches for heeled shoes.

Cutting heels of keg or handmade shoes:

1. The hot steel is placed in the middle of the half-round hardy instead of the side as would be done for a smaller foot. No attempt is made to cut the shoe on an angle with the width of the web. The heel is left round. This allows plenty of cover and expansion at the heel.
2. The heel may be cropped with the ground surface up instead of down as it is with light horses.
3. Heels are fit full to protect the bulbs and allow room for the frog. The shoe should follow a line created by a perpendicular line from the hair line to the ground on shallow, weak or low-heeled horses. The last inch or so of the heels may be turned out slightly on Scotch bottom shoes to provide lateral support at the heels. This places the heels or calks farther apart. However, the heel of the wall should remain completely covered and supported.

Turning calks on keg shoes:

1. Estimate the amount needed for the calk, mark and heat the heels.
2. Cut off the excess material with the straight hardy. Bend over the thickness of the shoe more than the amount desired as the height of the calk. This can be done in a vise or over the edge of the anvil. Calking vises are especially handy.
3. Upset the calk with the hammer to make it the desired height and thickness.
4. Rasp to finish, if necessary.

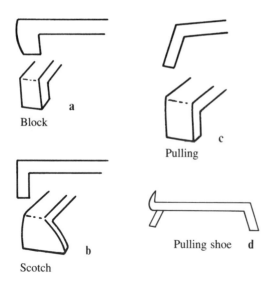

Block   a

Scotch   b

Pulling   c

Pulling shoe   d

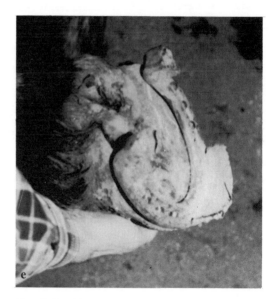

Fig. 42-12. Variations in draft horse heel calks: a) block (calkin), b) beveled (Scotch), c) and d) pulling, e) Draft horse foot shod with calks for pulling.

Calks for Scotch bottom shoes are made differently from those on farm work horse shoes. They may be made before the bar is bent or they may be made in the same heat as the branch is bent. The outside edge of the bar is placed over a rounded edge of the anvil about ¾ of an inch and is stepped down about ⅜ of an inch. The bar is then placed so the web is flat on the anvil with the step extending over the edge of the anvil the thickness of the stock. The calk is bent over the edge and then turned over and straightened on the anvil face.

While the end is still hot, the heel calk may be placed down in the step between the face and horn of the anvil. The outside edge of the calk can be hammered at a 45 degree angle to produce a bevel from the foot surface to the ground surface of the calk. Both calks must be made with the bevel on the outside edge of the shoe steel. The calk on the outside branch should be larger and more beveled than the one on the inside. Sometimes only one calk is put on the rear shoes. It goes on the outside branch and is extremely beveled.

Pulling clips may be done several different ways depending upon the tools available and individual preference. Consistently neat clips require a great deal of hammer control and prac-

tice. Large clips can be shaped by striking directly on the clip's edges after they are drawn. A flatter may be used to level the shoe around the clip after it is drawn.

1. Clips may be pulled from a clip horn on the anvil. The foot surface of the hot metal is driven into the clip horn and the clip is pulled from the toe metal sticking up.
2. Clips may be started by placing the hot shoe ground surface up on the anvil face and driving the projecting edge down the side of the anvil with a ball pein or cross pein hammer. Then the shoe is turned around and the clip is drawn using the edge of the anvil.
3. Clips can be drawn using a bob punch to start the metal down. This may be done in the hardy hole (if it is large enough) or it can be done over the edge of the anvil. Bob punching is a more accurate method and will usually result in a narrower neater looking clip. A handle should be added to the bob punch when using a striker.
4. Clips may be added by welding with an arc welder. This makes the poorest looking clip. However, when toe calks are attached with the arc welder, the arced-on clip may be the most practical.

Clips can be fit hot or cold. The nippers and rasp can be used to notch out for a clip when the foot is resting on a foot stand. A ½ inch wood chisel can be used to notch out when the foot is down resting on a board or mat.

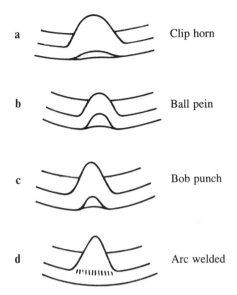

a — Clip horn

b — Ball pein

c — Bob punch

d — Arc welded

Fig. 42-13. Variations in draft horse toe clips: a) pulled on the anvil clip horn with a rounding hammer, b) pulled off the anvil edge with a ball pein hammer, c) started with a bob punch and pulled on the anvil face with the heel of the hammer, and d) arc welded clip.

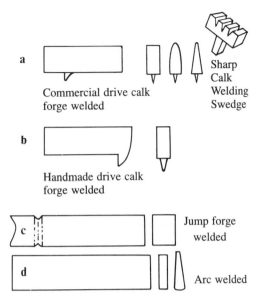

a — Commercial drive calk forge welded — Sharp Calk Welding Swedge

b — Handmade drive calk forge welded

c — Jump forge welded

d — Arc welded

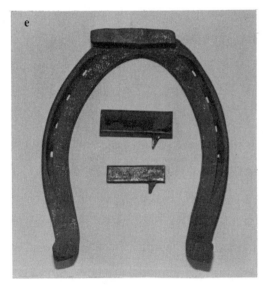

e

Fig. 42 14. Variations in draft horse welded toe calks: a) commercial calks with nubs, b) handmade calk with nub, c) calk prepared for jump welding, and d) arc welded sharp calk. (e) Keg shoe with forge welded blunt toe calk and commercial calks for forge welding.

Welding on toe calks may be done several ways. Consistent forge welding of toe calks requires extensive practice. Many horseshoers prefer to weld on toe calks with an arc welder.

Commercial drive-on toe calks have a little nub that holds the calk on the shoe until it is welded. The shoe is heated to a yellow heat and the calk is driven into place. Leave a little space between the calk and shoe. The nub holds the calk in place while it is taken to a welding heat in the forge. Drive-on calks can be made from bar stock by pulling a nub from a corner of the calk off the corner of the anvil. When the calk is in place, the toe is fluxed and brought to a welding heat. The toe calk is smashed into the toe of the shoe. Swedge blocks are necessary to protect sharp calks. Toes are welded on shoes with the calk down in these blocks. Usually a clip is drawn after welding. It is important to place the calk far enough back on the toe to allow for the clip.

Jump welding of toe calks is done using a long piece of steel the dimensions of the desired calk. The toe calk steel is heated (while the toe of the shoe is heating) and cut nearly all the way through on the straight hardy. The cut should be at the desired length for the calk. Both the calk and the shoe are fluxed and brought to a welding heat. The shoe is brought out and placed on the anvil and in the absence of a striker, the tongs

513

are dropped, the hammer picked up and the calk is stuck to the shoe. The handle on the calk is then twisted off. A second welding heat is taken and the toe calk is welded. The clip is then drawn in the same heat.

Screw calks require punching or drilling of the shoes. The holes must be tapped (threaded) to receive the screw calks. These calks have a hardened steel center and mild steel covering. They stay sharp as they wear. They are sometimes called neverslips. Usually, two are placed on the toe and one on each heel. The calks may be changed or replaced without reshoeing the horse. They come in a variety of sizes, the largest being for draft horses.

Drive calks or studs are also available which are similar to screw calks except they are driven into a punched hole which has been sized and tapered by a special punch (called a Morris taper) corresponding to the shank of the calk. These are available in sharp and blunt patterns for use at various times of the year.

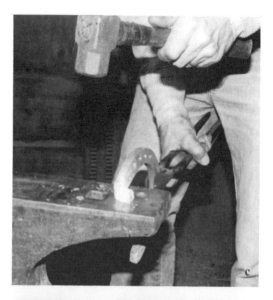

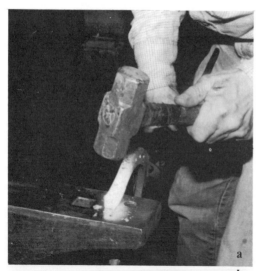

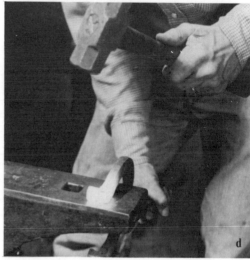

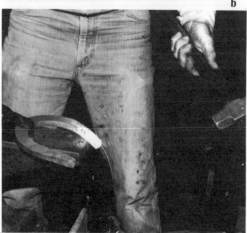

Fig. 42-15. *Steps in turning farm style heel calks:*
(a) Trailer the heel.
(b) Turn the heel of the shoe down over the heel of the anvil.
(c) Upset the calk on its side and end until it is the desired height and thickness.
(d) Turn the outside calk and trailer it.

Forging Draft Horse Shoes

Front shoes—farm or logging horse pattern can be made from ⅜ x 1 or ½ x 1 inch iron. These shoes are turned like a standard plate shoe. They may or may not be creased. They are usually clipped. Machine-made or keg shoes are available in size 6 and size 8. If heel calks are desired for increased traction, 1 inch may be added to each heel. The calks are turned over the edge of the anvil or in a vise and upset slightly. The shoe heels may be upset or tapered until square before turning. Less stock is required if this is done. Occasionally, they are turned over flat like a blocked heel. This gives a little height without traction and may be done when borium is to be applied to the shoe. Heel calks may be made before the toe bend is made or after the branches are bent on a handmade shoe. The outside calk is fit full with plenty of expansion. The inside calk is fit close with very little expansion to prevent treading on the coronary band of the opposite foot. Toe calks may be forge welded or arc welded. Borium may be applied to calks.

Hind shoes—farm horse pattern are made of the same stock as the front shoes. Flat toe calks are welded on about the same height as the heel calks. The toe piece can be extended laterally if the horse is extra base-narrow and moves its hocks outward excessively as it pulls.

Front and hind shoes—pulling horse pattern are usually made of ½ x 1 inch stock. The

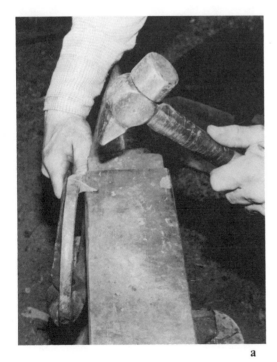

a

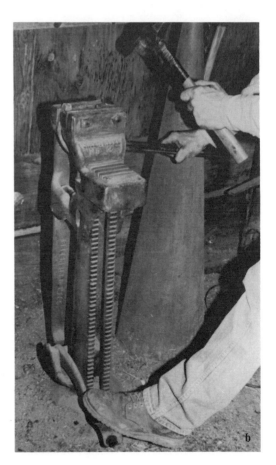

b

Fig. 42-16. Steps in sharp shoeing including forge welding on a toe calk:
(a) Calks are sharpened by drawing them to a point with a cross pein hammer on the anvil.
(b) Calks may be sharpened in a calking vise.

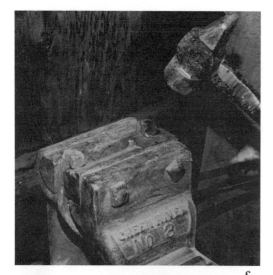

c

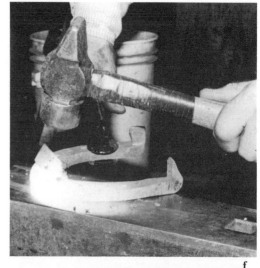

f

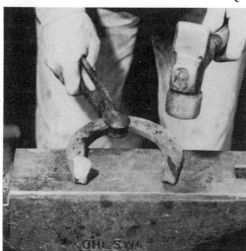

d

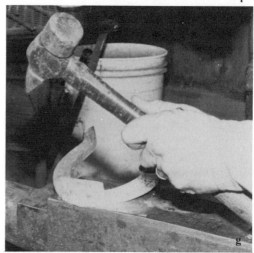

g

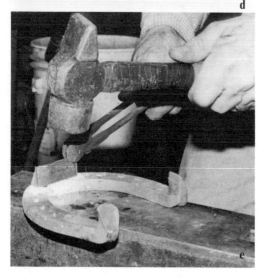

e

(c) Close-up of calking vise jaws.

(d) Sharp calks—outside is on left—inside is on right.

(e) The calk nub is driven into the hot shoe toe to hold in position for welding.

(f) The toe calk is fluxed and welded, sharp calks are finished in the swedge block on the calking vise or in a swedge that drops in the anvil hardy hole.

(g) The clip is started over the edge of the anvil while the toe is still hot.

(h) The clip is drawn on the heel of the anvil . . .

(i) . . . or, it may be drawn in the calking vise. Note the swedge block on the left for welding on sharp toe calks.

(j) The finished shoe showing blunt and sharp toe calks.

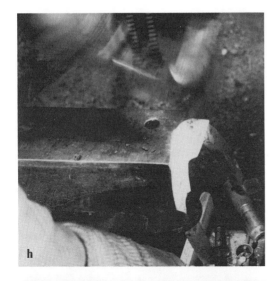

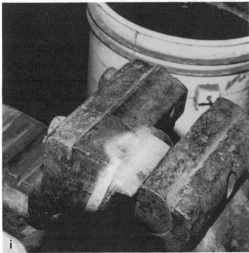

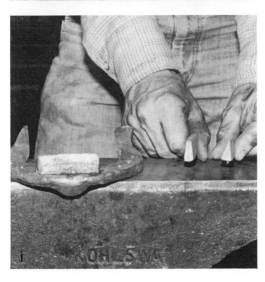

heels are turned down perpendicular to the shoe and may be 1 to 1½ inches or more in height. Some teamsters like the heel calks bent back away from the toe, especially on the hind feet. The toe calk should be a little lower than the heels. It should be fairly sharp and sloped slightly forward. The edge of an old grader blade or worn plow share (lay) makes a good toe calk. One-fourth by one inch stock welded on edge may be used. Toe pieces are arc welded on both sides. Borium or hard surfacing material applied to the toe and heel calks allows the shoes to stay sharp and be reset many times.

Front shoes—Scotch bottom pattern are usually made from ½ x 1¼ or 1½ inch iron. Today, most show horse shoes for any of the draft breeds are beveled or Scotched. The difference between breeds is primarily the hoof shape. Belgians and Percherons ideally have a round toe shape, Clydesdales and Shires have a more square toe shape. The outside branches of the shoes have more Scotch or bevel and are fit fuller than the inside branches. The last inch or so of the outside heels is turned out to emphasize the width of the foot and increase lateral support. The beveling may be done before the shoe is turned. Traditionally, Scotch bottom shoes are creased. Those that arc stamped only should be called bevel-edged show shoes. Some show horses are shod flat in front. Borium may be applied around the toes and on the calks (if used).

Hind shoes—Scotch bottom show pattern are usually made out of iron with the same dimensions as the front shoes. They usually have only one calk extremely beveled on the outside branch. The calk is placed behind the end of the heel and farther back than the end of the inside branch. A clip is drawn in the center of the curvature (closer to the inside) of the toe. The inside branch may be drawn to thin it out, is not beveled as much as the outside, is fit close and sometimes not creased. The outside branch is beveled to the extreme, creased and fit very full.

Hind shoes—Scotch bottom work pattern are made with two calks of equal height. The inside calk is lighter and follows the outline of the hoof wall at the heel. The outside calk is thicker and fit full. A broad and low toe calk is welded to the toe of the shoe. The majority of a horse's pulling power comes from its hind feet.

517

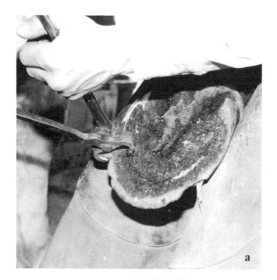
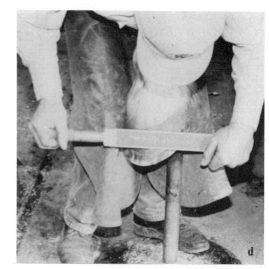
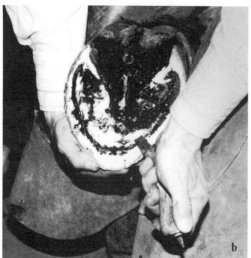
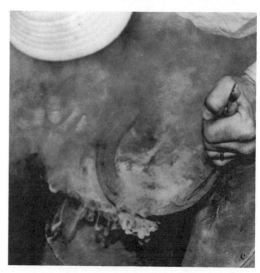
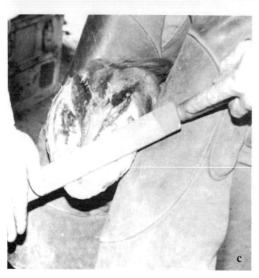

Fig. 42-17. Steps in shoeing a draft horse with handmade toe and heeled pulling shoes:
(a) Sight the foot and trim the wall level with the sole at the toe.
(b) Remove loose sole and ragged edges of the frog with the hoof knife.
(c) Level the hoof with the rasp sighting it frequently.
(d) Remove flares and shape the feet on a foot stand.
(e) Seat the clip and check the fit of the hot shoe.

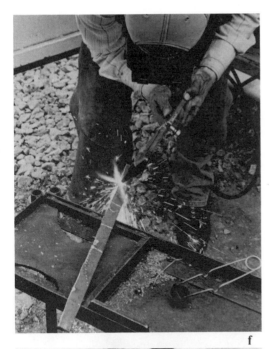

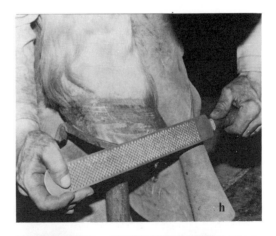

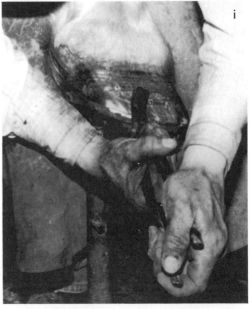

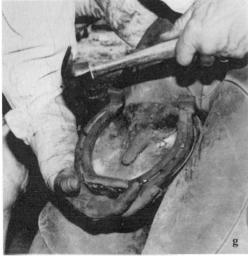

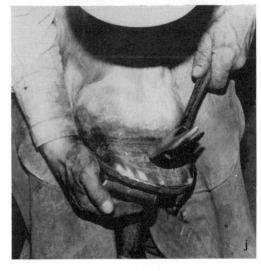

(f) Cut sharp toe calks from a piece of grader blade.
(g) Nail on shoe after arc welding on toe calk.
(h) Remove hoof burr from under blocked nails.
(i) Turn nails with clinchers.
(j) Seat clinches with hammer and block.

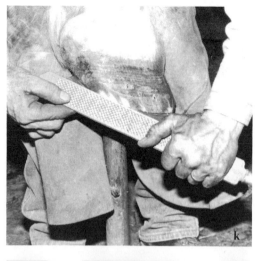
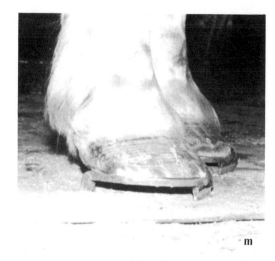
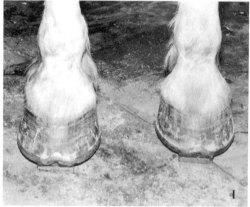
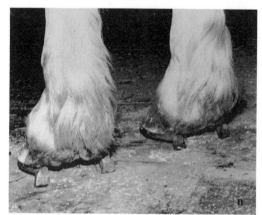

(k) Smooth wall with fine side of rasp and remove burr between hoof and shoe.
(l) Front, . . .
(m) . . . side, and. . .
(n) . . . rear views of completed job.

NOTES:

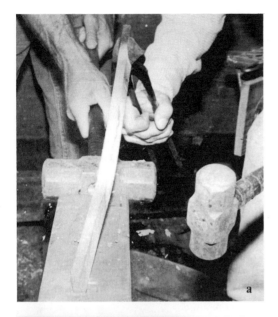

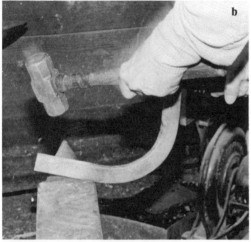

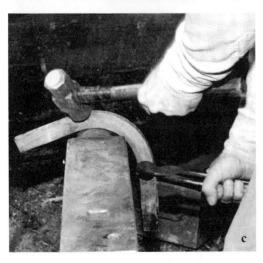

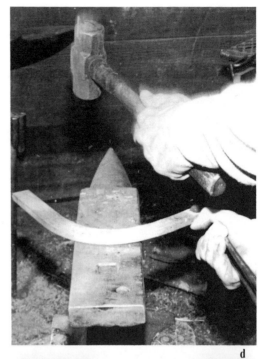

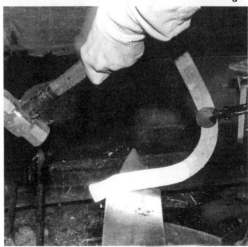

Fig. 42-18.   Steps in making a heeled Scotch bottom hitch horse show shoe:
(a) The sledge hammer and anvil hardy hole may be used to start the toe bend of a draft horse shoe.
(b) Make the toe of front shoes round.
(c) Use the horn as a fulcrum to finish the toe bend and put a bevel on the foot surface edge.
(d) Level the stock and reduce the thickened inside edge.
(e) Set down the end of the stock over a round edge to form the heel.

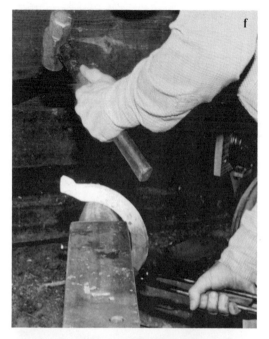

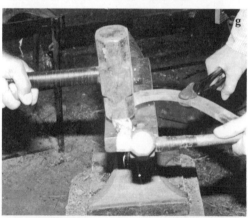

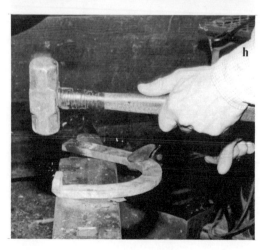

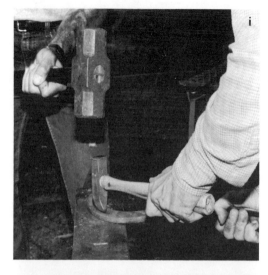

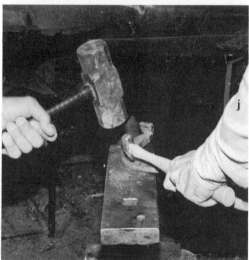

(f) Turn the branch over the anvil horn by striking next to the heel.

(g) Turn the heel of the shoe over the heel of the anvil using the sledge hammer to hold the shoe in place.

(h) Upset and straighten the heel calk.

(i) Strike the creaser with the sledge hammer handle in line with the creaser handle and over the center of the anvil.

(j) Strike the stamp with the sledge hammer handle perpendicular to the stamp handle.

(k) Pritchel out the holes with sharp blows at the angle of the wall at that point.

(l) Double strike the inside foot surface edge of the shoe to relieve sole pressure.

(m) Smooth up the crease if necessary.

(n) Taper the inside heel before setting it down over the round edge of the anvil.

(o) Turn the inside branch.

(p) Turn down the inside heel.

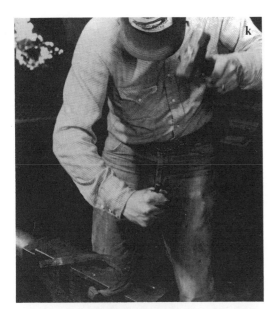

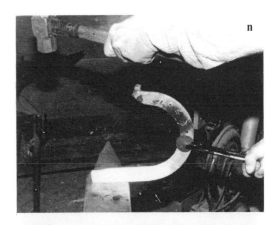

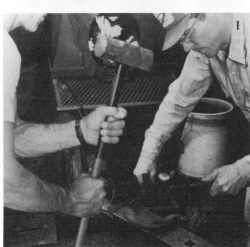

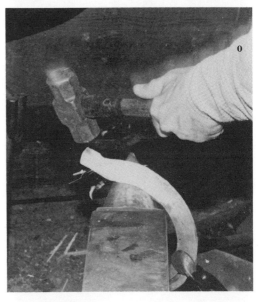

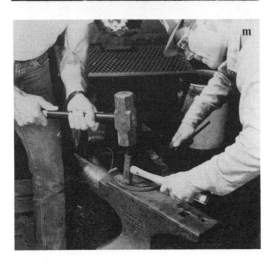

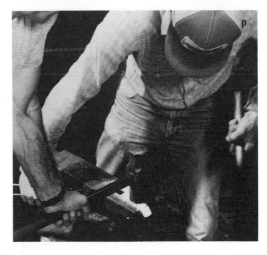

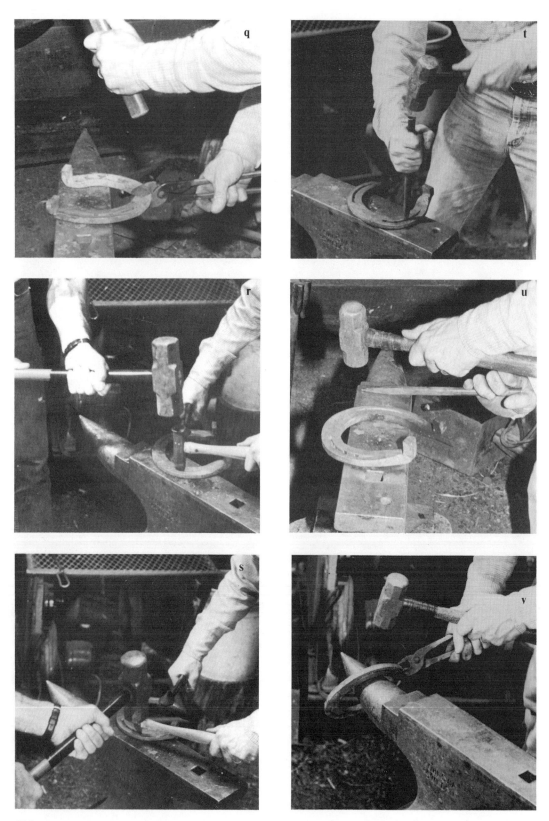

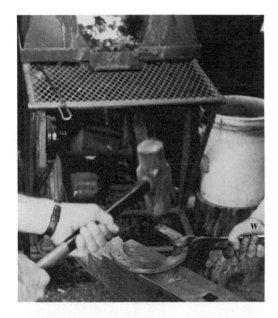

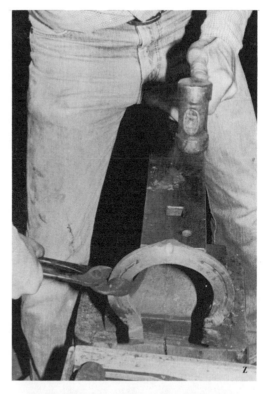

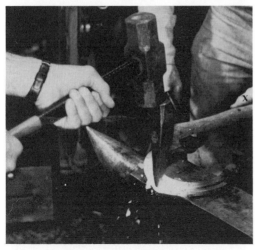

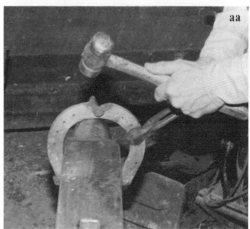

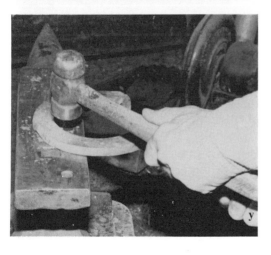

(q) Upset and straighten the calk.

(r) Run the crease.

(s) Stamp the nail holes.

(t) Pritchel out the nail holes at a steeper angle than the outside branch.

(u) Straighten the point of the pritchel as it becomes deformed.

(v) Bevel the foot surface edge.

(w) Concave the inside foot surface by double striking.

(x) Start the clip over the edge of the anvil with a bob punch.

(y) Cut down the bubble to the desired width of the clip.

(z) Pull the clip from the heel of the anvil.

(aa) Set the clip into the shoe and bevel the toe over the horn.

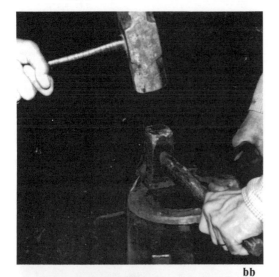

bb

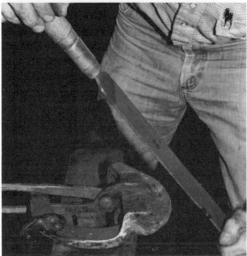

cc

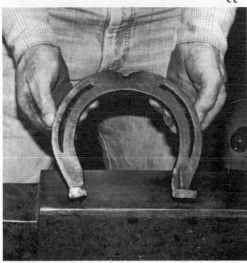

dd

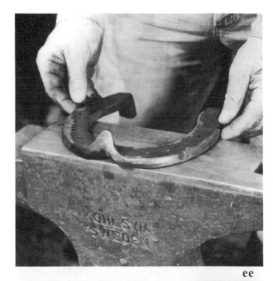

ee

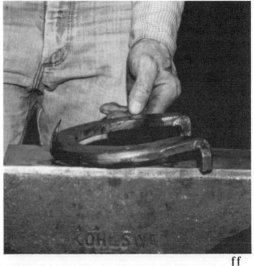

ff

(bb) Level the shoe around the clip with a flatter.
(cc) Finish the shoe with a hot rasp and file.
(dd) Ground surface, . . .
(ee) . . . foot surface, and . . .
(ff) . . . side view of the finished shoe.

Turning Scotch Bottom Show Shoes (Front-Calked)

A team of shoers works best for shoeing show draft horses. A team, where one acts as a striker and fire tender can shoe a draft horse with hand-made shoes in 2 to 3 hours. The system described has been used for centuries in Great Britain. Anyone that has been trained this way can interchange roles. However, by tradition, the old-

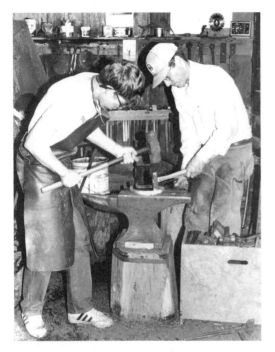

Fig. 42-15. *Draft horse shoes are best forged by two people working as a team.*

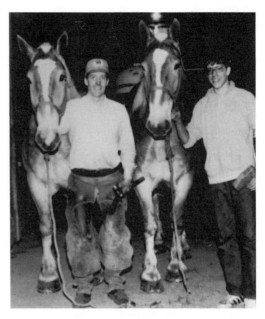

Fig. 42-20. *Shoeing a team of heavy horses with handmade shoes is satisfying but very hard work.*

est and therefore most experienced smith works behind the anvil. He makes decisions, directs the work and controls the hand hammer. The younger and less experienced person tends the fire, uses the sledge as requested (signaled), hands tools to the blacksmith and holds the filing tongs.

The fire should be kept going at a constant rate when a pair of shoes is turned. The striker should tend the fire and keep the iron properly positioned in it. Each heat (time the metal is taken from the fire) should be used efficiently. Practice is required to develop accuracy and timing. There are six or seven heats taken on each shoe for a total of 12 to 14 times the pair of shoes are taken from the fire and individually worked on the anvil. These are listed with the work to be done in each. The shoe would be taken to the horse for the first hot fitting after heat No. 4. Two extra heats may be required to accomplish the work in heats No. 2 and 3.

The sequence of hammer blows should be reviewed in the blacksmith's mind before the iron is brought to the anvil. At first, it may take two or more heats to do the work that is listed

to be done in one. Continually challenge yourself to work more efficiently. Work in haste while the iron is hot! Heavy iron is very unforgiving if you try to work it cold.

Work to be completed after each heating of the shoe:

1. Bevel the middle two-thirds of the straight iron toward the foot surface. Turn the toe to a rounded and predetermined shape.
2. Step down the outside heel and turn the outside branch. Bevel the foot surface outer edge. Turn the calk. Crease and stamp the branch. Pritchel the holes. Level the foot surface and concave it.
3. Turn the inside branch (as above).
4. Start the clip with a handled bob punch. Pull the clip. Shape the clip and toe. Go to the horse for the first fit check. Make minor adjustments.
5. Hot rasp the heel and foot surface edge of the branch using the vise or filing tongs held by helper.
6. Hot rasp the other heel and edge of the branch. File the clip, if necessary.
7. Check the general shoe shape and nail fit. Go to the horse for final check and fit before cooling.

References

Adams, J.W. 1903. Horseshoeing. USDA Farmer's Bull. #179.

Asmus, H. and J.O. Williams. 1927. Farm Horseshoeing. USDA Farmer's Bull. #1535.

Bashaw, B. and T. Bashaw. 1982. Shoeing stocks. Amer. Farriers' J. 8(3):164.

Bell, G.A. 1976. Breeds of draft horses. Small Farmer's J. 1(1):36.

Bjorck, G. 1958. Studies on the draught force of horses. Acta Agri. Scandinavica. Suppl. 4 p. 104.

Briggs, H.M. 1949. Modern Breeds of Livestock. The Macmillan Co., New York.

Buffus, D. 1977. Shoeing the horse. Small Farmer's J. 1(4):34.

Butler, D. 1982. Draft horseshoe making competition. Amer. Farrier's J. 8(3):154.

Butler, D. 1983. Train your own hammerman. Amer. Farrier's J. 9(4):294.

Daniels, B. 1980. Personal communication. Mullica Hill, NJ.

Daniels, B. 1983. Carriage horse shoeing. Amer. Farrier's J. 9(4):286.

DeMott, S. 1973. Wilma—the gentle giant that got away. Horseman. (Nov.):70.

Drew, J.M. 1979. Blacksmithing—horseshoeing. Small Farmer's J. 3(2):67.

Dyer, R. 1979. Personal communication. Tampa, FL.

Dykstra, R.R. 1977. When buying a horse. Small Farmer's J. 1(3):17.

Ensminger, M.E. 1977. Horses and Horsemanship (5th ed.) The Interstate, Danville, IL.

Farrell, B. 1980. Fitting draft horses for show. The Annual Clydesdale News. p. 9.

Flannigan, K.C. 1977. Those Magnificent Clydesdales. Crown Publishers, Inc., New York.

Garvan, F. and D. Reed. 1982. Pulling power: feet first. Amer. Farrier's J. 8(3):159.

Garvan, F. 1982. Shoeing with the Kriz brothers. Amer. Farriers' J. 8(3):167.

Gulley, J. 1983. Heavy horse shoeing competition. Amer. Farrier's J. 9(4):305.

Hamilton, S. 1980. 40 horses—how an Iowa farmer became a national celebrity with just a little help from his friends. Equus. 28:25.

Harris, F.S. 1972. Jake Posey and the forty-horse hitch. The Western Horseman. (Dec.):46.

Irons, R. 1983. Workhorse shoeing. Amer. Farrier's J. 9(4):270.

Johnstone, H. 1980. The draft horse. The Western Horseman. 45(10):47.

Kays, D.J. 1953. The Horse. Holt, Rinehart and Winston, New York.

Kraus, S. 1983. Scotch bottom shoes. Amer. Farrier's J. 9(4):280.

Lent, W. and L. Lent. 1983. Scotch bottom shoes—design and function. The Draft Horse Journal. (Autumn):70.

Lessiter, F. Horse Power. Reiman Publ., Inc., Milwaukee.

McHugh, F.T. 1968. Goliath. The Western Horseman. (Dec.):110.

Martin, E. 1982. Personal Communication. Valley Forge, PA.

Martin, E. 1982. Profile: Edward Martin remembers apprenticehood. Amer. Farrier's J. 8(3):174.

Miller, C. 1980. San Francisco ranch. Small Farmer's J. 4(3):38.

Miller, L.R. 1981. Work Horse Handbook. Mill Press, Inc., Reedsport, OR.

Nordby and Lattiz. 1977. Preparation of draft horses for show. Small Farmer's J. 1(3):64.

Plumb, C.S. 1917. Judging Farm Animals. Orange Judd Co., New York.

Reame, B. 1976. Draft horse shoeing. Michigan Horseshoer's Assn. Clinc. East Lansing, MI.

Rice, B. 1980. The making of a horseshoe. Small Farmer's J. 4(2):56.

Roberts, N. 1980. New England visit—Kriz bros. Small Farmer's J. 2(4):72.

Telleen, M. 1976. Draft horse pulling contests. The Western Horseman. (Aug.):44.

Telleen, M. 1977. The Draft Horse Primer. Rodale Press, Inc., Emmaus, PA.

Tew, N.C. 1945. The Safe and Scientific Method of Shoeing Horses and Mules. Published by the author.

The Shire: pulling his own weight. 1980. Equus. 35:57.

Thompson, D. 1978. Resurrection of the draft. Equus. 13:42.

Wade, G. 1982. Shoeing the big ones. Amer. Farrier's J. 8(3):150.

Weatherly, L. 1972. Heavy Horse Handbook. The Southern Counties Heavy Horse Assoc., Cranleigh, Surrey, ENGLAND.

Weber, P. 1968. How big is a horse? The Horseman's Courier. (June):27.

Wenk, B. 1980. Draft horse pull. Horseman. (Jan.):78.

Chapter 43

Road Horses

Many horse owners find it necessary to ride or drive their horses on hard-surfaced roads a good percentage of the time. Others must do their work and pleasure riding over icy or rocky terrain. Traction-increasing shoes are very desirable in such situations.

Carriage driving or coaching has undergone a dramatic comeback in recent years. Thousands of horsemen now drive horses in single or team hitches for pleasure and for sport. Driving marathons and three-day or combined driving competitions over obstacle courses are increasing in popularity. Teams of two, four or six or more horses may be used. The wheel horses are near the coach, the leaders are in front and the swing horses are in between. A four in hand is a hitch of two teams of carriage or coach horses. These horses are intermediate in size between riding horses and draft horses. Many are imported and most are valuable animals. They are often matched at great expense by breeding, selection and training. Carriage horses must be shod often due to the many miles they are driven over hard and slick roads.

Endurance and competitive trail riding are very popular in some parts of the U.S. Shoes for these mostly Arabian marathon runners must be light enough to prevent fatigue but heavy enough to provide resistance to wear and protection to the foot. A simple open plate self-cleaning shoe is best for the horse if its feet are gradually conditioned. Hard surfacing and/or traction increasing materials may be applied to the shoes. Light polyurethane plastic pads such as Farrier's Pride No. 1[1] are recommended on tender-footed horses to prevent sole injury. However, rules may prohibit full pads and limit the width and style of the shoes used in competition. Spooned heels may be used to protect the heel bulbs in rocky terrain.

Coach drivers (called whips) and others doing a lot of road work or long distance riding should be encouraged to carry a rubber or leather boot as a "spare tire." This may prevent injury to the hoof if a shoe is thrown when they are a long way from home. It will make repair much easier for the horseshoer and reduce the risk of lameness.

[1] *The Shoeing Shop, Yucaipa, CA*

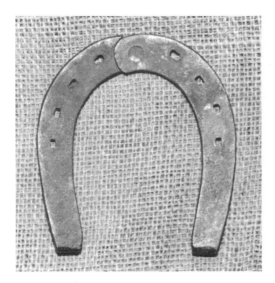

Fig. 43-1. "Spare tire" adjustable hinged shoe. Photo by J. Graves.

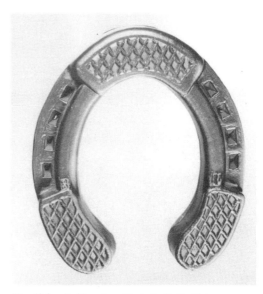

Fig. 43-2. Rubber shoe. Photo by G. Poellot.

Rubber Shoes and Pads

Rubber shoes are popular for horses used exclusively for slow road work. Rubber shoes are thicker than conventional shoes, are clipped, and have a steel center. They are fit cold. Rubber shoes have several disadvantages. They are expensive, they are difficult to fit and they keep the frog off the ground.

Rubber pads with traction risers in the heel area are called roadster or road pads. They are available in several styles and thicknesses. Some allow the use of a full shoe, others cover the entire heel and require only a three-quarter or short shoe. Two variations are the vacuum (suction cup) heel pad and the thinner x-ray racing pad with a leather pad bonded to the foot surface of the rubber pad. They are applied under a steel shoe.

Rubber shoes and pads absorb concussion as well as provide traction. Police, circus, parade, carriage and horses performing on stage use rubber shoes.

Pieces of tire tread cut the size of the horse's foot can be used when rubber shoes are not available. The tread is cut to half its thickness around the outside edge and nailed on. Small washers are slipped on the nails to prevent the heads from pulling through the rubber. A shoe can be nailed on to hold the outside edge leaving the tire insert (pad) next to the ground. A strip

of tire can be riveted across the shoe in front of the calks of draft horses used on roads.

Cast steel bar rope shoes were formerly used for traction on city streets. The tarred rope was removed while the shoe was fit and nailed. The rope was then laid in the groove and hammered into place. The rope was replaced each day, sometimes every few hours.

Hoof Cushions

A wide-webbed shoe may be all that is necessary on a road horse with a sound foot and a thick, well-arched sole. For others, pads may be necessary. Full pads have the disadvantage of covering the frog and keeping the sole soft.

Stromsholm hoof cushions[2] are thick rim pads made of alkathene plastic. They extend below the foot surface to the ground surface of the shoe. The thick inner rim has a foam center. Cushions absorb concussion and evenly distribute pressure over the sole and wall, but leave the frog uncovered. Cushions help prevent side bone and ringbone. These conditions are major problems in horses used on the road.

Studs

Studs, small calks with hardened centers, are driven or screwed into the shoe. They are preferred in Europe where borium application is prohibitively expensive. They are increasing in popularity in America. See Chapter 38.

[2] *Centaur Forge, Ltd., Burlington, WI*

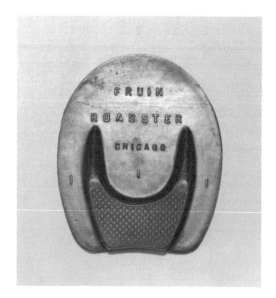

Fig. 43-3. Roadster pad. Photos by J. Graves.

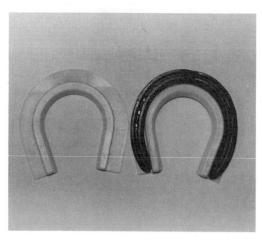

Fig. 43-4. Stromsholm hoof cushions.

In addition to price, studs have the advantage of allowing one to change the height of the calk to match the ground conditions encountered. This is very desirable for three-day event or combined driving horses since they compete on several types of ground in each competition. The weather can change ground condition rapidly. Studs are also good for road horses. Short studs are used in place of borium to create traction on hard roads. They may be replaced by tall studs when travel is to be across soft and slippery terrain.

Borium-coated rivets or bolts can be improvised and used in place of studs. They may be preferred on some surfaces. The tapped hole that is punched or drilled in the shoe heel may be filled with cork or a flush allen screw when a flat shoe is desired. Holes are easiest to drill and tap after a shoe has cooled slowly. Rapid quenching increases the hardness of a steel shoe. Self-tapping studs are now available[3]. Snow tire studs can be installed in shoes like Borium-coated rivets (Simpson, 1971).

Snow Shoes

Snow, especially wet snow, has a tendency to "ball up" or pack into the foot. A self-cleaning or concave pattern shoe (called a snow shoe by some manufacturers) is of some help. Smearing grease on the bottom of the sole was recommended for years. Formerly, each coach carried a small snowball hammer to assist in breaking the snow from the feet of the horses.

An effective short term solution to "snowballing" is spraying silicone or teflon spray on

[3] *Centaur Forge, Ltd., Burlington, WI*

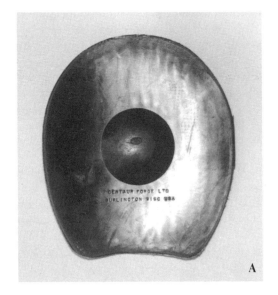

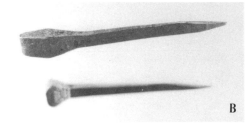

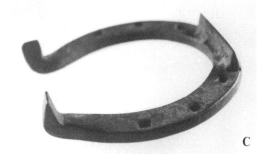

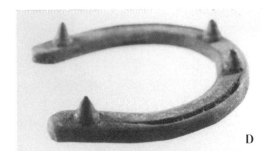

A

B

C

D

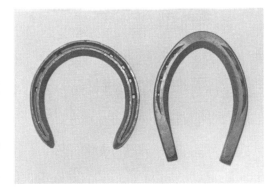

Fig. 43-5.   Snow, concave or self-cleaning shoe pattern.

Fig. 43-6.   Other winter shoeing aids: (A) anti-snowball pad, (B) frost head nail compared to city head nail, (C) sharp shoe—see Chapter 42, and (D) never-slip studs—see Chapter 38.

531

the bottom of the feet before traveling in snow. The bottom of the foot and shoe should be brushed clean and dried with alcohol first. This helps the silicone to stick.

Snow platform shoes made from wood and attached with metal bands have been used to prevent sinking in deep snow or boggy ground.

Anti-snowball pads[4], called pneumatic pads are made of resilient black rubber. The air-filled ball in the center compresses as the horse steps on it. When the foot is lifted, the ball pushes out the packed snow and ice. Ball height varies from 5/16 to 3/4 inch. Anti-snowball pads also prevent sole bruising by sharp ice. They do not crack when frozen as many plastic pads do. Foam rubber under plastic container material can be used as a substitute for rubber pneumatic pads.

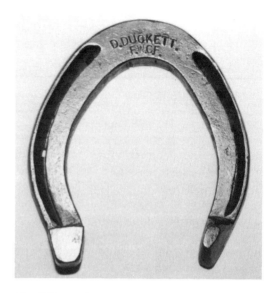

Fig. 43-7. English roadster shoe made by David Duckett. Photo by J. Graves.

Frost Nails

Borium spot build-up is best for creating traction on ice. However, a means of quickly creating traction on snow or ice covered surfaces is to use frost nails[5] instead of horseshoe nails. The old nails can be individually pulled and replaced by the frost nails without removing the shoe. Frost nails can be dangerous due to the possibility of treading on the opposite foot. They become dull and tend to work loose when left in the shoe for an extended period of time.

Roadster Shoes

Roadster shoes are a type used in the British Isles on horses that pull carts over roads. The front shoes are flat and creased from heel to heel. The hind shoe has a thickened toe, thinned branches and an outside caulkin (calk) and inside wedge. The hind shoes may be creased or stamped. Roadster shoes are made from 1/2 x 1 inch stock. These shoes make excellent competition shoes due to the variety of forging operations involved in making them.

Concave or heavy full swedged or fullered (creased) shoes are also used for road work. The crease fills with dirt and creates more traction than a flat shoe. "Cover" for the hoof heel and seat of corn area is especially important. Much

---

[4] *Centaur Forge Ltd., Burlington, WI*
[5] *O. Mustad and Son, Inc., Auburn, NY*
[6] *Stoody Company, Whittier, CA*

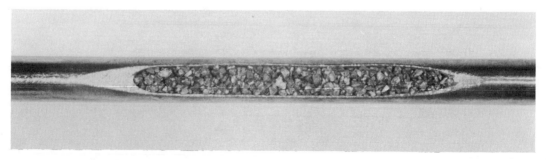

Fig. 43-8. Horseshoe borium—tungsten carbide particles in a mild steel filler rod. Photo from Stoody Co.

of the conditioning of heavy hunters is done on the roads in Great Britain.

Horseshoe Borium

Horseshoe Borium[6], pure tungsten carbide particles in a mild steel flux or matrix, is the most popular traction increasing substance for road horses in America. In most areas, its application has replaced the tall screw-type ice calk ("never slip") and traditional sharp shoeing with toed and heeled shoes. Borium may yet fall into disfavor in this country due to its rising cost, even though it is a superior traction-increasing substance.

Borium may be used to increase the life of a shoe. However, this practice is not generally recommended even though it may be a fringe benefit of its application for traction purposes. The use of Borium to extend the life of shoes usually proves to be disappointing since the shoe often wears out next to where the Borium has been placed, and the nail holes become too large to effectively hold the shoe in place for longer than the normal life expectancy of the shoe. People have a tendency to let horses that are shod with Borium go longer between shoeings, and thus these expensive shoes may be lost. Also, shoes with Borium on them are very hard to reshape and level, and are especially hard on tools and the anvil. A mild steel plate covering the anvil face and anchored in the hardy hole will protect the anvil.

Borium comes in several screen sizes. Horseshoe Borium, screen size 8 to 10, is made of large, uniformly-sized particles of pure tungsten carbide encased within a tubular mild steel rod. This type will provide some degree of traction on any surface. In some areas, Drill Tech or coarse borium particles (5 to 8 screen size) distributed in a bronze matrix is more popular than horseshoe borium. Shoes can be obtained made up with Borium or Drill Tech from some welding shops[7].

Acetylene-tube Borium and Electric-tube Borium, screen size 10 to 40, is made of very fine particles and is unsuitable for application to horseshoes to increase traction. It will reduce the rate of wear on a shoe but at the same time produces a very smooth surface. It is used mostly

for hard-surfacing the cutting edges of farm implements and cutting tools. The fine particle borium is manufactured in smaller diameter sticks (⅛ and 3/16 in.) than the regular (¼ in.) or coarse (⅜ in.) borium.

Horseshoe Borium is manufactured in mild steel rods ¼ inch in diameter and 14 inches long. Borium is very expensive, costing as much as $20.00 or more per pound wholesale in some areas. Leftover short pieces of Borium rods should be welded to the ends of new rods so there is no waste. Treat Borium like it was gold! A little goes a long way.

Borium Application

Borium is applied in several patterns to the shoe depending on the use of the horse. If the horse is to be ridden cross-country on turf and on roads occasionally, such as a hunter or jumper would be, two to three spots on the toe depending on the size of the shoe, and one on each heel, is recommended. When the horse is to be ridden on roads and other dry surfaces such as a parade or city horse would be, an application of a surface-facing pattern covering the heels and toe of the shoe is usually recommended.

Deposits of Borium should be placed on the outer edge of the ground surface at the toe to insure lateral support of the horse and uniform wear of the shoe. Occasionally, borium should be put on the branch of the shoe. Clips are recommended when borium is used to prevent shifting of the shoe. Wide and low clips or rolls on the rear shoes may be lightly coated with borium to prevent excessive toe wear in carriage horses. Borium creates so much traction that the nails have increased stress on them. Clips should always be used when a horse will not retain the shoes for at least four weeks.

Borium application must be applied with judgment. It is easily overdone. The borium will outwear the shoe no matter how applied. Put it where the shoe wears most. Light boned horses should not have as heavy an application as draft horses. Do not make calks out of borium. Build the calks from the shoe or added stock and then add the borium as a hard facing.

Horseshoe Borium is usually applied with an oxy-acetylene torch. It is very advisable to obtain training and practice in the use of the torch

[7] *D.L. Schwartz Co., Berne, IN*

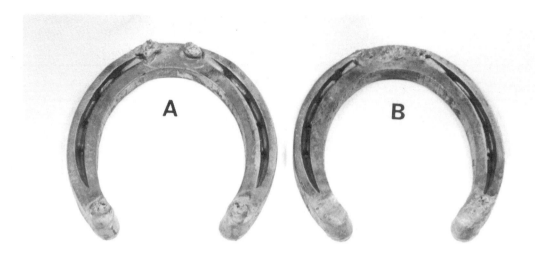

Fig. 43-9. Patterns of borium application: (A) spots—used mostly on cross country horses, (B) surface facing used mostly on road horses. Photo by G. Poellot.

before trying to apply borium to horseshoes. This should be done not only because of the danger involved in operating the equipment, but also because of the high cost of the Borium. Mistakes can be very costly.

Steps in applying Horseshoe Borium to horseshoes:

1. Secure the oxygen and acetylene tanks upright in your truck or shop so that they can not bounce around or be knocked over. The tank valves should be covered with screw-on caps during transport. Tank and valve connections should be checked for leaks with soapy water when you first set them up. Always wear welding goggles when applying Borium. Install flashback protection valves on your welding hoses or regulators.

2. Check both regulator screws to be sure they are backed off and loose. Turn on the acetylene tank valve about one-third of a turn. Leave the handle or key on the tank so it may be shut off in an emergency. Turn on the oxygen tank valve all the way open or about two turns. This prevents leakage from the top of the valve.

3. Set the regulator gauges at about 6 pounds pressure for acetylene and 12 pounds pressure for oxygen. Later, you can set the pressure lower and conserve gas. A No. 5 welding tip is about right for welding horseshoe size stock and applying borium.

4. Turn on the torch acetylene valve and light it with the striker.

5. Adjust the acetylene flame by slowly increasing the flow of gas until the flame jumps

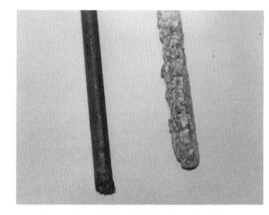

Fig. 43-10. Horseshoe borium rod (left) compared to a drill tech rod (right).

away from the tip; then slowly decrease the flow of the gas until the flame just starts to jump back to the tip. Another indicator of correct acetylene pressure is a flame that burns with no visible carbon.

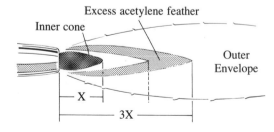

Fig. 43-11. Oxy-acetylene flame adjustment for applying horseshoe borium. Drawing by L. Sadler.

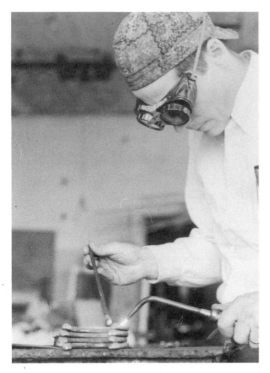

Fig. 43-12. *Preheating of shoes can be done in the forge or by stacking them. Photo by L. Butler.*

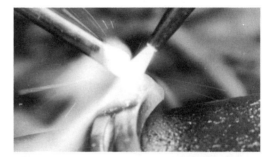

Fig. 43-13. *The shoe (and rod) must be heated until the surface melts or puddles before adding borium. Photos by G. Poellot.*

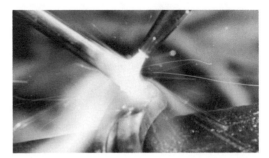

Fig. 43-14. *Borium is added or stacked to create spots by moving the torch tip up the rod.*

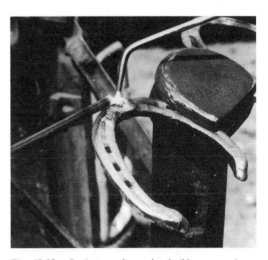

Fig. 43-15. *Borium can be used to build up worn shoes. Photos from Stoody Co.*

6. Turn on the torch oxygen valve and, by slowly increasing the flow of oxygen, adjust the flame to a 2X or 3X flame. A 3X flame has an excess acetylene adjustment that makes the greenish feather of the flame three times the length of the inner blue cone.

7. Preheat the area of the shoe to which the Borium is to be applied. This can be done with either the torch or the forge. If you have been using your forge, place all the shoes in the forge, one on top of the other, and preheat the toes or heels to an orange heat. The bottom one will get hot first. Remove it when it reaches the right temperature and turn the forge down low or off to avoid overheating of the remaining shoes. Apply Borium to the preheated shoe. Place the shoe back in the forge on top with the opposite end in the fire. Then pull the next bottom one from the forge and so on until Borium has been applied to all of them. This procedure will save a lot of time and welding gas.

8. Apply the torch flame to the specific place on the shoe where the Borium is to be placed until the surface of the shoe begins to "puddle" under the flame. Hold the tip of the Borium rod near the area being heated to allow it to preheat.

9. Place the preheated tip of the Borium rod in the puddle on the shoe and fuse the shoe and rod.

10. Transfer the flame to the rod and "stack" or drip the Borium particles in the melting metal rod matrix on top of the puddle spot.

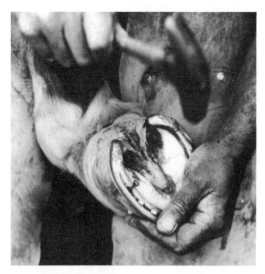

Fig. 43-16.   Shoes with borium applied can usually be reset many times.

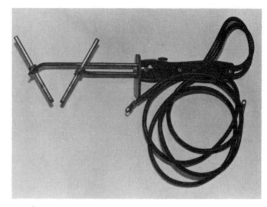

Fig. 43-18.   A carbon arc torch can be used in place of oxy acetylene equipment for borium application.

Do this until the deposit is about ¼ inch high or as high as desired. This method of deposit results in the spot type of pattern. The surface-facing type of pattern is applied by extending the puddle, much as one would when welding, and melting a small coating of the rod onto the puddle and spreading it over the surface of the web of the shoe.

11. "Wash" the Borium deposit, if necessary. This is done when instant traction on hard slick surfaces is desired. Continue heating the Borium deposit until the top layer of the matrix metal begins to flow slightly and leave the sharp Borium particles extending above it. The soft metal of the matrix will wear away with normal use and the same effect will be achieved in time.

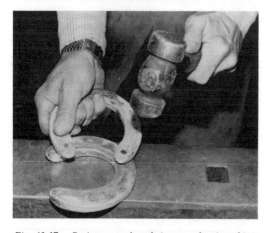

Fig. 43-17.   Borium coated steel rivets can be riveted into aluminum shoes to provide traction and reduce wear. Photos by J. Graves.

12. Allow the shoe to cool until it is only warm to the touch before placing it in water. If the shoe is placed in water before it is allowed to cool in the air, the Borium may chip or flake off if any minor alterations are made on the shoe, when it is nailed on, or in ordinary wear by the horse. In order to save time, nail on the first shoe to which Borium was applied while the others are cooling.

Welding Equipment

The carbon-arc torch attachment for the electric arc welder can be used to apply Horseshoe Borium. It allows a much faster application of Borium than the oxy-acetylene process but has required heavy and expensive equipment, a power source or gasoline-operated generator. Now, low amperage 115 volt welders are available. They are light and powerful enough for most horseshoeing uses. A carbon arc torch can also be used with these inexpensive portable units. Effective shielding of bystanders from the harmful rays of the electric arc is most important.

Extreme caution should always be exercised when using welding equipment, and training should be obtained by a horseshoer before attempting to use it. (Many high schools and colleges offer night school classes in welding.)

All horseshoers and blacksmiths should know how to use welding equipment safely and skillfully. Welding equipment can often save time and add versatility to the operations an expert horseshoer might perform with a forge, such as making bar shoes, clips, special corrective shoes, etc.

References

Atterbury, A.L. 1981. The horses wore wooden shoes. Amer. Farriers' J. 7(1):35.

Brown, B. and O. Lindholm. 1979. Shoeing for pavement. The Western Horseman. (Nov): 76.

Butler, D. 1977. The hoof's role in competitive trail riding. Saddle Action. 4(7):18.

Flock, K.D. 1968. Snowshoes for horses. The Western Horseman. (Dec):16.

Glass, N. 1977. Why not four? Saddle Action. 4(7):22.

Kennedy, G.A. 1975. Complete Book of Welding. J.W. Sams, Inc., Indianapolis.

Lungwitz, A. and J.W. Adams. 1913. A Textbook of Horseshoeing (11th ed.). Oregon State Univ. Press, Corvallis.

Mohr, N. 1977. On the trail of trax. Saddle Action. 4(7):22.

Rasmussen, M.I. 1975. Preventing snow from balling in the hoofs. The Western Horseman. (Jan):20.

Simpson, S. 1971. Studs on horseshoes. The Western Horseman. (Mar):90.

Simpson, S. 1972. Borium horseshoes. The Western Horseman. (Mar):147.

Simpson, S. 1977. Tips for winter shoeing. The Western Horseman. (Jan):78.

Smith, H.R.B. 1966. Blacksmiths' and Farriers' Tools at Shelburne Museum. The Shelburne Museum, Inc., Shelburne, VT.

Stockho, C. 1984. Coming to grips with ground grippers. Equus. 75:36.

Tellington, W. 1977. An analysis of horse shoes at the tevis cup ride. Saddle Action. 4(7):22.

Williams, T. 1981. Wedges and Cushions. Amer. Farriers' J. 7(3):134.

Winquist, B. 1969. Hoof pads. The Western Horseman. (Feb):84.

NOTES:

Chapter 44

Mules

Mules are different from horses. They have a different appearance, different behavior and different feet.

Draft mules are most common in the Southern states and the Midwest, especially Missouri. Saddle and pack mules are most common in the Rocky Mountains, the Southwest, and on the West Coast.

Mules are true hybrids, that is they are the product of a cross between two species. They have an odd chromosome number of 63 (between the mare's 64 and the jack's 62) which makes them sterile. Hybrids possess vigor or strengths greater than those of either parent. Thus, the mule has hardy qualities that make him preferred by many as a pack animal, a riding animal, a farm draft animal and a logging horse.

Mammoth jacks are a large breed of donkey or ass. A good jack will stand 15.3 hands and weigh 1200 pounds. They were made popular in the U.S. by George Washington. He began producing them as early as 1785. Mammoth jacks are bred to Thoroughbred and Quarter Horse mares to get riding mules. They are bred to Draft mares to get draft mules. Sorrel draft mules with light points (blonde) are especially popular.

Jennies carry their foals longer than mares, some as long as 13 months. Mule foals are very hardy. Mules live longer and are more active than horses at advanced ages. They are known to stand hot weather better than horses.

Ears and head are to a mule person what a silky smooth leg feather is to a Clydesdale enthusiast. Mules shed later than horses in the spring. They are usually clipped in a special way. The mane is always roached. The tail is roached down about 3 inches from the dock. In the West, the upper part of the tail is clipped in a bell pattern. The head and ears are clipped except for a little tuft of hair at the tip of each ear.

There is a difference of opinion regarding the disposition of mules. Some describe them as being stubborn and stoical or indifferent in temperament. Mules are said to be unpredictable

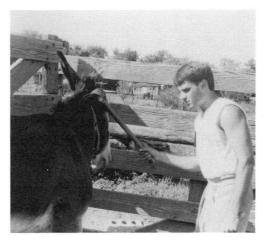

Fig. 44-1.   Mules and jack stock should be tied very short for trimming and shoeing.

Fig. 44-2.   An ear twitch or pressure at the base of the tail will restrain many mules.

and difficult to handle. It is said they will work patiently for 10 years for a chance to kick you once. Others say the mule's patience is due to his quiet temperament and docile habits. These people say mules aren't vicious, though they may be obstinate. Mules are said to have a more steady and reliable disposition than a horse.

Mules are less apt to injure themselves than horses. This is especially true when they are restrained properly. They develop fewer problems than horses since they stop before they are fatigued and rarely overeat. Even with self-feeding, laminitis is rare.

Mules are said to be less subject to various limb ailments than horses. Splints are almost unknown. Ringbone and spavin are less common than in horses worked under the same conditions. Mules are not as sensitive to fatigue from hard work as horses but are intolerant of abuse. The general conformation and structure of mules should closely resemble horses of a similar type (except the head and ears).

It has been said that mules can do more work on less food than a horse. However, in words of one stockman, "The mule was not consulted when that statement was made." The mule's ability to take care of itself and survive inexperienced handling has contributed to its longevity (they live longer than horses) and usefulness to man.

One must be cautious as well as patient when working with mules. Mules that kick are accurate. They possess a wide range of motion with their hind limbs. This ability has been referred to as cow kicking. Mules may also bite. Jacks are known to be worse than mules about this. In fact, a Missouri farmer once said, "If a jack bites you, you'll probably get your name in the paper!"

Mules have many regional nicknames. One of the most well known is "mountain canary" since mules bray or sing when they want to. Some names have to do with a mule's size and application. For example, there are draft, sugar, cotton, pack or mine mules.

Other mule names have to do with origin and sex. The donkey, or ass, is of the same genus but a different species than the horse. A male ass is called a jackass or jack. A female ass is called a jennet or jenny. A mule is the result of the mating of a jack to a mare. A hinny results from mating a stallion to a jenny. There are few hinnies. Jennies are used almost exclusively to produce good jack stock. Jacks should be raised with horses from the time they are weaned to prevent them from becoming jenny spoiled. A jenny spoiled jack prefers to breed only jennies. A horse mule is a male mule, a molly mule is a female mule. Male mules are usually castrated even though they are sterile.

Still other mule names refer to temperament. No examples!

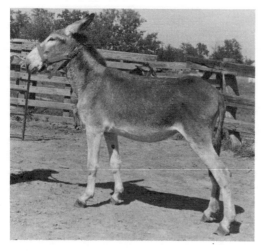

Fig. 44-3. An older jenny of the Mammoth breed showing high quality.

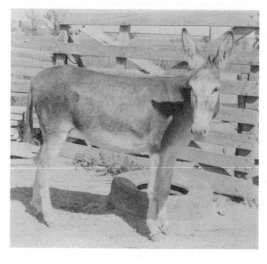

Fig. 44-4. A young high quality jenny.

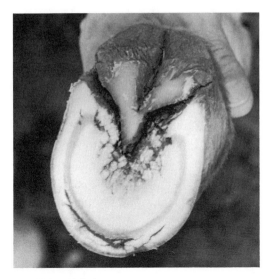

Fig. 44-5.   Mule foot.

to a size 6 or 8 on a similar sized draft horse. The foot has a peculiar, long, narrow shape. The frog fills the entire heel area and is proportionately larger in relation to the rest of the hoof than that of a horse. Weight is borne directly by the frog. The sole of the hoof is very concave.

The hoof wall is rounded and thick in the toe, pinched in and thinner at the quarter and flared out and thick at the heel. The bars are usually thick and prominent. The length of the hoof wall is relatively long and upright when compared to a horse's hoof. Mule hoofs are usually denser than horse hoofs and less subject to quarter cracks. The wall may have an almost vertical slope in the area where the toe nails are placed in a shoe. The angle of the wall may be more than 90 degrees in the area where the heel nails are placed. Mules are easily quicked in this area of the foot by inexperienced shoers.

Hoof Differences

Conformation of the ear and head is considered more important than the feet by most mule enthusiasts. Mules usually have sound feet and legs.

The mule's foot is smaller than that of a horse of equal body weight. A heavy draft mule may have a hoof that would be a size 1 or 2 compared

Shoeing Differences

Mules usually have a higher pastern angle than horses. Excessive trimming of the frog and bars should be avoided. The heels often grow faster than the toe and must be trimmed accordingly. The frog protrudes below the heels since the buttresses do not project as far back as they do on a horse.

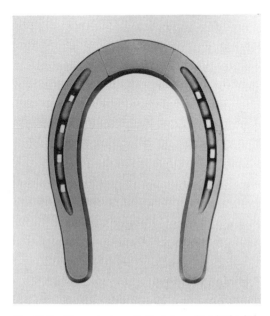 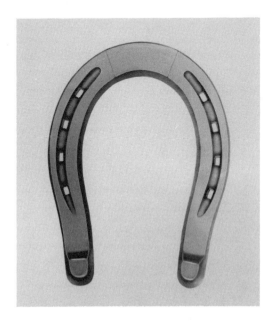

Fig. 44-6.   Keg mule shoes: (left) plain, and (right) heeled. Photos from Diamond.

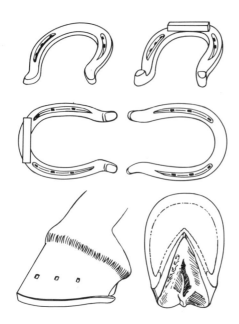

Fig. 44-7. Handmade mule shoe design and fit. Drawing by J. Hoffman and K. Burdette.

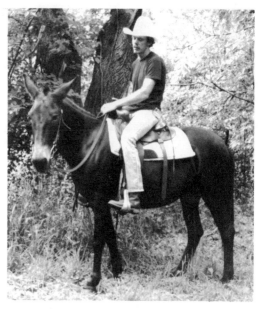

Fig. 44-8. A 5-year-old molly trail-riding mule sired by a Mammoth Jack and out of a Walking Horse mare. Photo by B. Bolling.

Shoes are fit to the outline of the hoof wall around to the quarter. The heels of the shoe are turned out, trailered or "muled" at the heels to follow the outward curvature of the hoof at the buttress and clear the frog. The shoe heels should extend beyond the buttresses ¼ inch or more depending on the hoof's conformation and slope at the heel.

Mule shoes should be lighter weight and not as thick as a horseshoe. Calks are popular. Low toe and heel calks are preferred. Borium is usually not needed, since mules are naturally very surefooted. Six nails per shoe are usually enough even for a large mule. Small mules or jacks need only four nails per shoe. Nail holes should be punched perpendicular to the shoe or as the wall slope indicates. Solid pieces of tire tread cut away to expose the frog may be nailed to the foot instead of shoes for traction in rough country or on roads. Small washers may be slipped over the nails to prevent them from being driven through the rubber.

Mule Shoeing Contests

Mule shoeing contests are an exciting part of Mule Days in several parts of the country. Trimming of the feet and preshaping of the shoes may be allowed. These contests are judged principally on speed. Times may be under 5 minutes.

References

Baumli, L. 1983. Personal communication. Barnard, MO.

Dollar, J.A.W. 1898. A Handbook of Horseshoeing. W.R. Jenkins, New York.

Ensminger, M.E. 1977. Horses and Horsemanship (5th edition). Interstate, Danville, IL.

Green, L. 1978. How to shoe a mule in six minutes. Amer. Farrier's J. 4(1):15.

Johnson, R. 1984. He who heehaws last heehaws best: the mule comeback. The Wall Street Journal. Feb. 9:1.

Lungwitz, A. and J.W. Adams. 1966. A Textbook of Horseshoeing. Oregon State University, Corvallis.

Mills, F.C. and H.L. Hall. 1980. The History of the American Jack and Mule. Helen L. Halls, Hutchinson, KS.

Plumb, C.S. 1917. Judging Farm Animals. Orange Judd Co., New York.

Riley, H. 1868. The Mule. Dick and Fitzgerald, New York.

Taylor, T. 1983. All you ever wanted to know about your ass but were afraid to ask. Anvil. 8(2):3.

Telleen, M. 1982. Ralph Chattin—Indiana mule man. The Draft Horse J. 19(4):23.

Telleen, M. 1982. What is a mammoth jack? The Draft Horse J. 19(4):30.

War Department. 1941. The Horseshoer. United States Government Printing Office, Washington, DC.

Youatt, W. and J.S. Skinner. 1843. The Horse, Ass and Mule. Porter and Coates, Philadelphia.

Chapter 45

Oxen

The trimming of dairy or beef cattle and the shoeing of oxen is discussed in all horseshoeing texts written on the continent of Europe. Most American and English texts ignore the subject. Some American farriers make most of their living caring for the feet of cattle. The detection and treatment of lameness in cattle is a significant part of the practice of a few large animal veterinarians.

Oxen or bullocks are steers used for draft purposes. Oxen were some of the first domesticated animals. Rarely do cattle need to be shod for any reason other than the correction of pathological foot problems. However, oxen often need to be shod to protect their feet from wear and to provide traction. Heavy aged oxen are most susceptible to foot ailments. The ox was considered superior to the horse for plowing and hauling for many centuries. Pound for pound a horse can out pull an ox, but ox teams may outweigh horse teams. Oxen are slower but less expensive than horses. Less expensive equipment is needed to work oxen.

Early American pioneers preferred oxen to horses for pioneering and the westward trek. Horses and harness were several times more expensive than oxen and a homemade neck yoke. The oxen could make do on poorer quality feed than a horse. They did not require an expert teamster, and were not as subject to stampeding and theft by Indians. Also, cattle could be eaten when they were no longer fit for draft use. Improvements in equipment and increased agricultural acreage caused oxen to be completely replaced by horses by the late 1800's in America. Oxen are still used in many parts of the world for draft purposes.

Anatomy of the Ox Claw

The ox claw is different from the horse's foot. There are two bones (and hoofs) for each one in the horse from the fetlock on down. The coronary band is wider and much flatter than that of a horse. The wall is comparatively thin and curved (convex). The ox does not have secondary laminae to strengthen the attachment of the hoof and foot bone. There are no lateral cartilages. The sole is flat and comparatively thicker than the hoof wall considering the weight the animals carry. The frog is nonexistent and appears as an enlarged heel bulb.

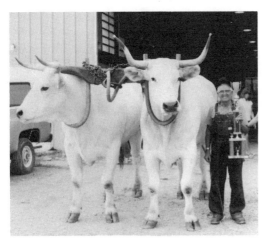

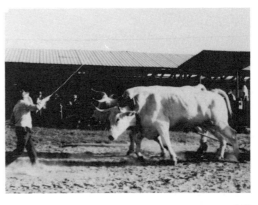

Fig. 45-1. (Left) Champion team of 8 year old Chianina oxen weighing 2850 pounds each owned by Frank Scruton of Rochester, NH. (Right) The same team in a pulling contest. Oxen used for competition pulling are often shod. Photos by D. Conroy.

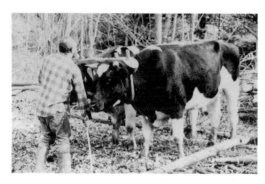

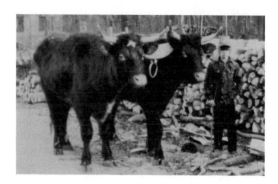

Fig. 45-2. (Left) Working in a woodlot with a team of 3 year old Holstein oxen weighing 1800 pounds each owned by Ed Ferguson of Deering, NH. Many teamsters shoe oxen that are worked in the woodlot to prevent slipping. (Right) Wood hauled by a team of 4 year old Milking Shorthorn oxen weighing 1100 pounds each owned by Richard Gordon of Weare, NH.

Draft Species	Developing Countries	Developed Countries
Cattle and Yaks (Oxen)	246 million	—
Buffaloes	60	—
Horses	27	62.5
Mules	10	—
Donkeys	40	—
Camels	16	—
Llamas	1	—
TOTAL	400	62.5

Fig. 45-3. Estimated world draft animal population (in millions). Figures from FAO (Fussner and Salterberg, 1984).

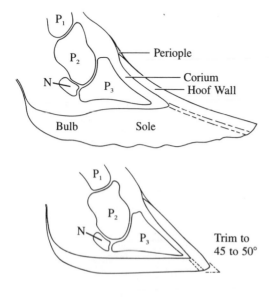

Fig. 45-4. (Top) Parts of the untrimmed ox claw. (Bottom) A trimmed ox claw. After Habel (1975).

The ox claw grows at the rate of about ⅕ inch per month. The claws of calves grow faster (¼ in. per mo.) than those of older cattle. Claws on the same digit may not grow at the same rate. Hoof growth (and soundness) is affected by weight distribution over the claws. The front medial claw and the hind lateral claw are most commonly diseased.

Trimming the Ox Claw

Untrimmed claws place excessive tension on the deep flexor tendons and cause inflammation of the corium of the bulbs. The ideal angle of a trimmed or worn claw is about 50 degrees. An animal may limp for several weeks due to a drastic change in hoof angle. Judgment in determining the amount to be trimmed can be developed by the study of bone and hoof specimens. The normal toe to heel ratio is about 2:1.

Practical experience is necessary to gain a feel for the correct trimming depth. Animals will limp for one or two weeks if they are cut too deeply. Abscesses may develop. Injured animals should be watched closely for a time. To avoid cutting too deeply, shave the sole from the bottom of the claw in slices ¹⁄₁₆ inch (or less) thick. The sole can be shaved until it yields slightly to firm thumb pressure. The faces between the claws should be parallel at the toe.

Sharp edges of the hoof should be rounded with a manual or power rasp. Power sanders must not be held on a foot continually. Alternate areas as you work to prevent overheating. The power tool is easier to use if the foot is stabilized by a rope or holder. Holders should wear heavy gauntlet type gloves.

Ideally, the animal should walk with uniform pressure on the hoof wall, sole and bulb.

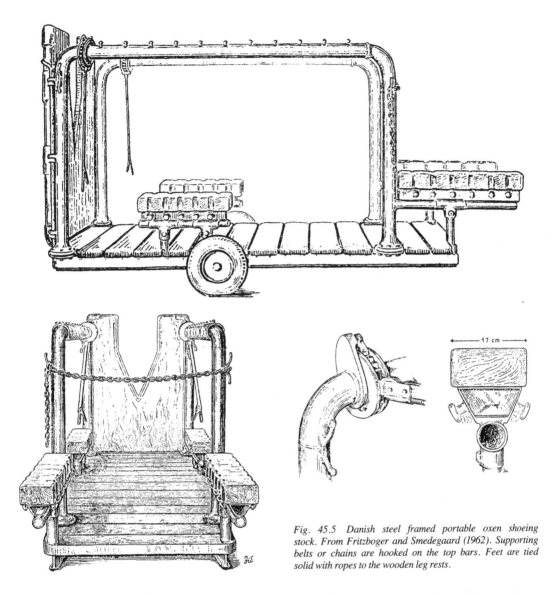

Fig. 45.5 Danish steel framed portable oxen shoeing stock. From Fritzboger and Smedegaard (1962). Supporting belts or chains are hooked on the top bars. Feet are tied solid with ropes to the wooden leg rests.

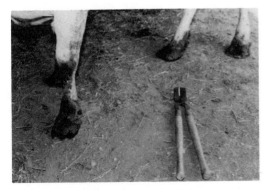

Fig. 45-6. Estimate the amount to be trimmed by studying bone and claw angles. Long handled hoof trimmers (foreground) may be used to trim a standing or a restrained animal.

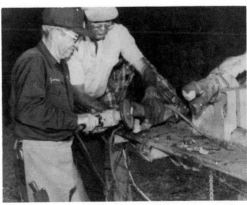

Fig. 45-7. Power sanders should not be held in one place for very long. Foot holders should wear heavy gloves.

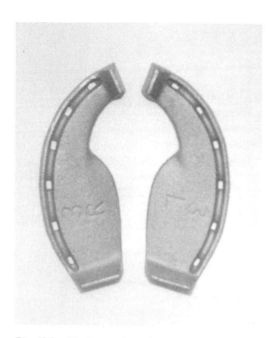

Fig. 45-8. Machine-made ox shoes.

Oxen Shoeing

Oxen are trained and shown in pulling contests in the Northeastern U.S. Heavy pulling oxen are shod with high calked shoes similar to those used on draft horse pulling teams. They can be made from ¼ x 1¼ to 1½ inch stock 4 to 5 inches long. The nail holes are punched very fine due to the thin hoof wall. Creasing of handmade shoes aids in the placement of nails. Size No. 3½ or 4 horseshoe nails are used in the hoof. Four to six nails are driven around the perimeter of each half-shoe. No nails should be placed in the rear one-fourth of the shoe. The heel nails must be pitched outward. The shoe should rest flat on the hoof wall and bulb.

Oxen are best shod in a rack or stocks designed for the purpose. A tilt table will work, but stocks are preferable. It is difficult to hold the foot when nailing on a table. Also, there is a chance of displacing the abomasum of a heavy, grain fed ox that is kept prone for more than a few minutes.

The shoes are fit full due to the natural inward curve of the claw wall. The shoe should cover the bulbs and give support at the heels. The toe third of the shoe should be shouldered and drawn. The shoe does not need to completely cover the toe. However, the outside edge of the toe may be fit full beyond the outer edge of the hoof. This gives the ox lateral support at the toe. The rear half of the shoe is fit close to the outer edge and beveled to the inside.

Cast keg shoes are available for oxen. These come in three sizes and can be fitted to most ox claws without alteration.[1]

Shoes are easiest to make from ¼ inch plate. The foot can be traced on heavy paper and the pattern cut out and transferred to the steel plate. A cutting torch is used to cut out the shoes. Nail holes can be drilled or stamped.

Some shoes are clipped on the outside of the toes. Clips are especially useful if an ox is walking on one side of a foot. Clips can also be drawn on the inside of the claws. This is especially useful when the claws wear extensively in this region or a wound between the claws may create a need to have the claws separated.

The texture of ox hoofs is different from that of horse hoof. Ox hoof is more leathery than horse hoof and less likely to split. Nails may be driven with a slight hook in them formed by the hammer claw. The nails should exit low on the wall.

Beef Show Cattle Trimming

Beef show cattle are trimmed to present a manicured appearance and to de-emphasize conformation faults. Much of show cattle trimming involves smoothing and sanding the feet. The horns are also smoothed and polished. Rarely will pasture or range cattle need trimming. Beef cattle are trimmed in the same way as dairy cattle.

Dairy Cattle Trimming

Dairy cattle trimming has become a big business with the growth in popularity of the free stall or pen stabling system. Free stalls or pipe frame pens are built higher than the floor in large ventilated sheds. The cows roam at will and eat together from automatically filled feed troughs. The cows select their own "stall" or bed to lay down in. Here they rest and ruminate.

Some persons make a full-time job of traveling from dairy to dairy to trim feet. The feet

[1] *William C. Plaisted, Plymouth, NH*

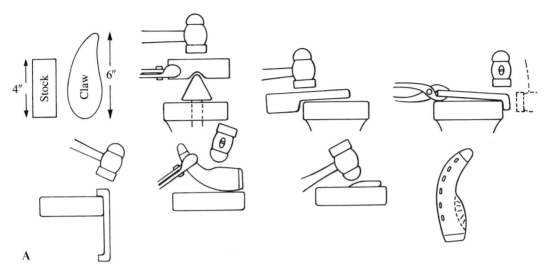

Fig. 45-9. (A) Steps in making a handmade calked ox shoe. (B) Handmade creased and clipped flat ox shoes fit to the foot.

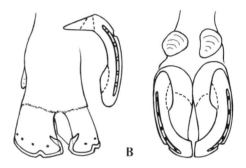

of pen stabled cattle should be trimmed at least twice a year. Those that are kept in stanchion barns (few now) can be trimmed once a year, usually right after calving. The ideal time to trim milk cows is a few weeks before the end of lactation before they go out on pasture.

Experienced teams of trimmers with a tilt table can do between 20 and 35 head per day between milkings. They may start around 9 o'clock and quit about 4 o'clock. Of course, this work is a little sloppier than horseshoeing, but it is just as lucrative and easier on your back.

The feet grow faster and don't wear as well in the free stall environment. The concrete becomes smooth due to frequent cleaning. The cows wade in the muck which keeps their feet soft and more subject to injuries and twisting (cork screw claws). Cows with upright or stumpy pasterns and steep hoof angles stay sound the longest. This type of conformation is most desirable in the hind legs. Few cows have trouble with soundness in the front legs. The old fashioned stanchion stabling is more likely to keep the feet dry. However, the lack of exercise eliminates normal wear and the toes become very long.

Dairy cattle are usually trimmed on a hydraulic tilt table. These can be made by the trimmer or purchased commercially. Most commercial tables must be modified to make them useful. High producing dairy cows must be handled gently. Rough handling may cause milk production to drop off for two to three weeks. However, regular trimming increases overall production. A power hoof rasp is used to shape and round the edges of the hoof. A small, flat board may be placed against the bottom of the foot to help detect high spots that need trimming while the cow is on its side.

Some say that high producing dairy cattle should not be laid down flat due to the possibility of causing an abortion or a displaced abomasum. They recommend tipping the cattle no more than 45 degrees. However, displaced abomasums are usually attributed to high concentrate feeding and excess gas formation due to fermentation in the abomasum. (The abomasum is the fourth stomach compartment or true stomach of the cow.)

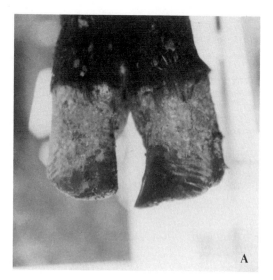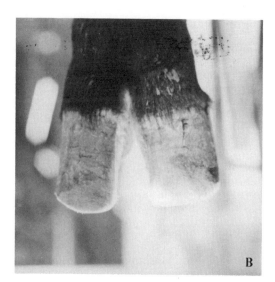

Fig. 45-10. Overgrown claws: (A) before trimming, (B) after trimming.

Dairy cattle can be trimmed in the standing position on a board (sheet of plywood) with a hammer and chisel and 30 inch wooden handled hoof trimmers. The bottom of the feet are trimmed by raising the leg and placing the dorsal surface of the foot down on a wooden block. The bottom of the hoof is trimmed with hoof nippers and a sharp push-type chisel. The cow's weight is supported by the trimmer's inside thigh under the cow's chest. The rear limbs can be raised by a rope run over a beam or pulley above a stanchion. This method of trimming is preferred for gentle cattle.

Calves can be thrown and tied down and trimmed with hoof shears. Sheep and goats can be held on their rumps with their back against the trimmer's legs while each foot is held with one hand and trimmed with the shears in the other hand.

Cattle Foot Diseases

Lameness severely limits the use and production of dairy or draft animals. An animal is predisposed to lameness by one or a combination of the following four factors (Greenough, *et al.*, 1972):

1. Inherited factors such as stance, weight and limb angles.
2. Nutritional factors such as protein, carbohydrate, vitamins, minerals and toxins.
3. Infectious factors such as bacteria or viruses.
4. Environmental factors such as housing, climate, and ground (road) conditions.

The most common problems with free-stalled cattle are deformed claws and bruises turning to abscesses. The feet are wet and don't wear off. There is often trouble with foot rot during the wettest times of the year. However, labor can be most efficiently managed with a free stall system.

Tie stall or stanchion barn housing keeps the cattles' feet dryer but they still have foot trouble due to lack of exercise. Pneumonia and foot rot are common problems. The system is comparatively labor intensive for milking and cleaning.

Foot rot, or interdigital necrobacillosis, is an infectious condition caused by *Fusiformis necrophorus*. The bacteria enter and create necrotic lesions between the claws that cause lameness. The condition is treated systemically with sulfa drugs administered by injection or orally in the feed. The type of bedding and ground conditions greatly influence an animal's susceptibility to the disease. It seems to be more common in the warm and wet months of the year. Bruising of the tissue between the claws by frozen ground, stones and stubble can predispose the animal to the disease.

Animals are made to pass through foot baths in areas of high incidence. Wet foot baths are

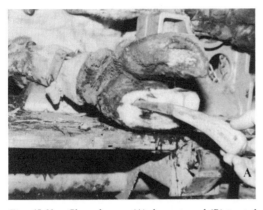
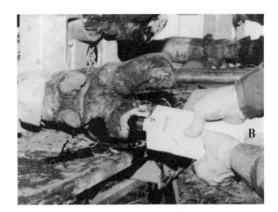

Fig. 45-11. Claw abscess: (A) dug out, and (B) treated with Kopertox.

made of copper sulfate or formalin solutions. Dry foot baths are made of a mixture of copper sulfate and slaked lime. Foot trimmers may carry Kopertox (copper sulfate) in a squeeze bottle to treat the foot after cleaning and trimming. The most important preventative measure is regular cleaning of the feet and pens of the cattle. Spraying the feet with water under pressure at milking time helps. Dry soil and bedding in the free stall is essential. A boot fastened to the digit and containing medication is sometimes used when treating foot rot. Shoeing a treated foot with a shoe closed at the toe may increase soundness.

Sole abscess or pododermatitis circumspecta is a lesion in the sole, especially at the sole-bulb junction. The condition may start as a bruise and progress to an abscess. The animal will show lameness, especially on hard ground, and abnormal stance to relieve pain. There will be an increased digital pulse and the foot may be hot. The horn over the sore area may be softer than usual and is discolored. Nails, glass or gravel may be found in the wound. However, their presence is not necessary to cause an abscess.

Abscesses may be caused by uneven weight bearing on the claws, excessive sole softening

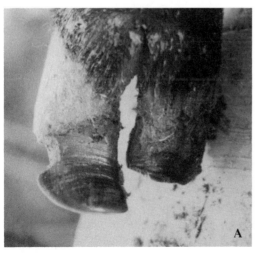
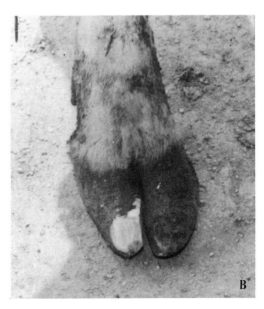

Fig. 45-12. Common problems: (A) untrimmed claw with uniform excess growth, (B) partially trimmed cork screw claw.

due to filthy housing conditions, small feet for the body size, excessive hoof length causing heel bruising and extra deep flexor tendon pressure. Both infrequent trimming and trimming too short may cause the condition. The sole should be pared to check for abscesses each time the feet are trimmed. An abscess should be allowed to drain and be dressed with Kopertox or Furacin. Deep, tender lesions should be protected by a bandage and pad or boot. Shoeing and elevation of the normal digit by shoeing or glueing on a wooden block will reduce lameness and prevent milk production loss. Occasionally, infections become gangrenous and the affected claw must be amputated.

Corkscrew claw is an abnormal inward-twisting of the lateral claw of the hind feet. It has been associated with pen stabling of dairy cattle. However, many scientists believe the condition is inherited. Corkscrew claw does not become evident until an animal is 3 years old. The lateral claw is noticeably narrower than the medial claw before it begins to twist. The heel of the claw grows faster than the rest of the wall. Lameness results if the claw is allowed to twist so that weight is borne on the side of the wall instead of the sole. Bony exostoses develop on the proximal or joint edge of the third phalanx. The increased blood circulation to the exostoses is thought to be responsible for increased growth of the lateral claw. The second phalanx is also deformed and becomes twisted.

Foot trimming greatly improves the gait and production of affected cows. Breeding of affected animals should be discouraged. However, there is some evidence this condition is associated with the traits of high producing cattle.

Laminitis or founder in cattle may result from overfeeding grain or from acute metritis (infection of uterus) or mastitis (infection of udder). It usually starts as an acute lameness but may develop into a chronic condition. Laminitis is said to be an inflammation of the sensitive laminae. The cow depends more on its sole to bear weight than the horse due to the absence of secondary laminae in the cow. Frequently, abscesses or sole ulcers are a serious consequence of both acute and chronic cases. The septic form (infected) may be a complicated combination of laminitis, punctures and foot rot. Affected animals tend to feed standing on their knees. They prefer to walk on soft ground.

A cow with laminitis will have a characteristic stiff gait and stance with an arched back and the hind feet up under the body. The toes will be long and curl up in chronic cases and there will be concavity at the toe. This conformation has been called slipper foot. Prominent ridges are visible in the wall. The ridges are noticeably farther apart in the heel region than at the toe. Radiographs reveal rotation of the third phalanx where it has torn away from the dorsal toe wall. The sole at the toe is thin and tender when pressed by hoof testers.

Laminitis may be treated in the acute stage by analgesics and antihistamine injections. Phlebotomy (bleeding) with removal of 3 to 5 liters of blood has been shown to improve many cases. The mechanism is not understood. Chronic cases should be slaughtered unless they are valuable breeding animals. These animals should be fed little grain. They can be maintained by frequent trimming of the heel and dorsal toe. The sole at the toe should not be trimmed. The sole may be protected with a wide plate shoe beveled (seated out) away from the foot.

Fractured Third Phalanx usually occurs in one or both medial claws of the front feet or, rarely, the lateral claw(s) of the hind feet. Some cases have been associated with flourine toxicity. Afflicted animals are suddenly and severely (three-legged) lame. Some cattle walk on their knees. Cattle with fractures in each medial claw may try to relieve pain by standing with the front legs crossed. Lame animals also arc their backs and place their hind legs up under the body. A radiograph is necessary for certain diagnosis. However, positive response from hoof tester pressure is a good evidence if other obvious possibilities have been ruled out. Treatment should consist of pain medication and therapeutic shoes. A shoe closed at the toe and fitted with a side clip on each side near the toe has been successful in some cases. However, glueing a wooden block to the claw with acrylic plastic is a superior treatment for this condition. Cows need only be kept recumbent for 15 minutes when using the acrylic. The animals can walk normally immediately after shoeing.

Interdigital Papillomatosis or interdigital skin

hyperplasia is an uncommon infectious condition that produces a finger-like projection that extends into the interdigital space. The cow is extremely lame, and drops off rapidly in milk production. The lesions are extremely tender and must be removed surgically by a veterinarian at the base of the papilloma. Shoeing with a shoe closed at the toe (like a horseshoe) may speed healing.

Therapeutic Shoes

Shoes may be applied to the claws of cattle for several reasons. Regular shoes are used only to prevent wear or increase traction. Therapeutic shoes may be applied to (after Greenough, *et al*, 1974):

1) Prevent or improve conformational defects.
2) Shift weight to a sound digit by raising the lame one off the ground.
3) Prevent the spread of the digits while interdigital injuries are healing.
4) Protect a sole or foot lesion from bruising or pressure.
5) Support a limb brace or prosthesis.

Polymerising resins such as Justi[2], Technovit[3] or 10X[4] Hoof Repair Material are suitable for many veterinary uses. They have been used to cover hoof wounds, replace missing hoof pieces and cast or immobilize the hoof (claws). A plywood block may be attached to the sound claw without shoeing in cases of digit amputation or fractured third phalanx until healing has taken place. The claw is cleaned and grooved with a grid pattern. The resin is placed between the hoof and block and up against the claw around the edges. The polymerising compounds harden in about 10 minutes after mixing. After healing has taken place, the block can be knocked off with a sharp blow from a hammer.

Therapeutic shoes can be constructed rapidly by tracing the claws, cutting the shoes out of steel plate with an oxy-acetylene torch or band saw and drilling holes for the nails. This technique prevents the problem of curve distortion encountered when making handmade shoes. The drilled holes can be shaped for the nail head by using a fore punch in the same heat that a clip is pulled. A wooden block can be attached to steel shoes by drilling and tapping for screws.

[2] *H.D. Justi Co., Oxnard, CA*
[3] *Jorgensen Labs, Loveland, CO*
[4] *Farriers, Inc., Wilmington, DE*

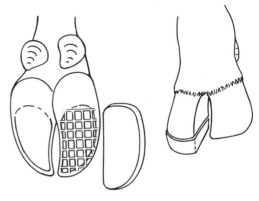

Fig. 45-13. A wooden block glued to a grooved sound claw promotes the healing of an adjacent damaged claw.

References

Andrist, F. 1954. Huf- horn- und klauenpflege. Deutsche Landwirtschafts-Gesellschaft, Frankfurt.

Barney, D.E. 1981. 4-H Working Steer Manual. Univ. of New Hampshire Ext. Service, Durham. No. 33.

Bates, A. 1982. The Clark clan. The Evener. 7(2):40.

Battaglia, R.A. and V.B. Mayrose. 1981. Handbook of Livestock Management Techniques. Burgess Publ. Co., Minneapolis.

Breuer, D. 1963. Technovit und klauenbeschlag. Tierarztl Umsch. 10:545.

Chew, K.H. 1972. Subacute/Chronic laminitis and sole ulceration in a dairy herd. Can. Vet. J. 13(4):90.

Eagle, M.L. 1982. Oxen shoeing. Amer. Farriers' J. 8(3):156.

Fowler, M.E. 1978. Restraint and Handling of Wild and Domestic Animals. Iowa State Univ. Press, Ames.

Frank, E.R. 1964. Veterinary Surgery. Burgess, Minneapolis.

Fritzboger, E. and H.H. Smedegaard. 1962. Kvaegets Klovpleje. Carl Fr. Mortensen, Kobenhaven.

Fussner, W. and S. Salterberg. 1984. Oxen—a part of our heritage. The Evener. 9(2):20.

Greenough, P.R., F.J. MacCallum and A.D. Weaver. 1972. Lameness in Cattle. J.B. Lippincott Co., Philadelphia.

Grossbauer, J. and F. Habacher. 1928. Der Huf- und Klauenbeschlag. Urban and Schwarzenberg, Berlin.

Habel, R.E. 1975. Applied Veterinary Anatomy. R.E. Habel, Ithaca, NY.

Holmstrom, J.G. 1902. Scientific Horse, Mule and Ox Shoeing. F.J. Drake and Co., Chicago.

Knezevic, P. 1966. Eine kombinierte untersuchungszange fur rinderklauen und pferdehufe. Wien. Tierarztl. Mona. 53:285.

Lungwitz, A. and J.W. Adams. 1966. A Textbook of Horseshoeing. Oregon State U. Press. Corvallis.

Maclean, C.W. 1966. Observations on laminitis in intensive beef units. Vet. Rec. 78(7):223.

Maclean, C.W. 1970a. A post-mortem x-ray study of laminitis in barley beef animals. Vet. Rec. 86(Apr.):457.

Maclean, C.W. 1970b. The haematology of bovine laminitis. Vet. Rec. 86(June 13):710.

Maclean, C.W. 1971. The long-term effects of laminitis in dairy cows. Vet. Rec. 89(July 10):34.

Nelson, D.R. and G.C. Petersen. 1984. Foot diseases in cattle. Part I. Examination and special procedures. The Compendium. 6(9):S543.

Nelson, M.E. 1955. 4-H Dairying—the Calf and Yearling. Univ. of Wisconsin Ext. Service, Madison. No. 79-A.

Nigam, J.M. and A.P. Singh. 1980. Radiography of bovine foot disorders. Mod. Vet. Practice. (July):621.

Nilsson, S.A. 1963. Clinical, Morphological and Experimental Studies of Laminitis in Cattle. ACTA Vet. Scand. Vol. 4 Suppl. 1.

Petersen, G.C. and D.R. Nelson. 1984. Foot diseases in cattle. Part II. Diagnosis and treatment. The Compendium. 6(10):S565.

Prentice, D.E. 1973. Growth rate and wear rates of hoof horn in Ayrshire cattle. Res. Vet. Sci. 14:285.

Prentice, D.E. and G. Wyn-Jones. 1973. A technique for angiography of the bovine foot. Res. Vet. Sci. 14(Jan):86.

Rebhun, W.C., R.M. Payne, J.M. King, M. Wolfe and S.N. Begg. 1980. Interdigital papillomatosis in dairy cattle. J.A.V.M.A. 177(5):437.

Ruthe, H. 1969. Der Huf. Fischer, Berlin.

Shaw, J. 1974. The Hoard's Dairyman Hoof Care Guide. W.D. Hoard and Sons, Co., Fort Atkinson, WI.

Staff. 1980. Hoard's Dairyman Hoof Care Guide. W.D. Hoard and Sons Co., Fort Atkinson, WI.

Staff, 1984. Their business moves forward one foot at a time. Hoard's Dairyman. (Jan 10):72.

Vaughan, L.C. and M.A.R. Osman.1967. Fracture of the third phalanx in cattle. Vet. Rec. 80(18):537.

Walker, D.F. 1979. Coaptation splinting of the bovine rear limb. Mod. Vet. Practice. (Aug):629.

Way, R.F. 1954. The Anatomy of the Bovine Foot. Univ. of Penn. Press, Philadelphia.

NOTES:

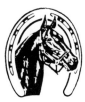

Index

INDEX

INDEX

O

Offset knees, 305
Offsetting, 228
Open, 43
Osselet, 106, 391
Osteochondrosis, 379
Osteolysis, 379
Osteum, 360
Out at the hocks, *see* bowlegged
Over at the knees, *see* buck-kneed
Overreach boots, 324
  padded, 326
Overreaching, 324
Owner responsibilities
  proper animal care, 175
Oxen
  anatomy of claw, 543
  definition, 543
  shoeing, 546
  trimming claw, 544

P

Pacer, 455
  free-legged, 456
  hobbled, 456
Paddling, *see* winging-out
Pads, 158, 447, 470, 530
  aluminum, 448
  anti-snowball, 532
  bonded rim, 442
  felt, 447
  full, 447
  leather, 447
  plastic, 447
  pneumatic, 532
  rim, 442, 447
  road, 530
  roadster, 530
  rubber, 530
  sorbothane, 448
Paint, 41
Palmar, 45
Palomino, 41, 494
Papillae, 145
Parade gait, 316, 495
Parade horse, 316, 492, 495
Parasite control, 53
Park
  pace, 316
  trot, 316
Park horse, 467, 499
  gaits, 499
Paso, 317
Paso corto, 317, 500
Paso Fino, 316, 317, 467, 499
  gaits, 499
Paso largo, 317, 500
Pastern, 41
  collar, 77
  conformation, 295
Patella, upward fixation of, 396
Pathological shoe, *see* therapeutic shoe
Pathological shoeing
  definition, 44
Patten shoe, 398, 411
Pawing, 42
Pedal osteitis, 354, 372
Penciled heel, 336

Pennsylvania, University of, 27
Percheron, 503
Performance horse, 421
Performance ratings, 205
Periople, 127, 129, 130
Perioplic ring, 127, 128, 145
Periosteum, 98
Peritendinitis, 109, 389
Peruvian Paso, 499
Phenylbutazone, *see* Bute
Phlebotomy, 550
Phoenix Horseshoe Company, 26
Physiological shoeing, 121
  definition, 44
Physis, 99
Pick, hoof, 158
Pigeon-toed, *see* toed-in
Pinto, 41, 494
Plaisted, William C., 547
Plantar, 45
Plantar cushion, 146
Plantation gait, 496
Plantation Walking Horse, 496
Plastic shoe, 459
Plate
  force, 358
  pressure, 358
  sole, 411
Plater, definition, 43
Pleasure Horse, 493
Pleasure walk, 498
Pliny, 20
Pododermatitis circumspecta, 549
Polo horse, 428
Polo plate, 424
Pony
  Hackney, 492
  Harness, 492
  harness racing, 456
  Shetland, 492
  Welsh, 492
Popped ankle, 391
Popped knee, 387
Popped sesamoid, 113, 391
Post-legged, *see* straight behind
Postle Industries, Inc., 508
Poultice, 359
Preakness, 441
Pritchel, 158, 226, 257
Pritcheling keg shoes, 243
Profession, characteristics, 7
Professional Rodeo Cowboys Association, 4
Proximal, 45
Pull off, 153, 158, 201
Pull tail, 41
Pulling back, 42
Pulling horse shoe, 516
Pulse rate, 349
Punch
  bob, 158
  center, 226
  handled, 226
Punching, 228
  nail hole, 262
Puncture wound, sole or frog, 176, 177
Purebred, 43
Putnam, Silas, 25

562

NOTES: